Current Issues in Heart Valve Disease

THROMBOSIS, EMBOLISM AND BLEEDING

Edited by

Eric G. Butchart and Endre Bodnar

ICR PUBLISHERS

THROMBOSIS, EMBOLISM AND BLEEDING
Published by ICR Publishers, London
First Edition, First Printing
ISBN: 1 872743 04 8

Printed in the United Kingdom
ISBN: 1 872743 04 8

CONTENTS

Preface xiii

PART 1: PATIENT RELATED AND SURGICAL FACTORS

1.1 Stroke and TIA in the general population 3
John Bamford and Charles P. Warlow

1.2 Atrial fibrillation without heart valve disease 16
Jonathan L. Halperin and Robert G. Hart

1.3 Abnormal cardiac anatomy and physiology 31
Dieter Horstkotte

1.4 Embolic complications of infective endocarditis 70
Lawrence R. Freedman

1.5 Hypercoagulability 81
George J. Miller and Thomas W. Meade

1.6 The influence of surgery on thromboembolic risk 93
Peter J.K. Starek

1.7 The effects of cardiopulmonary bypass and its pharmacological management. 105
Kenneth M. Taylor

PART 2: THE INFLUENCE OF PROSTHESIS-RELATED FACTORS

2.1 The influence of flow characteristics of prosthetic valves on thrombus formation 123
Agit P. Yoganathan, Timothy M. Wick and Helmut Reul

2.2 The haematological effects of non-physiological blood flow 149
Salvatore P. Sutera and J.Heinrich Joist

2.3 Interactions of blood with artificial surfaces 160
James M. Anderson and Frederick J. Schoen

2.4 Thrombogenicity, thrombosis and embolism 172
Eric G. Butchart

2.5 Scintigraphic and haematological detection of thrombosis and increased embolic risk 206
Jesse E. Adams III and Allan S. Jaffe

2.6 Ultrasonic detection of increased embolic risk. 223
Alan G. Fraser

PART 3: POSTOPERATIVE MANAGEMENT

3.1 Platelet inhibitor drugs after prosthetic heart valve replacement 247
Valentin Fuster and Douglas H. Israel

3.2 Pharmacology of anticoagulants 263
Philip A. Routledge and Hamsaraj G.M. Shetty

3.3 Standardisation of oral anticoagulation measurement and management 277
Antonius M.H.P. van den Bessalaar and Felix J.M. van der Meer

3.4 Prosthesis-specific and patient-specific anticoagulation 293
Eric G. Butchart

3.5 Patient-regulated anticoagulation 318
Ari Schachner, Ehud Deviri and Shai Shabat

3.6 Home prothrombin estimation 325
Angelika Bernardo, Carola Halhuber and Dieter Horstkotte

3.7 Computer-assisted anticoagulation 331
Hamsaraj G.M. Shetty and Philip A. Routledge

PART 4: ANTICOAGULATION IN SPECIAL CIRCUMSTANCES

4.1 Anticoagulation during pregnancy 339
Celia M. Oakley

4.2 Anticoagulation in children 346
Martin J. Elliott and Christopher Young

4.3 Anticoagulation in the elderly 356
Marc Verstraete, Raymond Verhaeghe and Philip A. Routledge

4.4 Anticoagulation in developing countries 362
Mervin A. Williams

4.5 Anticoagulation during non-cardiac surgical operations in patients with prosthetic valves 369
Mark H. Eckman

PART 5: MANAGEMENT OF THROMBOEMBOLIC AND BLEEDING COMPLICATIONS

5.1 Diagnosis and management of prosthetic valve thrombosis 387
Dirk Hausmann, Andreas Mügge and Werner G. Daniel

5.2 Recurrent embolism: significance and management 402
Albert Starr and Gary L. Grunkemeier

5.3 The management of stroke in patients with prosthetic valves 416
A. David Mendelow

5.4 Anticoagulant-related bleeding 425
Gordon D. O. Lowe and Isobel D. Walker

PART 6: FOLLOW-UP METHODS AND DATA ANALYSIS

6.1 Data collection and management 439
Peter A. Lewis

6.2 Analyses of thrombosis, embolism and bleeding as time-related outcome events 445
Eugene H. Blackstone

6.3 Reliability of comparative data from different sources 464
Gary L. Grunkemeier and Marla R. London

6.4 Critical assessment of thrombosis and embolism reporting methods 476
Endre Bodnar

CONTRIBUTING AUTHORS

James M. Anderson MD, PhD
Professor of Pathology
Macromolecular Science and Biomedical Engineering
Case Western Reserve University
Cleveland, Ohio, USA

Jesse E. Adams III MD
Fellow in Cardiology
Washington University School of Medicine
St. Louis, Minnesota, USA

John Bamford MD, MRCP
Consultant Neurologist and Physician in Cerebrovascular Medicine
St. James University Hospital,
Leeds, UK

Angelika Bernardo MD
Staff Member
Medical Rehabilitation Centre
Bad Berleburg, FRG

Antonius M.H.P. van den Besselaar PhD
Biochemist, Haemostasis and Thrombosis Research Unit
Department of Haematology
Leiden University Hospital
Leiden, The Netherlands

Eugene H. Blackstone MD
Professor of Cardiac Surgery
University of Alabama at Birmingham
Birmingham, Alabama, USA

Endre Bodnar MD
Editor
The Journal of Heart Valve Disease
London, UK

Eric G. Butchart FRCS
Consultant Cardiothoracic Surgeon
Clinical Director of Cardiac Surgery
University Hospital of Wales
Cardiff, UK

Werner G. Daniel MD, FACC
Professor of Internal Medicine and Cardiology
Department of Internal Medicine, Division of Cardiology
Hannover Medical School
Hannover, FRG

Ehud Deviri MD
Lecturer and Senior Staff Member
Department of Cardiovascular Surgery
Hadassa Ein Karem
Jerusalem, Israel

Mark H. Eckman MD, FACP
Assistant Physician
Divisions of Clinical Decision Making and General Medicine
New England Medical Center
Assistant Professor of Medicine
Tufts University School of Medicine
Boston, Massachusetts, USA

Martin J. Elliott MD, FRCS
Consultant Cardiac Surgeon
Hospital for Sick Children
Great Ormond Street
London, UK

Alan G. Fraser BSc, MRCP
Senior Lecturer in Cardiology
University of Wales College of Medicine
Cardiff, UK

Laurence R. Freedman MD
Professor of Medicine
Associate Chief of Staff for Education
University of California, Los Angeles
Los Angeles, California, USA

Valentin Fuster MD
Mallinckrodt Professor of Medicine
Harvard Medical School
Chief, Cardiac Unit
Massachusetts General Hospital
Boston, Massachusetts, USA

Gary L. Grunkemeier PhD
Director
Medical Data Research Center
St. Vincent Hospital and Medical Center
Assistant Professor
Division of Cardiopulmonary Surgery
Oregon Health Sciences University
Portland, Oregon, USA

Jonathan L. Halperin MD
Associate Professor of Medicine
Mount Sinai School of Medicine of the City University of New York
Attending Physician for Cardiology, Director of Clinical Services,
Division of Cardiology
Mount Sinai Medical Center
New York, USA

Carola Halhuber MD
Director
Medical Rehabilitation Centre
Bad Berleburg, FRG

Robert G. Hart MD
Associate Professor of Medicine
University of Texas Health Science Center at San Antonio
Staff Neurologist
Medical Center Hospital
San Antonio, Texas, USA

Dirk Hausman MD
Division of Cardiology
Department of Internal Medicine
Hannover Medical School
Hannover, FRG

Dieter Horstkotte MD, FESC
Department of Medicine
Division of Cardiology, Pneumology and Angiology
Heindrich-Heine-University
Düsseldorf, FRG

Douglas H. Israel MD
Clinical Instructor in Cardiology
Mount Sinai Medical Center
New York, USA

Allen S. Jaffe MD
Professor of Medicine
Washington University School of Medicine
St. Louis, Missouri, USA

J. Heinrich Joist MD, PhD
Professor of Internal Medicine and Pathology
Director, Division of Hematology
St. louis university School of Medicine
St Louis University Medical Center
St. Louis, Missouri, USA

Peter A. Lewis PhD
Senior Lecturer in Computing and Medical Statistics
University of Wales College of Medicine
Cardiff, UK

Marla R. London MA
Research Associate
Center for Outcomes Research and Education
St. Vincent Hospital and Medical Center
Portland, Oregon, USA

Gordon D. O. Lowe MD, FRCP (Edin., Glasg., Lond.)
Reader in Medicine, University of Glasgow
Honorary Consultant Physician and Co-Director, Haemophilia Centre
Glasgow Royal Infirmary
Glasgow, UK

Thomas W. Meade DM, FRCP
Director
MRC Epidemiology and Medical Care Unit
Wolfson Institute of Preventive Medicine
Medical College of St. Bartholomew's Hospital
London, UK

Felix J. M. van der Meer MD
Internist, Haemostasis and Thrombosis Research Unit
Department of Haematology
Leiden University Hospital
Leiden, The Netherlands

A. David Mendelow PhD, FRCS
Reader in Neurosurgery
Honorary Consultant Neurosurgeon
Head of Department
University of Newcastle-upon-Tyne
Newcastle-upon-Tyne, UK

George J. Miller MD, FRCP
Senior Clinical Scientific Staff
MRC Epidemiology and Medical Care Unit
Wolfson Institute of Preventive Medicine
Medical College of St. Bartholomew's Hospital
London, UK

Andreas Mügge MD, FACC
Division of Cardiology
Department of Internal Medicine
Hannover Medical School
Hannover, FRG

Celia M. Oakley MD, FRCP, FESC, FACC
Professor of Clinical Cardiology
Royal Postgraduate Medical School
London, UK

Philip A. Routledge MD, FRCP
Professor of Clinical Pharmacology
University of Wales College of Medicine
Consultant Physician
Llandough Hospital, South Glamorgan
Cardiff, UK

Helmut Reul PhD
Professor of Biomedical Engineering
Helmholtz Institute for Biomedical Engineering
Aachen, FRG

Ari Schachner MD
Chief, Department of Cardiac Surgery
Wolfson Medical Center
Professor of Surgery
Sackler School of Medicine
University of Tel-Aviv
Tel-Aviv, Israel

Frederick J. Schoen MD, PhD
Associate Professor of Pathology
Harvard-MIT Division of Health Sciences and Technology
Harvard Medical School
Vice-Chairman for Clinical Affairs (Anatomic Pathology)
Director, Cardiac Pathology
Brigham and Women's Hospital
Boston, Massachusetts, USA

Shai Shabat MD
Wolfson Medical Center
Sackler School of Medicine
University of Tel-Aviv
Tel-Aviv, Israel

Hamsaraj G.M. Shetty BSc, MRCP
Lecturer in Clinical Pharmacology and Therapeutics
University of Wales College of Medicine
Honorary Senior Registrar in Medicine,
Llandough Hospital, South Glamorgan
Cardiff, UK

Peter J.K. Starek MD
Professor of Surgery
Chief, Division of Cardiothoracic Surgery
University of North Carolina School of Medicine
Chapel Hill, North Carolina, USA

Albert Starr MD
Director, The Heart Institute
St Vincent Hospital and Medical Center
Professor of Surgery
Division of Cardiopulmonary Surgery
Oregon Health Sciences University
Portland, Oregon, USA

Salvatore P. Sutera MS, PhD
Professor and Chairman
Department of Mechanical Engineering
Washington University School of Engineering
St. Louis, Missouri, USA

Kenneth M. Taylor MS, FRCS
British Heart Foundation Professor of Cardiac Surgery
Department of Cardiac Surgery
Royal Postgraduate Medical School
London, UK

Raymond Verhaege MD
Professor of Medicine
University of Leuven
Consultant in Vascular Diseases
University Hospital, Gyasthuisberg
Leuven, Belgium

Marc Verstraete MD, PhD, FRCP(Edin.), FACP(Hon)
Professor of Medicine, University of Leuven
Centre for Thrombosis and Vascular Research,
Katholieke Universiteit
Leuven,Belgium

Isobel D. Walker MD, FRCPath, FRCP(Edin.)
Consultant Haematologist and Co-Director
Haemophilia Centre
Glasgow Royal Infirmary
Glasgow, UK

Charles P. Warlow MD, FRCP
Professor of Medical Neurology
Western General Hospital
Edinburgh, UK

Timothy M. Wick PhD
Assistant Professor
School of Chemical Engineering
Georgia Institute of Technology
Atlanta, Georgia, USA

Mervin A. Williams MD
Chief, Cardiothoracic Surgery
Greenacres Hospital
Port Elizabeth, South Africa

Agit P. Yoganathan PhD
Professor and Co-Director Bioengineering Center
Georgia Institute of Technology
Atlanta, Georgia, USA

Christopher P. Young MD, FRCS
Consultant Cardiothoracic Surgeon
St. Thomas' Hospital
London, UK

PREFACE

So often in medicine, research proceeds within the confines of one discipline and problems which overlap several specialities receive restricted, rather narrowly focused attention within each. A classical example of this phenomenon is the problem of thromboembolism in patients with heart valve disease. Traditionally cardiologists have focused their attention on abnormal anatomy and physiology within the heart whilst cardiac surgeons, materials scientists and prosthetic valve manufacturers have concentrated on technical issues and haematologists have directed their research efforts towards greater understanding of basic mechanisms of thrombosis and greater refinements of anticoagulation practice. At the same time pharmacologists have been developing new drugs for the prevention of thrombosis. Whilst each discipline has reported the results of its research efforts, until now there has been little attempt to co-ordinate these results in order to give a broader view of thrombosis and embolism in heart valve disease and answer some of the many questions which follow concerning causation, prevention and optimum management.

Thrombosis and embolism in patients with heart valve disease are determined by a complex interplay of patient-related, prosthetic-related and management-related factors. Together with anticoagulant-induced bleeding, they account for 75% of all complications after heart valve replacement. In no other situation is the pathophysiology of thrombosis and embolism confounded by so many variables and in few other situations is the need to solve these problems so great. By the end of this century, on current estimates, there will be two million patients world-wide with prosthetic heart valves. If present trends continue, 100,000 patients each year will suffer thromboembolic or bleeding complications, from which many will not recover or make only a partial recovery.

Despite the fact that oral anticoagulation has been available since the early 1940s, only in the last few years has any form of standardisation of measurement been available to allow comparison of one reported series with another and formulate meaningful recommendations. One legacy of this lamentable situation is that anticoagulant and antithrombotic prophylaxis has been flawed until recently by its arbitrary nature. As a consequence, many patients have received unnecessarily high levels of anticoagulation and suffered unnecessary bleeding complications.

The impetus for this book stemmed from the need to bring together acknowledged scientists and opinion leaders from all the disciplines which have an important bearing on the different aspects of thrombosis and embolism in patients with heart valve disease. In this way it was hoped to create a fresh perspective, weaving the various threads of the complex story into a consensus view, built up through a logical progression of ideas.

The challenge was to create a book that was developed around this common theme rather than being simply a compilation of loosely connected topics, possibly reflecting widely differing or even contradictory views. This was not an easy task to achieve and great credit must go to the contributing authors who understood the importance of creating a common understanding and common recommendations.

The final sculpturing of the book into its present shape was achieved with the collaboration of the contributing authors who spent two days together discussing each others' chapters in order to arrive at the necessary consensus. The editors believe that the result is a unique, logical, closely argued book that advances knowledge in this important field and creates a firm foundation for future research.

It is the editors' hope that this volume will prove a useful practical handbook for all those who, either directly or indirectly, care for patients with heart valve disease, and that it will also stimulate the reader to examine his or her own practice and initiate further investigation into the problems of thrombosis and embolism.

ERIC G. BUTCHART
ENDRE BODNAR

Part 1

Patient-related and surgical factors

Chapter 1.1

Stroke and TIA in the General Population

John Bamford and Charles Warlow

The enormous physical, psychological and economic burdens resulting from strokes are familiar to physicians in all developed countries. Indeed, few other conditions are capable of having such a devastating impact on patients, their careers and the community at large. It is for this reason that pathogenetic mechanisms such as cardiac valvular embolism, although by no means the most common cause of stroke, deserve detailed consideration. However, in order to put the specific problems of valvular embolism into context, it is important to appreciate the overall epidemiology of stroke and transient ischaemic attack (TIA) in the general population.

DEFINITIONS

In the past 30 years there have been a large number of epidemiological studies of stroke and TIA but it is often difficult to compare their results because of methodological differences that might introduce significant bias[1]. Several areas have become important because of the shift in focus of epidemiological studies towards considering pathological subgroups of stroke.

Stroke

To date, all epidemiological studies have used a clinical definition of cerebral stroke, usually along the lines suggested by the WHO[2]. According to this, stroke is the sudden onset of a focal neurological defect, the symptoms of which last for more than 24 hours or lead to prior death and are presumed to have a non-traumatic, vascular origin. Many studies have also included cases of subarachnoid haemorrhage (SAH) without focal signs. When the clinical diagnosis of 'stroke' has been compared with the results of computerised tomographic scanning (CTS) in relatively unselected populations, the false positive rates have been between 1% and 5%, although errors are more likely if the clinical details are incomplete, for example due to coma, dementia or dysphasia. In the Oxfordshire Community Stroke Project (OCSP), amongst 325 consecutive patients with a clinical diagnosis of first stroke, there were two cases with malignant cerebral glioma, one with cerebral metastasis and two with chronic subdural haematoma[3]. Since between 30% and 80% of acute CTS in patients with clinically definite ischaemic strokes will not show any relevant abnormality[4], using the clinical definition remains the method least likely to introduce bias.

Conversely, with the increased use of CTS for many neurological conditions, apparently asymptomatic areas of ischaemia are frequently found. For example, in a recent report from the NINCDS Stroke Data Bank study, 11% of patients presenting with a first stroke had CTS evidence of silent ischaemia in a different arterial territory[5]. The greater sensitivity of magnetic resonance imaging (MRI) combined with the present paucity of MRI-pathological correlation studies is likely to add further confusion. The prevalence of asymptomatic cerebral ischaemia visible by CTS in the general population is unknown. This is another reason, therefore, why studies based on CTS evidence of ischaemia should not be equated with studies which have used the clinical definition of stroke.

Completed stroke and TIA are arbitrarily distinguished by the persistence of symptoms for 24 hours. If the symptoms (but not necessarily asymptomatic signs such as an extensor plantar response) resolve within 1–3 weeks of onset, the terms "RIND" (reversible ischaemic neurological deficit) or "minor stroke" are sometimes used. These terms serve to identify a group of patients who have made a good physical recovery and in whom intensive measures to prevent further strokes may be appropriate, but there is no evidence that they identify a distinct pathogenetic group[6].

TIA

The differential diagnosis of TIA is somewhat wider than that for stroke. Metabolic disturbances such as hypoglycaemia and hyponatraemia can cause focal deficits and should be screened for routinely. Transient cardiac dysrhythmias causing reduced cardiac output are more likely to produce non-focal symptoms, but occasionally the symptoms may be lateralised if there is a haemodynamically significant stenosis of a major extra-cerebral artery. Perhaps the most difficult attacks to distinguish are those of focal epilepsy and migraine equivalents without headache. Care must be taken when eliciting the history of attacks with particular attention being paid to the time symptoms take to evolve and the presence of any positive phenomena such as jerking or visual scintillations.

A small proportion of patients who have a TIA will have areas of ischaemia in an area relevant to the symptoms when CTS is performed, suggesting that actual infarction has occurred[6]. However, there is no conclusive evidence that these are a group with a particularly distinctive underlying vascular pathology or prognosis.

Case ascertainment

The appearance in the last few years of reports from a number of well conducted, and very detailed, hospital-based stroke data banks[7,8] has highlighted the differences between hospital and community-based studies. The former are able to investigate patients in much more detail, but longer term follow up is rarely available. Claims that 'virtually all' patients in certain health care systems are admitted to hospital have not been substantiated. Even in the USA, between 20%[9] and 30%[10] of patients with acute stroke may not be admitted to hospital. Amongst the four hospitals in the NINCDS Stroke Data Bank, the proportion of cases of primary intracerebral haemorrhage (PICH) varied from 6% to 33%[7], a difference which is difficult to attribute to anything other than variation in case ascertainment. On the other hand, one has to be careful when extrapolating from community-based studies which may be based in rather atypical areas of a country.

Most authorities accept that for clinically orientated epidemiology (rather than that used for planning services) it is best to consider patients with a lifetime first-ever stroke since the rates of survival and recurrence are likely to differ between clinically important subgroups. A similar argument applies to TIA but the methodological issues are more complex and have recently been discussed in detail[11]. Even if one ignores the known errors in death certification, death rates are a relatively poor surrogate for incidence in a condition with a relatively low early fatality rate such as stroke. However, in the absence of incidence studies, a certain amount of information can be gleaned from them.

INCIDENCE OF STROKE AND TIA IN THE COMMUNITY

Crude incidence rates, even when standardised to a reference population are of much less value than those for age- and sex-specific groups. Figure 1.1–1 shows the almost exponential rise in stroke incidence with increasing age in the OCSP[12] and this pattern has been found in many studies world wide. In view of forthcoming demographic changes, it is important to note that the increase appears to continue even in the most elderly. The pattern is similar for both sexes. Although in many countries more females have strokes due to the greater number of elderly females, there is an overall excess risk of stroke in males of the order of 30% – 40%. This excess risk is age-dependent, the pattern being similar to, but less marked than, that for ischaemic heart disease[12]. There are fewer studies of TIA in the community. The pattern of incidence is similar to that revealed by the OCSP study (Fig. 1.1–1), although the smaller numbers result in more uncertainty about the rates in the most elderly.

There are very few longitudinal studies of stroke incidence, but there is little doubt that there has been a significant decline since the middle of this century. The reasons for this are unclear[13]. However, the recent data from Rochester, Minnesota[14] and Sonderham in Sweden[15] suggest that this decline may have ended. In passing, it is

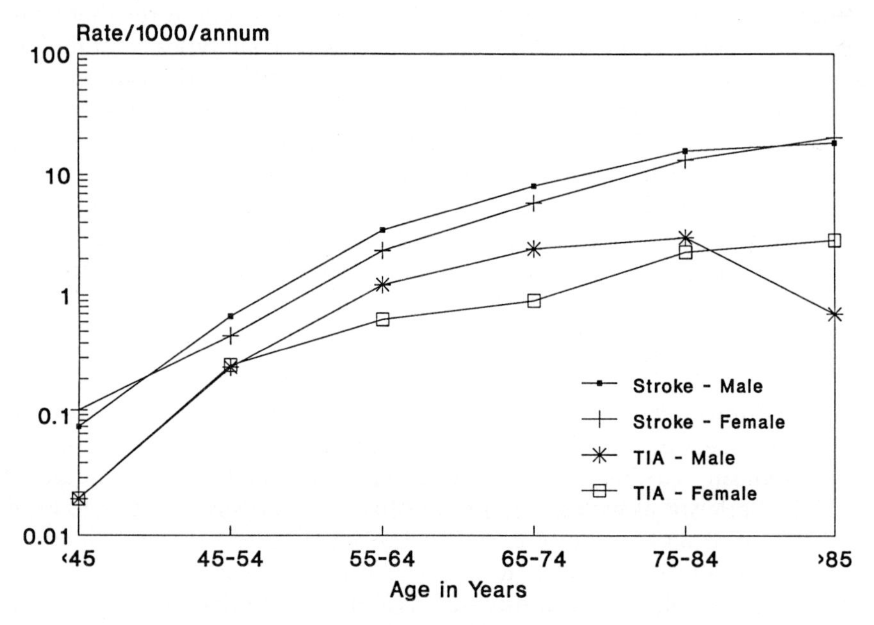

Figure 1.1–1. The age- and sex-specific incidence of first stroke and TIA in Oxfordshire, UK. (Note the logarithmic scale.)

worth noting that the incidence of primary intracerebral haemorrhage (PICH) actually increased in the mid 1960s in Rochester, against the overall trend at the time. This was attributed to the much greater use of anticoagulants at this time[16].

The paucity of good, prospective epidemiological studies makes geographical comparisons of stroke incidence difficult. In the USA, on the basis of mortality data, it was postulated that there was a 'stroke belt' in the south-eastern states, but a recent prospective study[17] failed to show convincingly that the rate was higher than in other areas of the USA. In that study, the annual age-adjusted incidence was 109/100,000 for whites and 208/100,000 for blacks and this difference has been found in other studies[9]. This difference may be a reflection of the higher prevalence of hypertension in the black community.

There is evidence that stroke is both quantitatively and qualitatively different in Japan. Pathological studies have shown a greater prevalence of intra-cranial vascular disease and, although the difference is probably not as great as was once thought, the Japanese also seem to have a greater proportion of haemorrhagic strokes. Of great interest was the comparison of Japanese residents of Japan, Hawaii and California, showing a substantial decline in incidence parallel to moving westwards[18]. In the UK, Acheson and Williams have pointed out that the death rate from stroke has a definite gradient between the North-West (high) and the South-East (low)[19] which seems to be independent of social class.

EPIDEMIOLOGY OF PATHOLOGICAL SUBGROUPS OF STROKE

The above mentioned limitations of CTS in diagnosing acute stroke do not apply to the distinction of cerebral infarction (CI) from PICH. In this matter, CTS is far superior to the clinical assessment and, in the individual case, one can argue that rational management is impossible without CTS information. Furthermore, there must be considerable doubt about the validity of data about stroke subtypes from the pre-CTS era unless there was a high autopsy rate as in Rochester[20,21] and Hisayama, Japan[22]. The proportions of stroke types in comparable studies world wide is relatively constant[21–26] (Fig. 1.1–2). Despite the reservations about earlier studies, the traditional view that the prognosis for survival and recovery is significantly poorer for PICH than CI has been confirmed. For example, in a recent community-based study in Oxfordshire, UK, the 30 day case fatality rate for PICH was 50% compared with 10% for CI, and the proportion who had recovered to functional independence one year later was 26% and 50%, respectively[23].

SUBTYPES OF CEREBRAL INFARCTION

In the community, about 80% of first strokes are due to CI. We know that the underlying pathogenetic mechanisms may include in-situ athero-thrombosis, artery-to-artery embolism, cardiogenic embolism, specific small artery vasculopathies, hypoperfusion, arteritis as well as other rarer causes. Intuitively, one would expect the natural history of strokes caused by each mechanism to differ, as would the treatments which might logically be expected to improve outcome. Unfortunately, one of the major continuing problems in the study of cerebrovascular disease is our inability to reliably distinguish these processes in the individual patient. Furthermore, if one considers the possible components of cardiogenic emboli (platelets, laminated fibrin-rich thrombi, calcific material, tumour), this dilemma increases further. The most recent report on the classification of stroke from the National Institute of Neurological Disorders and Stroke (NINDS) recognised this problem by having both pathophysiology and anatomy as bases for classifications[27].

The pathophysiological classification distinguishes cardioembolic from lacunar and atherothrombotic infarcts. Traditionally, cardioembolic strokes were thought to be of sudden onset and not to have had prior TIAs, but there is little evidence that these features are specific[28,29]. The classification places great emphasis on the results of investigations. Whilst they may give more information about *potential* sources of emboli, none is capable of demonstrating a definite pathogenetic link between cardiac pathology and the stroke. Furthermore, the determined investigator can often find evidence of more than one potential pathological mechanism in the individual patient. Indeed, the extra information from investigations may actually make classification more difficult; in the NINCDS Stroke Data Bank almost 40% of all infarcts had to be designated of 'undetermined cause' and the rate was highest in the centre that had investigated its patients most intensively[30]. The degree to which patients are investigated varies enormously. In part, this is because of predictable factors such as age, the severity of residual deficit and presence of co-existing illnesses. However, there are also less predictable factors such as the accessibility of diagnostic facilities, particularly when patients are not admitted to hospital, and perhaps most of all, the differing views of physicians about the value of any therapeutic interventions. These factors combine to make good community-based epidemiological data on these subtypes difficult to obtain.

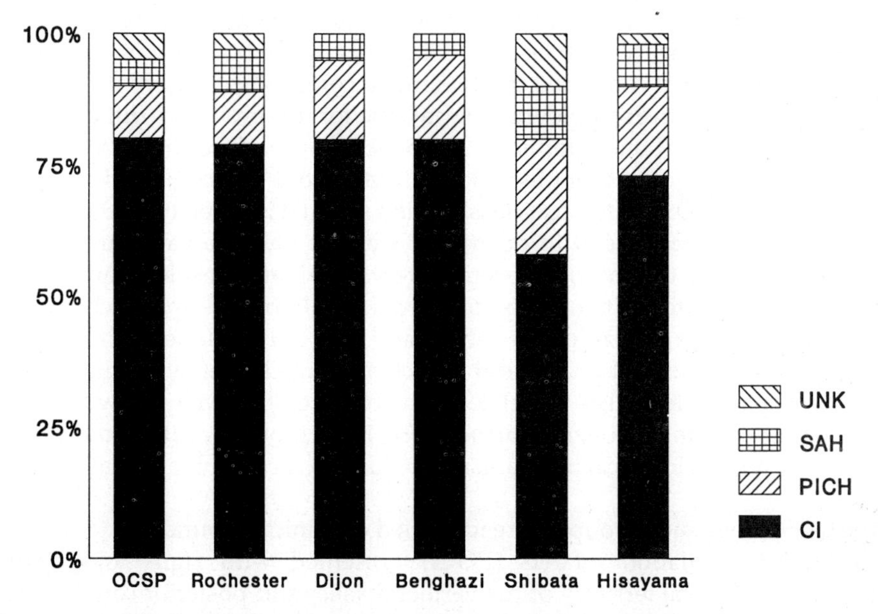

Figure 1.1–2. The distribution of the major pathological types of stroke in community-based studies worldwide. CI = cerebral infraction. PICH = primary intra-cerebral haemorrhage. SAH = subarachniod haemorrhage. UNK = unknown pathological type.

The large number of studies reporting rates of cardioembolic strokes was reviewed in detail by the Cerebral Embolism Task Force (CETF)[28,29]. In summary, it is generally thought that about 20% of ischaemic strokes are cardioembolic and a similar figure has been suggested for carotid territory TIAs. These proportions may well rise in younger patients as the a priori risk of degenerative vascular disease drops. The CETF concluded that about 12% of patients with a cardioembolic stroke would experience a recurrent stroke within 2 weeks (see also Chapter 4.2).

A further 20% of ischaemic strokes are thought to result from small infarcts deep in the cerebral substance which are caused by the occlusion of a single basal perforating artery: lacunar infarcts[31]. Considerable controversy surrounds this entity[32,33]. In part this is due to the varying use of the term lacune (which should probably only be used for a specific type of lesion seen at autopsy) and in part due to the relatively few detailed pathological studies which have ever been performed. Part of the debate surrounds the question of whether, in clinical practice, embolic particles travelling up the proximal middle cerebral artery are likely to enter one of the striate arteries which tend to branch at 90 degrees from the parent artery. Such a process has been reported in experimental animals[33] but, at present, it is thought that intrinsic vasculopathies such as microatheroma or lipohyalinosis, or perhaps less frequently atheroma at the mouth of the penetrating artery[34], are the most frequent causes. Certainly, a number of epidemiological studies have shown significantly fewer potential sources of cardiac embolism in this group than in strokes which have involved the cortical mantle[35]. Other epidemiological features are discussed later.

The remaining strokes are classed as atherothrombotic (this would include the 'infarcts of unknown origin' in the NINCDS Stroke Data Bank[30]). The mechanism is considered to be either hypoperfusion in the area of supply distal to an arterial stenosis or occlusion, or artery-to-artery embolism. The point is made that it is impossible to distinguish artery-to-artery embolism and cardiogenic embolism with certainty and other investigators have combined the two into a composite category of 'embolism'[7]. Not surprisingly, convincing epidemiological data for this group are difficult to find.

On the other hand, if one adopts an anatomical approach to the subclassification, then it is possible to obtain epidemiological data from the community. The main drawback of the NINDS anatomical classification is that it is based on the site of arterial occlusion. This can be difficult to determine without invasive vascular studies,, for example occlusion of the internal carotid artery (ICA) may result in anything from transhemispheric infarction to no infarction at all. An alternative approach is to classify according to the site and size of the infarct and this can be done with considerable accuracy using the classical anatomical associations of clinical symptoms and signs alone. These parameters also correlate with many of the well known prognostic features for survival and recovery. Furthermore, if the groupings are chosen carefully, one or two pathophysiological mechanisms are likely to predominate in any individual group.

In the OCSP, four such groups were identified on clinical grounds[36].

(a) Posterior circulation infarcts (POCI) presented with signs and symptoms confined to the classical territory of the vertebrobasilar and posterior cerebral arteries. Pathological evidence suggests that the majority of such infarcts are likely to be due to in situ thrombosis[37], although those confined to posterior cerebral artery territory are more likely to be embolic.

(b) Lacunar infarcts (LACI) presented with one of the four strictly defined lacunar syndromes[31] of pure motor stroke, pure sensory stroke, sensorimotor stroke or ataxic hemiparesis. In such cases there was *never* any evidence of a hemianopia or higher cerebral dysfunction. As noted before, embolism from any source seems to be an unlikely cause of these infarcts.

(c) Total anterior circulation infarcts (TACI) presented with an ipsilateral motor and/or sensory disturbance, *and* hemianopia *and* higher cerebral dysfunction. There is good pathological data to show that this clinical pattern is only likely to occur with occlusion of the proximal middle cerebral artery stem or the internal carotid artery by atherothrombosis or larger emboli[38].

(d) Partial anterior circulation infarcts (PACI) presented with more restricted deficits of cortical function and included all the cortical branch syndromes. The majority of such infarcts are probably embolic, although a proportion will be caused by boundary zone hypoperfusion secondary to more proximal arterial stenosis or occlusion. The embolic material is likely to be relatively small but this classification does not distinguish the site of origin.

In the OCSP, of all first cerebral infarcts, approximately 25% were POCI, 25% LACI, 17% TACI and 33% PACI. The outcome at one year after the stroke is shown in Figure 1.1–3. Although the overall stroke recurrence rate in the first year is about 10%, the majority of those in the PACI group had occurred within 3 months of the initial event (compatible with the notion of an active embolic source). In the LACI group however, recurrences tended to occur at a steady rate throughout the first year. This is what might be expected since, if our pathophysiological hypothesis is correct and the initial LACI was caused by the occlusion of a single perforating artery, then for further symptoms to occur another artery would have to become symptomatic.

Although the anatomical classification is relatively crude, its major advantage is that it can be applied to virtually all patients with stroke in the community and, therefore, reliable epidemiological data can be obtained. With this knowledge, it should be possible to assess to what extent hospital-based studies with detailed pathophysiological investigations are representative of the true situation.

CARDIAC DISEASE, CEREBRAL HAEMORRHAGE AND HAEMORRHAGIC INFARCTION

Even if it is difficult to be certain about the relationship between a cardioembolic source and areas of cerebral infarction in an individual patient, nevertheless, in the context of a patient with a prosthetic valve, the physician's response is likely to be the continued use of anti-haemostatic drugs. However the situation is quite different in someone who sustains a stroke whilst on anti-haemostatic drugs and whose CT scan shows evidence of intracerebral haemorrhage (ICH). In a minority of cases there will be underlying abnormalities of longstanding, such as angiomas, arteriovenous malformations and berry aneurysms, where the ICH is likely to be unrelated to the cardiac problem and may not even be related to anticoagulation. ICH secondary to an acute, non-infective cerebral arteritis is even less common. In patients who have had an episode of endocarditis, rupture of a mycotic aneurysm needs to be considered, even if the infective episode was months or years before and had been 'adequately' treated[39]. Until recently, traditional teaching has been that nearly all other spontaneous ICH results from chronic hypertensive damage to deep perforating arteries and, in particular, from the rupture of Charcot-Bouchard aneurysms. However in an era where the control of hypertension has been much improved, other vascular pathologies, such as cerebral amyloid angiopathy, are being recognised increasingly as a cause of ICH, particularly in the elderly. There have also been reports of ICH in association with drug abuse, cold weather and other situations in which there has been an acute increase in blood pressure. These have been reviewed recently by Caplan[40], who stressed that not all episodes of ICH could be explained by pre-existing vascular abnormalities.

In the context of cardiac embolism, a particular problem area is that of haemorrhagic transformation (HT) within areas of cerebral infarction. Traditionally HT was thought to occur when hypoxic capillaries were reperfused after the dissolution of a proximal arterial occlusion although there are cases in the literature where the vascular occlusion was still present at the time of HT[41]. The depth and duration of the ischaemia as well as the intensity of the reperfusion may be related to the risk of developing HT. It has been linked particularly to cardiogenic embolism[42], although it is certainly not confined to this group of strokes. Despite the fact that HT is being recognised more frequently, it is important to remember that CT scanning only detects areas of confluent haemorrhage in contrast to the small petechial haemorrhages commonly found at autopsy. Not all episodes of HT have clinically apparent sequelae. It is not clear whether HT is more likely to occur if anti-haemostatic drugs are given immediately after a cerebral infarct although it is probably more frequent in patients who are taking such drugs at the time of their stroke. About 20% of presumed cardioembolic infarcts may develop HT within 2 to 4 days of onset[28], but HT is a dynamic process and serial CT studies suggest that it

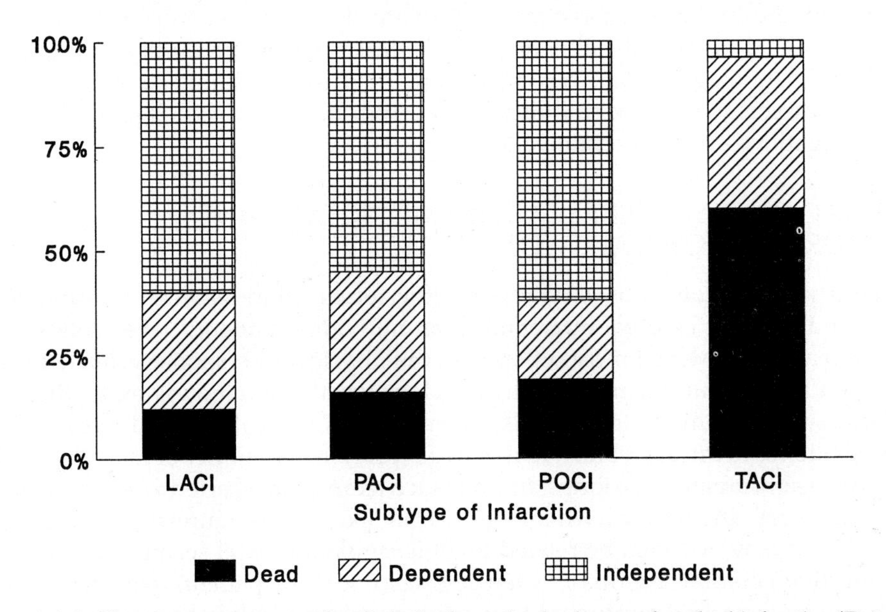

Figure 1.1–3. The outcome at one year for clinically determined subtypes of cerebral infarction (Data from the OCSP). LACI = lacunar infarcts. PACI = partial anterior circulation infarcts. POCI = posterior circulation infarcts. TACI = total anterior circulation infarcts.

can occur in up to 40% of supratentorial infarcts during the first 2 weeks post stroke[43]. HT secondary to cardiogenic embolism is probably more likely to occur early, and be more confluent, than when it is due to other mechanisms, particularly if the patients are on anticoagulants[28]. Recently, Bogousslavsky and others have shown that confluent HT indistinguishable from primary ICH may occur within 13 hours of the onset of symptoms[41] and one of the present authors (JMB) has seen a similar case within 9 hours of onset. The importance of these observations is that such cases may be misclassified as complications rather than failures of anticoagulant therapy and result in inappropriate management decisions being taken. The implication is that CT scans should be performed as a matter of urgency in anticoagulated patients with a valve prosthesis who develop sudden neurological symptoms. Trials are needed to determine whether the continuation of anticoagulant drugs will prevent the propagation of thrombi or early embolic stroke recurrence at the expense of increased HT, and if so, which is the more beneficial in terms of final functional outcome.

In the absence of large, well controlled clinical trials, the indications for surgical evacuation of intracranial haematoma are unclear and there are wide variations in individual practice worldwide from the ultra-aggressive to the ultra-conservative[44]. Similarly the risk/benefit ratio of patients remaining on anticoagulants is unknown.

RISK FACTORS

There are a large number of conditions, particularly those that have an effect on the coagulation system, which increase the risk of stroke in an individual (see Chapter 1.5). By and large, these factors are uncommon in the community and, therefore, the population attributable risk is very small. Here we have confined discussion to those factors which have a high population attributable risk. It is important also to distinguish true risk factors for stroke and TIA from factors which are simply markers of degenerative vascular disease and have no pathogenetic link (e.g. intermittent claudication).

Hypertension

After age, the most important risk factor for stroke is hypertension, and since it is common, it has the highest population attributable risk. This has been shown repeatedly in studies from all parts of the world. An overview of nine major prospective observational studies[45] clearly demonstrated the positive and continuous association between diastolic blood pressure (DBP) and stroke risk with prolonged differences in usual DBP of 5, 7.5 and 10 mmHg being respectively associated with at least 34%, 46% and 56% less strokes (Fig. 1.1–4). The Framingham study[46] has also demonstrated a relationship between stroke risk and systolic hypertension. This holds even if there is isolated systolic hypertension and the excess risk continues to be seen in the elderly.

A meta-analysis of 14 unconfounded, randomised trials of anti-hypertensive drugs[47] in a total of 37,000 individuals, with a mean treatment duration of 5 years and a mean reduction of DBP of 5–6 mmHg, showed a reduction in stroke of 42% (95% confidence interval 33% - 50%), a result that suggests that virtually all the epidemiologically expected stroke reduction appears rapidly.

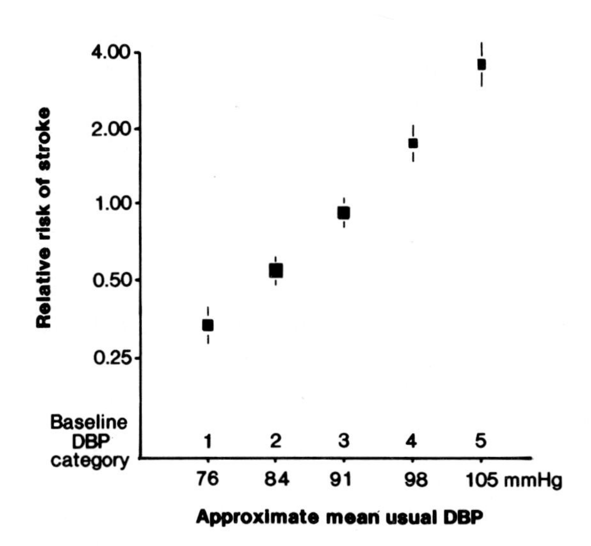

Figure 1.1–4 "The relative risk of stroke according to baseline diastolic blood pressure estimated from the combined results of seven prospective observational studdies" (reproduced with permission from Lancet 1990; 335:765–74)
The solid squares represent disease risk in each category relative to risk in the whole study population; sizes of squares are proportional to number of events in each DBP category; and 95% confidence intervals for estimates of relative risks are denoted by vertical lines.

Diabetes

Although the greatest atherosclerotic impact of diabetes is on the peripheral vascular tree, it is generally considered to increase the risk of ischaemic stroke by a factor of about two. In both the Honolulu Heart Program[48] and the Framingham study[46], this increase was independent of hypertension. In the study from Rochester[49] the same relationship held for TIAs but, for unknown reasons, not for stroke. The high prevalence of diabetes in the community means that there is a substantial population attributable risk. Despite advances in treatment, there is no clear evidence that controlling the diabetes reduces the stroke risk.

Cardiac disease

Cardiac disease will not be considered in detail here – suffice to say that up to 75% of patients with stroke may have evidence of either coronary artery disease, congestive heart failure or left ventricular hypertrophy on ECG or CXR (see Chapters 1.2 and 1.3).

Smoking

A number of recent studies have shown a clear association between smoking and risk of stroke. In a meta-analysis of 32 studies[50], the overall relative risk of stroke associated with cigarette smoking was 1.5 (95% CI 1.4 – 1.6). The excess risk was most marked in cases of subarachnoid haemorrhage (relative risk 2.9). For cerebral infarction the relative risk was 1.9 and for primary intracerebral haemorrhage 0.74. The excess risk was most notable in younger patients and was dose related. Although the risk in ex-smokers was less than in current smokers, they retained some excess risk over life-long non-smokers.

Lipids

The relationship between abnormal plasma lipids and cerebrovascular disease is much less clear than for coronary heart disease. It is probable that this reflects the heterogenicity of underlying pathogenetic mechanisms and further large studies on pathologically homogeneous subgroups are required. This will be especially important if the early promise of treatment-induced atheroma regression in coronary arteries is confirmed because disorders of lipid metabolism are common in the community (see Chapter 1.5).

SUMMARY

Once one goes beyond the basic division of stroke into cerebral infarction, primary intracerebral haemorrhage and subarachnoid haemorrhage, our epidemiological knowledge remains rudimentary. For this situation to change, we need more reliable and widely applicable ways of determining the underlying pathophysiological mechanisms that are operating in individual patients. With such knowledge, treatment trials could be focused on the patients who are most likely to respond.

REFERENCES

1. Malmgren R, Warlow C, Bamford J, Sandercock P. Geographical and secular trends in stroke incidence. Lancet 1987;2:1196–1200.
2. Hatano S. Experience from a multicentre stroke register: a preliminary report. Bull WHO 1976;54:541–553.
3. Sandercock P, Molyneux A, Warlow C. Value of computed tomography in patients with stroke. Br Med J 1985;290:193–197.
4. Lee DH. Investigation of stroke. Current Opinion in Neurology and Neurosurgery 1991;4:51–56.
5. Chodosh EH, Foulkes MA, Kase CS, Wolf PA, Mohr JP, Hier DB, Price TR, Furtadọ JG. Silent stroke in the NINCDS Stroke Data bank. Beurology 1988;38:1674–1679.
6. Dennis MS, Bamford JM, Sandercock PAG, Warlow CP. A comparison of risk factors and prognosis for transient ischaemic attacks and minor ischaemic strokes. Stroke 1989;20:1494–1499.
7. Kunitz SC, Gross CR, Heyman A et al. The Pilot Stroke Data Bank: Definition, Design, Data. Stroke 1984;15:740–746.
8. Bogousslavsky J, Van Melle G, Regli F. The Lausanne Stroke Registry: analysis of 1000 consecutive patients with first stroke. Stroke 1988;19:1083–1092.
9. Schoenberg BS, Anderson DW, Haerer AF . Racial differentials in the prevalence of stroke. Copiah County Mississippi. Arch Neurol 1986;43:565–568.
10. Schoenberg B, Schoenberg D, Whisnant J. Hospitalization for stroke: a population study in Rochester, Minnesota. Am J Epidemiol 1983;118:444 (abstract).
11. Dennis MS, Bamford JM, Sandercock PAG, Warlow CP. Incidence of Transient Ischaemic Attacks in Oxfordshire, England. Stroke 1989;20:333–339.
12. Bamford J, Sandercock P, Dennis M et al. A prospective study of acute cerebrovascular disease in the community: The Oxfordshire Community Stroke Project – 1981–1986. 1. Methodology, demography and incident cases of first-ever stroke. J Neurol Neurosurg Psychiatry 1988;51:1373–1380.
13. Garraway WM, Whisnant JP, Furlan AJ, Phillips LH, Kurland LT, O'Fallon WM. The declining incidence of stroke. N Engl J Med 1979;300:449–452.
14. Broderick JP, Phillips FJ, Whisnant JP, O'Fallon WM, Bergstralh EJ. Incidence rates of stroke in the 80s: The end of the decline in stroke? Stroke 1989;20:577–582.
15. Terent A. Increasing incidence of stroke among Swedish women. Stroke 1988;19:598–603.

16. Furlan A J, Whisnant JP, Elveback LR. The decreasing incidence of primary intracerebral haemorrhage: A population study. Ann Neurol 1979;5:367–373.
17. Gross CR, Kase CS, Mohr JP, Cunningham SC, Baker WE. Stroke in South Alabama: Incidence and diagnostic features – A population based study. Stroke 1984;15:249–255.
18. Kagan A, Popper J, Rhoads GG, Takaya Y, Kato H, Goode GB, Marmot M. Epidemiologic studies of coronary heart disease and stroke in Japanese men living in Japan, Hawaii and California: prevalence of stroke. In Scheinberg P, ed. Cerebrovascular Diseases, Tenth Princeton Conference. New York, Raven Press, 1976;267–277.
19. Acheson RM, Williams DRR. Epidemiology of cerebrovascular disease: some unanswered questions. In Rose FC, ed. Clinical Neuroepidemiology. Tunbridge Wells, Pitman Medical, 1980;88–104.
20. Whisnant JP, Fitzgibbons JP, Kurland LT, Sayre GP. Natural history of stroke in Rochester, Minnesota, 1945 through 1954. Stroke 1971;2:11–22.
21. Matsumoto N, Whisnant JP, Kurland LT, Okazaki H. Natural history of stroke in Rochester, Minnesota, 1955 through 1969: An extension of a previous study, 1945 through 1954. Stroke 1973;4:20–29.
22. Ueda K, Omae T, Hirota Y, Takeshita M, Katsuki S, Tanaka K, Enjoji M. Decreasing trend in incidence and mortality from stroke in Hisayama residents, Japan. Stroke 1981;12:154–160.
23. Bamford J, Sandercock P, Dennis M, Burn J, Warlow C. A prospective study of acute cerebrovascular disease in the community: The Oxfordshire Community Stroke Project – 1981–1986. 2. Incidence, case fatality rates and overall outcome at one year of cerebral infarction, primary intracerebral haemorrhage and subarachnoid haemorrhage. J Neurol Neurosurg Psychiatry 1990;53:16–22.
24. Ashok PP, Radhakrishnan K, Sridharan R, El-Mangoush MA. Incidence and pattern of cerebrovascular diseases in Benghazi, Libya. J Neurol Neurosurg Psychiatry 1986;49:519–523.
25. Tanaka H, Ueda Y, Date C et al. Incidence of stroke in Shibata, Japan:1976–8. Stroke 1981;12:460–466.
26. Giroud M, Beuriat P, Vion P, D'Athis PH, Dusserre L, Dumas R. Stroke in a French prospective population study. Neuroepidemiology 1989;8:97–104.
27. National Institute of Neurological Disorders and Stroke. Classification of Cerebrovascular Diseases III. Stroke 1990;21:637–676.
28. Cerebral Embolism Task Force. Cardiogenic Brain Embolism. The second report of the Cerebral Embolism Task Force. Arch Neurol 1989;46:727–743.
29. Cerebral Embolism Task Force. Cardiogenic brain embolism. Arch Neurol 1986;43:71–84.
30. Sacco RL, Ellenberg JH, Mohr JP, Tatemichi TK, Hier DB, Price TR, Wolf PA. Infarcts of undetermined cause: The NINCDS Stroke Data Bank. Ann Neurol 1989;25:382–390.
31. Bamford J, Sandercock P, Jones L, Warlow C. The natural history of lacunar infarction: The Oxfordshire Community Stroke Project. Stroke 1987;18:545–551.
32. Bamford J, Warlow C. The evolution and testing of the lacunar hypothesis. Stroke 1988;19:1074–1082.
33. Millikan C, Furtell N. The fallacy of the lacune hypothesis. Stroke 1990;21:1251–1257.
34. Caplan LR. Intracranial branch atheromatous disease. A neglected, understudied and underused concept. Neurology 1989;39:1246–1250.
35. Lodder J, Bamford JM, Sandercock PAG, Jones LN, Warlow CP. Are hypertension or cardiac embolism likely causes of lacunar infarction? Stroke 1990;21:375–381.
36. Bamford J, Sandercock P, Dennis M, Burn J, Warlow C. Classification and natural history of clinically identifiable subtypes of cerebral infarction. Lancet 1991;337:1521–1526.
37. Escourelle R, Poirier J. Manual of Basic Neuropathology. Philadelphia, W B Saunders, 1978.
38. Greenhall RCD. Pathological findings in acute cerebrovascular disease and their clinical implications. DM Thesis: University of Oxford, 1977.
39. Bamford JM, Hodges JR, Warlow CP. Late rupture of a mycotic aneurysm after 'cure' of bacterial endocarditis. J Neurol 1986;233:51–53.
40. Caplan LR, Intracerebral haemorrage revisited. Neurology 1988;38:624–627.
41. Bogousslavsky J, Regli F, Uske A, Maeder P. Early spontaneous haematoma in cerebral infarct. Neurology 1991;41:837–840.
42. Fisher CM, Adams RD. Observations on brain embolism with special reference to the mechanisms of hemorrhagic infarction. J Neuropathol Exp Neurol 1951;10:92–94.
43. Hornig CR, Dorndorf W, Agnoli AL. Hemorrhagic cerebral infarction. A prospective study. Stroke 1986;17:179–185.
44. Marshall J. Should spontaneous cerebral haematomas be evacuated and if so when? In Warlow CP, Garfield J (Eds.): Dilemmas in the Management of the Neurological Patient. Edinburgh, Churchill Livingstone. 1984:54–61.
45. MacMahon S, Peto R, Cutler J et al. Blood pressure, stroke and coronary heart disease. Part 1, prolonged differences in blood pressure: prospective observational studies corrected for the regression dilution bias. Lancet 1990;335:765–774.
46. Kannel WB, Wolf PA. Epidemiology of cerebrovascular disease. In: Russell RWR (Ed). Vascular Disease of the Central Nervous System. 2nd ed. Edinburgh, Churchill Livingstone, 1983:1–24.

47. Collins R, Peto R, MacMahon S et al. Blood pressure, stroke and coronary heart disease. Part 2, short-term reductions in blood pressure:overview of randomised drug trials in their epidemiological context. Lancet 1990;335:827–38.
48. Abbott RD, Donahue RP, Macmahon SW, Reed DM, Yano K. Diabetes and the risk of stroke:The Honolulu Heart Program. JAMA 1987;257:949–952.
49. Roehmholdt ME, Palumbo PJ, Whisnant JP, Elveback LR. Transient ischaemic attack and stroke in a community-based diabetic cohort. Mayo Clin Proc 1983;58:56–58.
50. Shinton R, Beevers G. Meta-analysis of relation between cigarette smoking and stroke. Br Med J 1989;298:789–94.

Chapter 1.2

Atrial Fibrillation Without Heart Valve Disease

Jonathan L. Halperin and Robert G. Hart

The estimated prevalence of atrial fibrillation in the absence of rheumatic heart disease or prosthetic heart valves is nearly 2% among adults over the age of 35 years. For example, in the USA there are more than 2 million such people[1]. While not as frequent a cause of brain ischaemia as cerebrovascular diseases, about half the strokes of suspected cardiac origin occur in patients with non-valvular atrial fibrillation. Epidemiological studies have estimated the risk of stroke and systemic embolism associated with atrial fibrillation as five to six events per 100 patient-years, well over five times the rate among comparable patients without this cardiac rhythm disturbance, and accumulating to a 35 per cent lifetime risk of stroke for patients with atrial fibrillation. The risk appears to rise with age, so that in nearly half of stroke victims over 85 years of age a history of atrial fibrillation can be found[4]. Clinically, these strokes are typically devastating events which leave survivors with lasting disability. However, there is an additional incidence of transient ischaemic attacks (TIAs) and subclinical 'silent' strokes, which may take an uncounted toll on cognitive function, possibly contributing to the problem of multi-infarct dementia among the elderly[1–7].

PATHOGENESIS OF THROMBOEMBOLISM

The pathogenesis of stroke in patients with atrial fibrillation has conventionally been related to thrombus formation in the left atrium or its appendage, with embolism of this material to the cerebral vascular tree. The mechanism of acute ischaemic stroke is usually difficult to ascertain, however, particularly when a number of stroke risk factors coexist. A triad of ingredients precipitating thrombus formation was outlined by the pathologist Rudolph Virchow over a century ago: endothelial injury, a zone of circulatory stasis and hypercoagulability[7]. Experimental[8] as well as clinical studies[9,10] have emphasised the importance of wall motion abnormalities in the development of left ventricular mural thrombi[11], and it seems clear that stasis of blood in regions of akinesia or dyskinesia is the essential factor. Similarly, stasis is important in the development of atrial thrombi[12] when effective mechanical atrial activity is impaired, as occurs in atrial fibrillation, atrial enlargement, mitral stenosis and cardiac failure. Stasis is tantamount to conditions of low shear rate, and activation of the coagulation system plays the predominant pathogenetic role in the development of intracavitary thrombi. One study of patients with atrial fibrillation found that alterations in coagulation may contribute to stroke[13], although laboratory changes were subtle and not studied serially.

The problem of thromboembolism originating from the cardiac chambers prompts consideration of the interaction between the effects of regional injury, stasis, and procoagulant factors that favour thrombus formation on the one hand and the dynamic forces of the circulation that are responsible for the migration of thrombotic material into the systemic circulation on the other. At post-mortem examination in patients with atrial fibrillation, thrombi are most frequently detected in the left atrial appendage. Stasis favours thrombus formation within this circulatory cul-de-sac, but isolation from dynamic circulatory forces protects against embolic migration[14,15]. Thus, factors leading to thrombus formation are not the same as those which produce systemic embolism.

MECHANISMS OF STROKE

The aetiology of ischaemic stroke in patients with non-valvular atrial fibrillation is diverse, ranging from emboli derived from distant, stasis-related thrombi in the left atrium or left ventricle, to thrombotic complications of associated cerebrovascular disease[2,5,16]. Abnormal endocardial tissue surfaces, including myxomatous or fibrotic mitral valve leaflets, mitral annular dilatation or calcification, damaged chordae tendineae or other lesions may stimulate platelet aggregation as well as the coagulation system. Alterations in haemostatic function have also been identified in patients with non-valvular atrial fibrillation whether or not they have sustained prior ischaemic stroke. Specifically, higher plasma concentrations of von Willebrand factor, factor VIIIc, fibrinogen, the fibrinolytic product D-dimer, beta-thromboglobulin and platelet factor 4 were found in one study comparing these measurements with those in age- and gender-matched patients with prior stroke and sinus rhythm as well as with healthy control subjects[17]. These biochemical changes may be either the cause or the effect of ongoing thrombosis in patients with atrial fibrillation, and the correlation with morphological evidence of thrombus formation or with clinical thromboembolic risk remains to be established.

Beyond these primary thrombotic mechanisms, coexisting atherosclerotic lesions in the aorta, extracranial or intracranial arteries may reduce cerebral perfusion by direct obstruction or as a result of thrombus formation provoked by exposure of lipid material and subintimal collagen[17]. The prevalence of atherosclerotic disease of the carotid arteries is twice as great in patients with atrial fibrillation as in age-matched controls[18], but less than one in four patients with atrial fibrillation and stroke has significant carotid disease apparent on ultrasound examination[19]. This is about half the prevalence in non-selected groups of stroke patients, supporting the view that stroke in patients with atrial fibrillation is mediated by a different mechanism. Clinical estimates of the frequency of cardiogenic embolism as the aetiology of stroke in patients with atrial fibrillation vary widely and are difficult to verify, but are generally in excess of fifty per cent[5,20,21].

Systemic emboli in patients with atrial fibrillation are suspected to originate as thrombi formed within the left atrial cavity or appendage[11]. To the extent that stasis-related thrombi are responsible for ischaemic stroke in patients with atrial fibrillation, administration of anticoagulant medication such as warfarin represents a logical preventive approach. The presence of endothelial lesions within the heart or blood vessels, which might be a nidus for thrombus formation, raises the likelihood of a response to platelet inhibitors such as aspirin[17]. The differential responses to warfarin and aspirin in recent clinical trials of antithrombotic therapy in patients with non-valvular atrial fibrillation may reflect, in part, the relative predominance of these aetiological factors.

ASYMPTOMATIC CEREBRAL INFARCTION

Clinical stroke in patients with atrial fibrillation is typically associated with substantial acute neurological deficit and often with lasting functional disability. A number of studies have suggested additionally that episodes of cerebral infarction may occur without symptoms. These clinically silent events are usually identified as small subcortical hypodense zones on computerised cerebral tomography, though cortical infarction or large deep areas of infarction have been reported in up to 10 per cent of patients[23]. Histopathological confirmation of the ischaemic nature of these infarcts is lacking, and there is as yet no proof that they are due to cardiogenic thromboembolism, though this seems a likely explanation. A series of studies in Denmark found minor cerebral infarcts in 48 per cent of 29 patients with chronic atrial fibrillation present for at least 1 year[24], but a lower rate among patients with paroxysmal atrial fibrillation[25]. Interpretation of these data is hampered by uncertainty about the prevalence of asymptomatic cerebral infarction in older persons without atrial fibrillation, though there is evidence of prior silent stroke in 10–11% of patients with acute stroke[26,27].

EXTRA-CEREBRAL SYSTEMIC EMBOLISM

While at least 75 per cent of symptomatic arterial emboli of cardiac origin involve the central nervous system, other regions of the systemic circulation are not spared, particularly the abdominal viscera and the extremities. Emboli to multiple sites occur in approximately one-fifth of cases of rheumatic heart disease[28], and a similar pattern is likely in patients with other conditions predisposing to thromboembolism derived from the cardiac chambers. Small emboli outside the central nervous system are detected at postmortem examination, in a distribution roughly proportionate to that of the cardiac output, but are usually asymptomatic.

ROLE OF ECHOCARDIOGRAPHY

Aside from the identification of mitral stenosis, specific echocardiographic features of patients with atrial fibrillation that predict greater or lesser thromboembolic risk have not been established (see also Chapter 2.6). Most studies have focused upon the diameter of the left atrium in the antero-posterior dimension, as measured by M-mode echocardiography. Enlargement of the left atrium appears related to thromboembolic risk in patients with prosthetic heart valves[29], but this relationship has not been confirmed for patients with rheumatic heart disease or non-valvular atrial fibrillation[30,31]. The left atrium appears to enlarge progressively as the duration and persistence of atrial fibrillation increases[32–34]. Any relationship between left atrial size and stroke risk in patients with atrial fibrillation may be difficult to interpret in view of a recent report, which suggests that left atrial diameter as determined from the M-mode echocardiogram may be an independent predictor of stroke risk among the elderly, even after adjustment for such factors as age, blood pressure and atrial fibrillation[35].

Transoesophageal echocardiography more frequently identifies potential sources of cerebral embolism in patients with acute brain infarction than transthoracic echocardiography[36]. This is particularly true for detection of thrombi in the left atrial appendage. This technique also appears more sensitive for the detection of spontaneous echo-contrast[37,38], which is seen most often in dilated cardiac chambers with reduced blood flow where it may relate to platelet and red cell aggregation within areas of blood stasis (see Chapter 2.6). This 'smoke sign' may be an early indicator of thrombus development[39,40] and in preliminary reports appears to correlate with the risk of embolism in patients with atrial fibrillation both with and without valvular heart disease[41–43]. Atherosclerotic lesions of the proximal aorta are relatively frequently discovered by transoesophageal ultrasound imaging, sometimes accompanied by the appearance of mobile echodensities protruding into the aortic lumen; potentially additional sources of atheroembolism and thromboembolism.

STRATIFICATION OF THROMBOEMBOLIC RISK

Recent thromboembolism

Among patients with non-valvular atrial fibrillation, the risk appears greatest when stroke or systemic embolism has occurred within the previous 2 years; in such cases the risk of recurrent stroke is even greater than 10 per cent per year[44–47](see also Chapter 5.2). The mechanism responsible for this incremental risk is not clear, but may be related either to the potential for the surface of freshly formed thrombus to stimulate additional coagulation[48], or to the association of other clinical factors, such as hypertensive or atherosclerotic vascular disease that may contribute to ischaemic events in these patients.

Thyrotoxicosis

Several reports have suggested that patients with atrial fibrillation in the setting of thyrotoxicosis, often associated with decompensated congestive heart failure, are also at particularly high risk (averaging 14 per cent over varying periods of observation)[49–51], though the exact mechanism underlying this enhanced embolic potential is not clear[50–52]. It remains controversial whether patients with atrial fibrillation associated with thyrotoxicosis are at higher risk of thromboembolic cerebrovascular events than those in whom this dysrhythmia accompanies forms of organic heart disease[53]. Nonetheless, consensus has emerged that thyrotoxic patients with atrial fibrillation should be treated with anticoagulant medication unless a contraindication to such therapy stands in the way, at least until a euthyroid state has been restored and congestive heart failure has been corrected.

Lone atrial fibrillation

At the other end of the spectrum of risk are patients younger than 60 years of age with 'lone' atrial fibrillation in the absence of clinical history, symptoms, signs or echocardiographic evidence of associated cardiopulmonary disease. These patients represented between 2.7% and 11.4% of cases of atrial fibrillation in the Framingham Heart Study[54]. Kopecky reported the findings of a cohort study involving 99 such patients extending over nearly 15 years in Olmstead County, Minnesota, in which the incidence of stroke was 0.4 per cent per year and the mortality was 0.1 per cent per year, not significantly greater than rates in patients with normal sinus rhythm[55]. Since lone atrial fibrillation is associated with such a low risk of stroke, it appears that the rhythm disturbance itself is not the cause of stroke but rather represents a marker of associated cardiovascular pathology, which is the true source of cerebral ischaemia. Older age, hypertension and congestive heart failure are among the factors that substantially increase the stroke risk in the presence of atrial fibrillation[54]. Another study by the Mayo Clinic investigators using the same criteria found that older patients were at increased risk of stroke[56].

Non-valvular atrial fibrillation associated with cardiac disease

Between these extremes are a large number of patients with non-valvular atrial fibrillation at intermediate risk of thromboembolism, which appears, according to older epidemiological data and more recently available results of randomised trials, to average about 5 per cent per year. The range of risks is relatively wide (at least 3% and perhaps more than 8% per year), reflecting the clinical diversity of this patient population and partially accounting for the controversy about anticoagulant therapy, particularly when this is contemplated for an extended period of time. It has long been suspected that, within this broad range of patients with atrial fibrillation, subgroups at relatively greater or lesser risk might be defined on the basis of clinical or echocardiographic features. Duration since the onset of atrial fibrillation, for example, has been suspected to relate to embolic risk[57]. Differences in rates of thromboembolic events have also been cited on the basis of the constant or paroxysmal character of atrial fibrillation[58,59], and the presence or absence of hypertension, congestive heart failure, or mitral regurgitation[5]. Enlargement of the left atrium, seemingly a correlate of stasis within the atrial appendage, has eluded validation as a particular marker of stroke

Table 1.2–1(A)
Randomised Trials of Antithrombotic Therapy in Non-valvular Atrial Fibrillation: Design

	SPAF	*AFASAK*	*BAATAF*	*CAFA*
Inpt/Outpt	both	outpt	both	both
Cnst/Int	both	cnst	both	both
PTR	1.5	1.7	1.3	1.3
INR	1.5-4.7	2.4-4.2	1.5-2.7	2.0-3.0
Dose ASA (mg/day)	325 mg/day	75 mg/day		–
blind	partial	partial	no	yes
control group	placebo	placebo	placebo	none/?aspirin

Abbreviations:

SPAF = Stroke Prevention in Atrial Fibrillation Study (U.S.A.)[64]
AFASAK = Atrial Fibrillation/Aspirin/Anticoagulation Study (Denmark)[65]
CAFA = Canadian Atrial Fibrillation Anticoagulation Study[66]
BAATAF = Boston Area Anticoagulation in Atrial Fibrillation Study (U.S.A.)[67]
Inpt = hospital inpatients
Outpt = ambulatory outpatients
PTR = prothrombin time ratio (patient/control)
INR = International Normalised Ratio
ASA = aspirin

risk[60–62], but the view is emerging that associated left ventricular dysfunction may contribute an important element of risk[15].

ANTITHROMBOTIC THERAPY

Before the availability of data from recently reported randomised trials, a consensus of the American College of Chest Physicians and the National Heart, Lung and Blood Institute issued a recommendation for long-term anticoagulant therapy (INR 3.0–4.5) in patients with a history of systemic embolism in the previous 2 years[44,45]. Other patients at substantial risk of embolism are those with atrial fibrillation associated with mitral stenosis or prosthetic heart valves. Data from numerous non-randomised and uncontrolled trials suggest that anticoagulation reduces the rates of embolism and death in patients with rheumatic valvular disease by 25 per cent[44].

At the lower end of the spectrum of embolic risk in patients with atrial fibrillation are those without evidence of associated organic heart disease. The natural history of lone atrial fibrillation suggests that for patients under the age of 60 years with atrial fibrillation but no evidence of organic heart disease the hazards of chronic anticoagulation outweigh its potential benefits[55].

RANDOMISED CLINICAL TRIALS

Over the past several years, no fewer than six prospective trials, aimed at the primary prevention of stroke and systemic embolism in patients with atrial fibrillation have been undertaken. The results from four have been reported[64–67]. While these share certain features, there are sufficient differences in the demographics of the populations investigated, specific trial designs and results to leave some issues still in dispute. Salient features of those studies from which results are available are summarised in Tables 1.2–1(A), 1.2–1(B) and 1.2–1(C).

The Copenhagen Atrial Fibrillation-Aspirin-Anticoagulation (AFASAK) study [64] involved 1,007 patients with constant atrial fibrillation randomly assigned to therapy

Table 1.2–1(B)
Randomised Trials of Antithrombotic Therapy in Non-valvular Atrial Fibrillation: Patient Characteristics

	SPAF	*AFASAK*	*BAATAF*	*CAFA*
number	1330	1007	420	378
age	67	74	68	68
% male	71	64	72	75
% CHF	19	51	26	22
% prior MI	8	8	12	13
% HTN	52	33	51	39
LA dia (mean,mm)	46	–	41	46

Additional abbreviations:

CHF = congestive heart failure
MI = myocardial infarction
HTN = hypertension
LA dia = left atrial diameter

Table 1.2–1(C)
Randomised Trials of Antithrombotic Therapy in Non-valvular Atrial Fibrillation: Outcome†

	SPAF	*AFASAK*	*BAATAF*	*CAFA*
Control				
event rate	6.3	5.5	3.0*	4.6
Warfarin				
event rate	2.3	2.6	0.4	3.0
% reduction	67	53	86	35
Aspirin				
event rate	3.6	5.0	–	–
% reduction	42	9		
Control mortality				
% year	6.5	6.1	6.0*	3.3

†intention-to-treat analysis
*not placebo-controlled; values refer to control group, nearly half of which used aspirin for unspecified periods
Event rates expressed per cent per patient/year

with warfarin (INR 2.8–4.2), aspirin (75 mg daily) or placebo, followed on treatment for a mean of 11 months by a single investigator using the primary endpoint events: stroke (both ischaemic and haemorrhagic), transient cerebral ischaemia and systemic embolism. The mean patient age was 74 years and the prevalence of congestive heart failure (51 per cent) was greater than in the other trials[65–67]. The proportion of women was more evenly balanced with men than in the other trials. Although 38 per cent of patients assigned to anticoagulant therapy were withdrawn, warfarin seemed to be protective ($p < 0.05$) while aspirin did not. Of 57 primary events, 25 occurred among those given placebo, 21 in the aspirin group and 11 in those assigned to warfarin; three during periods of subtherapeutic anticoagulation and six after anticoagulant medication was withdrawn[59]. The incidence of events increased with the duration of atrial fibrillation. Only one patient with a primary event had a history of thyrotoxicosis. The dimension of the left atrium, determined by M-mode echocardiography at the time of patient enrolment, did not correlate with thromboembolic risk, but a history of myocardial infarction appeared to represent a significant risk factor for development of a primary event during follow-up for a maximum of two years[68].

In the United States, the Stroke Prevention in Atrial Fibrillation (SPAF) Study[65,69] randomised 1,330 patients with either intermittent (34%) or constant atrial fibrillation who were candidates for anticoagulation (Group I) to receive warfarin (INR 1.7–4.5), aspirin (325 mg/day) or placebo, and those ineligible for warfarin (Group II) to receive either aspirin or placebo. Only the aspirin and placebo were blinded. The mean age in this study was 67 years, and only 10.9% of patients assigned to warfarin were withdrawn. The primary events were ischaemic stroke and systemic embolism. Patients were followed for a mean of 1.3 years, after which placebo administration was terminated because the event rate with active therapy (1.6%/year) was less than with placebo (7.4%/year) in Group I (risk reduction 81%).

An insufficient number of events were observed in the active treatment arms of group I to detect a difference between warfarin and aspirin. The results with warfarin (primary event rate 2.3%/year; risk reduction 67%; 95% confidence interval 27–85%; p=0.01) were not significantly different from those with aspirin because of the small total number of events in patients treated with active antithrombotic medication in Group I. Compared with placebo, the risk of primary event or death was reduced by 58% with warfarin (95% confidence interval 20–78%; p=0.01). Among all patients given aspirin (Groups I and II combined), the rate of primary events was 3.6%/year, compared with 6.3%/year in those given placebo (risk reduction 42%; 95% confidence interval 9–63%; p< 0.02). The reduction in primary events or death was 32% (95% confidence interval 7–50%; p=0.02). Aspirin appeared particularly effective in those 75 years or younger (p=0.0042), with reduction in risk of stroke or systemic embolism of 65% (95% confidence interval 34% to 81%) for event rates of 2.2%/year in those treated with aspirin and 6.2%/year with placebo. Conversely, the benefit of aspirin seemed to evaporate in patients over the age of 75 years; for the limited number of patients over 75 years (n=238) the rate of stroke was identical in patients assigned to aspirin and placebo, each 7.4%/year.

In the Boston Area Anticoagulation Trial for Atrial Fibrillation (BAATAF)[66] 420 patients (35% with paroxysmal rather than constant atrial fibrillation) were randomly assigned to warfarin (INR 1.5–2.7) or control groups. Aspirin was permitted in the control group, and reportedly taken by 46%. Follow-up extended over a mean of 2.2 years, and the primary endpoint event was ischaemic stroke. The incidence of stroke was very low in the group given warfarin (0.41%/year) compared with the control group (3.0%/year; risk reduction 86%). The mortality rate was also lower in patients assigned to warfarin (2.3%/year) than to placebo (6.0%/year), particularly for death attributed to non-cardiac causes. The mean age was 68 years and only 10% of warfarin patients stopped therapy. Twenty-six percent of patients had a history of congestive heart failure and 13% had previously sustained myocardial infarction, prevalences similar to those in the SPAF study[65]. Mitral annular calcification (present in 30% of patients) and age were significantly related to stroke risk. Patients in the control group

Table 1.2–2
Randomised Trial of Antithrombotic Therapy in Non-valvular Atrial Fibrillation: Complications of Anticoagulation

	SPAF	*AFASAK*	*BAATAF*	*CAFA*
anticoagulation (duration (pt-yr))	260	407	487	235
mean dose warfarin (mg/d)	4.8	–	4.3	4.1
rate of major haemorrhage (%/yr)	1.5	0.8	0.8	2.5
mean INR (approximate)	3.0	3.3	2.1	2.4
intracerebral haemorrhage (events)	1	1	1	1

were permitted to take aspirin, and nearly half of this group acknowledged doing so in a non-randomised manner. Although the authors indicate that there was no correlation between aspirin intake and thromboembolic risk, this factor could account for the low overall rate of stroke in this trial.

The results of the Canadian Atrial Fibrillation Anticoagulation (CAFA) Study have been reported only in preliminary form[67]; the trial was terminated before statistically meaningful endpoints were reached because of convincing results in other trials favouring antithrombotic therapy. Of all the published studies, however, this was the only one to incorporate a double-blind design for administration of warfarin, and as such is of particular value as it avoids potential bias in event detection.

In none of these studies was the incidence of major haemorrhagic complications significantly increased with anticoagulant therapy, even though the average patient age was nearly 70 years (Table 1.2–2). Taken together, these trials confirm observations in epidemiological studies that the risk of ischaemic stroke in patients with non-valvular atrial fibrillation is about 5%/year, approximately 5–7 times that of the general population of comparable age and gender. Each study provides support for the view that anticoagulation with warfarin is effective in comparatively low intensity (INR 1.5–4.5) for reducing the risk of stroke in patients with non-valvular atrial fibrillation by about 3%/year (Table 1.2–3A and 1.2–3B). This benefit offsets the increased risk of bleeding sufficiently severe to require hospitalisation, transfusion or surgery (about 1–2%/year). Aspirin is also effective in reducing the incidence of ischaemic stroke in patients with atrial fibrillation, but the results of the two studies that included aspirin arms differed on the basis of aspirin dose and patient population. Secondary analysis of data from the SPAF study[65] suggested reduced aspirin efficacy in older patients and this might account, in part, for the minimal beneficial effect of aspirin in the AFASAK study[64]. The lower incidence of stroke in the control group of the BAATAF study[66] than

Table 1.2–3(A)
Randomised Trials of Antithrombotic Therapy in Non-valvular Atrial Fibrillation: Meta-analysis of Anticoagulant Efficacy*

	All events		*Disabling Ischaemic Stroke*	
	control	*warfarin*	*control*	*warfarin*
SPAF	18	6	7	2
AFASAK	22	9	12	6
BAATAF**	13	2	6	1
CAFA	11	7	4	2
	64	24	29	11
Aggregate % reduction	**63**		**62**	
Control event rate%/yr**	**5.8**		**2.6**	

*intention-to-treat analysis including all ischaemic strokes and systemic emboli, but excluding primary intracerebral haemorrhages and transient ischaemic attacks.

**not controlled in BAATAF; about half of control patients received aspirin in various doses in a nonrandomized manner and are not included in aggregate control event rate calculation.

Table 1.2–3(B)
Randomised Trials of Antithrombotic Therapy in Non-valvular Atrial Fibrillation: Meta-analysis of Aspirin Efficacy*

	All events		*Disabling Ischaemic Stroke*	
	placebo	*aspirin*	*placebo*	*aspirin*
SPAF	46	26	18	13
AFASAK	22	19	12	8
	68	45	30	21
Aggregate % reduction	**34**		**30**	

*intention-to-treat analysis including all ischaemic strokes and systemic emboli, but excluding primary intracerebral haemorrhages and transient ischaemic attacks.

in the SPAF and AFASAK studies may be due to the use of aspirin in nearly half the patients.

As ischaemic stroke in patients with atrial fibrillation may involve any of a number of mechanisms, the disparate antithrombotic actions of aspirin (platelet inhibitor) and warfarin (anticoagulant) may prevent strokes of entirely different aetiologies. Indeed, the relative efficacy of warfarin and aspirin for prevention of disabling ischaemic cerebral events in patients with atrial fibrillation remains an unsettled issue and a priority for continued research. At this point, however, it seems reasonable to conclude that most patients with non-rheumatic cardiac disease associated with atrial fibrillation who can safely tolerate these antithrombotic medications should be given either aspirin or warfarin to prevent stroke and systemic embolism.

ABOLITION OF ATRIAL FIBRILLATION

Anticoagulation during cardioversion

The notion that the risk of stroke should be greater proximate to chemical or electrical attempts to restore sinus rhythm in patients with atrial fibrillation is fraught with conjecture, particularly since spontaneous termination of episodes of atrial fibrillation among patients in whom fibrillation is paroxysmal is not associated with increased risk[58]. Nevertheless, several reports cite an unexpectedly high incidence of stroke within the first several days following successful electrical reversion to sinus rhythm by direct-current countershock, and suggest that the risk may be lowered by anticoagulant therapy[71]. It is difficult to interpret these reports, however, because of the relatively high incidence of rheumatic heart disease subtending atrial fibrillation in many of the cases studied.

In the largest study, 437 patients with a variety of atrial arrhythmias, 58% of whom had underlying rheumatic heart disease, underwent electrical cardioversion procedures with or without anticoagulant medication depending upon the practice of the referring physicians. Those receiving anticoagulants had presumed embolic events at a rate of 0.8 incidents per 100 successful conversions, compared with 5.3% in those not anticoagulated (p=0.016), despite the greater prevalence of rheumatic heart disease, congestive heart failure, prior embolism and cardiac enlargement among those receiving anticoagulants[72–73]. Half of the thromboembolic events occurred in patients with non-rheumatic cardiac disorders. This study is mentioned not so much for its implications regarding therapy, which involved long-term rather than short-term anticoagulation, but because it illustrates the limitations imposed by non-randomised design and other issues[70].

Undoubtedly, a heightened awareness of danger may contribute to event detection under these circumstances. Alternatively, patients at greater intrinsic risk of thromboembolism, such as those with left ventricular dysfunction, may be more frequent candidates for cardioversion. As there should be no difference in rates of thromboembolism associated with spontaneous, chemical or electrical means of cardioversion, the risk of stroke at the time of cardioversion is probably linked with the intrinsic cardiovascular factors which contribute to risk on a chronic basis. More aggressive use of anticoagulant medication may be justified for a period of 3–4 weeks prior to and another 3–4 weeks after cardioversion because of the reduced cumulative danger of haemorrhage when the intensity of anticoagulation is closely controlled over a relatively short period of time. The need for therapy over this interval is based upon the latency of the onset of cerebral ischaemic symptoms in some patients, which has been attributed to delayed activation of the left atrial contractile function that retards the embolic propulsion of thrombus across the mitral orifice and into the circulation[74–77].

Maintenance of sinus rhythm with antiarrhythmic medication

Successful treatment which maintains sinus rhythm might suspend the need for antithrombotic therapy. A meta-analysis of six randomised, placebo-controlled, double-blind trials incorporating 800 patients with chronic atrial fibrillation evaluated quinidine maintenance of normal sinus rhythm following electrical cardioversion[78]. Although quinidine was more effective than placebo in preventing recurrent atrial fibrillation (50% at 1 year vs. 25%/year in the control groups) the risk of death was threefold greater among drug-treated patients (2.9% vs. 0.8% with placebo; odds ratio 2.89, $p < 0.05$). The mechanism by which mortality occurs is speculative, but pro-arrhythmic drug toxicity is one possible mechanism[79]. The risk of the latter (approximately 5%/year) might seem to outweigh a 3%/year annual risk from quinidine, pointing to the advantage of elimination or prevention of atrial fibrillation. On the other hand, atrial fibrillation may be more important as a marker of thromboembolic risk rather than the primary cause of stroke. Elimination of the dysrhythmia as a means of preventing ischaemic stroke remains an untested hypothesis.

PREVENTION OF STROKE AND SYSTEMIC EMBOLISM

Atrial fibrillation is now recognised as a major risk factor for the development of ischaemic stroke, particularly among elderly patients. However, the rhythm disturbance is better viewed as a clinical marker of associated cardiovascular pathology which is more directly at the root of stroke than atrioembolic mechanisms alone. The effectiveness and relative safety of chronic anticoagulant therapy with warfarin has now been validated in four separate clinical trials, supporting a thrombotic mechanism for most of the strokes which occur in patients with atrial fibrillation. The success of therapy with aspirin in younger individuals in one of the studies suggests that administration of this platelet inhibitor may be sufficient for some patients with non-valvular atrial fibrillation.

The dimensions of the left atrium as determined by M-mode or two-dimensional transthoracic echocardiography do not appear to predict ischaemic stroke or systemic thromboembolic events in patients with non-valvular atrial fibrillation, though left atrial enlargement has been identified as a risk factor for embolism among patients with rheumatic or prosthetic valvular heart disease associated with atrial fibrillation. Whether more comprehensive analyses of atrial volume, that take into account the extent and pattern of mitral regurgitation, will show such a relationship in other patients with atrial fibrillation, remains an unresolved issue. Presently available data suggest a great predictive value for the finding of left ventricular dysfunction which, along with clinical features of congestive heart failure, appears to identify a group of patients at higher thromboembolic risk. The exact role of transoesophageal echocardiography for risk stratification and identification of patients requiring therapy with an anticoagulant rather than a platelet inhibitor has not yet been clarified.

Among the other pressing clinical questions is whether subgroups of patients at such increased risk as to justify long term anticoagulant therapy can be identified and, conversely, whether there are others at comparatively low risk for whom aspirin alone will prove sufficient. At this juncture, the proportion of ischaemic strokes in patients with atrial fibrillation that have a cardioembolic mechanism has not been defined and it is possible that warfarin and aspirin exert differential benefit related to stroke mechanism and severity. In addition, the significance of associated cerebrovascular disease and its implications for selection of optimum antithrombotic agents are unresolved as well. The slightly different intensities of anticoagulant therapy employed in various randomised trials lead to speculation that even lower warfarin doses may prove effective with still less risk of bleeding. Nevertheless, it remains to be established that the low rates of bleeding in patients given anticoagulant medication in these trials will apply in general clinical practice, particularly among older patients treated for longer periods of time.

Goals for the future include collaborative analysis by investigators involved with ongoing and recently completed trials to further stratify patients in terms of the relative risk of stroke based upon the aetiology of the dysrhythmia and associated clinical conditions. Such an effort would greatly enlarge the available data pool, allowing inferences about the optimal therapeutic range for warfarin anticoagulation and selection of some patients for alternative therapy with aspirin. A longer-range view includes the development and testing of more effective strategies of antithrombotic therapy. The present challenge is for physicians to identify patients with atrial fibrillation who might benefit from antithrombotic therapy and to supervise treatment closely to avoid both haemorrhage and stroke.

REFERENCES

1. Phillips SJ, Whismant JP, O'Fallon WM, et al. Prevalence of cardiovascular disease and diabetes in residents of Rochester, Minnesota. Mayo Clin Proc 1990;65:344–359.
2. Cerebral Embolism Task Force. Cardiogenic brain embolism. Arch Neurol 1986;43:71–84.

3. Cerebral Embolism Task Force. Cardiogenic brain embolism: The second report of the Cerebral Embolism Task Force. Arch Neurol 1989;46:727–743.
4. Kannel WB, Abbott RD, Savage DD, McNamara PM. Epidemiologic features of chronic atrial fibrillation: the Framingham Study. N Engl J Med 1982;306:1018–1022.
5. Wolf PA, Abbott RD, Kannel WB. Atrial fibrillation: a major contributor to stroke in the elderly: The Framingham Study. Arch Intern Med 1987;147:1561–1564.
6. Halperin JL, Hart RG. Atrial fibrillation and stroke: New ideas, persisting dilemmas. Stroke 1988;19:937–941.
7. Candelise L, Pinerdi G, Morabito A and the Italian Acute Stroke Study Group. Mortality in acute stroke with atrial fibrillation. Stroke 1991;22:169–174.
8. Virchow R. Gesammelte Abhandlungen zur Wissenschaftlichen Medicine. Frankfurt, Meidinger Sohn & Co, 1856, pp 219–732.
9. Mikell FL, Asinger RW, Elsperger KJ, Anderson WR, Hodges M. Regional stasis of blood in the dysfunctional left ventricle: echocardiographic detection and differentiation from early thrombosis. Circulation 1982;66:755–763.
10. Asinger RW, Mikell FL, Elsperger J, Hodges M. Incidence of left ventricular thrombosis after acute transmural myocardial infarction: serial evaluation by two-dimensional echocardiography. N Engl J Med 1981;305:297–302.
11. Weinrich DJ, Burke JF, Pauletto FJ. Left ventricular mural thrombi complicating acute myocardial infarction: long term follow-up with serial echocardiography. Ann Intern Med 1984;100:789–794.
12. Shresta NK, Moreno FL, Narciso FV, Torres L, Calleja HB. Two-dimensional echocardiographic diagnosis of left atrial thrombus in rheumatic heart disease: a clinicopathologic study. Circulation 1983;67:341–347.
13. Kumagai K, Fukunami M, Ohmori M, Kitabatake A, Kamada T, Hoki N. Increased intravascular clotting in patients with chronic atrial fibrillation. J Am Coll Cardiol 1990;16:377–380.
14. Fuster V, Badimon L, Cohen M, Ambrose JA, Badimon JJ, Chesebro JH. Insights into the pathogenesis of acute ischemic syndromes. Circulation 1988;77:1213–1220.
15. Cabin HS, Roberts WC. Left ventricular aneurysm, intra-aneurysmal thrombus and systemic embolus in coronary heart disease. Chest 1980;77:586–590.
16. Chesebro JH, Fuster V, Halperin JL. Atrial fibrillation – risk marker for stroke. N Engl J Med 1990;323:1556–1558.
17. Gustafsson C, Blomback M, Britton M, Hamsten A, Svensson J. Coagulation factors and the increased risk of stroke in non-valvular atrial fibrillation. Stroke 1990;21:47–51.
18. Stein B, Fuster V, Halperin JL, Chesebro JH. Antithrombotic therapy in cardiac disease: An emerging approach based on pathogenesis and risk. Circulation 1989;80:1501–1513.
19. Tegeler CH. Stroke Prevention in Atrial Fibrillation Study: Carotid Stenosis Study Group: Carotid stenosis in atrial fibrillation. Neurology 1989;39 (Suppl):159 (Abs).
20. Weinberger J, Rothlauf EB, Materese E, Halperin JL. Non-invasive evaluation of the extracranial carotid arteries in patients with cerebrovascular events and atrial fibrillation. Arch Intern Med 1988;148:1785–1788.
21. D'Olhaberriague L, Hernandez-Vidal A, Molina L et al. A prospective study of atrial fibrillation and stroke. Stroke 1989;20:1648–1652.
22. Bogousslavsky J, vanMelle G, Regli F, Kappenberger L. Pathogenesis of anterior circulation stroke in patients with non-valvular atrial fibrillation: The Lausanne Stroke Registry. Neurology 1190;40:1046–1050.
23. Feinberg WM, Seeger JF, Carmody RF, Anderson DC, Hart RG, Pearce LA. Epidemiologic features of asymptomatic cerebral infarction in patients with non-valvular atrial fibrillation. Arch Intern Med 1990;150:2340–2344.
24. Petersen P, Madsen EB, Brun B, Pedersen F, Glydensted C, Boysen G. Silent cerebral infarction in chronic atrial fibrillation. Stroke 1987;18:1098–1100.
25. Petersen P, Pedersen F, Johnsen A, et al. Cerebral computed tomography in paroxysmal atrial fibrillation. Acta Neurol Scand 1989;79:482–486.
26. Chodosh EH, Foulkes MA, Kase CS, et al. Silent stroke in the NINCDS Stroke Data Bank. Neurology 1988;38:1674–1679.
27. Kase CS, Wolf PA, Chodosh EF, et al. Prevalence of silent stroke in patients presenting with initial stroke: the Framingham Study. Stroke 1989;20:850–852.
28. Coulshed N, Epstein EJ, McKenrisk CS, Galloway RW, and Walker E. Systemic embolism in mitral valve disease. Br Heart J 1970;32:26–34.
29. Burchfiel CM, Hammermeister KE, Krause-Steinrauf H, et al. Left atrial dimension and risk of systemic embolism in patients with a prosthetic heart valve. J Am Coll Cardiol 1990;15:32–41.
30. Sherrid MR, Clark RD, Cohn K. Echocardiographic analysis of left atrial size before and after operation in mitral valve disease. Am J Cardiol 1979;43(II):171–178.

31. Moss AJ. Atrial fibrillation and cerebral embolism. Arch Neurol 1984;41:707.
32. Presti CF, Asinger RW, Goldman ME. Comparative measurements of the left atrium in patients with constant vs. intermittent non-valvulopathic atrial fibrillation. Circulation 1988;78(II):600 (Abs).
33. Ruocco NA, Most AS. Clinical and echocardiographic risk factors for systemic embolization in patients with atrial fibrillation in the absence of mitral stenosis. J Am Coll Cardiol 1986;7:165A.
34. Sanfilippo AJ, Abascal V, Sheehan M, Oertel LB, Harrigan P, Hughes RA, Weyman AE. Atrial enlargement as a consequence of atrial fibrillation. Circulation 1990;82:792–797.
35. Benjamin EJ, Levy D, Plehn JF, Belanger AJ, D'Agostino RB, Wolf PA. Left atrial size: an independent risk factor for stroke. The Framingham Study. Circulation 1989;80 (IV):615 (Abs).
36. Nellessen U, Daniel WG, Matheis G, Oelert H, Depping K, Lichtlen PR. Impending paradoxical embolism from atrial thrombus: correct diagnosis by transesophageal echocardiography and prevention by surgery. J Am Coll Cardiol 1985;5:1002–1004.
37. Aschenberg W, Schluter M, Kremer P, Schroder E, Siglow V, Bleifeld W. Transesophageal two-dimensional echocardiography for the detection of left atrial appendage thrombus. J Am Coll Cardiol 1986;7:163–166.
38. Meltzer RS, Visser CA, Fuster V. Intracardiac thrombi and systemic emolization. Ann Intern Med 1986;104:689–698
39. Visser CA, Kan G, Meltzer RS, Lie KI, Durer D. Long-term follow-up of left ventricular thrombus after acute myocardial infarction: a two-dimensional echocardiographic study of 96 patients. Chest 1984;86:532–536.
40. Stratton JR, Lighty GW, Pearlman AS, Ritchie JL. Detection of left ventricular thrombus by two-dimensional echocardiography: sensitivity, specificity and causes of uncertainty. Circulation 1982;66:156–166.
41. Malone SA, Palac RT, Imus, et al. Prevalence of left atrial thrombi in symptomatic versus asymptomatic patients with non-valvular atrial fibrillation. Circulation 1989;80 (Suppl II):1 (Abs).
42. DeBelder MA, Tourikis L, Leech G, et al. Spontaneous contrast echoes are markers of thromboembolic risk in patients with atrial fibrillation. Circulation 1989;80 (Suppl II):1.
43. Hirabayashi T, Terahisli J, Mikami T et al. Spontaneous contrast echoes (SCE) are associated with an increased risk of cerebral infarction in patients with non-valvular chronic atrial fibrillation. Circulation 82 (Suppl II): 108.
44. Dunn M, Alexander J, de Silva R, et al. Antithrombotic therapy in atrial fibrillation. Chest 1989;95 (Suppl):118S–127S.
45. Sherman DG, Dyken ML, Fisher M, et al. Antithrombotic therapy for cerebrovascular disorders. Chest 1989;95 (Suppl):140S–155S.
46. Sage JI, Van Uitert RL. Risk of recurrent stroke in patients with atrial fibrillation and non-valvular heart disease. Stroke 1983;14:537–540.
47. Hart RG, Coull BM, Hart PD. Early recurrent embolism associated with non-valvular atrial fibrillation. Stroke 1983;14:688–693.
48. Fuster V, Badimon L, Coehn M, et al. Insights into the pathogenesis of acute ischemic syndromes. Circulation 1988;77:1213–1220.
49. Hurley DM, Hunter AN, Hewett MJ, et al. Atrial fibrillation and arterial embolism in hyperthryroidism. Aust NZ J Med 1981;11:391–393.
50. Yuen RWM, Gutteridge DH, Thompson PL, et al. Embolism in thyrotoxic atrial fibrillation. Med J Aust 1979;1:630–631.
51. Staffurth JS, Gibberd MC, Tang Fui SN. Arterial embolism in thyrotoxicosis with atrial fibrillation. Br Med J 1977;2:688–690.
52. Bar-Sela S, Ehrenfeld M, Eliakim M. Arterial embolism in thyrotoxicosis with atrial fibrillation. Arch Intern Med 1981;141:1191–1192.
53. Petersen O, Hansen JM. Stroke in thyrotoxicosis with atrial fibrillation. Stroke 1988;19:15–18.
54. Brand FN, Abbott RD, Kannel WB, et al. Characteristics and prognosis of lone atrial fibrillation: 30-year follow-up in the Framingham Study. JAMA 1985;254:3449–3453.
55. Kopecky SL, Gersh BJ, McGoon MD, et al. The natural history of lone atrial fibrillation: a population-based study over three decades. N Engl J Med 1987;317:669–674.
56. Kopecky SL, Gersh BJ, McGoon MD, et al. Lone atrial fibrillation in the elderly: a population-based long term study. Circulation 1989;80 (Suppl II):409 (Abs).
57. Wolf PA, Kannel WB, McGee DL, et al. Duration of atrial fibrillation and imminence of stroke: The Framingham Study. Stroke 1983;14:664–667.
58. Petersen P, Godtfredsen J. Embolic complications in paroxysmal atrial fibrillation. Stroke 1986;17:622–626.
59. Petersen P. Thromboembolic complications in atrial fibrillation. Stroke 1990;21:4–13.
60. Wiener I, Hafner R, Nicolai M, et al. Clinical and echocardiographic correlates of systemic embolism in non-rheumatic atrial fibrillation. Am J Cardiol 1987;59:177.

61. Caplan LR, D'Cruz I, Hier DB, et al. Atrial size, atrial fibrillation and stroke. Ann Neurol 1986;19:158–161.
62. Tegeler CH, Hart RG. Atrial size, atrial fibrillation and stroke. Ann Neurol 1987;21:315–316.
63. Roy D, Marchand E, Gagne P, Chabot M, Cartier R. Usefulness of anticoagulant therapy in the prevention of embolic complications of atrial fibrillation. Am Heart J 1986;112:1039–1043.
64. Petersen P, Boysen G, Godtfredsen J, Andersen ED, Andersen B. Placebo controlled, randomised trial of warfarin and aspirin for prevention of thromboembolic complications in atrial fibrillation: The Copenhagen AFASAK study. Lancet 1989;1:175–179.
65. Stroke Prevention in Atrial Fibrillation Study Group Investigators. Preliminary report of the Stroke Prevention in Atrial Fibrillation study. N Engl J Med 1990;322:863–868.
66. The Boston Area Anticoagulation Trial for Atrial Fibrillation Investigators. The effect of low-dose warfarin on the risk of stroke in patients with non-rheumatic atrial fibrillation. N Engl J Med 1990;323:1505–1511.
67. Connolly SJ. Canadian atrial fibrillation anticoagulation (CAFA) study. Circulation 1990;82 (Suppl III):108 (Abs).
68. Petersen P, Kastrup J, Helweg-Larsen S, Boysen G, Godtfredsen J. Risk factors for thromboembolic complications in chronic atrial fibrillation: The Copenhagen AFASAK study. Arch Intern Med 1990;150:819–821.
69. Stroke Prevention in Atrial Fibrillation Investigators. Design of a multi-centre randomised trial for the Stroke Prevention in Atrial Fibrillation Study. Stroke 1990;21:538–45.
70. Stroke Prevention in Atrial Fibrillation Investigators. The Stroke Prevention in Atrial Fibrillation Study: Patient characteristics and final results. Circulation 1991;84: 527–539.
71. Stein B, Halperin JL, Fuster V. Should patients with atrial fibrillation be anticoagulated prior to and chronically following cardioversion? In Dilemmas in Clinical Cardiology, Cheitlin MD, ed. Philadelphia: F.A. Davis Co;1990;231–247.
72. Bjerkelund CJ, Orning OM. An evaluation of DC shock treatment of atrial arrhythmias: Immediate results and complications in 437 patients, with long term results in the first 290 of these. Acta Med Scand 1968;184:481–491.
73. Bjerkelund CJ, Orning OM. The efficacy of anticoagulant therapy in preventing embolism related to DC electrical conversion of atrial fibrillation. Am J Cardiol 1969;23:208–216.
74. Mancini GBJ, Goldberger AL. Cardioversion of atrial fibrillation: Consideration of embolization, anticoagulation, prophylactic pacemaker, and long-term success. Am Heart J 1982;104:611–621.
75. Ikram H, Nixon PGF, Arcan T. Left atrial function after electrical conversion to sinus rhythm. Br Heart J 1968;30:80–83.
76. Rowlands DJ, Logan WFWE, Howitt E, et al. Atrial function after cardioversion. Am Heart J 1967;74:149–160.
77. Manning WJ, Leeman DE, Gotch PJ, et al. Pulsed Doppler evaluation of atrial mechanical function after electrical cardioversion of atrial fibrillation. J Am Coll Cardiol 1989;13:617–623.
78. Coplen SE, Antmann EM, Berling et al: Efficacy and safety of quinidine therapy for maintenance of sinus rhythm after cardioversion: a meta-analysis of randomised controlled trials. Circulation 1990;82:1106–1116.
79. Feld GK: Atrial fibrillation: Is there a safe and highly effective pharmacological treatment? Circulation 1990;82:2248–2250.

Chapter 1.3

Abnormal cardiac anatomy and physiology

Dieter Horstkotte

A variety of pathophysiological conditions, so far not fully explained, have been linked with intracardiac thrombosis and consequent cardioembolism. In these conditions, thrombogenesis may be connected with specific cardiac morphology or physiology resulting in a potential for local activation of the coagulation system. In the presence of various life-style influences or metabolic changes or when antithrombotic therapy is ineffective, such prothrombotic situations may lead to local thrombus formation.

As the risk of thrombosis cannot be decreased without an increased risk of bleeding complications if anticoagulants or antithrombotic drugs are used, the indication for such treatment requires careful consideration. Calculation of the thrombotic and thromboembolic hazard in a given patient has to be based on the evaluation of individual cardiac morphology and physiology and on comparison with known thromboembolic rates for comparable patient populations.

A major problem for risk/benefit calculations remains the lack of sensitive and specific diagnostic criteria on which to establish the diagnosis of intracardiac thrombus formation[1]. In many cases, transthoracic 2D-echocardiography (TTE) is suitable to detect intracardiac thrombi or at least to contribute to the evaluation in the presence of proven predisposing factors[2–4]. For the demonstration of intracardiac sources of systemic emboli, transoesophageal echocardiography (TEE) is superior and is today the diagnostic tool of choice[5]. Scintigraphic methods, using for example indium–111-labelled platelets, may contribute further to diagnosis in the future[6,7] (see also Chapters 2.5, 2.6 and 5.1).

Consensus in cost/benefit terms has not yet been reached on the routine use of TTE or TEE in all patients with systemic thromboembolism. Before the mid 1980s, TTE and TEE were reserved for patients presenting with a combination of clinically manifest embolism and a suspected cardiovascular source[8–13]. Recently the indications for the use of TEE particularly have been greatly widened[14–17]. Using TEE, potential cardiac sources of embolism in otherwise unexplained stroke may be identified in more than 50% of cases, as compared to not more than 15% using TTE[16].

One result of the rapid development of TEE has been the identification of spontaneous echo contrast in the left atrium as a phenomonon associated with an increased risk of thromboembolic complications[18]. It was found initially in patients after valve replacement with devices that had unfavourable haemodynamic characteristics[18,19]. Images provided by the current, high resolution echocardiography equipment suggest that the echogenicity of flowing blood is probably the consequence of corpuscular element aggregation, which is greatest at low flow velocities or within non-physiological flow patterns[20–22]. Since the introduction of high frequency transducers[16,23], such spontaneous echoes have been demonstrated in various cardiac conditions, such as dissecting aortic aneurysm[21,24], mitral valve disease[25,26], right ventricular failure[27], atrial fibrillation[16] or immediately following cardiac surgery[28].

It has been established that patients with intracardiac spontaneous echoes have a significantly increased risk of arterial embolism, especially cerebral embolism, and a similarly increased incidence of left atrial thrombus formation[10,25,29]. Whether this echo contrast is an independent risk factor for thromboembolic complications, or is only coincidentally present in a highly thrombogenic state due to the underlying cardiac pathology and physiology has not yet been demonstrated in a prospective study. Spontaneous echo contast is discussed further in Chapter 2.6.

The true incidence of embolism of cardiac origin (cardioembolism) is considerably underestimated. *Small* emboli from intracardiac sources do not cause clinical symptoms unless they involve the brain, hence the apparently high percentage of central nervous embolism from cardiac sources (35–65%). In fact, the involvement of the carotid arteries, as compared to the rest of the arterial tree, is proportionately not more than the relevant percentage of the total cardiac output. Autopsy studies show that cerebral embolism accounts for only about 20% (11–23%) of all cardioembolic events[30,31]. In these cases, the central arteries are often involved[32–37].

FREQUENCY AND PREVALENCE OF RISK FACTORS FOR CARDIOEMBOLISM.

The frequency of cardioembolism in the total population appears to be increasing. In a stroke registry of 1964, 3% of all cerebrovascular events were ascribed to cardioembolism[38], while in a series published in 1984, this proportion was 17%[39]. Other series in the period 1978–1983, have reported cardioembolism as the causative factor in 11–23% (mean 15.7%) of all cerebrovascular accidents[40–44]. Although some of this apparent increase may be due to improved diagnostic methods, a proportion may be due to the increase in life expectancy, because diseases that predispose to intracardiac thrombosis become more frequent with advanced age; these include arteriosclerotic ischaemic heart disease, hypertensive heart disease, calcific aortic sclerosis and stenosis, mitral annular calcification and sick-sinus syndrome[45].

In populations with a high prevalence of symptomatic atherosclerosis, multifocal calcific deposits are found with an increasing frequency that parallels the increase in age; the so-called 'senile cardiac calcification syndrome'[46]. Generalised arteriosclerosis is the common aetiological factor in the development of such calcium deposits, which involve with decreasing frequency the epicardial coronary arteries, the mitral valve annulus, the aortic valve annulus or cusps and the apical portions of the left ventricular papillary muscles[47–50]. Calcification in each of the aforementioned entities has been linked with an increasing risk of thromboembolic events. An increase in left atrial size and in the incidence of atrial fibrillation with advancing age is also well documented [51–55]. Moreover, rheumatic heart disease is associated with a higher incidence of cardioembolic complications in the elderly[56].

A number of published studies document the frequency of cardiogenic cerebral embolism in different patient populations. However, only a few report the frequency of clinically evident peripheral embolism. In the author's own experience between 1981 and 1990, a total of 529 consecutive cases with suspected cardioembolism were admitted to hospital. In all these cases, the diagnosis of a thromboembolic event was confirmed by cerebral computed tomography (CCT), angiography and/or convincing clinical findings (whenever peripheral embolism was suspected). Cardiac sources of embolism were suspected if there were no pathological findings in Doppler studies of the carotid arteries in patients with embolic stroke and no pathological findings with Doppler or peripheral angiographic studies in patients with acute peripheral ischaemia. The aetiology could not be identified in 138 of these cases with suspected cardioembolism, despite the use of routine clinical examination, phono-mechanocardiography, X-ray, fluoroscopy, standard ECG, Holter ECG for at least 24 hours, transthoracic and transoesophageal echocardiography (Table 1.3–1). The most frequent aetiology in the remaining 391 patients was ischaemic, followed by valvular heart disease (Table 1.3–2) and idiopathic or 'lone' atrial fibrillation. Lone atrial fibrillation was defined as atrial fibrillation in the absence of precipitating illness or overt cardiovascular disease, including systemic hypertension. All other aetiologies accounted individually for less than 5% and together for only 14.2% of all events[57].

The lack of validated criteria on which to base a diagnosis of cardioembolism casts doubt on the accuracy of any prevalence estimates[45,58,59]. Nevertheless, the relatively large number of cases in the Düsseldorf experience, the thorough evaluation of these patients using all appropriate techniques and the inclusion of all potential sources[1,59] suggest that the figures in Table 1.3–1 are close to the true distribution of sources

Table 1.3–1
Abnormal cardiac anatomy and physiology in consecutive patients[1] with cerebral (n=447)[2] or major peripheral (n=82) embolism of suspected cardiac origin (Düsseldorf 1981–1990)

Aetiology	*n*	(%)[3]	(%)[4]
– Ischaemic heart disease[5]	121	22.9	30.9
– Valvular heart disease[1]	117	22.1	29.9
– Idiopathic atrial fibrillation	98	18.5	25.1
– Paradoxical embolism[6]	19	3.6	4.9
– Cardiomyopathy – dilated	11	2.1	2.8
– hypertrophic	2	0.4	0.5
– Non-infective endocarditis[7]	9	1.7	2.3
– Congenital heart disease[8]	7	1.3	1.8
– Acute myocarditis	3	0.6	0.8
– Cardiac tumors	3	0.6	0.8
– Atrial septal aneurysm	1	0.2	0.3
– No aetiology identified	138	26.1	

1 patients with proven/suspected infective endocarditis excluded
2 no pathological findings with Doppler of the carotid vessels in patients with embolic stroke (CCT)
3 % of all cases
4 % of all cases with an aetiology identified
5 incl. acute myocardial infarction and left ventricular aneurysm
6 right-to-left shunts in congenital heart disease (n=12) and patent foramen ovale (n=7)
7 marantic, Libman-Sacks, endomyocardial fibrosis, carcinoid heart disease, scleroderma, rheumatoid arthritis
8 pre- and postoperative without right-to-left shunts

Table 1.3–2
Underlying valve pathology in 117 consecutive patients (1981–1990) with cerebral or major peripheral embolism[1]. In addition there were 23 embolic episodes in patients with proven (n=22) or suspected acute bacterial/fungal endocarditis during the same period.

Valve lesion	*n*	%[2]	%[3]
– rheumatic heart valve disease			
– mitral	35	29.9	
– aortic	6	5.1	
– multivalvular	15	12.8	
– degenerative heart valve lesion			
– mitral valve prolapse	8	6.8	
– mitral annulus calcification	4	3.4	
– calcific aortic stenosis	2	1.7	
– prosthetic heart valves	47	40.2	83.6
– acute infective endocarditis	23		16.4

[1] for more details see Table 1.3–1
[2] % of all cases with non-infective valve lesions
[3] % of all cases.

predisposing to cardioembolism in an unbiased German patient population referred to hospital. Other countries, particularly those with large third world populations, may encounter different proportions of aetiological factors (vide infra).

The prevalence of risk factors for cerebral cardioembolism in representative samples of patients in case-controlled studies ranges from 15 to 65% for non-valvular atrial fibrillation or other forms of supraventricular arrhythmias, from 22 to 27% for ischaemic heart disease, from 10 to 19% for rheumatic heart disease without atrial fibrillation, from 4 to 10% for patients with prosthetic valves or any other kind of valve surgery, from 5 to 9% for patients with cardiomyopathy or congestive heart failure and is approximately 5% for mitral valve prolapse as well as for infective endocarditis (for references, see the relevant sections of this chapter). The prevalence of calcific aortic stenosis, congenital heart disease and mitral anulus calcification in these samples are reported to be approximately 1% [1,30,60–66].

There are considerable differences in the literature regarding the underlying aetiology in cases of systemic embolism. The reasons for the widely different data are mainly ethnic and/or geographical. In those parts of the world where rheumatic fever, Chagas' disease or tropical endomyocardial fibrosis are endemic, these may be the predominant causes of cardioembolism. In industrialised countries and in temperate climates arteriosclerosis, ischaemic or degenerative valvular heart disease will predominate.

The high percentage of cerebral as compared to peripheral events (84% vs. 16%) in the Düsseldorf patient population is confirmed by other investigators reporting a five- to sixfold predominance of cerebral over peripheral embolism in atrial fibrillation[67,68]. Considering only peripheral events, a probable cardiac source was found in 74% of 248 consecutive patients with peripheral arterial emboli observed during 1964–84, in 77% of consecutively admitted patients with peripheral arterial emboli in the years

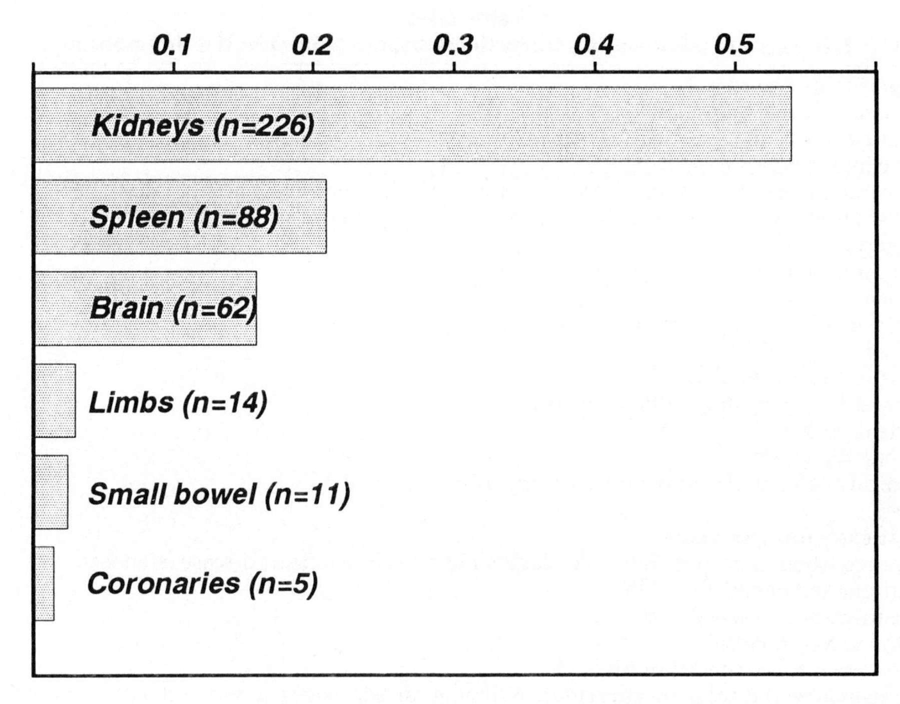

Fig. 1.3–1 Arterial beds affected by cardioembolism in patients with Chagas' heart disease (adapted from Oliviera et al. Amer. J. Cardiol. 1983;52:147)

1970–81[69] and in 77% of 201 consecutive patients with acute limb ischaemia admitted to hospital during 1975–81[70].

The true incidence of cardioembolic events is, however, difficult to define. While most of the clinical studies suggest that less than 20% of strokes arise from cardiac emboli, autopsy studies show the presence of an intracardiac thrombus in up to 50% of fatal strokes[71–73]. Moreover, it is evident that non-cerebral events are often associated with few or absent clinical signs and symptoms and therefore remain undiagnosed in the majority of cases.

Of 636 thromboembolic events verified by autopsy in Chagas' heart disease[74,75], 227 were pulmonary and 407 systemic. The arteries affected by the latter are shown in Figure 1.3–1. It is apparent in this study that, in Chagas' heart disease, peripheral embolism is more than five times more frequent than cerebral embolism but the peripheral events remain undiagnosed in a high proportion of cases.

In the same study, the total incidence of cardiac thrombosis confirmed at autopsy was 27.4% (369/1345 patients). The chambers affected by thrombus were the left ventricle (59.6%), right atrium (57.7%), followed by the right ventricle (20.1%) and the left atrium (14.6%). The low proportion of left atrial thrombi is especially remarkable and contrasts with the commonly observed findings in valvular heart disease or in atrial fibrillation.

PATHOPHYSIOLOGY OF INTRACARDIAC THROMBUS FORMATION

In the presence of sinus rhythm, physiological flow conditions and normal

Table 1.3–3
Diseases and interventions likely to predispose to intracardiac thrombosis

temporarily increased risk
- acute myocardial infarction[82–93]
- stunned/hibernating myocardium of any origin[94–97]
- acute infective endocarditis[80, 98–102]
- intermittent atrial fibrillation or other supraventricular/ventricular arrhythmias[103–108]
- first three months following any open heart surgery (especially after valve replacement surgery)[109–111]
- first three months following balloon valvuloplasty[112, 113]
- cardiac tamponade[114]
- non-penetrating chest trauma (myocardial contusion)[115]
- acute myocarditis[116–120]
- heart catheterisation[121]
- intracardiac indwelling catheters[122–127]
- acute diphtheria[128]
- chest radiation[129]
- medical or electrical cardioversion of atrial fibrillation[111, 130, 131]

permanently increased risk
- acquired (rheumatic, post-infective, degenerative) valvular heart disease (stenosis, regurgitation or both)[121, 132–140]
- prosthetic heart valves[141–154]
- mitral valve prolapse[155–160]
- history of infective endocarditis[129, 161]
- congenital heart disease (in particular: involving cardiac valves, associated with intracardiac shunts or shunts near the heart, after palliative surgery or incomplete repair)[162, 163]
- isolated mitral/aortic annular calcification[164, 165]
- left ventricular dysfunction in ischaemic heart disease[82, 93, 166–169]
- non-ischaemic cardiomyopathies
  - rheumatic myocarditis[170]
  - cardiac involvement in neuromuscular disorders[171]
  - Chagas' disease[74]
  - dilated cardiomyopathy of alcoholic[172], peripartum[173–175] or unknown origin[176–179]
  - induced by chemotherapy (Adriamycin)[180]
  - hypereosinophilic syndrome (Löffler's endocarditis, tropical endomyocardial fibrosis, Becker's disease)[181–184]
  - right ventricular dysplasia (Uhl's anomaly)[185]
  - storage disease[186]
- atrial septal aneurysm[16, 188–192]
- primary cardiac tumors (e.g. myxoma, papillary fibroelastoma)[193–203]
- inflammatory valvulitis
- systemic lupus erythematosus (Libman-Sacks endocarditis)[204–206]
  - carcinoid heart disease[129]
  - Bechet's disease[207]
  - hypertensive heart disease[208]
- rheumatic heart disease with apparent valve lesion[209–215]
- hypertrophic cardiomyopathy[216–219]
- chronic atrial fibrillation or other superventricular/ventricular arrhythmias[108, 220–230]
- pacemaker leads[231]
- intracardiac thrombi in the absence of underlying heart disease
  - non-bacterial (marantic) endocarditis[232–238]
  - polycystic disease[239]
  - myeloproliferative disorders[240, 241]

endocardium, intracardiac thrombus formation is an extreme rarity in humans. Conversely arrhythmia, pathological blood flow and endocardial damage are the major mechanisms associated with increased risk of intracardiac thrombosis (Fig. 1.3–2)[76–78]. This risk may be constant or may be increased temporarily, as is the case in the first weeks after heart valve replacement or after acute myocardial infarction. For the latter, the incidence of cardioembolism is reported to be 2–5%[1,30,79] with the greatest hazard occurring after anterior wall infarction involving the left ventricular apex[1].

Acute infective endocarditis is associated with the highest risk of cardioembolism. The hazard is reported to be 9–37% within 30 days[80] and bears little relationship to the size of vegetations as measured by echocardiography. This may be due to the fact that the size of the vegetation depends on the causative organism as well as on patient related factors[80,81] (see also Chapter 1.4). Other diseases and interventions temporarily predisposing to intracardiac thrombosis are listed in Table 1.3–3.

A permanently increased risk is present in chronic and progressive cardiovascular diseases, like rheumatic heart disease, dilated cardiomyopathy, chronic non-valve related atrial fibrillation, mitral valve prolapse syndrome and in conditions associated with hypercoagulability (Table 1.3–3 – see also Chapter 1.5).

Endocardial damage

The endocardial surface is the key to understanding the generation of intracardiac thrombosis (Fig 1.3–2). In a number of cardiac or systemic diseases, which are

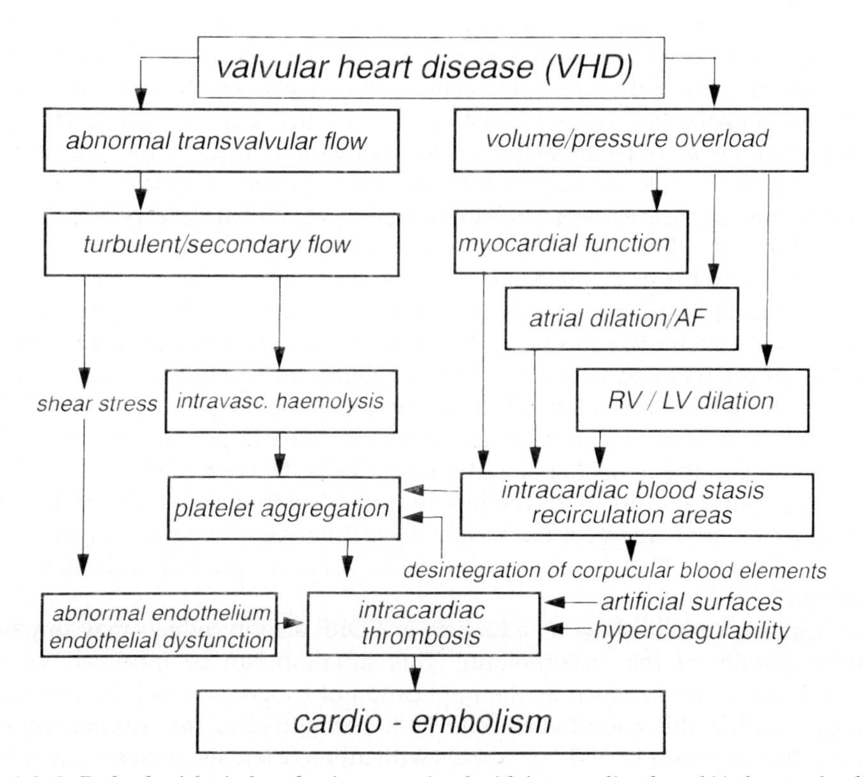

Fig. 1.3–2. Pathophysiological mechanisms associated with intracardiac thrombi in heart valve disease.

associated with a high intracardiac thrombosis rate, concomitant structural alterations of the endothelium are present. Knowledge regarding the physiology and biochemistry of the endocardium and the interaction between endocardium and corpuscular blood elements, especially platelets, has increased dramatically in recent years.

The endocardial endothelium is a structural and metabolic barrier between the blood and the sub-endothelial tissue, and consists of a single continuous layer of flat cells[241,242]. The normal endocardium does not activate the coagulation cascade and does not promote adhesion of platelets or other cellular blood components. Its considerable biosynthetic capability and storage of von Willebrand factor within the Weibel-Palade bodies further contribute to the maintenance of a highly non-thrombogenic surface[339]. Usually, the endothelial cells of the endocardium are interlocked by well developed junctions and anchored to the subendothelial cells by myoendothelial junctions[243].

It is a difficult task to maintain viable endocardial endothelium cells in tissue culture, and this has been a major setback in research directed at the role of the endothelium in intracardiac thrombus formation. Nevertheless, considerable knowledge regarding the interaction between endothelium and corpuscular blood elements has accumulated during the past few years[244,245].

Endothelial cells synthesise nitric oxyde (NO) from the amino acid L-arginine through a chain of enzyme reactions. Different isoforms of endothelial NO-synthase have been isolated from the cytosolic compartment and from cell membranes[244]. NO-synthase, the principal enzyme responsible for the conversion of L-arginine to NO, exists primarily in two forms; a constitutive form and a non-constitutive form. The constitutive form, constantly present in cells, is responsible for the variable release of NO from endothelial cells. The non-constitutive or inducible form is generated by cells (including endothelial cells) in response to stimulation, usually by endotoxins or certain cytokines. Its role in endothelium becomes important mainly in endotoxic shock. In macrophages, the release of NO by this enzyme is partly responsible for their bacteriocidal activity. Both constitutive and non-constitutive enzymes can exist in different isoforms in the particulate and cytosolic fractions of cells.

The constitutive endothelial NO-synthase is calcium-calmodulin-dependent whereas the non-constitutive form is not. The NO produced by the constitutive form is responsible for the biological activity of endothelium-derived relaxing factor, usually abbreviated as EDRF. The major effect of the endothelium produced NO/EDRF is relaxation of vascular smooth muscle via activation of its target enzyme, the soluble guanylate cyclase in the cytosol of smooth muscle cells. However, NO is also released on the luminal surface of the endothelium in quantities that are sufficient to prevent platelet adhesion and aggregation locally by activating the same target enzyme within the platelets. This biochemical reaction inhibits platelet adhesion to the endothelium[247,248].

Atherosclerotic vessels show a reduction in EDRF activity which may impair the antiplatelet activity of the endothelium. This situation can be modified by pharmacological interventions, such as the application of exogenous NO donors that are metabolised within the endothelial cells[246]. Experimentally, the administration of L-arginine, the precursor of NO, to animals with atherosclerosis prevents the reduced EDRF activity seen in these animal models[244].

Apart from the endothelium/platelet interaction, circulating neutrophils may also influence thrombus formation through the same L-arginine-NO pathway. Once neutrophils adhere to the endothelial surface, they are capable of invading the endothelium and producing a cascade of various enzymes that generate cytotoxic oxygen-derived radicals and release several digestive enzymes. It has been demonstrated recently, that this cell type can also synthesise NO from L-arginine. The physiological and/or pathological importance of this finding awaits further clarification[244]. However, recent experimental results have demonstrated that both endogenous and drug-released NO are capable of inhibiting neutrophil adhesion to the vascular wall with concomitant inhibition of the cascade of inflammatory events[244].

In spite of the lack of any corroborating evidence from tissue culture studies yet, it is possible that decreased endocardial NO synthesis may contribute to the development of intracardiac thrombosis. Thus the recent findings in vascular endothelium, if equally applicable to endocardium, offer new therapeutic possibilities in the modulation of endogenous NO release or the application of exogenous NO to reduce platelet and/or neutrophil adhesion to the endocardium, thereby influencing a crucial step in the initial phase of intracardiac thrombus formation. Further research work in this important area is clearly required.

The cellular morphology of the endocardium is strongly influenced by the characteristics of the neighbouring blood flow. Different flow patterns are likely to modify the structure as well as the function of the endocardial endothelium[245–247]. With

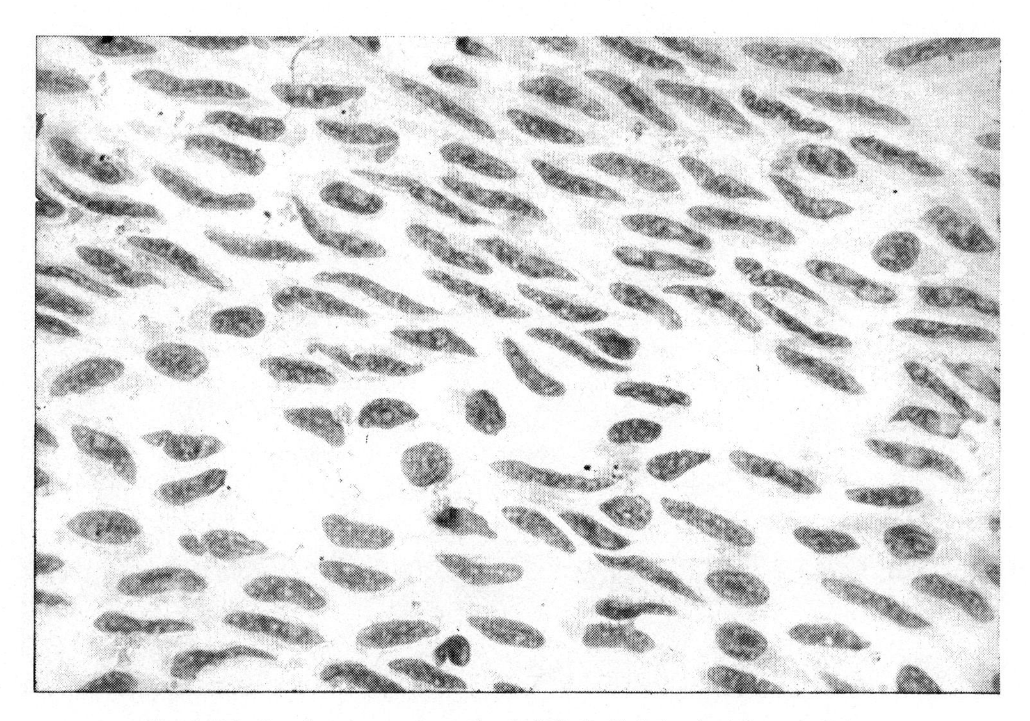

Fig. 1.3–3. Regular arrangement of endothelial cells in laminar flow conditions.

laminar flow, the endothelial nuclei are uniformly arranged parallel to the axis of the direction of flow (Figure 1.3–3). The blood flow not only modifies, but in a sense creates the specific directional arrangements of the endothelial cells, since monolayers of these cells in tissue culture never show any characteristic pattern of arrangement[241].

If the direction of laminar local blood flow is changed, the endothelial cells respond to the altered condition and rearrange themselves within days according to the new flow direction [246]. In vitro studies likewise suggest a blood-borne shear stress effect on nucleus and cell orientation. When exposed to a laminar shear stress of 5–10 dynes/cm^2, confluent monolayers undergo a time dependent change in cell shape from polygonal to ellipsoidal and become uniformly orientated[245].

With disturbed flow involving rapidly changing flow directions, the pattern of the endothelial cell arrangement becomes irregular (Fig. 1.3–4). A similar pattern is seen in the normal carotid sinus, where the orientation of the endothelium is different according to the level of cross section of the artery under investigation[248,249]. While in the common and internal carotid arteries the endothelial nuclei are aligned parallel and the cell shape is fusiform without irregularities, at the outer wall of the carotid sinus, opposite the flow divider, the nuclei are less orientated and the cytoplasm is polygonal, indicating secondary flow conditions. At the point of the highest shear stress, the flow divider, the nuclei and the cytoplasm are extremely elongated[248–250].

In the valvular endocardium, the orientation and shape of the endothelial nuclei vary from one position to another. On the atrial surface at the base of the mitral valve and on its mid-portion, for instance, the nuclei are rather elongated and usually

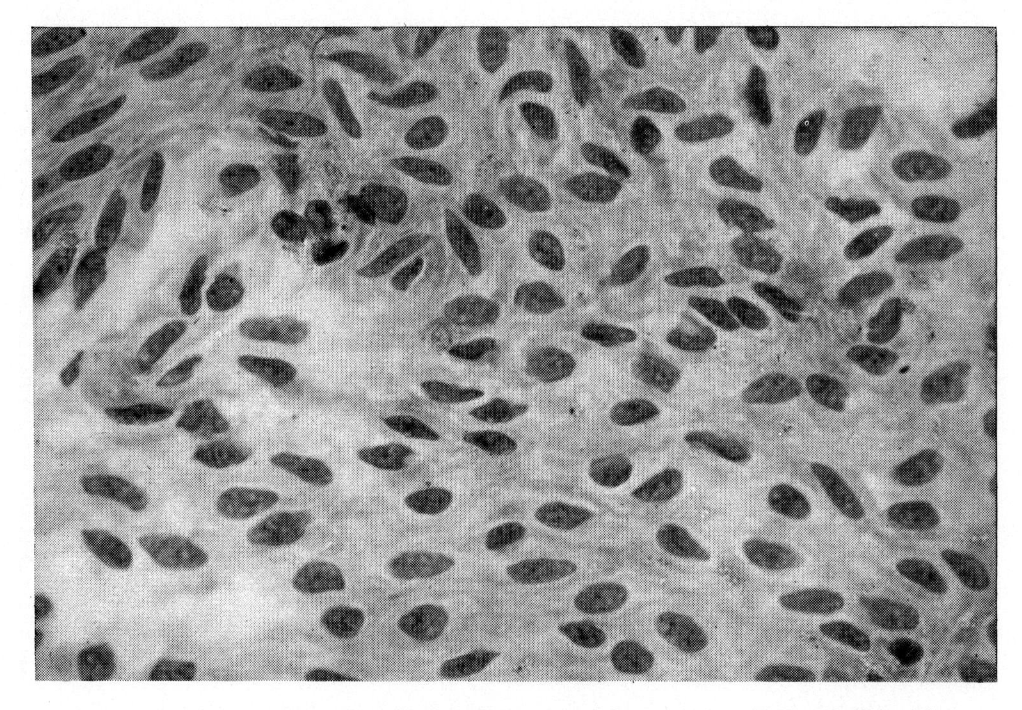

Fig. 1.3–4. Irregular pattern of endothelial cell arrangement in conditions of disturbed blood flow.

aligned in parallel[241]. In contrast, at the line of closure of the valve, there is irregularity and the nuclei are less orientated, in keeping with the different local flow conditions.

With heart valve lesions and consequent disturbed flow, the endothelial cells lose their orientation and rearrange in a random way. This can be demonstrated by exposure of cultured endothelial cells to turbulent flow, which results uniformly in cell-cell retraction and cell loss[245]. True turbulence rarely occurs under physiological conditions (see Chapter 2.2), but with severely damaged heart valves or following heart valve replacement it may be an important factor in the increased risk of thrombus formation in these situations. Moreover, in many valvular and non-valvular cardiac abnormalities including hypertension, disturbed flow can occur, in which flow separation and vortices are superimposed on laminar flow. Prolonged exposure to disturbed flow significantly increases endothelial turnover, probably causes endothelial injury or dysfunction and is accompanied by enhanced adherence of leukocytes to the endothelium[249].

Heart valve disease can also produce gross damage to the endocardium as seen in the well known jet lesions of the left ventricular outflow tract in aortic incompetence or McCallum's patch in mitral regurgitation. With scanning electron microscopy, endothelial denudation can be found in these lesions[101,251].

In the first two days after myocardial infarction, leukocyte infiltration lifts off the endocardium[259], exposing the subendothelial tissue. The circulating blood therefore comes into contact with thrombogenic subendothelial tissues. It is not surprising that thrombi are often present in these areas four to five days after an acute myocardial infarction[260]. The endocardial abnormalities persist if a left ventricular aneurysm develops, perpetuating the risk of embolism[261]. Endocardial abnormalities may also be seen in patients with cardiomyopathy[262].

The thrombi which develop as the consequence of an acute myocardial infarction are almost always found in areas of hypokinetic, akinetic or dyskinetic myocardium[263], pointing to the significance of the combination of a thrombogenic surface and disturbed flow conditions. In some of these cases spontaneous swirling, smoke-like echos can be seen on 2D-echocardiography, as evidence of relatively stagnant flow conditions[264,265].

In severe left ventricular hypertrophy, especially when associated with aortic regurgitation or severe aortic stenosis, the subendocardial blood supply/demand ratio is often adversely affected to such an extent that angina[266,267], an ischaemic electrocardiogram and disseminated subendocardial necrosis develop[268,269]. Impaired subendocardial blood supply is the explanation for stress-induced (by isoprenaline or pacing) subendocardial ischaemia leading to elevated lactate levels in patients with advanced aortic valve disease and apparently normal coronary angiograms[270–272]. The causative factor is decreased coronary vasodilatory capacity, which develops because the total cross-section of the coronary microvessels cannot expand sufficiently to match the increased myocardial mass. The result is increased basal coronary vascular resistance and a corresponding decrease in the capacity to dilate in response to stress[273,274]. This chronic subendocardial ischaemia predisposes to endocardial damage and consequent thrombosis[275].

Myocardial contusion is the most common form of cardiac injury following non-penetrating chest wall trauma[276]. Mural thrombi and thromboembolism may complicate severe myocardial contusion, because the endocardium suffers damage

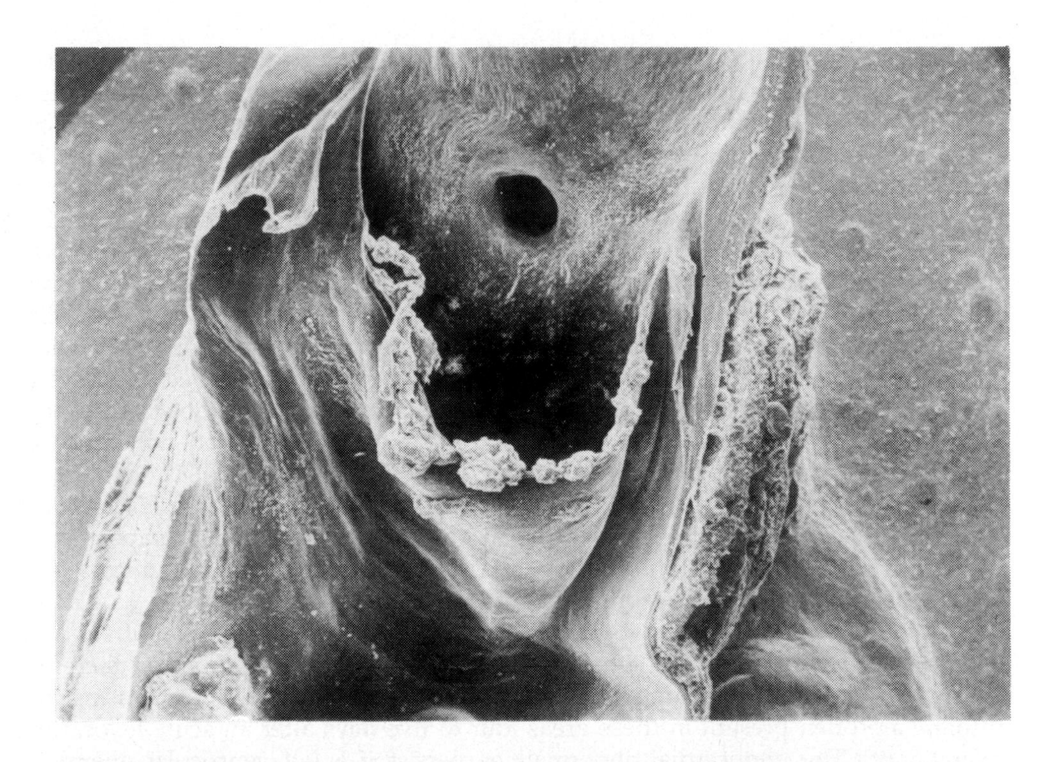

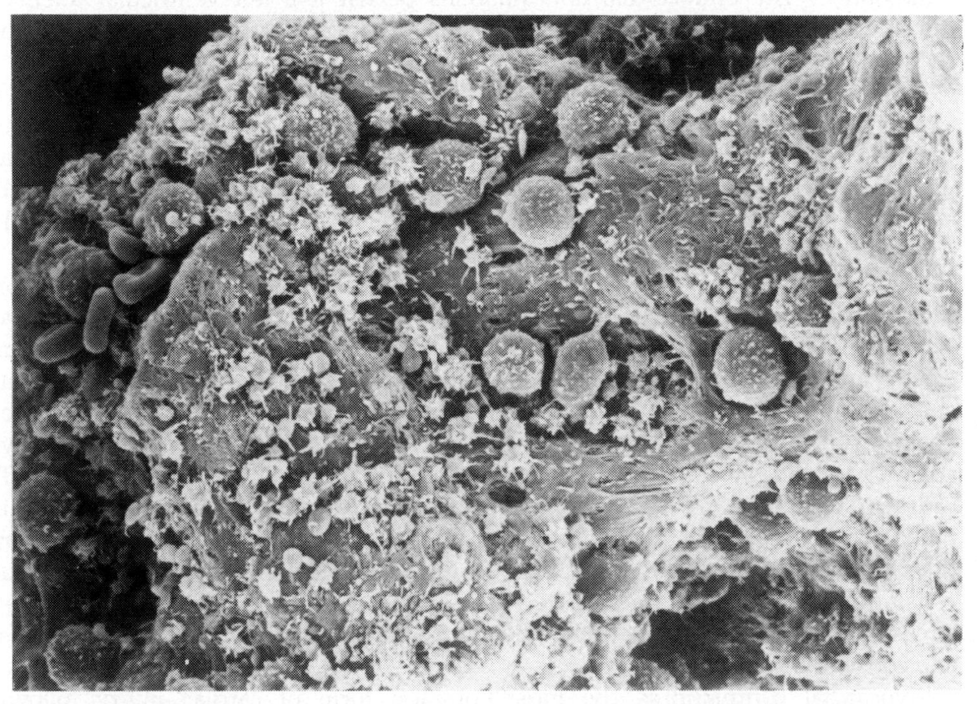

Fig. 1.3–5 Photograph and scanning electron micrograph of bacterial vegetation on the free edge of an aortic cusp, induced experimentally by an indwelling catheter for 24 hrs in a rat.

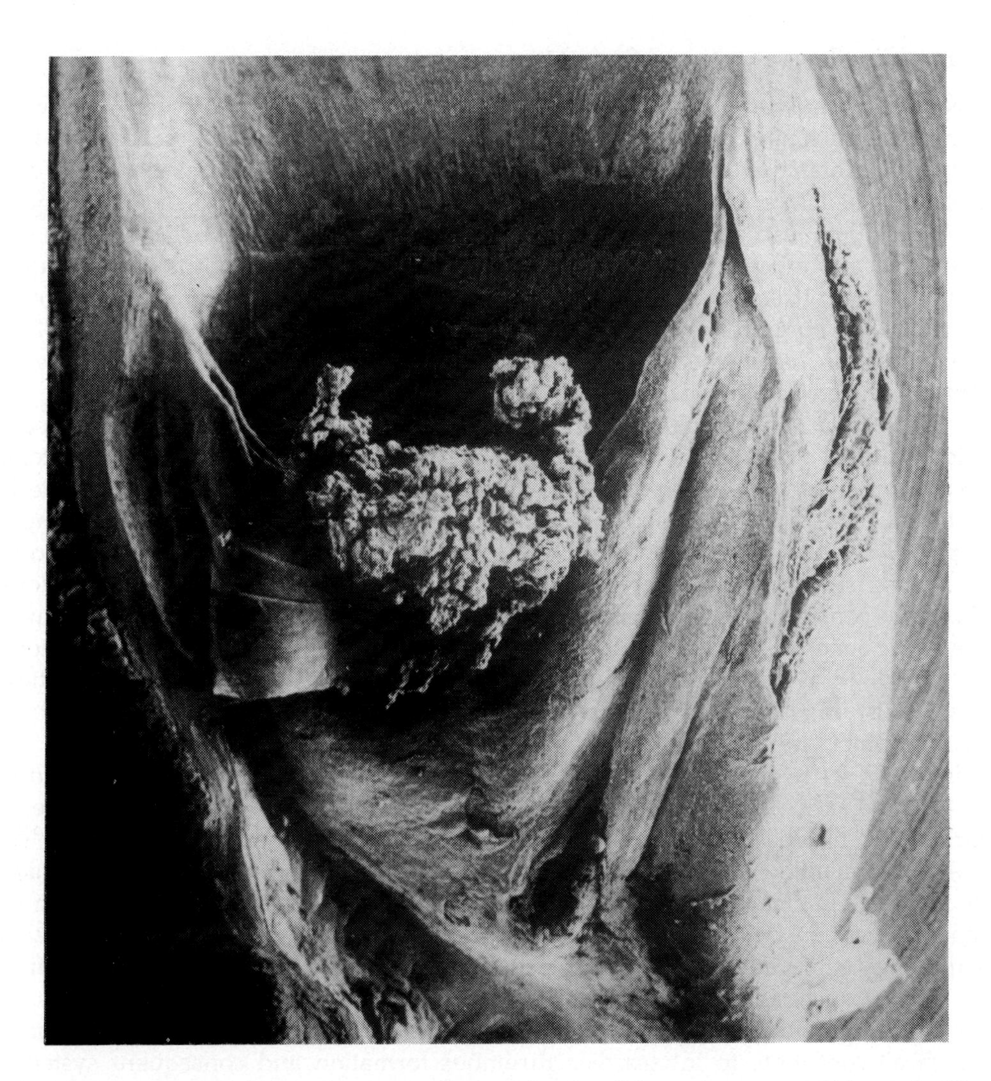

Fig. 1.3–6. Large bacterial vegetation surrounding a perforation of the aortic cusp caused by an indwelling catheter in a rat.

very similar to that in acute myocardial infarction (vide supra)[277–282]. Internal trauma may be caused by pacemaker leads, and endothelial defects are easily produced in both man and experimental animals by indwelling catheters with consequent generation of platelet/fibrin thrombi (Fig. 1.3–5 and 1.3–6).

Mural thrombi have been found in cardiac amyloidosis[283,284] and in experimental viral myocarditis[285]. However, although one publication documents a high incidence of mural thrombus formation in clinical viral myocarditis[116], most publications record a low incidence unless the illness is complicated by cardiac failure[117–120]. Cardiac oxalosis[286] and malignancies with concomitant hypercoagulability[287–290] may also initiate mural thrombus formation.

Intracardiac flow velocity and flow patterns

Neither corpuscular elements of the blood nor micro-organisms can adhere to normally functioning endothelium. Apart from the conditions discussed above, like myocardial infarction and the tropical disease endomyocardial fibrosis, endocardial damage is usually related to blood flow disturbances[291], although dietary influences have been demonstrated in animals (see Chapter 2.4). Abnormal flow conditions are created by a number of anatomical variants or pathological conditions of the cardiac valves without haemodynamically significant stenosis or regurgitation. The congenitally bicuspid but non-stenotic aortic valve, an anatomical variant present in 1–2% of the population, is an especially important clinical example of progressive endothelial damage caused by abnormal flow conditions across the valvular orifice[135,162,264,292]. As the bicuspid valve is unable to open fully, resistance is created, which is not present under normal conditions. The consequence is leaflet stretching during systole, accompanied by a high frequency vibration of the free margin. The flow profile is distorted by turbulence and secondary flow patterns, resulting in endothelial damage. Repeated cycles of platelet and fibrin deposition with subsequent organisation lead to thickening, fibrosis and ultimately leaflet calcification[139]. The abnormal flow conditions should be considered as the predisposing factor leading to early tissue deterioration of the aortic cusps, a process not usually seen until old age if normal flow conditions prevail[132,133,138,293]. The pathogenesis of infective endocarditis shows great similarities; it is the disturbed flow associated with an abnormal valve that results in platelet/fibrin microthrombi, the initial foci of the infection[161].

In the presence of replacement heart valves, where the flow is always abnormal due to high velocity, turbulence, recirculation and diminished or stagnant flow areas, thrombotic, fibrotic and occasionally calcified endocardial lesions are often seen[111,294].

As abnormal flow conditions within the cardiac chambers are usually accompanied by a change in chamber diameter, the presence of a prosthesis, atrial fibrillation or other factors, the demonstration of intracardiac stasis alone cannot be accepted as a satisfactory explanation of thrombus formation[8]. It is more likely to be a combination of factors, such as those already discussed coupled with the relative stasis in the atrial appendage exaggerated by the lack of contraction in atrial fibrillation, which all contribute to intracardiac thrombus formation and consequent systemic embolism[147,148,209].

Intracardiac artificial material

This important factor influencing intracardiac thrombus formation is discussed in detail in chapter 2.3.

Arrhythmias

The majority of intracardiac thrombi occur in the presence of a discernible endocardial abnormality affecting cardiac valves, atrial or ventricular endocardium. Nevertheless, there are a few physiological and morphological factors capable of causing intracardiac thrombus formation without apparent structural or functional damage to the endocardium, such as arrhythmias (particularly atrial fibrillation), gross dilatation of one or more cardiac chambers and impaired myocardial contractility. It is, however, difficult to demonstrate the independent role of these factors in thrombus formation, because typically they present as part of the underlying valvular, rheumatic or ischaemic heart disease, which may have an effect on the endothelium[293,294].

The ever widening application of Holter-monitoring in the diagnosis of paroxysmal arrhythmias has provided proof that both permanent and paroxysmal atrial fibrillation as well as sinus-atrial disorders are associated with intracardiac thrombus formation and consequent embolism[295]. The clinical picture may be obscured because these arrhythmias alone can cause temporary cerebral ischaemia with symptoms very similar to transient ischaemic attack (TIA) caused by minor cerebral embolism. Furthermore, cardiac dysrhythmias can be the consequence rather than cause of brain damage[296,297].

The relatively high cost limits the application of Holter-monitoring as a routine procedure in cerebral ischaemic attacks of unknown origin; in most cases the patient's history and standard electrocardiography are capable of establishing the diagnosis[298,299]. However, Holter-monitoring is the diagnostic method of choice if sick-sinus syndrome is suspected[300].

Atrial fibrillation

Before the 1970s, atrial fibrillation was most commonly associated with rheumatic and ischaemic heart disease. Parallel to the decline of rheumatic fever in industrialised countries, the prevalence of atrial fibrillation as a consequence of rheumatic heart disease has diminished during the last two decades. Currently, in these countries it is usually associated with ischaemic heart disease or arterial hypertension or alternatively occurs as 'lone' (idiopathic) atrial fibrillation.

Apart from 'lone' atrial fibrillation and atrial fibrillation secondary to hyperthyroidism, all other aetiological categories of atrial fibrillation are associated with organic cardiac disease in which there is a potential endocardial abnormality which could predispose to thrombus formation. Such diseases include cardiomyopathies with blood stagnation, mitral valve prolapse with abnormal systolic leaflet movement and myxomatous degeneration causing endothelial damage, and mitral stenosis with significantly impaired emptying of the left atrium.

Using data from the Düsseldorf heart valve database, no correlation could be demonstrated between left atrial size and thromboembolic complications in 314 consecutive patients with isolated mitral incompetence of comparable haemodynamic severity (Grade II angiocardiographic classification). In non-anticoagulated patients, the embolic rate was 0.7%/patient-year with sinus rhythm and 2.2%/patient-year with atrial fibrillation in those whose left atrial diameter was 35–39mm/m^2 body surface area. In the group where the left atrial diameter was 40–45mm/m^2, the respective rates were 0.6%/patient-year and 2.6%/patient-year (Fig. 1.3–7). Thus in this patient population, none of whom had giant left atria, the rhythm was an independent predictor of thromboembolism, whereas left atrial dimension was not.

The importance of atrial fibrillation is further enhanced by the recent finding that established atrial fibrillation is accompanied by significantly elevated plasma levels of D-dimer, irrespective of the presence or absence of organic cardiac disease[301] (see also Chapter 2.5). This suggests that atrial fibrillation itself may be a more important factor in the development of intracardiac thrombosis than factors predisposing to atrial

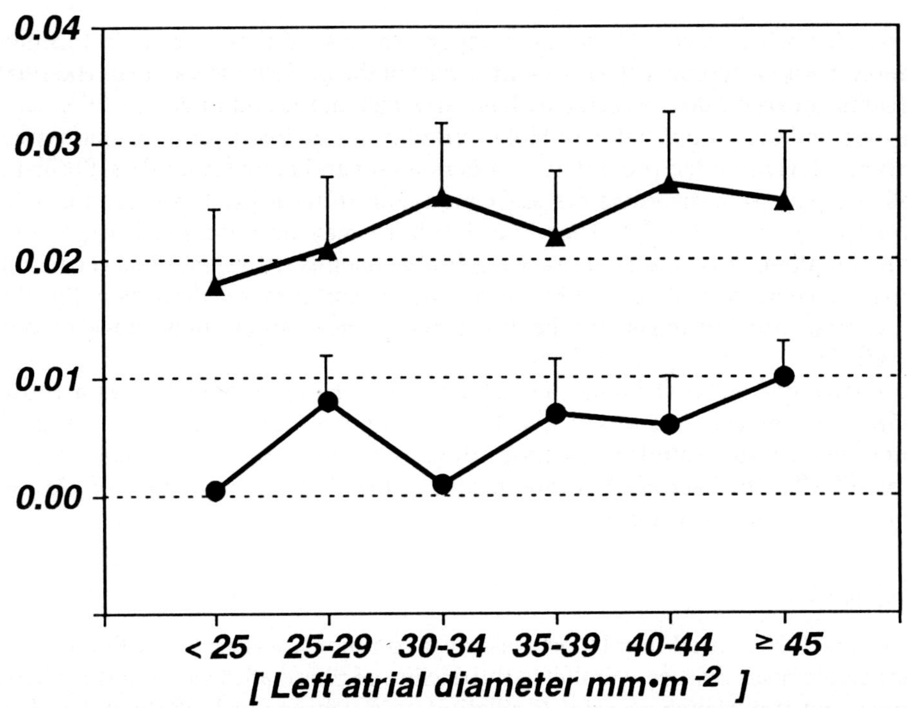

Fig. 1.3–7 Frequency of thromboembolic events in 314 consecutive non-anticoagulated patients with mitral regurgitation (grade 2). (Prospective follow-up, Düsseldorf 1976–1990). ▲—▲ atrial fibrillation (n=127); follow up months=9,119 ●—● sinus rhythm (n=187); follow up months=13,745

fibrillation. Embolism in atrial fibrillation is a common clinical experience even in the absence of any detectable rheumatic or ischaemic heart disease. In one atrial fibrillation study[225], 14 patients had morphologically normal hearts at autopsy; nevertheless emboli were recorded in three (21%) during their life time. In 35 patients in whom left ventricular hypertrophy was the only cardiac finding at autopsy, emboli occurred in eight (23%). According to the Framingham study, the risk of stroke is increased 7-fold in rheumatic heart disease and 5-fold in the presence of atrial fibrillation without any additional risk factors[57]. Chronic or paroxysmal atrial fibrillation unaccompanied by any recognisable heart disease is thus associated with a substantial increase in embolic incidence (see also Chapter 1.2).

'Lone' atrial fibrillation, usually transient and often associated with emotional or physical exhaustion, over-indulgence in alcohol or vomiting[221] is discussed in detail in Chapter 1.2; thromboembolic risk appears to be low in this condition[302–312].

The prognosis regarding thromboembolic complications is worse in chronic than in intermittent atrial fibrillation in patients who do not have coexistent cardiovascular disease. Retrospective clinical assessment shows a 7 to 8-fold increase in morbidity with chronic atrial fibrillation as compared to sinus rhythm, whereas the morbidity is only doubled if the atrial fibrillation is paroxysmal[307]. In the Framingham study, the stroke risk was five times higher in chronic than in intermittent atrial fibrillation[313]. It has also been demonstrated that embolic events cluster shortly after the onset of atrial fibrillation or after the transition from paroxysmal to chronic atrial fibrillation[221,314–316].

Atrial fibrillation accompanying valvular heart disease is a complex clinical condition in which, unlike 'lone' atrial fibrillation, atrial enlargement is common and significant morphological changes occur in the atrial wall. Fibrosis, calcification or elongation of the myocardial fibres take place (see Fig. 1.6–1) due to the underlying pathological process rather than the atrial fibrillation per se or any elevation of intracavitary pressures[317,318]. In this respect it is perhaps relevant that long term atrial fibrillation cannot be induced in animal experiments as long as the atria remain structurally normal[317–321].

Fibrillation leads to ineffective atrial muscle contraction and to further atrial dilation[317,319,320,322]. A dilated left atrium with patchy fibrosis tends to perpetuate atrial fibrillation, setting the scene for stasis and thrombus formation[317,320]. In this situation, loosely attached mural thrombi are often found within the atrial appendage.

The response of atrial fibrillation to therapy in patients with heart valve disease correlates closely with left atrial size and the underlying aetiology of the valve disease[322–326]. Atrial fibrillation is found in approximately 40% of all patients with mitral stenosis (regardless of the severity of obstruction) and in 75% of patients with mitral insufficiency[319,327], but is unusual in aortic valve disease, even in its advanced stages.

Supraventricular arrhythmias

In addition to atrial fibrillation, other supraventricular arrhythmias are also associated with embolic events. This is especially true in sick-sinus syndrome[103,299,300]. The cumulative risk of thromboembolism in these patients is about 15% and the annual risk about 1.3%[105,106,223,328,329]. Pacing in AAI-mode appears to reduce the risk significantly[198,202,203,206,207], whereas VVI-stimulation hardly has any effect[107,330–334].

There is no valid information available on thromboembolic risk in other forms of supraventricular arrhythmia, which are usually transient in nature.

Ventricular arrhythmias

It is not known whether ventricular arrhythmias constitute an independent risk factor for thrombus formation, or whether the association between these arrhythmias and intracardiac thrombus formation is only coincidental. One can speculate that changes in intracardiac flow conditions, due to the altered contraction pattern in ventricular ectopics or ventricular tachycardia, create a situation predisposing to thrombus formation. However, there is no evidence to prove that patients with left bundle branch block are exposed to a higher thromboembolic risk, despite the grossly abnormal left ventricular flow pattern in this condition. Since ventricular arrhythmias are almost always the consequence of underlying organic heart disease, it is impossible to establish the independent causative role of these arrhythmias in the development of thromboembolic complications. Ventricular tachycardia without other cardiac anomaly (automatic type) does not impose an increased thromboembolic risk.

Cardiac chamber dimension

Enlargement of one or more cardiac chambers is a common finding in many types of heart diseases, including myocardial ischaemia, myocarditis, dilated cardiomyopathy and pressure or volume overload. All these conditions carry an elevated risk of thromboembolism[253–258,335]. It is, however, difficult to prove that cardiac chamber enlargement alone acts as an independent determinant of increased thromboembolic risk, because with the exception of some forms of dilated cardiomyopathy, concomitant endocardial damage is usually present. This is particularly the case in myocardial ischaemia[259–262]. Furthermore, chamber dilation is accompanied by functional impairment in the majority of cases.

Right atrium and right ventricle

The possible relationship between right atrial and ventricular cavity size and thromboembolic risk has not yet been investigated. The vast majority of pulmonary emboli are of peripheral venous origin[336–338]. There are only sporadic case reports in the literature concerning right atrial thrombus detected by echocardiography either as an incidental finding or after pulmonary embolism[193,338–344]. However, data to clarify the potential relationship between right atrial size and thrombotic risk do not exist. The problem is further complicated by the fact that right atrial enlargement is practically always accompanied by atrial fibrillation. Finally, echocardiographic imaging of the right atrium, even using the transoesophageal approach, is much more difficult than visualising the left atrium. The frequency of left and right atrial mural thrombi was found to be identical in one autopsy study[345], underlining the point that right atrial thrombi are probably underdiagnosed clinically and may be more relevant as sources of pulmonary emboli than commonly thought. Right ventricular mural thrombus is usually the consequence of organic disease and secondary to endocardial damage (Table 1.3–3).

Although thrombus is sometimes present in right ventricular failure, the thrombogenic influence of increased cavity size per se has not yet been established. In the Düsseldorf experience, 62 adult patients with secundum ASD, associated with a left-to-right shunt greater than 35% of the left ventricular output and right ventricular diameter larger than 35±4 (29–42) mm as assessed by 2D-echocardiography, were followed up for five consecutive years. The total follow up information was 3,813 months. Only two right ventricular thrombi were identified during this period. From this data it appears that right ventricular dilation without myocardial failure does not impose an increased thrombotic risk.

Left atrium

Left atrial enlargement is frequently found at autopsy, because the cavity size increases not only according to increase in body surface area[346] but also with advancing age[346,347]. The strong correlation between atrial fibrillation and left atrial size is well known (vide supra). In rheumatic heart disease, atrial fibrillation and left atrial enlargement are accompanied by pathological changes in the left atrial wall, including myocardial degeneration and fibrous tissue proliferation. Ultimately calcification may occur but this develops on the endocardium in organised thrombus[317]. Similar changes in the left atrial muscle occur in cardiomyopathy, mitral incompetence caused by chordal rupture and in papillary muscle dysfunction[319]. In all these conditions, loose platelet/fibrin thrombus on the atrial wall, particularly within the atrial appendage, is a common finding[317,319–321]. Atrial fibrillation results in ineffective atrial contractions which in turn leads to further increase in left atrial dilation[317,320,322]. A dilated left atrium, with irregularly distributed fibrous replacement of the myocardium and ineffective atrial contractions, creates a thrombogenic milieu, especially within the left atrial appendage[317,320]. Left atrial size in different cardiac anomalies has been well documented in the literature[319,322–326,348], using M-mode or 2D-echocardiography[327].

It is probable that local blood stasis may create conditions for thrombus formation in a large left atrium even during sinus rhythm, because the flow velocity may drop to extremely low levels at the periphery of a slow moving stream. Unfortunately, this is difficult to prove because the increase in left atrial diameter usually triggers the development of atrial fibrillation[349], making it difficult to separate left atrial size per se as an independent source of thrombus formation.

The Düsseldorf experience with 314 consecutive patients with angiographically estimated grade II mitral regurgitation, divided into two groups on the basis of normal or mildly increased left atrial dimension (vide supra), failed to identify mild left atrial enlargement as an independent risk factor for thromboembolism (Fig. 1.3–7), in keeping with the results of others[350]. However, a slight elevation of the embolic rate is usually observed with increasing left atrial size both in sinus rhythm and in atrial fibrillation. A further confounding factor is that some patients apparently in stable sinus rhythm are in fact subject to frequent episodes of atrial fibrillation between consecutive follow-up visits.

The Düsseldorf experience of 795 consecutive patients with *moderate* mitral stenosis (mitral valve area 2.5–1.5 cm^2) revealed a very small incidence of embolism in patients in sinus rhythm, irrespective of anticoagulant usage or left atrial diameter. However, in

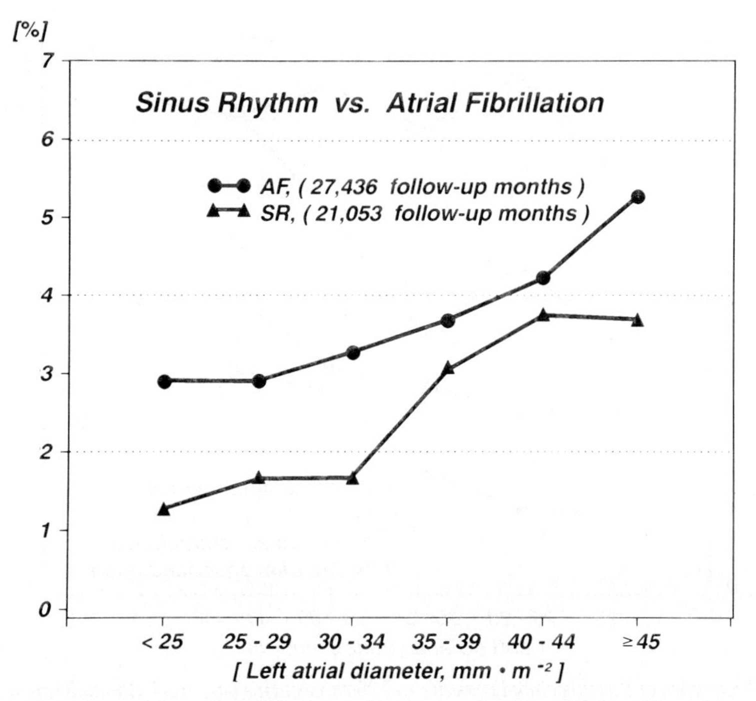

Fig. 1.3–8. Frequency of thromboembolic events in 795 consecutive patients with moderate mitral valve stenosis (mitral valve area 2.5–1.5cm²): effect of rhythm. (Prospective follow-up, Düsseldorf 1975–1990)

patients in atrial fibrillation on oral anticoagulation, the embolic rate increased with increasing left atrial size, underlining the important difference between moderate mitral stenosis (Fig. 1.3–8 and 9) and moderate mitral incompetence (Fig. 1.3–7). Thus, atrial size appears to be an independent predictor of embolism in moderate mitral stenosis. The opportunity to follow the natural history of severe mitral stenosis or incompetance in terms of embolic risk factors is of course lost nowadays, because these patients are almost always referred for surgical treatment.

Left ventricle

Using the Düsseldorf heart valve database, no relationship could be demonstrated between the left ventricular end-diastolic volume index and thromboembolism in patients who had aortic incompetence of varying severity, but whose ejection fraction was larger than 55% and left atrial diameter less than 25mm/m^2 body surface area (Fig. 1.3–10). Furthermore, in 43 patients with aortic incompetence and 52 with mitral incompetence who experienced embolic events, decreasing left ventricular ejection fraction seemed to correlate better with embolism than the end-diastolic volume index (Fig. 1.3–11). Similarly it was not possible to relate evidence of thrombosis or embolism to the endsystolic or enddiastolic volume index in patients with advanced aortic stenosis. It seems therefore that the propensity for thrombosis and embolism is influenced more by deteriorating myocardial function than by the size of the left ventricular cavity.

Thus in heart valve disease, it is unlikely that increasing left ventricular size per se

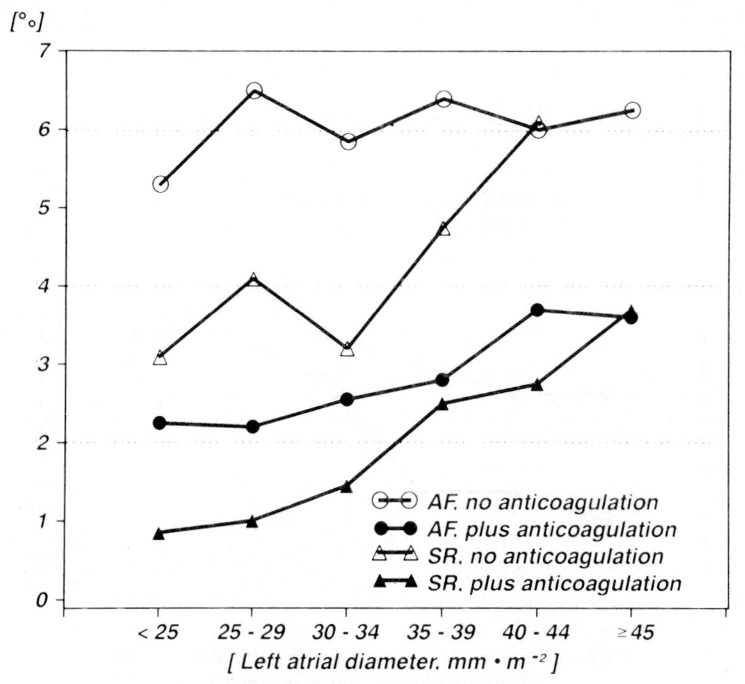

Fig. 1.3–9. Frequency of thromboembolic events in 795 consecutive patients with moderate mitral valve stenosis (mitral valve area 2.5–1.5cm^2): effect of anticoagulation and rhythm. (Prospective follow-up, Düsseldorf 1975–1990)

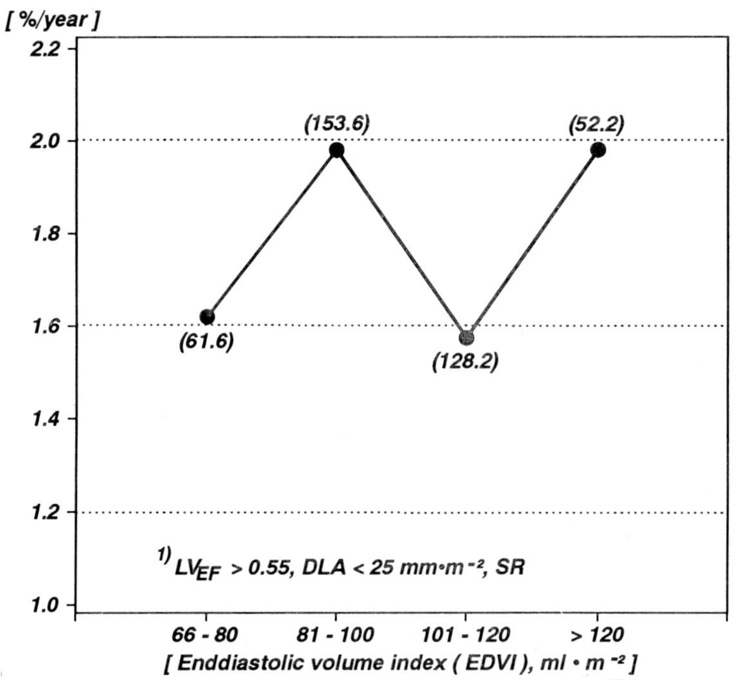

Fig. 1.3–10. Incidence (% per year) of thromboembolic events in 174 consecutive patients with aortic regurgitation according to the enddiastolic volume index (EDVI). LV_{EF}=left ventricular ejective traction; DLA=left atrial diameter; SR=sinus rhythm (Prospective follow-up, Düsseldorf 1976–1990)

adversely affects thromboembolic risk. This is probably also the case in left ventricular enlargement of other aetiology. For example, in dilated cardiomyopathy, where mural thrombi are found in about 50% of cases at autopsy, endocardial damage is invariably present[202,351–353]. The conclusion appears to be that abnormal wall excursion together with endocardial damage rather than ventricular enlargement promote left ventricular thrombus formation[252,262,352,354–357].

Myocardial function

Although in the vast majority of cases of intracardiac thrombus formation there is a discernible abnormality of the endocardium, injury of the endocardium does not seem to be a necessary prerequisite in all instances of cardiac thrombosis. Another important pathogenetic factor is blood stasis due to local or global myocardial injury, especially if it affects systolic function. If stasis and endocardial injury co-exist, thrombus formation may take place rapidly. This is the case with acute myocardial infarction, left ventricular aneurysm, valve prostheses, mitral stenosis and atrial fibrillation.

In contrast, stasis alone does not lead to thrombus formation so quickly[357–359], requiring additional factors that create hypercoagulability[360,361], for example endo- or exotoxins[362–364] or ellagic acid[365,366]. Bacterial toxins may cause severe, temporary myocardial failure by activating macrophages, granulocytes and endothelial cells and eventually provoking the release of sepsis-mediators[367–370].

Locally occurring low flow conditions often co-exist with endothelial damage in heart valve disease and after heart valve replacement. The resulting thrombus is

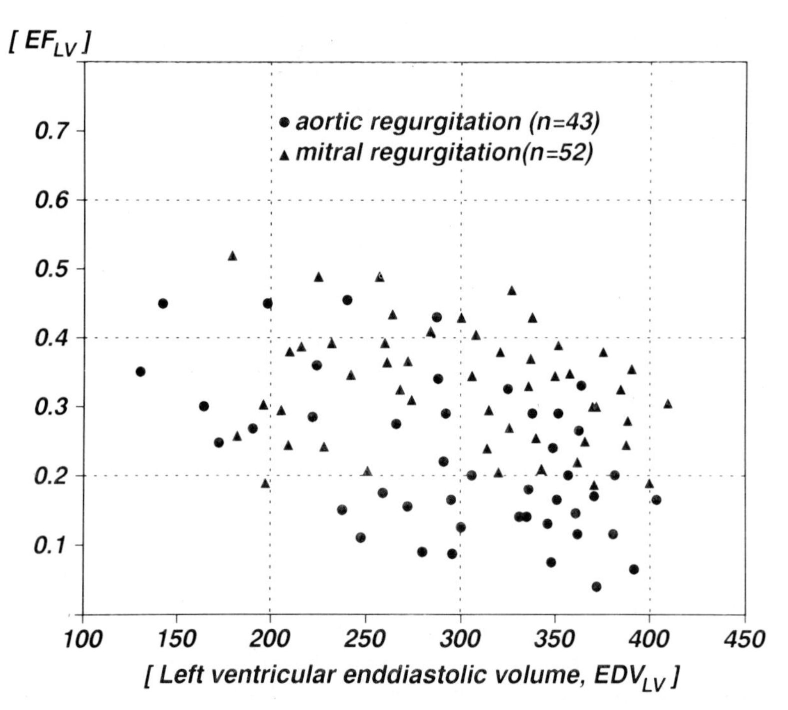

Fig. 1.3–11. Thromboembolic episodes in patients with mirtal or aortic regurgitation: relation to EDV_{LV} and EF_{LV}

brought about by the activation of the coagulation system rather than platelets; it is dark red and composed mainly of red blood cells incorporated in a fibrin network with relatively few platelets[360]. This type of thrombus occurs in conditions of local hypercoagulability in which the balance of procoagulant and anticoagulant influences are disturbed[361,371–374].

Loss of atrial contraction

Loss of atrial contraction is not necessarily the consequence of atrial fibrillation. Effective atrial contraction may be lost even in the presence of electrophysiologically normal sinus rhythm. Therefore, when comparing thromboembolic rates in atrial fibrillation with those in sinus rhythm, it is essential to confirm the presence of *mechanical* atrial activity as well as *electrical* activity in patients in sinus rhythm, by visualising the atrial contraction pressure wave either echocardiographically or manometrically.

The loss of atrial contraction has particularly important consequences in mitral stenosis or elevated left ventricular end-diastolic pressure, especially if the lack of blood propulsion through the mitral valve is aggravated by tachycardia which shortens the diastolic filling period. This mechanism leads eventually to the decreased cardiac output typical of significant mitral stenosis[111,374]. In mitral patients who have lost effective mechanical contraction of the atrium whilst in sinus rhythm, the onset of atrial fibrillation does not have additional haemodynamic consequences.

The Düsseldorf experience with 795 consecutive patients with moderate mitral stenosis (mitral valve area 2.5 – 1.5 cm^2) demonstrates the effect of atrial contraction. The patients were regularly followed by echocardiography, occasionally by repeat cardiac catheterisation, and were removed from further data analysis if the orifice area decreased to less than 1.5 cm^2. The mean follow up was 55 months with a range of 38–166 months. If sinus rhythm changed to atrial fibrillation or mechanically effective atrial contractions could no longer be demonstrated, the patient was re-allocated to the respective group.

In 351 patients with sinus rhythm, 33 thromboembolic episodes were reported during a total follow up of 21,053 months (1.88%/patient-year). In the remaining 444 cases in atrial fibrillation, 72 embolic episodes were reported during a total follow up of 27,436 months (3.15%/patient-year). The respective cumulative rates are depicted in Fig. 1.3–8.

The gradual increase in left atrial size was followed by a parallel increase in embolic risk in both the sinus rhythm and the atrial fibrillation groups (Fig. 1.3–9). Ignoring the presence or absence of anticoagulation, the embolic rate was 1.49% vs. 3.74% in sinus rhythm and 2.84% vs. 6.38% in atrial fibrillation, depending on whether the left atrial diameter was less than 25mm or more than 44 mm per m2 body surface area, respectively. The differences in both groups were statistically significant ($p<0.025$; $p<0.02$).

In total, 706 of the 795 patients (72.1% of those in sinus rhythm and 82.2% of those in atrial fibrillation) received oral anticoagulation with phenprocoumon according to the relevant recommendations for mitral stenosis[111] to achieve an INR between 3.0 and 4.0. When the atrial fibrillation group was stratified according to the presence or absence of anticoagulation, it was found that an increase in left atrial diameter from less than 25 mm to more than 44 mm continued to have an influence on embolic incidence; in patients with the smaller left atria, the embolic rates were 2.38% and 3.56%, with and without anticoagulation respectively, versus 5.42% and 6.58% in patients with the larger left atria. Identical stratification of patients in stable sinus rhythm according to anticoagulation demonstrated a considerable increase of the embolic rate parallel to the gradual enlargement of the left atrium. Furthermore, if the atrial diameter was larger than 36 mm, the difference between embolic rates in sinus rhythm and atrial fibrillation diminished (Fig. 1.3–9).

A further analysis was performed, stratifying patients in 'electro-physiological' (ECG) sinus rhythm according to M-mode echocardiographic evidence of the presence or absence of mechanically effective atrial contraction. The increase in the rate of thromboembolism parallel to the progressive left atrial dilatation was almost exclusively limited to those who did not have mechanically effective atrial contractions. It appears therefore that the lack of mechanically effective atrial contraction rather than the increase in atrial diameter is the primary cause of the increased thromboembolic risk under these circumstances (Fig. 1.3–12).

Ineffective atrial contraction may be the explanation for the persistence of an increased embolic risk in the period immediately following electrical or pharmacological conversion of atrial fibrillation to sinus rhythm. It is possible that in some patients restoration of normal electrical activity does not coincide with the return of mechanically effective atrial contraction. If this is the case, it provides additional justification for continuing the anticoagulation of these patients following successful cardioversion, at least until there is evidence of the return of effective atrial contraction.

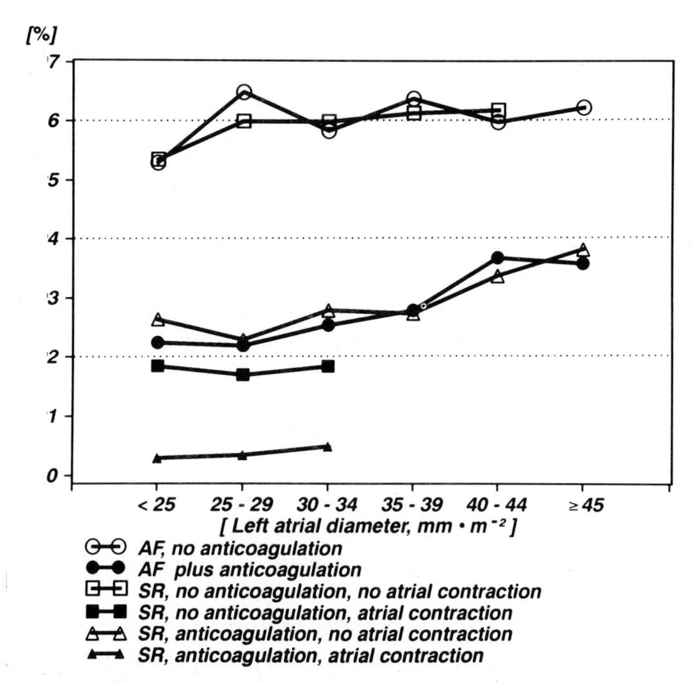

Fig. 1.3–12. Frequency of thromboembolic events in 795 consecutive patients with moderate mitral valve stenosis (mitral valve area 2.5–1.5cm^2): effect of atrial contraction. (Prospective follow-up, Düsseldorf 1975–1990)

Right ventricular function

Right ventricular thrombi, unlike those in the left ventricle, do not necessarily develop within the ventricular cavity. Thrombi formed in the venous system can embolise to the right ventricle and become anchored within the subvalvar apparatus of the tricuspid valve (pulmonary emboli in transit)[374]. It may be difficult to distinguish between this type of thrombus and that associated with impaired right ventricular contraction. The configuration of the thrombus may provide some guidance; a wormlike, longitudinal shape suggests a venous origin, whereas a flat, broadly based shape is more indicative of right ventricular origin[374–378]. The distinction is important because the latter type of thrombus probably has less tendency to embolise.

Although clearly plausible on theoretical grounds, there is currently no definite evidence that impaired right ventricular function is associated with an increased incidence of pulmonary embolism. However, there are case reports of pulmonary embolism in congestive cardiac failure[193] or right ventricular dysplasia[185]. In dilated cardiomyopathy involving the right ventricle, the increase in diameter is always accompanied by endocardial injury, making it difficult to separate these two pathological changes as aetiological factors in pulmonary embolism[379]. An increased rate of pulmonary embolism has also been reported in cases of Friedrich's ataxia with severe myocardial involvement[380].

The pathophysiology of right ventricular thrombus formation is basically identical to that in the left ventricle, with the only difference being the lower incidence of thrombus development on the right side[381,382].

Left ventricular function

Impaired left ventricular function is associated with an increased risk of systemic embolism in a number of diseases. In dilated cardiomyopathy the reported incidence of clincally evident thrombosis and embolism varies considerably[205,383–391], but both thrombus and emboli are found in a large percentage of autopsy cases irrespective of the presence or absence of atrial fibrillation[392–404]. A number of publications report the thrombogenic role of endocardial injury in different forms of cardiomyopathy well in advance of the development of clinically important left ventricular failure[399,403,405–408].

Mural thrombus frequently develops in left ventricular aneurysm[252,254,354,409]. In the majority of cases the thrombus formation commences in the acute phase of myocardial infarction when, due to the loss of endocardium, blood comes into direct contact with thrombogenic subendocardial tissues[410]. The local stasis, secondary to loss of contraction, acts as an additional thrombogenic factor.

Typically ventricular thrombus forms at a site of regional reduction of wall motion. This localised wall motion abnormality was originally thought not to occur in global left ventricular failure, such as that seen in cardiomyopathy or heart valve disease. Recently however angiographic, isotope imaging and echocardiographic evidence has been accumulating to show that regional wall motion abnormalities are not an infrequent finding in these conditions[411–414]. The apical region of the left ventricle is particularly predisposed to thrombus formation due to local flow abnormalities[74,414]. Doppler-echocardiography reveals that the ventricular apex, the centre of the left ventricle and the neighbourhood of the ventricular septum are particularly susceptible to flow abnormalities[205,414,415].

Information from the Düsseldorf heart valve database has provided confirmatory evidence that embolic risk in heart valve disease increases as left ventricular function deteriorates. The findings in patients with mitral regurgitation and aortic regurgitation have already been described earlier in this chapter and are illustrated in Figure 1.3–11. However, when interpreting data on left ventricular function in mitral regurgitation, it is important to remember that imaging techniques cannot provide quantitative information on the severity of left ventricular dysfunction in mitral regurgitation, because the left ventricle can eject a major part of its enddiastolic volume into the low resistance left atrium, thereby 'artificially' maintaining its ejection fraction irrespective of myocardial contractility.

In aortic stenosis, most systemic embolism probably originates from the valve, either as thrombus or calcium, rather than from the left ventricular cavity[416,417]. Nevertheless, 410 consecutive patients with aortic stenosis studied in Düsseldorf between 1971–1990 revealed a significant correlation between left ventricular function and thromboembolism (Figure 1.3–13).

CONCLUSION

Normal anatomical and physiological conditions within the heart secure a non-thrombogenic environment. This milieu, however, can be disturbed by relatively trivial changes affecting the endocardial surface or local wall motion. Endocardial damage, cardiac dilatation and myocardial failure can each promote intracardiac thrombus formation. The predominance of one or the other is difficult to ascertain under clinical conditions, because they rarely occur independently. Although there is

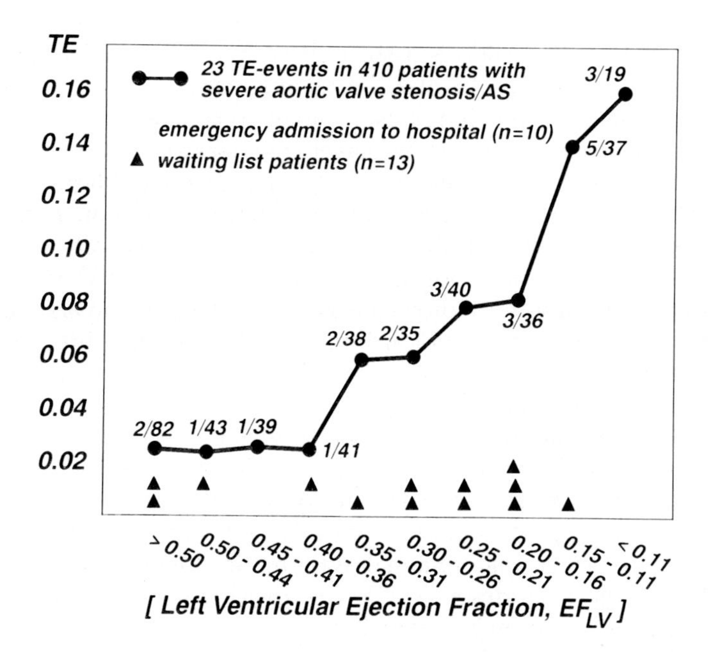

Fig. 1.3–13. Influence of left ventricular pump function [EF_{LV}] on the frequency of thromboembolism in advanced aortic stenosis.

proven correlation between deteriorating global myocardial function and embolic risk, recent evidence using modern imaging techniques suggests that thrombus formation is not a random process in global cardiac failure, because there are usually predilection points where the local conditions create a particularly thrombogenic situation.

The same principles apply after heart valve replacement. The introduction of artificial surfaces into the blood stream does not diminish the importance of the role played by abnormal cardiac morphology and physiology in the development of thromboembolic complications after valve replacement.

REFERENCES

1. Cerebral embolism task force. Cardiogenic brain embolism. Arch Neurol 1986;43:71–84
2. Bogousslavsky J, Hachinsky VC, Boughner DR et al. Cardiac and arterial lesions in carotid transient ischaemic attacks. Arch Neurol 1986;43:223–228
3. Kinney EL. The significance of left ventricular thrombi in patients with coronary heart disease: a retrospective analysis of pooled data. Am Heart J 1985;109:191–194
4. Fogelholm R, Melin J. Echocardiography in ischaemic cerebrovascular disease. Br Med J 1987;295:305–306
5. Pop G, Sutherland GR, Koudstaal PJ, et al. Transesophageal echocardiography in the detection of intracardiac embolic sources in patients with transient ischemic attacks. Stroke 1990;21:560–565
6. Kessler Ch, Henningsen H, Reuther R, et al. Identification of intracardiac thrombi in stroke patients with Indium–111 platelet scintigraphy. Stroke 1987;18:63–67
7. Ezekowitz MD, Burrow RD, Heath PW, et al. Diagnostic accuracy of indium–111 platelet scintigraphy in identifying left ventricular thrombi. Am J Cardiol 1983;51:1712–1716
8. Bergeron GA, Shah PM. Echocardiography unwarranted in patients with cerebral ischemia events (letter). N Engl J Med 1981;304:489
9. Lighty GW, Pearlman AS. Cardiac source of emboli: clinical/echocardiographic correlations (abstract). Circulation 1981;64[suppl IV]:19

10. Fanning WJ, Vaccaro PS, Satiani B, et al. The role of echocardiography in patients with acute peripheral arterial embolization. Ann Vasc Surg 1986;1:316–320
11. Herzog CA, Bass D, Kasse M, Asinger R. Two-dimensional echocardiographic imaging of left atrial appendage thrombi. J Am Coll Cardiol 1984;3:1340–1344
12. Greenland P, Knopman DS, Mikell FL, et al. Echocardiography in diagnostic assessment of stroke. Ann Intern Med 1981;95:51–53
13. Lovett JL, Sandok BA, Giuliani ER, Nasser FN. Two-dimensional echocardiography in patients with focal cerebral ischemia. Ann Intern Med 1981;95:1–4
14. Aschenberg W, Schlüter M, Kremer P, et al. Transesophageal two-dimensional echocardiography for the detection of left atrial appendage thrombus. J Am Coll Cardiol 1986;7:163–166
15. Kronzon I, Tunick PA, Glassman E, et al. Transesophageal echocardiography to detect atrial clots in candidates for percutaneous transseptal mitral balloon valvuloplasty. J Am Coll Cardiol 1990;16:1320–1322
16. Pearson AC, Labovitz AJ, Tatineni S, Gomez CR. Superiority of transesophageal echocardiography in detecting cardiac source of embolism in patients with cerebral ischemia of uncertain etiology. J Am Coll Cardiol 1991;17:66–72
17. Zenker G, Erbel R, Kramer G, et al. Transesophageal two-dimensional echocardiography in young patients with cerebral ischemic events. Stroke 1988;19:345–348
18. Schuchman H, Feigenbaum H, Dillon JC, Shang S. Intracavitary echoes in patients with mitral prosthetic valves. J Clin Ultrasound 1975;3:111–115
19. Preis LK, Hess JP, Austin JL, et al. Left ventricular microcavitations in patients with Beall valves [abstract]. Am J Cardiol 1980;45:402
20. Machi J, Sigel B, Beitler JC, Coelho JCU, et al. Relation of in vivo blood flow to ultrasound echogenicity. J Clin Ultrasound 1983;11:3–8
21. Mikell FL, Asinger RS, Elsperrer KJ, et al. Regional stasis of blood in the dysfunctional left ventricle: echocardiographic detection and differentiation from early thrombosis. Circulation 1982;66:755
22. Wolverson JK, Nouri S, Joist HJ, et al. The direct visualization of blood flow by real-time ultrasound: clinical observations and underlying mechanisms. Radiology 1981;140:443–448
23. Erbel R, Stern H, Ehrenthal W, et al. Detection of spontaneous echocardiographic contrast within the left atrium by transesophageal echocardiography: spontaneous echocardiographic contrast. Clin Cardiol 1986;9:245–252
24. Panidis JP, Kotler MN, Mintz GS, Ross J. Intracavitary echoes in the aortic arch in type III aortic dissection. Am J Cardiol 1984;54:1159–1163
25. Daniel WG, Nellessen U, Schröder E, et al. Left atrial spontaneous echo contrast in mitral valve disease: an indicator for an increased thromboembolic risk. J Am Coll Cardiol 1988;11:1204–1211
26. Vandenbosche JL, van Kuyk M, Englert M. Echocardiographic detection of blood stasis pattern in the left atrium. J Cardiovasc Ultrasonogr 1983;2:341–345
27. Arora RR, Teichholz LE, Meltzer RS. Spontaneous echocardiographic contrast in the inferior vena cava. J Cardiovasc Ultrasonogr 1984;3:27–30
28. Topol EJ, Humphrey LS, Borkon AM, et al. Value of intraoperative left ventricular microbubbles detected by transesophageal two-dimensional echocardiography in predicting neurologic outcome after cardiac operations. Am J Cardiol 1985;56:773–775
29. Castello R, Pearson AC, Labovitz AJ, Wallace P. Atrial spontaneous contrast in patients undergoing transesophageal echocardiography: prevalence and clinical implications. Am J Cardiol 1990;65:1149–1153
30. Nadeau SE. Stroke due to cardiogenic embolism. Semin Neurol 1986;6:277–284
31. Barnett HJ. Heart in ischemic stroke: a changing emphasis. Neurol Clin 1983;1:291–315
32. Brockmeier LB, Adolph RJ, Gustin BW, et al. Calcium emboli to the retinal artery in calcific aortic stenosis. Am Heart J 1981;101:32–36
33. Caltrider ND, Irvine AR, Kline HJ, Rosenblatt A. Retinal emboli in patients with mitral valve prolapse. Am J Ophthalmol 1980;90:534–538
34. Hallermann D, Singh G. Iatrogenic central retinal artery embolization. A complication of cardiac catheterization. Ann Ophthalmol 1984;16:1025–1029
35. Holley KE, Bahn RC, McGoon DC, Mankin HT. Spontaneous calcific embolization associated with calcific aortic stenosis. Circulation 1963;27:197–200
36. Rush JA, Kearns TP, Danielson GK. Cloth-particle retinal emboli from artificial cardiac valves. Am J Ophthalmol 1980;89:845–847
37. Stefánsson E, Coin JT, Lewis WR, et al. Central retinal artery occlusion during cardiac catheterization. Am J Ophthalmol 1985;95:586–589
38. Aring CD. Differential diagnosis of cerebrovascular stroke. Arch Intern Med 1964;113:195–199
39. Kunitz SC, Gross CR, Heyman A, et al. The pilot stroke data bank: definition, design, and data. Stroke 1984;15:740–746

40. Caplan LR, Hier D, D'Cruz I. Cerebral embolism in the Michael Reese Stroke Registry. Stroke 1983;14:530–537
41. Chambers BR, Donnan GA, Bladen PF. An analysis of the first 700 consecutive admissions to the Austin Hospital Stroke Unit. Aust NZ J Med 1983;13:57–64
42. Herman B, Leyten ACM, Luijk JH, et al. Epidemiology of stroke in Tilburg, The Netherlands. Stroke 1982;13:629–634
43. Mohr JP, Caplan LR, Melski JW, et al. The Harvard Cooperative Stroke Registry: A prospective registry. Neurology 1978;28:745–762
44. Wolf PA, Kannel W, McGee DL, et al. Duration of atrial fibrillation and imminence of stroke: The Framingham Study. Stroke 1983;14:664–667
45. Wenger NK. Cardiovascular disease in the elderly. In: Wiley A, Chichester C (eds): Research and the Ageing Population. Ciba Foundation Symposium 1988;134:106–128
46. Roberts WC. The senile cardiac calcification syndrome. Am J Cardiol 1986;58:572–574
47. Roberts WC, Perloff JK, Costantino T. Severe valvular aortic stenosis in patients over 65 years of age. A clinicopathologic study. Am J Cardiol 1971;27:497–506
48. Roberts WC, Cohen LS. Left ventricular papillary muscles. Description of the normal and a survey of conditions causing them to be abnormal. Circulation 1972;46:138–154
49. Savage DD, Garrison RJ, Castelli WP, et al. Prevalence of submitral (anular) calcium and its correlates in a general population-based sample (The Framingham Study). Am J Cardiol 1983;51:1375–1378
50. Waller BF, Roberts WC. Cardiovascular disease in the elderly. Analysis of 40 necropsy patients aged 90 years or older. Am J Cardiol 1983;51:403–421
51. Flegel KM, Shipley MJ, Rose G. Risk of stroke in nonrheumatic atrial fibrillation. Lancet 1987;1:526–529
52. Kelley RE, Berger JR, Altar M, Kovacs AG. Cerebral ischemia and atrial fibrillation: prospective study. Neurology 1984;34:1285–1291
53. Onundarson PT, Thorgeirsson G, Jonmundsson E, et al. Chronic atrial fibrillation: epidemiologic features and 14 year follow-up: a case-control study. Eur Heart J 1987;8:521–527
54. Tanaka H, Hayashi M, Date C, et al. Epidemiologic studies of stroke in Shibata, a Japanese provincial city: preliminary report on risk factors for cerebral infarction. Stroke 1985;16:775–780
55. Wolf PA, Abbott RD, Kannel WB. Atrial fibrillation: a major contributor to stroke in the elderly: The Framingham Study. Arch Intern Med 1987;147:1561–1564
56. Mahapatra RK, Agarwal JB, Chopra P. Systemic thromboembolism in rheumatic heart disease. Jpn Heart J 1980;21:773–777
57. Wolf PA, Dawber TR, Thomas HE. Epidemiologic assessment of chronic atrial fibrillation and risk of stroke: The Framingham Study. Neurology 1978;28:973–976
58. Kutzke JF, Kurland LT. The epidemiology of neurologic disease. In: Baker AB, Baker LH (eds): Clinical Neurology, Vol. 4. Philadelphia: Harper & Row, 1984;pp 1–143
59. Cerebral Embolism Task Force. Cardiogenic brain embolism. Arch Neurol 1989;46:727–743
60. Caplan LR, Hier D, D'Cruz I. Cerebral embolism in the Michael Reese Stroke Registry. Stroke 1983;14:530–537
61. Cerebral Embolism Study Group. Immediate anticoagulation of embolic stroke: a randomized rial. Stroke 1983;14:668–676
62. Joubert J, van Gelder AL, Pilloy WC. The cardiovascular status of the black stroke patient. S Afr Med J 1989;76:657–664
63. Kittner SJ, Sharkness CM, Price TR, et al. Infarcts with a cardiac source of embolism in the NINCDS stroke data bank: clinical features. Neurology 1990;40:281–284
64. Mohr JP, Caplan LR, Melski JW, et al. Harvard Cooperative Stroke Registry: a prospective registry. Neurology 1978;28:754–762
65. Sandercock PAG, Warlow CP, Jones LN, et al. Predisposing factors for cerebral infarction: the Oxfordshire community stroke project. Br Med J 1989;298:75–80
66. Wolf PA, Dawber TR, Thomas HE, Kannel WB. Epidemiologic assessment of chronic atrial fibrillation and risk of stroke: the Framingham Study. Neurology 1978;28:973–977
67. Cabin HS, Clubb KS, Hall C, et al. Risk for systemic embolization of atrial fibrillation without mitral stenosis. Am J Cardiol 1990;65:1112–1116
68. Flegel KM, Hanley J. Risk factors for stroke and other embolic events in patients with nonrheumatic atrial fibrillation. Stroke 1989;20:1000–1004
69. Baxter-Smith D, Ashton F, Slaney G. Peripheral arterial embolism. J Cardiovasc Surg 1988;29:453–457
70. Jivegard L, Holm J, Schersten T. Acute limb ischemia due to arterial embolism or thrombosis: influence of limb ischemia versus pre-existing cardiac disease on postoperative mortality rate. J Cardiovasc Surg 1988; 29:32–36
71. Blackwood N, Hallpike JF, Kocen RS, Mair WGP. Atheromatous disease of the carotid arterial system and embolism from the heart in cerebral infarction: a morbid anatomical study. Brain 1969;92:897–901

72. Humphrey PRD, Harrison MJG. How often can en embolic stroke be diagnosed clinically? A clinicopathological correlation. Postgrad Med J 1985;61:1039–1042
73. Torvik A, Jorgensen L. Thrombotic and embolic occlusions of the carotid arteries in an autopsy material. Journal of Neurologic Sciences 1964;1:24–29
74. Oliviera JSH, Correa de Araujo RR, Navarro MA, Muccillo G. Cardiac thrombosis and thrombembolism in chronic Chagas' heart disease. Am J Cardiol 1983;52:147–151
75. Torres CM. Endocardite pariétale dans la maladie de Chagas (Trypanosmiase Américaine) CR Soc Biol (Paris) 1928;99:886–888
76. Fry DL. Acute vascular endothelial changes associated with increased blood velocity gradients. Circ Res 1968;22:165–197
77. Hinze JO. Turbulence. New York:McGraw-Hill,1959;354–355
78. Mustard JF, Murphy EA, Rowsel HC, Downie HG. Factors influencing thrombus formation in vivo. Am J Med 33:621–647
79. Resnekov L, Chediak J, Hirsh J, et al. Antithrombotic agents in coronary artery disease. Chest 1988;89 [suppl 2]:54–67S
80. Horstkotte D, Schulte HD, Bircks W. Factors influencing prognosis and indication for surgical intervention in acute native-valve endocarditis. In: Horstkotte D, Bodnar E (eds): Infective Endocarditis. London: ICR Publishers, 1991; 171–197
81. Pruitt AA, Rubin HH, Karchmer AW, et al. Neurologic complications of bacterial endocarditis. Medicine (Baltimore) 1978;57:329–343
82. Asinger RW, Mikell FL, Elsperger J, Hodges M. Incidence of left ventricular thrombosis after acute transmural myocardial infarction. N Engl J Med 1981;305:297–302
83. Bhatnager SK, Hudak A, Al-Yusuf AR. Left ventricular thrombosis, wall motion abnormalities, and blood viscosity changes after first transmural anterior myocardial infarction. Chest 1985;88:40–44
84. Ezekowitz MD. Acute infarction, left ventricular thrombus and systemic embolization: an approach to management. J Am Coll Cardiol 1985;5:1281–1282
85. Hellerstein HK, Martin JW. Incidence of thrombo-embolic lesions accompanying myocardial infarction. Am Heart J 1947;33:443–452
86. International Collaborative Study Group. Reduction of infarct size with the early use of timolol in acute myocardial infarction. N Engl J Med 1984;310:9–15
87. Johannessen KA, Nordehaug JE, v d Lippe G. Left ventricular thrombosis and cerebrovascular accident in acute myocardial infarction. Br Heart J 1984;51:553–556
88. Johannessen KA, Nordrehaug JE, von der Lippe G, Vollset SE. Risk factors for embolization in patients with left ventricular thrombi and acute myocardial infarction. Br Heart J 1988;60:104–110
89. Komrad MS, Coffey E, Coffey KS, et al. Myocardial infarction and stroke. Neurology 1984;34:1403–1409
90. Puletti M, Cusmano E, Testa MG, et al. Incidence of systemic thromboembolic lesions in acute myocardial infarction. Clin Cardiol 1986;3:331–333
91. Puletti M, Morocutti C, Borgia C, et al. Acute myocardial infarction and brain. Ital J Neurol Sci 1987;8:245–248
92. Visser CA, Kan G, Meltzer RS, et al. Embolic potential of left ventricular thrombus after myocardial infarction: a two-dimensional echocardiographic study of 119 patients. J Am Coll Cardiol 1985;5:1276–1280
93. Weinrich DJ, Burke JF, Pauletto FJ. Left ventricular mural thrombi complicating acute myocardial infarction: long-term follow-up with serial echocardiography. Ann Intern Med 1984;100:789–794
94. Bateman TM, Czer LSC, Gray RJ, et al. Transient pathologic Q-waves during acute ischemic events: an electrocardiographic correlate of stunned but viable myocardium. Am Heart J 1983;106:1421–1427
95. Burch GE, Giles TD, Colcolough HL. Ischemic cardiomyopathy. Am Heart J 79:291–288
96. Manley JC, King JF, Zeft HF. The "bad" left ventricle. Results of coronary surgery and effect on late survival. J Thorac Cardiovasc Surg 1976;72:841–848
97. Yattlou RF, Peter RH, Behar VS, et al. Ischemic cardiomyopathy: the myopathy of coronary artery disease. Natural history and results of medical versus surgical treatment. Am J Cardiol 1974;34:520–525
98. Davenport JG, Foster JW, Hart RG. Prosthetic valve endocarditis: antibiotics, anticoagulation and stroke. Stroke 1988;19:145
99. Hart RG, Kagen-Hallet K, Joerns SE. Mechanisms of intracranial hemorrhage in infective endocarditis. Stroke 1987;18:1048–1056
100. Horstkotte D, Schulte HD, Bircks W. Factors influencing prognosis and indication for surgical intervention in acute native-valve endocarditis. In: Horstkotte D, Bodnar E (eds): Infective Endocarditis. London: ICR;1991;pp 171–197
101. Horstkotte D. Prosthetic valve endocarditis. In: Horstkotte D, Bodnar E (eds): Infective Endocarditis. London: ICR;1991;pp 229–261

102. Salgado AV, Furlan AJ, Keys TF, Nichols TR, Beck GJ. Neurological complications of native and prosthetic valve endocarditis: a 12-year experience. Neurology 1989;39:173–178
103. Abdon NJ, Zettervall O, Carlson J, et al. Is occult atrial disorder a frequent cause of non-hemorrhagic stroke? Long-term ECG in 86 patients. Stroke 1982;13:832–837
104. Kannel WB, Abbott RD, Savage DD, et al. Epidemiologic features of chronical atrial fibrillation. The Framingham study. N Engl J Med 1982;306:1018–1022
105. Kaul T, Kumar EB, Thomson RM, Bain WH. Sinoatrial disorders:the "sick sinus" syndrome. Experience with implanted cardiac pacemakers. J Cardiovasc Surg 1978;19:261–265
106. Radford DJ, Julian DG. Sick sinus syndrome. Experience of a pacemaker clinic. Br Med J 1974;3:504–507
107. Susaki S, Takeuchi A, Ahzaki M, et al. Long-term follow-up of paced patients with sick sinus syndrome. In: Steinbach K (ed): Cardiac Pacing. Proceedings of the VIIth World Symposium on Cardiac Pacing. Darmstadt: Steinkopff-Verlag, 1983;pp 85–90
108. Takahashi N, Seki A, Imatake K, et al. Clinical features of paroxysmal fibrillation, an observation of 94 patients. Jpn Heart J 1981;22:143–149
109. Forbes CD, Prentice CR. Thrombus formation and artificial surfaces. Br Med Bull 1978;34:201–207
110. Harke H, Schwarz EW, Stambolis C, Bernhard A. The influence of increased clotting reactions as shown by thrombosis formation in the immediate postoperative period on aortic valve prosthesis. Thorax-chirurg 1975;23:422–426
111. Horstkotte D, Loogen F. Erworbene Herzklappenfehler. München-Wien-Baltimore: Urban & Schwarzenberg, 1987;112
112. Davidson CJ, Skelton TN, Kisslo KB, et al. The risk of systemic embolization associated with percutaneous balloon valvuloplasty in adults. Ann Intern Med 1988;108:557–560
113. Safian RD, Berman AD, Diver DJ, et al. Balloon aortic valvuloplasty in 170 consecutive patients. N Engl J Med 1988;319:125–130
114. Spodick DH. The normal and diseased pericardium: current concepts of pericardial physiology, diagnosis and treatment. JACC 1983;1:240–251
115. Dugani BV, Higginson LAJ, Beanlands DS, Akyurekli Y. Recurrent systemic emboli following myocardial contusion. Am Heart J 1984;108:1534–1537
116. Daly K, Monaghan M, Richardson P, et al. Significant incidence of mural thrombi in acute myocarditis. Indication for early anticoagulation [abstract]. J Am Coll Cardiol 1983;1:584
117. De la Chapelle CE, Kossmann CE. Myocarditis. Circulation 1954;10:747–751
118. Desa'Neto A, Bullington JD, Bullington RH, et al. Coxsackie B5 heart disease: demonstration of inferolateral wall myocardial necrosis. Am J Med 1980;68:295
119. Fish M, Barton HR. Heart involvement in infectious mononucleosis. Arch Int Med 1958;101:636–642
120. Obeyesekere I, Hermony Y. Arbovirus heart disease: myocarditis and cardiomyopathy following dengue and chikungunya fever. A follow-up study. Am Heart J 1973;85:186–189
121. Kapila A, Hart RG. Calcific cerebral emboli and aortic stenosis: detection by computed tomography. Stroke 1986;17:619–621
122. Elliott CG, Zimmerman GA, Clemmer TP. Complications of pulmonary artery catheterization in the care of critically ill patients – a prospective study. Chest 1979;76:647–650
123. Foote GA, Schabel SI, Hodges M. Pulmonary complications of the flow directed balloon tipped catheter. N Engl J Med 290:927–930
124. Greene JF, Cummings KC. Aseptic thrombotic endocardial vegetations – a complicaton of indwelling pulmonary artery catheters. JAMA 1973;225:1525–1528
125. Hoar PF, Wilson RM, Mangano DT, et al. Heparin bonding reduces thrombogenicity of pulmonary artery catheters. N Engl J Med 1981;305:993–997
126. Pace NL, Horton W. Indwelling pulmonary artery catheter their relationship to aseptic thrombotic endocardial vegetations. JAMA 1975;233:893–895
127. Yorra FH, Oblath R, Jaffe H, et al. Massive thrombosis associated with use of a Swan-Ganz catheter. Chest 1974;65:682–685
128. Riley HD, Weaver TS. Cardiovascular and nervous system complications of diphtheria. Am Pract 1952;3:536–539
129. Horstkotte D. Endokarditis. In: Hornborstel D, Kaufmann W,Siegenthaler W (eds). Innere Medizin in Praxis und Klinik, Vol. I, 1992; 295–329
130. Goldman MJ. The management of chronic atrial fibrillation: indications for and method of conversion to sinus rhythm. Prog Cardiovasc Dis 1960;2:465–471
131. Lown B. Electrical reversion of cardiac arrhythmias. Br Heart J 1967;29:469–472
132. Braunwald E, Goldblatt A, Aygen MM. Congenital aortic stenosis: clinical and hemodynamic findings in 100 patients. Circulation 1963;27:426–432
133. Campbell M. Calcific aortic stenosis and congenital bicuspid aortic valve. Brit Heart J 1968;30:606–610
134. Edwards JE. The congenital bicuspid aortic valve. Circulation 1965;23:485–489

134. Edwards JE. The congenital bicuspid aortic valve. Circulation 1965;23:485–489
135. Horstkotte D, Loogen F. Histoire naturelle des cardiopathies valvulaires acquises. In: Acar J (ed): Cardiopathies Valvulaires Acquises. Paris: Flammarion, 1985; 225–252
136. Levine JH, Pauker S, Salzman EW. Antithrombotic therapy in valvular heart disease. Chest 1989;95 [suppl]:98–106
137. Lombard JT, Selzer A. Valvular aortic stenosis. Ann Intern Med 1987;106:292–298
138. Mills P, Leech G, Davies M. The natural history of a non-stenotic bicuspid aortic valve. Brit Heart J 1978;40:951–954
139. Rapaport E. Natural history of aortic and mitral valve disease. Am J Cardiol 1975;35:221–228
140. Seigel R, Tresch DD, Keelan MH, Brooks HL. Effects of anticoagulation on recurrent systemic emboli in mitral stenosis. Am J Cardiol 1987;60:1191–1192
141. Arom KV, Nicoloff DM, Kersten TE, et al. St.Jude Medical prosthesis: valve-related deaths and complications. Ann Thorac Surg 1987;43:591–598
142. Bloomfield P, Kitchin AH, Wheatley DJ, et al. A prospective evaluation of the Bjørk-Shiley, Hancock, and Carpentier-Edwards heart valve prostheses. Circulation 1986;73:1213–1222
143. Butchart EG, Lewis PA, Grunkemeier GL, et al. Low risk of thrombosis and serious embolic events despite low-intensity anticoagulation: experience with 1,004 Medtronic Hall valves. Circulation 1988;78 [suppl 1]:I-66 – I-I77
144. Chesebro JH, Adams PC, Fuster V. Antithrombotic therapy in patients with valvular heart disease and prosthetic heart valves. J Am Coll Cardiol 1986;8:41B – 56B
145. Duveau D. Anticoagulation is necessary in all patients with mechanical prostheses in sinus rhythm. Z Kardiol 1986;75 [suppl 2]:326–331
146. Edmunds LH. Thrombotic and bleeding complications of prosthetic heart valves. Ann Thorac Surg 1987;44:430–445
147. Gonzalez-Lavin L, Chi S, Blair TC, et al. Thromboembolism and bleeding after mitral valve replacement with porcine valves: influence of thromboembolic risk factors. J Surg Res 1984;36:508–515
148. Hill JD, LaFollette L, Szarnicki RJ, et al. Risk-benefit analysis of warfarin therapy in Hancock mitral valve replacement. J Thorac Cardiovasc Surg 1982;83:718–723
149. Horstkotte D, Haerten K, Herzer JA, et al. Preliminary results in mitral valve replacement with the St. Jude Medical prosthesis. Comparison with the Bjørk-Shiley valve. Circulation 1981;64 [suppl III]:203–209
150. Horstkotte D, Körfer R, Seipel L, et al. Late complications in patients with Bjørk-Shiley and St. Jude Medical heart valve replacement. Circulatioan 1983;68 [suppl II]:175–184
151. Horstkotte D, Loogen F. Thrombogenicity of different mechanical heart valve prostheses and the risk of anticoagulation therapy. Eur Heart J 1983;4 [suppl I]:7
152. Horstkotte D. Prosthetic valves or tissue valves – a vote for mechanical prostheses. Z Kardiol 1985;74 [suppl 6]:19–37
153. Kuntze CE, Ebels T, Eijgelaar A, v d Heide JNH. Rates of thromboembolism with three different mechanical heart valve prostheses: randomised study. Lancet 1989;1 :514–517
154. Olesen KH, Rygg IH, Wennevold A, Nyboe J. Long-term follow-up in 185 patients after mitral valve replacement with the Lillehei-Kaster prosthesis: overall results and prosthesis-related complications. Eur Heart J 1987;8:680–688
155. Bisset GS, Schwartz DC, Meyer RA, et al. Clinical spectrum and long-term follow-up of isolated mitral valve prolapse in 119 children. Circulation 1980;62:423–429
156. Duren DR, Becker AE, Dunning AJ. Long-term follow-up of idiopathic mitral valve prolapse in 300 patients: a prospective study. J Am Coll Cardiol 1988;11:42–47
157. Egeblad H, Hesse B. Mitral valve prolapse with mobile polypoid cul-de-sac thrombus and embolism to brain and lower extremity. Am Heart J 1987;114:648–650
158. Kelly RE, Pina I, Lee SC. Cerebral ischemia and mitral valve prolapse: case-control study of associated factors. Stroke 1988;19:443–446
159. Nishimura RA, McGoon MD, Shub D, et al. Echocardiographically documented mitral valve prolapse: long-term follow-up of 237 patients. N Engl J Med 1985;313:1305–1309
160. Wolf PA, Sila CA. Cerebral ischemia with mitral valve prolapse. Am Heart J 1987;113:1308–1315
161. Freedman LR. Role of non-bacterial thrombotic vegetations in the pathogenesis of endocarditis. In: Horstkotte D, Bodnar E (eds): Infective Endocarditis. London: ICR Publishers, 1991;pp 10–14
162. Keith JD. Biscuspid aortic valve. In: Keith JD, Rowe RD, Vlad P (eds): Heart Disease in Infancy and Childhood. New York: Macmillan, 1978;pp 728–735
163. Kratz JM, Usher BW, Sade RM, Gaddy JE. Systemic thromboembolism from a ventricular septal patch. Chest 1980;78:744–745
164. Jespersen CM, Egeblad H. Mitral anulus calcification and embolism. Acta Med Scand 1987;222:37–41
165. Lin CS, Schwartz IS, Chapman I. Calcification of the mitral anulus fibrosus with systemic embolization. Arch Pathol Lab Med 1987;111:411–414

166. Keating EC, Gross SA, Schlamowitz RA, et al. Mural thrombi in myocardial infarction: prospective evaluation by two-dimensional echocardiography. Am J Med 1983;74:989–995
167. Lepeyre AC, Steele PM, Kazmier FJ, et al. Systemic embolism in chronic left ventricular aneurysm: incidence and the role of anticoagulation. J Am Coll Cardiol 1985;6:534–538
168. Turpie AGG, Robinson JG, Doyle DJ, et al. Comparison of high-dose with low-dose subcutaneous heparin to prevent left ventricular mural thrombosis in patients with acute transmural anterior myocardial infarction. N Engl J Med 1989;320:352–357
169. Tramarin R, Pozzoli M, Febo O, et al. Two-dimensional echocardiographic assessment of anticoagulant therapy in left ventricular thrombosis early after acute myocardial infarction. Eur Heart J 1986;7:482–492
170. Nespeca MP, Townsend JJ. Multiple cerebral emboli in a young man. West J Med 1987;146:589–595
171. Biller J, Ionasescu V, Zellweger H, et al. Incidence of cerebral infarction in inherited neuromuscular conditions. Stroke 1987; 81:805–807
172. Kyrle PA, Korninger C, Gossinger H, et al. Prevention of arterial and pulmonary embolism by oral antiocoagulants in patients with dilated cardiomyopathy. Thromb Haemost 1985;54:521–523
173. Homans DC. Peripartum cardiomyopathy. N Engl J Med 1985;312:1432–1437
174. Julian DG, Szekely P. Peripartum cardiomyopathy. Prog Cardiovasc Dis 1985;27:223–240
175. Knobel B, Melamud E, Kishon Y. Peripartum cardiomyopathy. Isr J Med Science 1984;20:1061–1063
176. Fuster V, Gersh BJ, Giuliani ER, et al. The natural history of idiopathic dilated cardiomyopathy. Am J Cardiol 1981;47:525–531
177. Gottdiener JS, Gay JA, Van Voorhees L, et al. Frequency and embolic potential of left ventricular thrombus in dilated cardiomyopathy: assessment by two-dimensional echocardiography. Am J Cardiol 1983;52:1281–1285
178. Takamoto T, Kim D, Urie PM, et al. Comparative recognition of left ventricular thrombi by echocardiography and cine-angiography. Br Heart J 1985;53:36–42
179. Taliercio CP, Seward JB, Driscoll DJ, et al. Idiopathic dilated cardiomyopathy in the young: clinical profile and natural history. J Am Coll Cardiol 1985;6:1126–1131
180. Schachter S, Freeman R. TIA and Adriamycin cardiomyopathy. Neurology 1982;32:1380–1381
181. Becker BJP, Chatgidakis CB, Lingen B van. Cardiovascular collagenosis with parietal endocardial thrombosis. Circulation 1953;7:345–356
182. Davies JNP. Pathology and pathogenesis of endocardial disease. Cardiologia 1963;42:161–175
183. Gottdiener JS, Maron BJ, Schooley RT, et al. Two-dimensionalechocardiographic assessment of the idiopathic hypereosinophilia snydrome: anatomic basis of mitral regurgitation and peripheral embolization. Circulation 1983;67:572–578
184. Niehues R, Klein RM, Horstkotte D, Schultheiss HP, Strauer BE. Löffler'sche Endokarditis: Seltene Ursache einer biventrikul○ren Herzinsuffizienz. Diagnostik und Therapie bei drei Patienten. Intensivmed 1991;28:336–337
185. Marais FI, Fontaine GH, Guiraudou G. Right ventricular dysplasia: a report of 24 adult cases. Circulation 1982;65:384–398
186. Botker HE, Rasmussen OB. Recurrent cerebral embolism in cardiac amyloidosis. Int J Cardiol 1986;13:81–83
187. Belkin RN, Hurwitz BJ, Kisslo KB. Atrial septal aneurysm:association with cerebrovascular and peripheral embolic events. Stroke 1987;18:856–862
188. Di Pasquale G, Andreoli A, Grazi P, et al. Cardioembolic stroke from atrial septal aneurysm. Stroke 1988;19:640–543
189. Gallet B, Malergue MC, Adams C, et al. Atrial septal aneurysm: potential cause of systemic embolism: an echocardiographic study. Br Heart J 1985;53:292–297
190. Hanley PC, Tajik AJ, Hynes JK, et al. Diagnosis and classification of atrial septal aneurysm by two-dimensional echocardiography: report of 80 consecutive cases. J Am Coll Cardiol 1985;6:1370–1382
191. Roberts WC. Aneurysm (redundancy) of the atrial septum (fossa ovale membrane) and prolapse (redundancy) of the mitral valve. Am J Cardiol 1984;54:1153–1154
192. Silver MD, Dorsey JS. Aneurysms of the septum primum in adults. Arch Pathol Lab Med 1978;102:62–65
193. Armstrong WF, Feigenbaum H, Dillon JC. Echocardiographic detection of right atrial thromboembolism. Chest 1985;87:801–806
194. Heath D. Pathology of cardiac tumors. Am J Cardiol 1968;21:315–325
195. Kasarskis EJ, O'Connor W, Earle G. Embolic stroke from cardiac papillary fibroelastomas. Stroke 1988;19:1171–1173
196. Markel ML, Waller BF, Armstrong WF. Cardiac myxoma: a review. Medicine 1987;66:114–126
197. Larrieu AJ, Jamieson WRE, Tyers GFO, et al. Primary cardiac tumors. J Thorac Cardiovasc Surg 1982;83:339–348

198. Pomerance A. Papillary "tumours" of the heart valves. J Pathol Bacteriol 1961;81:135–139
199. Marvaste MA, Obeid AI, Potts IL Approach to the management of atrial myxoma with long-term follow-up. Ann Thorac 1984;38:53–56
200. Topol EJ, Bierm RO, Reitz BA. Cardiac papillary fibro-elastoma and stroke. Am J Med 1986;80:129–131
201. Roeltgen DP, Weimer GR, Patterson LF. Delayed neurologic complications of left atrial myxoma. Neurology 1981;31:8–13
202. Sandok BA, v Estorff I, Giuliani ER. CNS embolism due to atrial myxoma. Arch Neurol 1980;37:485–488
203. Tsuchija F, Kohno A, Saitoh R, et al. CT findings of atrial myxoma. Radiology 1984;151:139–148
204. Gorelik PB, Rusinowitz MS, Tiku M, et al. Embolic stroke complicating systemic lupus erythematosus. Arch Neurol 1985;42:813–815
205. Fowler NO, Geuron M. Primary myocardial disease. Circulation 1965;32:830
206. Fox IS, Spence AM, Wheelis RF, Healey LA. Cerebral embolism in Libman-Sacks endocarditis. Neurology 1980;30:487–491
207. Huycke EC, Robinosiwtz M, Cohen IS, et al. Granulomatous endocarditis with systemic embolism in Bechet's disease. Ann Intern Med 1985;102:791–793
208. Seneviratne BI, Reiners J. Nonvalvular atrial fibrillation associated with cardioembolic stroke: the role of hypertensive heart disease. Aust NZ J Med 1990;20:127–134
209. Askey JM, Bernstein S. The management of rheumatic heart disease in relation to systemic arterial embolism. Prog Cardiovasc Dis 1960;3:220–232
210. Calandre L, Ortego JF, Berbemo F, et al. Anticoagulation and hemorrhagic infarction in cerebral embolism secondary to rheumatic heart disease. Arch Neurol 1984;41:1152–1154
211. Daly R, Mattingly TW, Holt CT, et al. Systemic arterial embolism in rheumatic heart disease. Am Heart J 1951;42 :566–581
212. Darling RC, Austin WC, Linton RR. Arterial embolism. Surg Gynecol Obstet 1967;124:106–114
213. Fleming HA, Bailey SM. Mitral valve disease, systemic embolism and anticoagulants. Postgrad Med J 1971;47 :599–604
214. Guberman BA, Fowler NO, Engel PJ, et al. Cardiac tamponade in medical patients. Circulation 1981;64:633–640
215. Santamaria J, Graus F, Peres J. Cerebral embolism and anticoagulation. Neurology 1983;33:1104–1107
216. Furlan AJ, Craciun AR, Raju NR, Hart N. Cerebrovascular complications associated with idiopathic hypertrophic subaortic stenosis. Stroke 1984;15:282–284
217. Glancy DL, O'Brien KP, Gold HK, et al. Atrial fibrillation in patients with idiopathic hypertrophic subaortic stenosis. Br Heart J 1970;32:652–659
218. Koga Y, Itaya K, Toshima H. Prognosis in hypertrophic cardiomyopthy. Am Heart J 1984;108:351–355
219. Kogure S, Yamamoto Y, Tomono S, et al. High risk of systemic embolism in hypertrophic cardiomyopathy. Jpn Heart J 1986;27:475–480
220. Alpert H. Atrial fibrillation. Acta Med Scand 1968;185 :373–379
221. Algart JS, Peterson P, Godtfredsen J. Atrial fibrillation: natural history, complications, and management. Ann Rev Med 1988;39:41–52
222. Beer DT, Ghitman B. Embolization from the atria in arteriosclerotic heart disease. JAMA 1961;177:287–290
223. Fairfax AJ, Lambert CD, Leatham A. Systemic embolism in chronic sinoatrial disorder. N Engl J Med 1976;295:190
224. Cerebral Embolism Study Group. Immediate anticoagulation of embolic stroke: a randomized trial. Stroke 1983;14:668–676
225. Hinton RC, Kistler JP, Fallon JT, et al. Influence of etiology of atrial fibrillation on incidence of systemic embolism. Am J Cardiol 1977;40:509–513
226. Fisher CM. Reducing risks of cerebral embolism. Geriatrics 1979;34:59–66
227. Phillips StJ. Is atrial fibrillation an independent risk factor for stroke? Can J Neurol Sci 1990;17:163–168
228. Sage JI, van Uitert RL. Risk of recurrent stroke in atrial fibrillation: differences between rheumatic and arteriosclerotic heart disease. Stroke 1983;14:537–540
229. Sherman DG, Hart RG, Easton JD. The secondary prevention of stroke in patients with atrial fibrillation. Arch Neurol 1986;43:68–70
230. Wolf PA, Darsber TR, Thomas HE, et al. Epidemiologic assessment of chronic atrial fibrillation and risk of stroke. The Framingham Study. Neurology 1978;28:973–977
231. Zager J, Berberich SN, Eslova R, et al. Dynamic tricuspid valve insufficiency produced by a right ventricular thrombus from a pacemaker. Chest 1978;7:455–456
232. Cammarosano C, Lewis W. Cardiac lesions in acquired immune deficiency syndrome (AIDS). J Am Coll Cardiol 1985;5:703–706
233. De Groat TS, Parameswaran R, Popper P, Kotler MN. Left ventricular thrombi in association with normal left ventricular wall motion in patients with malignancy. Am J Cardiol 1985;56:827–828

234. Garcia I, Fainstein V, Rios A, et al. Non-bacterial thrombotic endocarditis in a male homosexual with Kaposi's sarcoma. Arch Intern Med 1983;143:1243–1244
235. Graus F, Rogers LR, Posner JB. Cerebrovascular complications in patients with cancer. Medicine 1985;64:16–35
236. Lim SP, Hakim SZ, Schoenhoff DD. Non-bacterial thrombotic endocarditis: two-dimensional echocardiographic features in an autopsy-proven case. Chest 1987;92:176–177
237. Lopez JA, Ross RS, Fishbein MC, Siegel RJ. Nonbacterial thrombotic endocarditis: a review. Am Heart J 1987;113 :773–784
238. Rogers LR, Cho ES, Kempin S, Posner JB. Cerebral infarction from nonbacterial thrombotic endocarditis: clinical and pathological study including the effects of anticoagulation. Am J Med 1987;83:746–756
239. Schmaler AH, Denenberg B. Left ventricular thrombus with normal left ventricular function and hyperaggregable platelets in a patient with polycystic disease of multiple organs. Am J Med Sci 1984;288:223–227
240. Stoddard MF, Pearson AC, Kanter KR, Labovitz AJ. Left ventricular thrombus with normal left ventricular wall motion in a patient with myelofibrosis. Am Heart J 1989;117:966–968
241 Bürrig KF, Schulte-Terhausen J, Hort W. Special role of the endocardium in the pathogenesis of endocarditis. In: Horstkotte D, Bodnar E (eds): Infective Endocarditis. London: ICR Publishers, 1991; 3–9
242. Thorgeirsson G, Robertson AL. The vascular endothelium – pathobiologic significance. A review. Am J Pathol 1978;93:803–848
243. Davies PF. Biology of disease. Vascular cell interactions with special reference to the pathogenesis of atherosclerosis. Lab Invest 1986;55:5–24
244. Moncada S, Palmer RMJ, Higgs EA. Nitric oxide: physiology, pathophysiology, and pharmacology. Pharm Rev 1991;43:109–142
245. Ogawa SK, Yurberg ER, Hatcher VE, et al. Bacterial adherence to human endothelial cells in vitro. Infect and Immunity 1985;50:218–224
246. Berenger FP, Cano JP, Rolland PH. Antithrombogenic endothelial cell defense. Basal characteristics in cultured endothelial cells and modulation by short-term and long-term exposure to isosorbide nitrates. Circ Res 1987;60:612–618
247. Kelm M, Schrader J. Control of coronary vascular tone by nitric oxide. Circ Res 1990;66:1561–1575
248. Pohl U, Busse R. EDRF increases cyclic GMP in platelets during passage through the coronary vascular bed. Circ Res 1989;64:1798–1806
249. Bürrig KF, Diefenbach C, Jacob B, Hort W. Arteriosklerose, Endothelausrichtung und Mediastruktur im Sinus caroticus des Menschen [abstract]. Verh Dtsch Ges Pathol 1978;71:545
250. Langille BL. Integrity of arterial endothelium following acute exposure ot high shear stress. Biorheology 1984;21:333–346
251. Davies PF, Remuzzi A, Gordon EJ, et al. Turbulent fluid shear stress induces vascular endothelial turnover in vitro. Proc Natl Acad Sci USA 1986;83:2114- 2117
252. Adams PC, Cohen M, Chesebro JH, Fuster V. Thrombosis and embolism from cardiac chambers and infected valves. J Am Coll Cardiol 1986;8:76B – 87B
253. Arvan S. Mural thrombi in coronary artery disease: recent advances in pathogenesis, diagnosis, and approaches to treatment. Arch Intern Med 1984;144:133–116
254. Cabin HS, Roberts WC. Left ventricular aneurysm, intraaneurysmal thrombus and systemic embolus in coronary heart disease. Chest 1980;77:586–590
255. Chesebro JH, Ezekowitz MD, Badimon L, Fuster V. Intracardiac thrombi and systemic thromboembolism: detection, incidence and treatment. Ann Rev Med 1985;36:579–605
256. Meltzer RX, Visser CE, Fuster V. Intracardiac thrombi and systemic embolization. Ann Intern Med 1986;104:689–698
257. Nixon JV. Left ventricular mural thrombus. Arch Intern Med 1983;143:1567–1571
258. Stratton JR. Mural thrombi of the left ventricle. Chest 1983;83:166–168
259. Johnson RC, Crissman RS, DiDio LJA. Endocardial alterations in myocardial infarction. Lab Invest 1979;40:183–193
260. Mallory GK, White PD. Salcedo-Salgar J. The speed of healing of myocardial infarction: a study of the pathologic anatomy in seventy two cases. Am heart J 1939;18:647–671
261. Hochman JS, Platia EB. Bulkley BH. Endocardial abnormalities in left ventricular aneurysms: a clinicopathologic study. Ann Intern Med 1984;100:29–35
262. Roberts WC, Ferrans VI. Pathological aspects of certain cardiomyopathies. Circ Res 1974;34/35 [suppl II]:II–128-II–144
263. Asinger RW, Mikell EL, Elsperger J, Hodges M. Incidence of left ventricular thrombosis after acute transmural myocardial infarction. Serial evaluation by two-dimensional echocardiography. N Engl J Med 1981;305:297–302

264. Haughland JM, Asinger RW, Mikell FL, et al. Embolic potential of left ventricular thrombi detected by two-dimensional echocardiography. Circulation 1984;70:586–598
265. Mikell FL, Asinger RW, Elsperger KJ, Anderson WJ, Hodges M. Regional stasis of blood in the dysfunctional left ventricle: echocardiographic detection and differentiation from early thrombosis. Circulation 1982;66:755–763
266. Bertrand ME, Le Blanche JM, Tilmant PY, et al. Coronary sinus blood flow at rest and during isometric exercise in patients with aortic valve disease: mechanism of angina pectoris in presence of normal coronary arteries. Am J Cardiol 1981;47:199–205
267. Fallen EL, Elliott WC, Gorlin R. Mechanism of angina in aortic stenosis. Circulation 1967;36:480–484
268. Hoffman JIE, Buckberg GD. The myocardial supply/demand ratio – a critical review. Am J Cardiol 1978;41:327–331
269. Nadell R. Myocardial oxygen supply/demand ratio in aortic stenosis: hemodynamic and echocardiographic evaluation of patients with and without angina pectoris. J Am Coll Cardiol 1983;2:258–261
270. Neill WA, Fluri-Lundeen JH. Myocardial oxygen supply in left ventricular hypertrophy and coronary heart disease. Am J Cardiol 1979;44:747
271. Thormann J, Schlepper M. Comparison of myocardial flow, hemodynamic changes, and lactate metabolism during isoproterenol stress in patients with coronary heart disease and severe aortic stenosis. Clin Cardiol 1979;2:437–441
272. Trenouth RS, Phelps NC, Neill WA. Determinants of left ventricular hypertrophy and oxygen supply in aortic valve disease. Circulation 1976;53:644–648
273. Marcus ML. Decreased coronary reserve: a mechanism for angina pectoris in patients with aortic stenosis and normal coronary arteries. N Engl J Med 1982;307:1362–1365
274. Tauchert M, Hilger HH. Application of the coronary reserve concept to the study of myocardial perfusion. In: Schaper W (ed): The Pathophysiology of Myocardial Perfusion. Amsterdam: Elsevier, 1979;pp 141–167
275. Attarian DE. Characteristics of chronic left ventricular hypertrophy induced by subcoronary valvular aortic stenosis: II: Response to ischemia. J Thorac Cardiovasc Surg 1981;81:389–392
276. Watson JH, Bartholomae WM. Cardiac injury due to nonpenetrating chest trauma. Ann Intern Med 1960;52:871–880
277. Harthorne JW, Kantrowitz PA, Dinsmore RE, Sanders CA. Traumatic myocardial infarction: report of a case with normal coronary angiogram. Ann Intern Med 1967;66:341–344
278. Kertes P, Westlake G, Luxton M. Multiple peripheral emboli after cardiac trauma. Br Heart J 1983;49:187–189
279. Kessler KM, Mallon SM, Bolooki H, Myerburg RJ. Pedunculated right ventricular thrombus due to repeated blunt chest trauma. Am Heart J 1981;102:1064–1066
280. Mackintosh AF, Fleming HA. Cardiac damage presenting late after road accidents. Thorax 1981;36:811–813
281. Oren A, Bar-Shlomo B, Stern S. Acute coronary occlusion following blunt injury to the chest in the absence of coronary atherosclerosis. Am Heart J 1976;92:501–505
282. Parmley LF, Manjon WC, Mattingly TW. Nonpenetrating traumatic injury of the heart. Circulation 1958;18:371–396
283. Botker HE, Rasmussen OB. Recurrent cerebral embolism in cardiac amyloidosis. Int J Cardiol 1986;13:81–83
284. Rice GPA, Ebers GC, Newland F, Wysocki GP. Recurrent cerebral embolism in cardiac amyloidosis. Neurology (NY) 1981;31:904–906
285. Tomioka N, Kishimoto C, Matsumori A, Kawai C. Mural thrombi in mice with acute viral myocarditis. Jpn Circ J 1985;49:1277–1279
286. DiPasquale G, Ribani M, Andreoli A, et al. Cardioembolic stroke in primary oxalosis with cardiac involvement. Stroke 1989;20:1403–1406
287. Acharya G, Garik E. Arterial emboli and malignant disease. Vasc Surg 1977;11:26–28
288. Green WH, Benjamin RS, Glusman S, et al. Arterial embolism of tumor causing fatal organ infarction. Arch Int Med 1974;134:545–548
289. Lieberman JS, Borrero J, Urdaneta E, Wright IS. Thrombophlebitis and cancer. JAMA 1961; :542–545
290. Waterbury LS, Hampton JW. Hypercoagulability with malignancy. Angiology 1967;18:197–203
291. Langille BL. Integrity of arterial endothelium following acute exposure to high shear stress. Biorheology 1984;21:333–346
292. Roberts WC. The structure of the aortic valve in clinically isolated aortic stenosis. An autopsy study of 162 patients over 15 years of age. Circulation 1970;42:91
293. Pape LA. Pathogenesis and etiology of valvular heart disease. In: Dalen JE, Alpert JS (eds): Valvular Heart Disease. Boston: Little, Brown & Co., 1981;p 1
294. Wallach JB, Lukash L, Angrist AA. The mechanism of formation of left auricular mural thrombi. Am J Med 1954;16:543–548

295. Abdon NJ, Jönsson BM. High risk of systemic embolization in episodic sick sinus syndrome. In: Meere C (ed): Proceedings of the VIth World Symposium on Cardiac Pacing. Montreal Pace Symposium. Pace 1979;2:A50
296. Norris JW, Frogatt GM, Hachinski VC. Cardiac arrhythmias in acute stroke. Stroke 1978;9:392–396
297. Wallach JB, Lukash L, Angrist AA. An interpretation of the incidence of mural thrombi in the left auricle and appendage with particular reference to mitral commissurotomy. Am Heart J 1953;45:252–254
298. Come PC, Riley MF, Bivas NK. Roles of echocardiography and arrhythmia monitoring in the evaluation of patients with suspected systemic embolism. Ann Neurol 1983;13:527–531
299. Sutton R, Kenny RA. The natural history of sick sinus syndrome. Pace 1986;9:1110–1114
300. Koudstaal PJ, van Gijn J, Klootwijk APJ, et al. Holter monitoring in patients with transient and focal ischemic attacks of the brain. Stroke 1986;17:192–195
301. Kumagai U, Kukunami M, Ohmori M, et al. Increased intra-cardiovascular clotting in patients with chronic atrial fibrillation. J Am Coll Cardiol 1990;16:377–380
302. Close JB, Evans DW, Bailey SM. Persistent lone atrial fibrillation: its prognosis after clinical diagnosis. J R Coll Gen Pract 1979;29:547–549
303. Kopecky SL, Gerah BJ, McGoon MD, et al. The natural history of lone atrial fibrillation. N Engl J Med 1987;317:669–674
304. Wipf JE, Lipsky. Atrial fibrillation – thromboembolic risk and indication for anticoagulation. Arch Int Med 1990;150:1598–1603
305. Brand FN, Abbott RD, Kannel WB, Wolf PA. Characteristics and prognosis of lone atrial fibrillation. JAMA 1985;254:3449–3453
306. Davidson E, Rotenberg Z, Weinberger I, et al. Diagnosis and characteristics of lone atrial fibrillation. Chest 1989;95:1048–1050
307. Gajewski J, Singer RB. Mortality in an insured population with atrial fibrillation. J Am Med Assoc 1981;245:1540–1544
308. Boston Area Anticoagulation Trial for Atrial Fibrillation Investigators. The effect of low-dose warfarin on the risk of stroke in nonrheumatic atrial fibrillation. N Engl J Med 1990;323:1505–1511
309. Cairns JA, Connolly SJ. Nonrheumatic atrial fibrillation. Risk of stroke and role of antithrombotic therapy. Circulation 1991;84:469–481
310. Conolly SJ, Laupaucis A, Gent M, et al. Canadian Atrial Fibrillation Anticoagulation Study. Circulation 1990;82 [suppl IV]:366–372
311. Petersen P, Boysen G, Godtfredsen J, Andersen ED, Andersen B. Placebo-controlled, randomized trial of warfarin and aspirin for prevention of thromboembolic complication in chronic atrial fibrillation. The Copenhagen AFASAK Study. Lancet 1989;1:175–179
312. Stroke Prevention in Atrial Fibrillation Investigators. Stroke prevention in atrial fibrillation study: final results. Circulation 1991;84:527–539
313. Kannel WB, Abbott RD, Savage DD, McNamara PM. Coronary heart disease and atrial fibrillation. Am Heart J 1983;106:389–396
314. Friedman HZ, Goldberg SF, Boneman JD, et al. Acute complications associated with new-onset atrial fibrillation. Am J Cardiol 1991;67:437–439
315. Petersen P, Godtfredsen J. Embolic complications in paroxysmal atrial fibrillation. Stroke 1986;17:62–66
316. Wolf PA, Kannel WB, McGee DL, et al. Duration of atrial fibrillation and imminence of stroke: The Framingham Study. Stroke 1983;14:664–667
317. Bailey G, Braniff B, Hancock E, Cohn K. Relation of left atrial pathology to atrial fibrillation in mitral valve disease. Ann Intern Med 1968;69:13–20
318. Moe G, Abildskov J. Atrial fibrillation as a self-sustaining arrhythmia independent of local discharge. Am Heart J 1991;58:59–70
319. Caplan LR, D'Cruz I, Hier DB, et al. Atrial size, atrial fibrillation, and stroke. Ann Neurol 1986;19:158–161
320. Katz L, Pick A. Current status of theories of mechanisms of atrial tachycardias, flutter, and fibrillation. Prog Cardiovasc Dis 1960;2:650–662
321. Pollard JH. A Handbook of Numerical and Statistical Techniques. Cambridge University Press, 1977
322. Probst P, Goldschlager N, Selzer A. Left atrial size and atrial fibrillation in mitral stenosis. Circulation 1983;48:1282–1287
323. Ewy G, Ulfers R, Hager W, et al. Response of atrial fibrillation to therapy: role of etiology and left atrial diameter. J Electrocardiol 1980;13:119–124
324. Goldman M. The management of chronic atrial fibrillation: indications for and method of conversion to sinus rhythm. Prog Cardiovasc Dis 1960;2:465–484
325. Henry W, Morganroth J, Pearlman A, et al. Relation between echocardiographically determined left atrial size and atrial fibrillation. Circulation 1976;53:273–279

326. Mancini GB, Goldberger AL. Cardioversion of atrial fibrillation: consideration of embolization, anticoagulation, prophylactic pacemaker and long-term success. Am Heart J 1987;104:617–621
327. Sahn DJ, DeMaria A, Kisslo J, Weyman A. Recommendations regarding quantitation in M-mode echocardiography: results of a survey of echocardiographic measurements. Circulation 1978;58:1072–1083
328. Breivik K, Ohm OJ, Segadal L. Sick sinus syndrome treated with permanent pacemaker in 109 patients. A follow-up study. Acta Med Scand 1979;206:153
329. Stone JM, Bhakta RD, Lutgen J. Dual chamber sequential pacing management of sinus node dysfunction: advantages over single chamber pacing. Am Heart J 1982;8 :1319–1322
330. Areosty JM, Cohen SL, Morkin E. Bradytachycardia syndrome. Results in twenty-eight patients treated by combined pharmacologic therapy and pacemaker implantation. Chest 1974;66:257–261
331. Curzi GF, Mocchegianni R, Ciempani N, et al. Thromboembolism during VVI permanent pacing in cardiac pacing. Gomez FP (ed): Electrophysiology and Tachyarrhythmia. Editorial Grouz, Madrid, 1985;pp 1203–1206
332. Krishnaswami V, Geraci AR. Permanent pacing in disorders of sinus node function. Am Heart J 1975;69:579–583
333. Rosenqvist M, Brandt J, Schüller H. Atrial versus ventricular pacing in sinus rhythm disease. A treatment comparison study. Am Heart J 1986;111:292–296
334. Santini M, Messina G, Porto MP. Sick sinus syndrome: single chamber pacing in cardiac pacing. In: Gomez FP (ed): Electrophysiology and Tachyarrhythmias. Editorial Grouz, Madrid, 1985;pp 144–152
335. Komrad MS, Coffey CEW, Coffey KS, et al. Myocardial infarction and stroke. Neurology 1984;34:1403–1409
336. Corman C, Roudaut R, Gosse P, et al. Right atrial thrombosis: echocardiographic features and management. Results in eight cases. Arch Mal Coeur 1986;79:464–471
337. Grollier G, Gerard JL, Commeau P, et al. Right cardiac cavity thrombi: echocardiographic diagnosis and therapeutic indications. Report of two cases and review of the literature. Can J Cardiol 1986;2:68–75
338. van Kuyk M, Mols P, Englert M. Right atrial thrombus leading to pulmonary embolism. Br Heart J 1984;51:462–464
339. Brown AK, Anderson V. Resolution of right atrial thrombus shown by serial cross sectional echocardiography. Br Heart J 1985;53:659–601
340. Come PC. Transient right atrial thrombus during acute myocardial infarction: diagnosis by echocardiography. Am J Cardiol 1983;51:1226–1228
341. Kushwada S, Jepson EM. Resolution of right atrial thrombus following anticoagulation. Int J Cardiol 1990;27:269–271
342. Manno BV, Panidis IP, Kotler MV, et al. Two-dimensional echocardiographic detection of right atrial thrombi. Am J Cardiol 1983;51:615–616
343. Redish GA, Anderson AL. Echocardiographic diagnosis of right atrial thromboembolism. J Am Coll Cardiol 1983;1:1167–1169
344. Riggs T, Paul MH, DeLeon S, Ilbawi M. Two dimensional echocardiography in evaluation of right atrial masses: five cases in pediatric patients. Am J Cardiol 1981;48:961–966
345. Garvin CF. Mural thrombi in the heart. Am Heart J 1941;21 :713–720
346. Henry WL, Ware J, Gardin JM, et al. Echocardiographic measurements in normal subjects: growth-related changes that occur between infancy and early adulthood. Circulation 1978;57:278–285
347. Gardin JM, Henry WL, Savage D, et al. Echocardiographic measurements in normal subjects: evaluation of an adult population without clinically apparent heart disease. J Clin Ultrasound 1979;7:439–447
348. Selzer A, Katayama M. Mitral regurgitation: clinical patterns, pathophysiology and natural history. Medicine 1972;51:337–366
349. Henry WL, Morganroth J, Pearlman AS, et al. Relation between echocardiographically determined left atrial size and atrial fibrillation. Circulation 1976;53:273–279
350. Sherrid MV, Clark RD, Cohn K. Echocardiographic analysis of left atrial size before and after operation in mitral valve disease. Am J Cardiol 1979;43:171–178
351. Johnson RA, Palacios I. Dilated cardiomyopathy in the adult (part I). N Engl J Med 1982;307:1051–1058
352. Stratton JR, Nemanich JW, Johanessen KA, Resnick AD. Fate of left ventricular thrombi in patients with remote myocardial infarction or idiopathic cardiomyopathy. Circulation 1988;78:1388–1393
353. Hatle L, Örjavik O, Storstein O. Chronic myocardial disease. I: Clinical picture related to long-term prognosis. Acta Med Scand 1976;199:399–405
354. Cooley DA, Hanman GL. Surgical treatment of left ventricular aneurysm: experience with excision of post infarction lesions in 80 patients. Prog Cardiovasc Dis 1968;11:222–228
355. Lapeyre AC III, Steele PM, Kazmier FJ, et al. Systemic embolism in chronic left ventricular aneurysm: incidence and the role of anticoagulation. J Am Coll Cardiol 1985;6:534–538

356. Reeder GS, Lengyel M, Tajik AJ, et al. Mural thrombus in left ventricular aneurysm: incidence, role of angiography, and relation between anticoagulation and embolization. Mayo Clin Proc 1981;56:77–81
357. Sherman DG, Dyken ML, Fisher M, et al. Cerebral embolism. Chest 1986;89 [suppl]:82S – 98S
358. Hewson W. Experimental inquiries. I. An inquiry into the properties of the blood, with some remarks on some of its morbid appearances: and an appendix relating to the discovery of the lymphatic system in birds, fish, and the animals called amphibians. London, T Cadell, 1771
359. Wessler S. Thrombosis in the presence of vascular stasis. Am J Med 1962;33:648–652
360. Wessler S, Reiner L, Freiman DG, et al. Studies of its induction and evolution under controlled conditions in vivo. Circulation 1959;20:864–869
361. Wessler S, Yin ET. On the mechanism of thrombosis. Prog Haematol 1969;6:201–209
362. Bussolino F, Breviario F, Tetta C, et al. Interleukin 1 stimulates platelet-activating factor production in cultured human endothelial cells. J Clin Invest 1986;77:2027–2033
363. McIntyre TM, Zimmerman GA, Satoh K, Prescott SM. Cultured endothelial cells synthesize both platelet-activating factor and prostaclyclin in response to histamine, bradykinin, and adenosine triphosphate. J Clin Invest 1985;76:271–280
364. Thomas DP, Wessler S. Stasis thrombi induced by bacterial endotoxin. Circ Res 1964;14:486–489
365. Botti RE, Ratnoff OD. Studies on the pathogenesis of thrombosis: an experimental "hypercoagulable" state induced by the intravenous injection of ellagic acid. J Lab Clin Med 1964;64:385–391
366. Nordöy A, Chandler AB. Formation of platelet-fibrin thrombi by ellagic acid and adenosine diphosphate in the rat. Lab Invest 1967;16:3–8
367. Auclair MC, Vernimmen C, Lechat P. Influence of prostacyclin and two metabolites on the contractility of cultured rat heart cells. Prostaglandins Leukotrienes and Essential Fatty Acids 1988;32:33–38
368. Carmona RH, Tsao T, Dae M, Trunkey DD. Myocardial dysfunction in septic shock. Arch Surg 1985;120:30–35
369. Lefer AM. Myocardial depressant factor and circulatory shock. Klin Wochenschr 1974;52:358–370
370. Parrillo JE. Pathogenesis of cardiovascular dysfunction in septic shock. In: Vincent JL (ed): Update in Intensive Care and Emergency Medicine. Heidelberg-New York: Springer, 1989; 317–321
371. Deykin D. Thrombogenesis. N Engl J Med 1967;276:622
372. Size HS, Moschos CB, Becker R. On the nature of hypercoagulability. Am J Med 1962;33:667–671
373. Glas-Greenwalt P, Dalton BC, Astrup T. Localization of tissue plasminogen activator in relation to morphologic changes in human saphenous veins used as coronary artery bypass autografts. Ann Surg 1975;181:431–435
374. Farfel Z, Shechter M, Vered Z, et al. Review of echocardiographically diagnosed right heart entrapment of pulmonary emboli in transit with emphasis on management. Am Heart J 1987;113:171–178
375. European Working Group on Echocardiography. The European Cooperative Study on the clinical significance of right heart thrombi. Eur Heart J 1989;10:1040–1059
376. Ouyang P, Camara EJ, Jain A, et al. Intracavitary thrombi in the right heart associated with multiple pulmonary emboli. Chest 1983;84:296–299
377. Shiu MF, Abrama LD. Echocardiographic features of free floating thrombus mimicking right ventricular myxoma. Br Heart J 1983;49:612–614
378. Stowers SA, Leiboff RH, Wasserman AG, et al. Right ventricular thrombus formation in association with acute myocardial infarction: diagnosis by two-dimensional echocardiography. Am J Cardiol 1983;52:912–913
379. Ferrer JM, Harvey R. Some hemodynamic aspects of cardiac arrhythmias in man. Am Heart J 1964;68:153–158
380. Berg RA, Kaplan AM, Jarrett PB, Mothan ME. Friedreich's ataxia with acute cardiomyopathy. Am J Dis Child 1980;134:390–393
381. Basmadijan D. The hemodynamic forces acting on thrombi, from incipient attachment of single cells to maturity and embolization. J Biomechanics 1984;17:287–298
382. Basmadijan D. The hemodynamic and embolizing forces acting on thrombi - II.: The effect of pulsatile blood flow. J Biomechanics 1986;19:837–845
383. Adams PC, Cohen M, Chesebro JH, Fuster V. Thrombosis and embolism from cardiac chambers and infected valves. J Am Coll Cardiol 1988;8:76B–87B
384. Gottdiener JS, Maron BJ, Schooley RT, et al. Two-dimensional echocardiographic assessment of the idiopathic hypereosinophilia syndrome: anatomic basis of mitral regurgitation and peripheral embolization. Circulation 1983;67:572–578
385. Kyrle PA, Korninger C, Gossinger H, et al. Prevention of arterial and pulmonary embolism by oral anticoagulants in patients with dilated cardiomyopathy. Thromb Haemost 1985;54:521–523
386. Robert WC, Ferrans VJ. Pathological aspect of certain cardiomyopathies. Circ Res 1974;34/35 [suppl II]:128–133
387. Stoddard MF, Pearson AC, Kanter KR, Labovitz AJ. Left ventricular thrombus with normal left ventricular wall motion in a patient with myelofibrosis. Am Heart J 1989;117:966–968

388. Taliercio CP, Seward JB, Driscoll DJ, et al. Idiopathic dilated cardiomyopathy in the young: clinical profile and natural history. J Am Coll Cardiol 1985;6:1126–1131
389. Takamoto T, Kim D, Urie PM, et al. Comparative recognition of left ventricular thormbi by echocardiography and cineangiography. Br Heart J 1985;53:36–42
390. Tobin R, Slutsky RA, Higgins CB. Serial echocardiograms in patients with congestive cardiomyopathies: lack of evidence for thrombus formation. Clin Cardiol 1984;7:99–101
391. Verma AK, Alam M, Rossman HS, Brymer J, Keith F. Systemic embolization from thrombus in normal left ventricles. Chest 1988;93:441–442
392. Demakis JG, Proskey A, Rahimtoola SH, et al. The natural course of alcoholic cardiomyopathy. Ann Intern Med 1974;80:293–297
393. Fuster V, Gersh BJ, Guiliani ER, et al. The natural history of idiopathic dilated cardiomyopathy. Am J Cardiol 1981;47:525–531
394. Gottdiener JS, Gay JA, Van Voorhees L, et al. Frequency and embolic potential of left ventricular thrombus in dilated cardiomyopathy: Two-D echocardiography. Am J Cardiol 1983;52:1281–1285
395. Gottdiener JA, Maron BJ, Schooley RT, et al. Two-dimensional echocardiographic assessment of the idiopathic hypereosinophilic syndrome. Circulation 1983;67:572–575
396. Hodgman MT, Pessin MS, Homans DC, et al. Cerebral embolism as the initial manifestation of peripartum cardiomyopathy. Neurology 1982;32:668–671
397. Johnson RA, Palacios I. Dilated cardiomyopathies of the adult. N Engl J Med 1982;307:1051–1058
398. Parameswaran R, Meadows WR, Sharp JT. Coronary embolism in primary myocardial disease. Am Heart J 1969;78:682–687
399. Rice GPA, Ebers GC, Newland F, et al. Recurrent cerebral embolism in cardiac amyloidosis. Neurology 1981;31:904–906
400. Schachter S, Freeman R. TIA and adriamycin cardiomyopathy. Neurology 1982;32:1380–1381
401. Segal JP, Harvey P, Gurel T. Diagnosis and treatment of primary myocardial disease. Circulation 1965;27:837–845
402. Shafii A. Chagas' disease with cardiomyopathy and hemiplegia. NY State J Med 1977;77:418–419
403. Thomas WA, Randall RV, Bland EF, et al. Endocardial fibroelastosis: a factor in heart disease of obscure etiology. N Engl J Med 1954;251:327–338
404. Arita M, Ueno Y, Masuyama Y. Detection of intracardiac thrombi in a case of cardiomyopathy by two-dimensional echoardiography. Br Heart J 1982;47:397–399
405. Cosnett JE, Pudifin J. Embolic complications of cardiomyopathy. Br Heart J 1964;26:544–548
406. Gould L, Gopalaswamy C, Chandy F, et al. Congestive cardiomyopathy and left ventricular thrombus. Arch Intern Med 1983;143:1472–1473
407. Kramer NE, Rathod R, Chawla KK, et al. Echocardiographic diagnosis of left ventricular mural thrombi occurring in cardiomyopathy. Am Heart J 1978;96:381–383
408. Segal JP, Stapleton JF, et al. Idiopathic cardiomyopathy: clinical features, prognosis, and therapy. Curr Probl Neurol 1978;3:1–45
409. Cabin HS, Roberts WC. Left ventricular aneurysm, intra-aneurysmal thrombus and systemic embolus in coronary heart disease. Chest 1980;77:586–590
410. Simpson MT, Oberman A, Kouchoukos NT, Roger WJ. Prevalence of mural thrombi and systemic embolization with left ventricular aneurysm. Chest 1980;77:463–469
411. Kreulen TH, Gorlin R, Herman MV. Ventriculographic patterns and hemodynamics in primary myocardial disease. Circulation 1973;47:299–304
412. Mather P, Delius W, Sebening H, et al. Regional left ventricular wall motion in congestive cardiomyopathy. In: Kaltenbach M, Loogen F, Olsen EGJ (eds): Cardiomyopathy and Myocardial Biopsy. Berlin-Heidelberg-New York: Springer, 1978;pp 192–195
413. Wallis D, O'Connell JB, Henkin RE, et al. Segmental wall motion abnormalitities in dilated cardiomyopathy: a common finding and good prognostic sign. J Am Coll Cardiol 1984;4:674
414. Yokota Y, Kawaniski H, Hayakawa M, et al. Cardiac thrombus in dilated cardiomyopathy. Relationship between left ventricular pathophysiology and left ventricular thrombus. Jpn Heart J 1989;30:1–11
415. Stein PD, Subbah HN. Measured turbulence and its effect on thrombus formation. Circ Res 1974;35:608–610
416. Holley KE. Spontaneous calcific embolization associated with calcific aortic stenosis. Circulation 1963;27:197
417. Soulié P. Les embolies calcaires des orificielles calcif÷es du coeur gauche. Arch Med Coeur 1969;62:1657–1660

Chapter 1.4

Embolic Complications of Infective Endocarditis

Lawrence R Freedman

The importance of embolism as a consequence of infective endocarditis was recognised by Samuel Wilks in 1868 as arterial pyaemia, well before Osler's classic description of "malignant endocarditis" in 1885[1,2]. Jürgensen in 1900 and Königer in 1903 called attention to the possibility that infection was established in thrombotic lesions within the heart[3,4]. By 1909, Horder's paper entitled "Infective Endocarditis" clearly identified the bacteria usually responsible for the disease, the frequency with which they were recovered from the blood stream and the importance and distribution of embolic phenomena[5]. Osler had emphasised the preponderance of infection on the left side of the heart and this was fully supported by Horder's observations[2,5].

The vegetations to which bacteria attach were believed by Mönckeberg to form as a consequence of mechanical injury[6]. Grant, Wood and Jones later demonstrated the presence of microscopic thrombi on valves damaged by rheumatic or congenital heart disease. They cited the evidence indicating that these vegetations were the site of attachment of bacteria, and that the ease with which bacteria were able to attach was related to the stage of development of the vegetation[7]. Furthermore, these authors emphasised that bacteria within a valve thrombus "will be protected from leukocytes, since in the platelet thrombi very few are present" . It is useful to think of bacteria within vegetations as multiplying in a zone of localised agranulocytosis. By 1929 it was well established that microscopic thrombi at the site of valve injury were the site of attachment of bacteria, and that these vegetations were easily dislodged, resulting in emboli capable of being distributed to any portion of the vascular system.

The aspects of infective endocarditis which will be emphasised in this chapter are the development of the lesions that serve as the point of attachment for infecting bacteria and the dislodgement of fragments of the vegetations resulting in the dissemination of emboli throughout the body.

THE VEGETATION

Initiation of endocardial infection

In their study that identified fibrin thrombi on the surface of heart valves susceptible to developing infective endocarditis, Grant, Wood and Jones employed a binocular microscope since they found that "many of the details of surface roughening or irregularity are too small to be seen clearly with the unaided eye"[7]. Stein and co-workers identified microthrombi histologically in 10 of 19 valve specimens from persons with aortic stenosis, only one of which was grossly visible[8]. These authors reviewed the role of turbulent blood flow in the production of fibrin deposits on heart valves (see also Chapter 2.2). Whereas bacteria injected intravenously do not stick to normal heart valves, the trauma of a polyethylene catheter within the heart is sufficient to produce a non-bacterial thrombotic vegetation that serves easily as the site of initiation of the infection[9]. Durack, Beeson and Petersdorf found that five minutes trauma of cardiac catheterisation was sufficient to produce endothelial damage that permitted the initiation of infective endocarditis[10]. Since it is not likely that a visible lesion would have resulted from such a short period of mechanical insult by a polyethylene catheter, these experiments support the view proposed by Grant, Wood and Jones, that endothelial lesions too small to be seen by unaided vision are capable of serving as sites of attachment for circulating bacteria, thereby initiating infective endocarditis.

This view finds further support in the studies of Hook and Sande and Valone and Freedman[11,12]. Anticoagulants given to rabbits with catheters in their hearts prevented the development of grossly visible endothelial lesions. When bacteria were inoculated into such rabbits the outcome was rapidly lethal. Yet the injection of bacteria into anticoagulated rabbits without catheters in their hearts was well tolerated and infection did not develop. These experiments suggest that the "grossly invisible" endothelial lesion was sufficient to permit circulating bacteria to initiate an endovascular infection that, in the anticoagulated rabbit, was lethal. Ferguson and co-workers have conducted similar experiments in rabbits[13]. They have demonstrated the initiation of staphylococcal colony formation on the surface of the aorta 72 hours after infection, which was not evident macroscopically.

These observations indicate that infection of the vascular endothelium can be established in animals without a macroscopical vegetation being evident. If this type of endovascular infection also occurs in man, it suggests that any effort aimed at preventing the development of endothelial lesions, capable of serving as the site of origin of endovascular infection, would have to focus on early phenomena, which preceed the development of the fibrin clot[14].

It has long been recognised in animals that the longer the interval following valve injury the less the valve is susceptible to bacterial infection[14]. Pujadas-Capmany and co-workers have associated this decreased susceptibility to infection with progressive endothelialisation of the vegetation[15]. However it remains to be determined whether this change in susceptibility results from the endothelialisation itself or from other changes in the vegetation that permit or encourage endothelialisation.

Anticoagulants after endocardial injury to inhibit initiation of infection

As long as the visible vegetation was considered the structure critical to the initiation of infective endocarditis, efforts to influence the development of the disease were directed at preventing the appearance of visible vegetations. This view gained support from the finding that the larger the infected vegetation, the more difficult it was to sterilise it with antibiotics[11,11a]. Experimentally, it was logical therefore, after providing the trauma that ultimately resulted in vegetation formation, to prevent the development of a vegetation with anticoagulants hoping that the susceptibility of the provocative lesion to infection would thereby be diminished[11,12]. The experiments were unsuccessful. Indeed, the combination of an endocardial lesion, anticoagulants and the intravenous inoculation of bacteria was lethal to a high percentage of rabbits so tested. In contrast, the intravenous inoculation of bacteria in anticoagulated rabbits without an endocardial lesion was well tolerated. Ferguson and co-workers subsequently demonstrated the colonisation of the endothelium (examined microscopically) in rabbits prior to the development of a grossly visible vegetation[13].

Efforts to prevent the development of infective endocarditis, by making the endocardial lesion less susceptible to bacterial colonisation, might profitably be directed to those factors that operate immediately after endothelial injury, before the development of a vegetation. Studies of antithrombin III, proteins C and S, and fibronectin are providing the information that offers promise of such an approach[16–21]. Other factors such as bacterial dextran production, the influence of subinhibitory antibiotic effects and host factors, like laminin and type 4 collagen are also under active investigation[22](see also section on Embolism below).

Antiphospholipid antibodies

Other factors that have been recognised in recent years and are found sufficiently frequently to deserve careful scrutiny, comprise a family of antiphospholipid antibodies, such as the lupus 'anticoagulant', antibodies to cardiolipin, the false positive test for syphilis and the VDRL. The clinical findings associated with these autoantibodies include venous and arterial occlusions, recurrent abortions, thrombocytopenia, pulmonary hypertension and several expressions of neurological dysfunction.

A review of publications through 1988 by Love and Santoro[23] revealed that 28–34% of patients with systemic lupus erythematosus had the lupus anticoagulant. Anticardiolipin was found in about 44% of these patients. Approximately 50% of patients with antiphospholipid antibodies (aPL) had no evidence of systemic lupus erythematosus or autoimmune disease and surprisingly, there were percentages of aPL antibodies in various patient categories, (acute viral infections, healthy elderly) that were approximately as high as in patients with systemic lupus erythematosus. The authors of this careful review of series published through 1988 were unable to satisfy themselves that the clinical consequences, so clearly associated with aPL antibodies in patients with systemic lupus erythematosus, were also associated with patients not suffering from that disease.

Nevertheless, cases continue to be reported since this large review was written, lending support to the association between the finding of antiphospholipid antibodies and the thrombotic lesions resulting in non-bacterial thrombotic vegetations (Libman-Sacks verrucous endocarditis), strokes and multinfarct dementia[24–29].

That antiphospholipid antibodies appear to be responsible for the development of non-bacterial thrombotic vegetations on heart valves in persons without identifiable underlying disease is a most interesting finding. It offers a possible explanation for the bacterial endocarditis which develops in drug addicts with no evidence of underlying heart valve disease to explain their susceptibility to bacterial infection. It has recently been shown that in drug addicts there are a variety of immunological abnormalities that are independent of HIV antibody status[30]. Although no determination was made of antiphospholipid antibodies in this study, the alteration of the number of several lymphocyte subsets and their responses to phytohaemagglutinin and pokeweed mitogen raise the question as to whether there might also be autoantibody formation favouring intravascular coagulation and non-bacterial thrombotic vegetation formation on heart valves[30].

EMBOLISM

Dislodgement of fragments of the infected valve vegetation with dissemination to vessels anywhere in the body has long been recognised as a serious risk in infective endocarditis. As early as 1909, Horder had called attention to embolism as the initial phenomenon, announcing the presence of infective endocarditis: "The first event to direct attention to the real state of affairs (in patients with bacterial endocarditis) may be embolism, thus a hemiplegia may be the first warning, or, ... the patient may first of all complain of an aneurysmal swelling at some part of his body"[5].

The frequency with which embolism is said to occur varies with the probability of the embolus evoking clinical signs and symptoms and the extent to which thorough autopsies are conducted to search for silent emboli. In animals with intracardiac vegetations, scattered systemic emboli are often found upon autopsy examination[9]. Weinstein and Rubin have summarised the differences in the frequency of embolism detected during life and at autopsy[31].

The consequences of emboli arising from intracardiac vegetations are obviously dependent upon the size of the embolus and the effectiveness of collateral circulation at the point where the embolus occludes an artery. Questions that arise frequently are whether the risk of embolism is proportional to the size of the vegetation, as visualised by echocardiography (see Chapter 2.6), and whether size alone is a sufficient indication for surgical treatment. An important study of patients with native valve endocarditis, who had a two-dimensional echocardiogram performed within 72 hours of starting antimicrobial treatment, was carried out to determine the factors contributing to the risk of embolism[32]. The observation period began with the initiation of effective antimicrobial therapy and ended with the successful completion of therapy, an embolic event, surgical valve replacement, death or hospital discharge.

Vegetations were seen more commonly in patients with infections due to fastidious gram-negative coccobacilli and nutritional variant viridans streptococci than among patients with infections due to staphylococci and other streptococci. During the period of observation 13% of patients had an embolic event (CNS – 16 patients, viscera - seven patients, peripheral arteries – two patients, retinal and coronary arteries - one patient each). The risk of embolism was 1.4 times greater in those with vegetations that were visualised, but this difference was not statistically significant. The incidence of embolism was 13 per 1000 patient-days during the first week of antimicrobial therapy and fell to less than 1.2 per 1000 patient-days after the second week of therapy.

There was no correlation between the risk of embolism and the size of the vegetation, which ranged from three to 30mm with a median of 10mm. However, there were important correlations with the nature of the infecting micro-organism. Emboli were 2.4 times more common with Staphylococcus aureus than with Streptococcus viridans infections. In patients with Staphylococcus aureus infection, there was no difference in the frequency of embolism whether vegetations were detected by echocardiography or not. However, in patients with Streptococcus viridans infection, echocardiographically detectable vegetations were associated with a sevenfold increase in the risk of embolism as compared with patients without detectable vegetations.

Patients with viridans streptococcal infection and echocardiographically documented vegetations were at approximately the same risk of clinically manifest embolism as were all patients with Staphylococcus aureus endocarditis.

The factors which are known to be important in determining the size of the endocarditis vegetation include the specific bacteria responsible, platelet aggregation[32a] and particularly the procoagulant activity resulting from the interaction of bacteria with monocytes[33] and endothelial cells[34,35]. These factors operating to increase vegetation size are opposed by fibrinolytic activity as well as the tendency for the endothelium to cover the vegetation. The contribution of living bacteria to vegetation growth is evident in the usually rapid disappearance of vegetations in both man and animals after cure of infection. The study of Steckelberg and co-workers[32] is pertinent in this regard, illustrating the rapid fall in the risk of embolism in the first weeks of effective antibiotic therapy.

Spleen

In a recent study, splenic infarcts were found in over half the cases of bacterial endocarditis autopsied in the active phase of the disease. Curiously however, it appeared that "infection or abscess formation was not significantly associated with the site (right or left side) of endocarditis"[36]. Embolism to the spleen in patients with infective endocarditis has three important implications. (a) Splenic abscess has long been recognised as a cause of persistent infection despite apparently effective antibiotic treatment. Splenectomy has been necessary to control infective endocarditis in such instances[37]. (b) Rupture of the spleen can occur as a complication of abscess formation, and has even been the event leading to the diagnosis of endocarditis in some cases[38,39,40]. (c) In cases where cardiac surgery is indicated, preoperative CT imaging of the spleen to exclude abscess formation is a wise precaution, since the risk of a splenic abscess serving as the source of reinfection of a subsequent prosthetic valve can be avoided by timely splenectomy[37,41]. In a series of 20 patients with septic splenic embolism, only two had localising abdominal symptoms or physical signs, illustrating the importance of CT screening[41].

Kidney

Renal embolism is as common as splenic embolism[5]. It usually presents with haematuria rather than pain, since the renal capsule with its independent blood supply is less susceptible to embolism causing pain than the capsule of the spleen. However haematuria is a symptom of many pathophysiological processes in the kidney and cannot be considered diagnostic of embolism in patients with endocarditis. Even gross haematuria, long considered a good indication of renal infarction, may occur for example in focal and diffuse glomerulonephritis[42].

Central nervous system

Embolism to the central nervous system is the greatest embolic danger threatening the lives of patients with infective endocarditis. The risk of embolic stroke and the consequent disability that results are important elements of the powder keg, upon which all patients with infective endocarditis are sitting prior to the establishment of the diagnosis and the introduction of antibiotic therapy. The physician is constantly balancing himself on a narrow line between the urgent need to start antibiotic treatment and the necessity of ascertaining the nature of the infecting micro-organism in order to ensure optimal effectiveness of the antibiotic treatment.

Cerebral embolism was noted in 15% of Horder's 1909 patient series[5]. It has been noted recently in 14% of patients as the presenting sign of infective endocarditis[43]. In another recent series, where the rates of embolism were similar to those cited above, the frequency was similar in both native and prosthetic endocarditis[44].

The CNS complication of infective endocarditis that remains a source of controversy is mycotic aneurysm, both in terms of its incidence and its management. Mycotic aneurysms are believed to result from infected emboli eroding the vessel wall from the lumen or from the vasa vasorum[45]. Recent work has demonstrated factors that complicate our interpretation of the details of these studies. Nevertheless, the principle appears to hold that mycotic aneurysms result from embolic events[46]. Mycotic aneurysms have been reported to occur in cerebral vessels in 2%–10% of patients with infective endocarditis[31].

The principal controversy concerns the management of patients with such aneurysms. Some restrict arteriography to patients with subarachnoid haemorrhage or severe headache persisting after control of infection[47,48,49], while others[50] recommend:

"1. that careful neurological examination, computed tomography and (unless contraindicated) lumbar puncture be performed on any patient with endocarditis;

2. that those with neurological abnormalities not attributable to systemic toxicity, including pleocytosis in the cerebrospinal fluid or apparent infarction on CT scans, undergo four-vessel cerebral angiography;

3. that a single accessible mycotic aneurysm in medically stable patients be promptly excised, with individualisation of multiple or proximal aneurysms; and

4. that repeat angiography be performed at the conclusion of antibiotic therapy in patients requiring long term anticoagulation."

The risks of anticoagulant therapy in patients with endocarditis have been reviewed by Jones and Siekert[51]. Ting, Silverman and Levitsky have examined the question of valve replacement in patients with endocarditis and cerebral septic emboli[52]. Of those who underwent valve replacement for endocarditis, 42% had suffered cerebral emboli, although only two thirds of these were symptomatic. The presence of a haemorrhagic infarct preoperatively predisposed to a further perioperative stroke but anticoagulation in the patients with non-haemorrhagic ischaemic infarcts did not lead to haemorrhagic transformation perioperatively (see also Chapter 1.1).

Another factor influencing the decision to investigate for mycotic aneurysm is the occurrence of late rupture. Bamford reported rupture of an occult mycotic aneurysm six months after the diagnosis of infective endocarditis in a patient who was given warfarin[53]. Indeed, mycotic aneurysms are said to be possible even several years after infection on the valve has been eliminated and embolic strokes have been noted to occur as long as two years following successful treatment of infective endocarditis[31,54]. Current practice in the USA is to perform cerebral angiography in most patients with infective endocarditis who have either a prominent headache, focal cerebral symptoms or an indication for anticoagulant treatment[51,55]. However a recent publication employing decision analysis techniques recommended non-invasive screening (CT scan) for cerebral mycotic aneurysms in patients with infective endocarditis[56]. The assumptions employed were: 1) 10% aneurysm incidence, 2) 30% spontaneous resolution rate, 3) angiography is 100% sensitive, 100% specific, 4) CT scan is 95% sensitive, 95% specific. Angiography could only be justified as preferable to CT scan if the frequency of aneurysms were more than 43%, CT sensitivity less than 65% or the angiographic risk was less than 0.4%.

Paradoxical embolism

Emboli passing from the right to the left side of the circulation are thought to traverse a patent foramen ovale. This is found at autopsy in 25%–35% of cases but the use of two-dimensional contrast echocardiography during life suggests that the true incidence may be higher[57]. There have been several instances where attention was directed to the finding of systemic arterial emboli in patients with right sided endocarditis. Eknoyan refers to the presence of renal infarcts in 10%–15% of patients with endocarditis on the right side of the heart[42]. However, in the studies he cites, if one were to exclude those with simultaneous lesions on the left side of the heart and those with abnormal communications between the two sides of the heart, very few cases remain, for example only one of 41 patients considered by Barker[58]. Cates and Christie refer to four cases in their series of 442 patients[59]. Pruitt and co-workers discuss 10 patients with infections of the tricuspid valve, of whom three had neurological complications and six had non-cerebral arterial emboli[54]. Du and others found no difference in the frequency of splenic emboli if the valvular lesion was on the right or the left side of the heart[36].

The difficulty in interpreting these data is that the identification of the location of the cardiac lesion is, in the majority of instances, presumptive[54]. Even modern imaging techniques are not able to rule out the presence of a vegetation. On the other hand, there are some carefully examined cases, where there can be little doubt that an arterial embolus occurred in a patient with right sided disease. In the case discussed by Eknoyan, the patient also had disseminated intravascular coagulation, raising the possibility that other thrombotic phenomena might participate in the development of 'emboli'[42].

Other sites of embolism

Arterial emboli in endocarditis have been reported in many situations including the coronary arteries (60,61), intra-abdominal vessels (62), extremities (62) and gall bladder and liver (63).

Prevention of embolism

Anticoagulants

Anticoagulants were first employed in the treatment of infective endocarditis in the early 1940s in the hope of increasing the effectiveness of sulphonamides[64] but the frequent occurrence of cerebral haemorrhage led to the abandonment of this approach[65]. Subsequently, anticoagulants were used to prevent the formation of the vegetation after endocardial injury in the rabbit model of infection[11,12,66]. The goal was to prevent the ability of bacteria to initiate infection. Although there was some diminution of susceptibility to infection with Staphylococcus epidermidis, the susceptibility of Streptococcus sanguis and Streptococcus viridans was not altered[11,12,66]. In fact, the course of the disease was explosive in these latter experiments, similar to what had previously been noted in man[65]. Aspirin and fibrinolytic enzymes have also been used in experimental models without any benefit having been noted[67,68].

There is no convincing evidence that prophylactic anticoagulation reduces the risk of embolism in native valve endocarditis[69]. Opinion is divided on the effectiveness of anticoagulation in reducing the number of embolic events in prosthetic valve endocarditis. However, since these patients require long-term anticoagulation in any case, it is generally agreed that anticoagulants should be maintained along with the administration of effective antibiotics. The recommendations for anticoagulation in patients with infective endocarditis are similar to those in patients with heart valve disease without infective endocarditis[71]: (a) in patients in normal sinus rhythm with uncomplicated native or bioprosthetic valve endocarditis : no anticoagulation, and (b) in patients with mechanical prostheses: continue anticoagulation.

When systemic embolism occurs during the course of infective endocarditis, the indications for anticoagulant therapy are uncertain[69]. The decision is often influenced by other factors, for example atrial fibrillation, evidence of left atrial thrombus, perhaps vegetation size as well as the site and severity of the embolism. Cerebral embolism requires special consideration[69,73], but the recommendations for the prevention of recurrent embolic stroke in patients with infective endocarditis are largely arbitrary. Anticoagulation should be introduced providing there is no evidence of haemorrhagic transformation on CT or MRI scan (see Chapter 1.1) and the patient is not hypertensive. The literature provides no clear guidelines on the optimum intensity or duration of anticoagulation.

Early diagnosis of infective endocarditis

It is difficult to document with precision, but there is an impression gained from the literature that embolic phenomena have decreased in frequency as the index of suspicion and effectiveness of blood culture techniques have improved[31]. The recognition that duration of disease has an effect on outcome and on the effectiveness of antibiotic therapy has been a major factor promoting an increased index of suspicion of infective endocarditis[73]. Nevertheless undue delay in thinking of infective endocarditis as a diagnostic possibility is encountered regularly. Osler and Horder emphasised in the earliest days of our awareness of this disorder that the "typical" clinical picture of fever, heart murmur, skin and embolic phenomena were frequently absent at the time the patient first seeks medical advice. Fever may be absent on presentation and throughout the course of the illness[2]. A heart murmur may be absent throughout or interpreted as "functional" and thus ignored[74]. Embolic phenomena may be the first indication of the disease that brings the patient to the physician. In addition, the wide variety of symptoms that are found in infective endocarditis often misdirect physicians to search for explanations other than infective endocarditis. Patients with infective endocarditis have been found undergoing gastrointestinal investigations for their loss of appetite and weight loss. Orthopaedic explorations of back pain and neuropsychiatric disorders have been managed without a thought to the possibility of infective endocarditis. One patient mentioned by Greenlee and Mandell received electroshock therapy for a neuropsychiatric disturbance before infective endocarditis was recognised as the underlying problem[75]. Tan and others have emphasised that "bacterial endocarditis should be suspected in any elderly patient who has not been feeling well"[76]. This suspicion should not be restricted to the elderly.

REFERENCES

1. Wilks S. Pyaemia as a result of endocarditis. Br Med J 1868;1:297–298.
2. Osler W. Malignant endocarditis. Br Med J 1885;1:467–470, 522–526, 577–579.
3. Jürgensen V. Erkrankungen der Kreislauforgane Endocarditis. Alfred Holder, Wien, 1900. In: Libman E, Friedberg CK [Eds]: Subacute Bacterial Endocarditis. Oxford Medical Publications, 1941.
4. Königer. Histologische Untersuchungen uber Endokarditis. Leipzig, 1903. Cited by Grant, Wood, Jones (Ref 7).
5. Horder TJ. Infective endocarditis. Quart J Med, 1909;2:289–324.
6. Mönckeberg. Virch Arch 1904;176:472. Cited by Grant, Wood, Jones (ref 7).
7. Grant RT, Wood JE, Jones TD. Heart valve irregularities in relation to subacute bacterial endocarditis. Heart 1927–29;14:247–251.
8. Stein PD, Sabbah HN, Pitha JV. Continuing disease process of calcific aortic stenosis. Role of microthrombi and turbulent flow. Am J Cardiol 1977;39:159–163.
9. Freedman LR. Infective endocarditis and other intravascular infections. In Current Topics in Infectious Disease. New York, Plenum Press, 1982;243.
10. Durack DT, Beeson PB, Petersdorf RG. Experimental bacterial endocarditis III. Production and progress of the disease in rabbits. Br J Exp Path 1973;54:142–151.
11. Hook EW, Sande MA. Role of the vegetation in experimental Streptococcus viridans endocarditis. Infect Immun 1974;10:1433–1438.
11a. Robbins MJ, Frater RWM, Soeiro R, Frishman WH, Strom JA. Influence of vegetation size on clinical outcome of right sided infective endocarditis. Am J Med 1986;80:165–171.
12. Freedman LR, Valone J. Experimental endocarditis. Prog Cardiovasc Dis 1979;22:169–180.
13. Ferguson DJP, McColm AA, Savage TJ, Ryan DM, Acred PA. A morphological study of experimental rabbit staphylococcal endocarditis and aortitis. I: Formation and effect of infected and uninfected vegetations on the aorta. Br J Exp Path 1986;67:667–678.
14. Freedman LR. Role of non-bacterial thrombotic vegetations in the pathogenesis of endocarditis. In: Horstkotte D, Bodnar E [Eds]: Current Issues in Heart Valve Disease; Infective Endocarditis. London, ICR Publishers, 1991;10–14.
15. Pujadas-Capmany R, Permanyer-Miralda G, Fox-Sala M, et al. Reduction of the susceptibility to infective endocarditis with time in animals with endocavitary catheters. Br J Exp Path 1984;65:683–690.
16. Becker RC, DiBello PM, Lucas FV. Bacterial tissue tropism: an in vitro model for infective endocarditis. Cardiovasc Res 1987;21:813–820.
17. Hamill RJ. Role of fibronectin in infective endocarditis. Rev Inf Dis 1987;9(suppl 4):S360-S371.
18. Esmon CT. The regulation of natural anticoagulant pathways. Science 1987;235:1348–1352.
19. Bevilacqua MP, Pober JS, Wheeler ME, Cotran RS, Gimbrone MA Jr. Interleukin I acts on cultured human vascular endothelium to increase the adhesion of polymorphonuclear leukocytes, monocytes, and related leucocyte cell lines. J Clin Invest 1985;76:2003–2011.
20. Mohr JP. Cryptogenic stroke. N Eng J Med 1988;318:1197–1198.
21. Lafeullade A, Alessi MC, Poizot-Martin I, et al. Protein S deficiency and HIV infection. N Eng J Med 1991;324:1220.
22. Scheld WM, Sande MA. Endocarditis and intravascular infections. In Mandell GL, Douglas RG, Bennett JE (Eds): Principles and Practice of Infectious Diseases, 3rd Edition. Churchill Livingstone 1990;672–700.
23. Love PE, Santoro SA. Antiphospholipid antibodies: anticardiolipin and the lupus anticoagulant in systemic lupus erythematosus (systemic lupus erythematosus) and in non-SLE disorders. Ann Intern Med 1990;112:682–698.
24. Chartash EK, Lans DM, Paget SA, Qunar T, Lockshin MD. Aortic insufficiency and mitral regurgitation in patients with systemic lupus erythematosus and the antiphospholipid syndrome. Am J Med 1989;86:407–412.
25. Asherson RA, Hughes GRV. The expanding spectrum of Libman Sacks endocarditis: the role of antiphospholipid antibodies. Clin Exp Rheum 1989;7:225–28.
26. Asherson RA, Khamashta MA, Gil A, et al. Cerebrovascular disease and antiphospholipid antibodies in

systemic lupus erythematosus, lupus-like disease, and the primary antiphospholipid syndrome. Am J Med 1989;86:391–399.
27. Pope JM, Canny CLB, Bell DA. Cerebral ischemic events associated with endocarditis, retinal vascular disease, and lupus anticoagulant. Am J Med 1991;90:299–309.
28. Olsen ML, O'Connor S, Arnett FC, Rosenbaum D, Grotta JC, Warner NB. Autoantibodies and rheumatic disorders in a neurology inpatient population: a prospective study. Am J Med 1991;90:479–488.
29. Espinoza LR, Jara LJ, Silveira LH, et al. Anticardiolipin antibodies in polymyalgia rheumatic giant cell arteritis: association with severe vascular complications. Am J Med 1991;90:474–478.
30. Klimas NG, Blaney NT, Morgan RO, Chitwood D, Milles K. Lee H, Fletcher MA. Immune function and anti-HTLV–I/II status in anti-HIV–1-negative intravenous drug users receiving methadone. Am J Med 1991;90:163–170.
31. Weinstein L, Rubin RH. Infective endocarditis, 1973. Prog Cardiovasc Dis 1973;16:239–302.
32. Steckelberg JM, Murphy JG, Ballard D, et al. Emboli in infective endocarditis: the prognostic value of echocardiography. Ann Intern Med 1991;114:635–640.
32a. Dankert J, Hess J, Joldersma W, van der Werff J, Durack D. Pathogenesis of experimental viridans streptococcal endocarditis. Presented at the 30th Interscience Conference on Antimicrobial Agents and Chemotherapy, Atlanta, GA, 1990.
33. Buiting AGM, Thompson J, van der Keur D, Schmal-Bauer WC, Bertina RM. Procoagulant activity of endocardial vegetations and blood monocytes in rabbits with Streptococcus sanquis endocarditis. Thromb Haemost 1989;62:1029–1033.
34. Drake TA, Rodgers GM, Sande MA. Tissue factor is a major stimulus for vegetation formation in enterococcal endocarditis in rabbits. J Clin Invest 1984;73:1750–1753.
35. Drake TA, Pang M. Staphylococcus aureus induces tissue factor expression in cultured human cardiac valve endothelium. J Inf Dis 1988;157:749–756.
36. Du LTH, Wechsler B, Cabane J, Herson S, Godeau P, Chomette G. Splenic abscess and infectious endocarditis. Arch Intern Med 1984;144:414.
37. Lingeman CJ, Smith EB, Battersby JS, Behnke RH. Subacute bacterial endocarditis; splenectomy in cases refractory to antibiotic therapy. Arch Int Med 1956;97:309–314.
38. Gonin A, Berthou JD, Simonin C, Delaye J, Roques JC, Dufoix V. Ruptures spontanees de rate au cours de l'endocardite infectieuse, a propos de 3 nouvelle observations. Lyon Med 1973;229:1269–1271.
39. Gallavardin P, Coiffier B, Tissot E, Brun F. Abces de la rate revelant une endocardite infectieuse. A propos d'un cas. Lyon Med 1979;242:297–300.
40. Haiat R, Gabarre J, Desoutler P, Stoltz JP, Halphen Ch. Abces splenique revelateur d'une endocardite. Am Cardiol Angeiol 1985;34:625–627.
41. Ting W, Silverman NA, Arzouman DA, Levitsky S. Splenic septic emboli in endocarditis. Circulation 1990;82(suppl IV):IV105–1V109.
42. Eknoyan G. Discussion in Feinstein EI. Renal complications of bacterial endocarditis. Am J Nephrol 1985;5:457–469.
43. Le Cam B, Guivarch G, Boles JM, Garre M, Cartier F. Neurologic complications in a group of 86 bacterial endocarditis Eur Heart J 1984;5(suppl C):97–100.
44. Salgado AV, Furlan AJ, Keys TF, Nichols TR, Beck GJ. Neurologic complications of endocarditis: A 12-year experience. Neurology 1989;39:173–178.
45. Molinari GF, Smith L, Goldstein MN, Satran R. Pathogenesis of cerebral mycotic aneurysms. Neurology 1973;23:325–332.
46. Foote RA, Reagan TJ, Sandok BA. Cerebral arterial lesions resulting from inflammatory emboli. Stroke 1978;9:498–503.
47. Hart RG, Kagan-Hallet K, Joerus SE. Mechanisms of intracranial hemorrhage in infective endocarditis. Stroke 1987;18:1048–1056.
48. Kanter MC, Hart RG. Cerebral mycotic aneurysms are rare in infective endocarditis. Ann Neurol 1990;28:590–591.
49. Hart RG, Foster JW, Luther MF, Kanter MC. Stroke in infective endocarditis. Stroke 1990;21:695–700.
50. Brust JCM, Dickinson PCT, Hughes JEO, Holtzman RNN. The diagnosis and treatment of cerebral mycotic aneurysms. Ann Neurol 1990;27:239–246.
51. Jones HR Jr, Siekert RG. Neurological manifestations of infective endocarditis. Brain 1989;112:1295–1315.
52. Ting W, Silverman N, Levitsky S. Valve replacement in patients with endocarditis and cerebral septic emboli. Ann Thorac Surg 1991;51:18–22.
53. Bamford J, Hodges J, Warlow C. Late rupture of a mycotic aneurysm after "cure" of bacterial endocarditis. J Neurol 1986;233:51–53.
54. Pruitt AA, Rubin RH, Karchmer AW, Duncan GW. Neurologic complications of bacterial endocarditis. Medicine 1978;57:329–343.

55. Salgado AV, Furlan AJ, Keys TF. Mycotic aneurysm, subarchnoid hemorrhage, and indications for cerebral angiography in infective endocarditis. Stroke 1987;18:1057–1060.
56. Westman EC, Hagen MD. Screening for cerebral mycotic aneurysms in infective endocarditis: a cost-utility analysis. Clin Res 1991;39:589A.
57. Lechat Ph, Mos JL, Lascault G, et al. Prevalance of patent foramen ovale in Patients with stroke. N Eng J Med 1988;318:1148–1152.
58. Barker PS. A clinical study of subacute bacterial infection confined to the right side of the heart or the pulmonary artery. Am Heart J 1949;37:1054–1068.
59. Cates JE, Christie RV. Subacute bacterial endocarditis. Quart J Med 1951;20:93–130.
60. Feder HM Jr, Chameides L, Diana DJ. Bacterial endocarditis complicated by myocardial infarction in a pediatric patient. JAMA 1982;247:1315–1316.
61. Herzog CA, Henry TD, Zimmer SD. Bacterial endocarditis presenting as acute myocardial infarction: a cautionary note for the era of reperfusion. Am J Med 1991;90:392–397.
62. Dean RH, Meacham PW, Weaver FA, Waterhouse G, O'Neil JA Jr. Mycotic embolism and embolomycotic aneurysms: neglected lessons of the past. Ann Surg 1986;204:300–307.
63. Henrich WL, Huehnergarth RJ, Rosch J, Melnyk CS. Gallbladder and liver infarction occurring as a complication of acute bacterial endocarditis. Gastroenterology 1975;68:1602–1607.
64. Katz LN, Elek SR. Combined heparin and chemotherapy in subacute bacterial endocarditis. JAMA 1944;124:149–152.
65. Kanis JA. The use of anticoagulants in bacterial endocarditis. Postgrad Med J 1974;50:312–313.
66. Thorig L, Thompson J, Eulderink F. Effect of warfarin on the induction and course of experimental Staphylococcus epidermidis endocarditis. Infect Immun 1977;17:504–509.
67. Levison ME, Carrizosa J, Tanphaichitro D, Schick PK, Rubin W. Effect of aspirin on thrombogenesis and on production of experimental aortic valvular Streptococcus viridans endocarditis in rabbits. Blood 1977;49:645–650.
68. Parker BM, Andresen DC, Thomas WA, Smith JR. Effect of intravenous fibrinolytic enzymes on the vegetations of experimental bacterial endocarditis. J Lab Clin Med 1958;52:588–595.
69. Levine HJ, Parker SG, Salzman EW. Antithrombotic therapy in valvular heart disease. Chest 1989;95(suppl 2):98S–106S.
70. Stein PD, Kantrowitz A. Antithrombotic therapy in mechanical and biological prosthetic heart valves and saphenous vein bypass grafts. Chest 1989;95(suppl 2):107S–117S.
71. Delahaye JP, Poncet Ph, Malquarti V, Beaune J, Gare JP, Mann JM. Cerebrovascular accidents in infective endocarditis: role of anticoagulation. Eur Heart J 1990;11:1074–1078.
72. Sherman DG, Dyken ML, Fisher M, Harrison MJG, Hart RG. Antithrombotic therapy for cerebrovascular disorders. Chest 1989;95(suppl 2):140–155.
73. Phair JP, Tan J, Venezio F, Westenfelder G, Reisberg B. Therapy of infective endocarditis due to penicillin-susceptible streptococci: duration of disease is a major determinant of outcome. In Bisno AL (Ed): Treatment of Infective Endocarditis. New York, Grune and Stratton, 1981;75–79.
74. Osler W. Chronic infectious endocarditis. Quart J Med 1909;2:219–30.
75. Greenlee JE, Mandell GL. Neurological manifestations of infective endocarditis: a review. Stroke 1973;4:958–963.
76. Tan JS, Watanakunakorn C, Terhune CA Jr. Streptococcus viridans endocarditis: favorable prognosis in geriatric patients. Geriatrics 1973;28:68–73.

Chapter 1.5

Hypercoagulability

George. J. Miller and Thomas. W. Meade

Arterial thromboembolic complications are an important cause of morbidity and mortality after heart valve replacement. In a review of the literature up to 1989, Grunkemeier and Rahimtoola arrived at annual linearised embolism rates of about 1.5 and 2.5 events/100 valve-years for aortic and mitral valve replacement respectively[1]. These smoothed estimates obscure the fact that, although an embolic event can occur many years after surgery, the risk is much higher in the early postoperative months (see Chapters 3.4 and 6.2). The additional finding that there is considerable variability in embolic rates between different groups of patients with the same prosthesis (Chapter 6.3), coupled with the fact that embolism cannot be totally eliminated by anticoagulation (Chapter 3.4), suggests that some patients are more susceptible than others for reasons unrelated to their surgery, and that it should be possible to distinguish this sub-group prior to operation. This problem is similar to that in preventive medicine, namely the identification of those ostensibly healthy adults who are at high risk of myocardial or cerebral infarction. Recent progress in the development of markers of hypercoagulability may therefore have some relevance in the construction of a preoperative risk profile for patients about to undergo heart valve surgery. By comparison with the long-standing endeavour to unravel the aetiology and pathogenesis of the atheromatous component of coronary heart disease, interest in the thrombotic component has been relatively recent. In the mid–1970s the debate focused on whether coronary thrombosis preceded or followed transmural myocardial infarction and whether thrombus formation contributed in any way to sudden coronary death. With the advent of thrombolytic therapy and the need to establish its rationale, angiographic studies soon demonstrated a high frequency of total coronary occlusion during the initial phase of myocardial infarction[2]. The significance of acute thrombosis in transmural myocardial infarction is now undoubted[3], though the evidence for its involvement in subendocardial infarction is less clear[3].

A series of careful autopsy studies during the 1980s, the best example being that of Davies and Thomas[4], has demonstrated the almost universal occurrence of at least a degree of thrombosis in sudden coronary death. The minority of fatal events in which thrombosis is not apparently associated with plaque rupture[4,5] raises the possibility that the coagulability and fibrinolytic potential of the blood per se may have a role in the precipitation of some arterial thrombi; a central theme of this chapter. The fact that thrombi associated with sudden coronary death are frequently found only to partially occlude the arterial lumen at autopsy may be due to the intense fibrinolytic activity accompanying sudden death, with consequent partial lysis of the thrombus post mortem[3,6].

HAEMOSTATIC FUNCTION AND ARTERIAL THROMBOSIS

Given the major thrombotic contribution to myocardial infarction and sudden coronary death, an obvious question for the clinician and epidemiologist is the extent to which those at high risk of coronary heart disease can be characterised by changes in the coagulation system indicative of a thrombotic tendency. Prospective population surveys have now demonstrated that, expressed in comparable terms, high levels of certain clotting factors are associated with coronary heart disease risk at least as strongly as other well-known characteristics such as serum cholesterol concentration and blood pressure.

In 1980, Meade and others[7] published preliminary results suggesting that high levels of factor VII coagulant activity (VII_c), plasma fibrinogen concentration and possibly also factor VIII activity, were associated with a high subsequent mortality from cardiovascular disease (principally coronary heart disease) in middle-aged men. At completion of this study[8] there had been 148 deaths from all causes during the follow up, of which 68 were due to coronary heart disease. In addition, there were 60 non-fatal episodes of myocardial infarction. High levels of VII_c and of fibrinogen were associated significantly with mortality from all causes. Furthermore, the relations of both haemostatic indices with the 5-year incidence of coronary heart disease were positive, statistically highly significant and, if anything, stronger than that of cholesterol, although the latter association was also apparent. Neither VII_c, nor fibrinogen were related to cancer incidence, so that the associations appear specific for vascular disease.

The Northwick Park Heart Study is so far the only prospective survey to report on VII_c, but several others have published similar results with respect to plasma fibrinogen. In the Göteborg Study, Wilhelmsen and others[9] showed a positive association between fibrinogen levels and the incidence of both coronary heart disease and, in particular, stroke, in 792 men born in 1913. There also appeared to be an interaction between fibrinogen and systolic blood pressure with respect to stroke; men with high levels of both being at considerably higher risk than expected from the sum of their separate effects. However, the relatively small number of events on which this analysis was based needs to be taken into account.

In 1985, Stone and Thorp[10] found a high fibrinogen concentration to be associated with an increased coronary heart disease risk in a group of men aged 40–69 years whom they followed for up to 20 years. This relation was stronger than that for cholesterol, blood pressure or smoking. In this study, too, there was evidence suggestive of interaction between blood pressure and fibrinogen with respect to risk. Thus, men whose systolic pressure and fibrinogen level were in the top third of the respective distributions had a coronary heart disease incidence 12 times that of men whose levels fell in the low third.

In the same year, Kannel and co-workers[11] reported a positive association between fibrinogen concentration and the incidence of cardiovascular disease (coronary heart disease, stroke, heart failure or peripheral vascular disease) in 554 men and 761 women aged been 47 and 79 years and free of these disorders at recruitment. Subsequent publications[12,13] established a clear relation between fibrinogen concentration and coronary heart disease incidence in both sexes, and between fibrinogen and stroke in men but not women. More recently, in a follow-up of 4860 men, Yarnell and others[14] found that the incidence of major coronary heart disease events was strongly and positively related to plasma fibrinogen concentration, viscosity and white cell count. Together with the results of the Northwick Park Heart Study on VII_c, these studies suggest that the biochemical disturbances leading to myocardial infarction and sudden coronary death reside at least as much in the coagulation pathway as in the metabolism of cholesterol. These disturbances can be interpreted as a pre-morbid coronary thrombotic state. Studies have been undertaken in the past decade to explore the basis of these changes in the haemostatic pathway.

BASAL PRO-COAGULANT ACTIVITY

The pro-coagulant system consists of a series of interdependent proteolytic reactions. At each step, a zymogen is converted to its corresponding serine protease, the primary function of which is to activate the next zymogen in the sequence of reactions that leads ultimately to thrombin generation. At several stages in this pathway, for example in the conversions of factors IX, X and prothrombin to IXa, Xa and thrombin respectively, an activation peptide is released into the circulation. These peptides are without coagulant activity, but they are stable by-products of serine protease generation that have been shown to have finite half-lives in vivo.

The ultimate step in the pro-coagulant pathway is the conversion of prothrombin to thrombin. In vivo, this transformation is achieved by the assembly of the substrate prothrombin, the serine protease factor Xa, and its co-factor Va on the platelet surface. Cleavage at Arg 273-Thr 274 releases the activation peptide fragment F_{1+2} ($F_{1.2}$) for which a specific radio-immunoassay has been developed[15,16]. The presence of basal concentrations of circulating $F_{1.2}$ in all healthy individuals[16] indicates continuous pro-coagulant activity within the haemostatic pathway, though at an extremely low flux. This basal activity may well have more to do with vascular repair processes than haemostasis per se. The latter is only required when the vessel wall endothelial lining has been breached.

Free thrombin is rapidly neutralised by natural anticoagulant mechanisms, especially the heparin sulphate/antithrombin III mechanism, but not before there has been some conversion of fibrinogen to fibrin I at the site of thrombin generation. Hence under basal conditions, fibrinopeptide A (FPA) is liberated from fibrinogen by thrombin, albeit at an extremely low rate, and thrombin conjugates with antithrombin III (ATIII) as thrombin-ATIII complex. As with $F_{1.2}$, FPA and thrombin-ATIII are detectable in the plasma of healthy individuals, providing more evidence of continuous physiological turnover within the haemostatic pathway. Further evidence for a basal flux throughout the system is the recent demonstration of basal levels of factor IX activation peptide[17] and factor X activation peptide[18] in the plasma of healthy adults.

Classically, the haemostatic pathway has been described as a cascade[19] or waterfall[20], in which each molecule of enzyme activates many molecules of its zymogen substrate at each stage, so that the system functions as a biochemical amplifier. This is undoubtedly the case in situations where there is a need for rapid clot formation. However, at other times each zymogen-enzyme transformation is tightly regulated to control the extent of amplification and, if necessary, prevent it completely. This control is achieved by natural anticoagulant mechanisms[21]. The heparin sulphate/ATIII system effectively neutralises excess thrombin and Xa activity. The activation of protein C by thrombin within the thrombomodulin-protein C system leads to the destruction of the co-factors VIIIa and Va, employed in the generation of factor Xa and thrombin respectively. Self-damping, a control mechanism originally proposed by Nemerson and others[22], may also have a role to play. For example, the activation peptide $F_{1.2}$ may compete with prothrombin for binding to the platelet surface, thereby reducing substrate availability for further thrombin generation. It is important to appreciate that, in vivo, these pro-coagulant reactions occur on cell surfaces and not in the fluid phase.

THE HYPERCOAGULABLE STATE

Between the extremes of the basal level of activity in the coagulant pathway found in healthy individuals, and the explosive generation of serine protease activity during clot or thrombus formation, there is a state of increased flux termed a hypercoagulable state. This state is defined by the presence of raised concentrations of one or more activation peptides in an asymptomatic individual. When plasma FPA levels are also slightly increased, thrombosis is presumably being averted by enhanced fibrinolytic activity that prevents the conversion of soluble fibrin I to an insoluble fibrin polymer.

One category of the hypercoagulable state is found in the asymptomatic phases of a number of inherited thrombotic diseases. In antithrombin III deficiency, for example, Bauer and co-workers[23] reported a significant increase in mean F_{1+2} concentration in 22 asymptomatic patients, in whom plasma FPA levels were not substantially higher than those found in healthy individuals. Clearance studies with $^{131}I - F_{1+2}$ indicated that the elevation in F_{1+2} was due to excessive activation of prothrombin rather than impaired removal of the fragment from the circulation. Infusion of purified antithrombin III concentrate led to a temporary reduction in F_{1+2} concentration. Raised F_{1+2} concentrations were also found in some asymptomatic patients with protein C deficiency[24], again with only minimal elevation in FPA concentration. The processes by which an asymptomatic hypercoagulable state is converted to a symptomatic thrombotic episode in these inherited deficiency states are not understood.

In addition to deficiencies within the natural anticoagulant mechanisms, a second category of the hypercoagulable state probably arises when normal blood is exposed to surfaces that have lost their normal anticoagulant properties. Endothelial cells have a strongly anticoagulant luminal surface, which can rapidly acquire procoagulant properties when injured physically, chemically or immunologically. Normally, heparin-like proteoglycans on the cell surface form complexes with, and act as a co-factor for, antithrombin III. Additionally, surface-bound thrombomodulin forms a 1:1 complex with locally-generated thrombin. This complex activates protein C, which in turn destroys activated factors VIII_a and V_a[25]. A smaller form of thrombomodulin is also present in human blood and urine[26]. Neither form of thrombomodulin has been measured in substantial numbers of human subjects, but it is conceivable that diseased endothelium, as perhaps occurs over an atheromatous plaque, will lose its ability to synthesise heparin-like substances and thrombomodulin and thereby become more pro-coagulant in nature. Exposure of vascular endothelial cells to the cytokines interleukin I and tumour necrosis factor (TNF) released by macrophages has been shown to down-regulate thrombomodulin expression[27] and up-regulate tissue factor (the co-factor for factor VII)[28]. Resultant imbalance between the procoagulant and anticoagulant mechanism at the vessel wall surface would then induce a hypercoagulable state, with acquired deficiencies in antithrombin III and protein C activity (see also Chapter 2.4).

Advancing vascular disease may be one explanation for the gradual increases in indices of thrombin generation (F_{1+2} and FPA) and protein C activation found with ageing in clinically healthy men[29], evidence for an acquired and evolving hypercoagulable state. The existence of a continuous though basal rate of zymogen-enzyme transformation within the coagulant pathway, which can be elevated at times without inducement of thrombosis, affords an explanation for a high VII_c in men at high risk of coronary thrombosis.

FACTOR VII AND HYPERCOAGULABILITY

Factor VII is secreted by the liver as a single-chain zymogen which can be cleaved to a 2-chain species (consisting of 2 disulphide-linked polypeptides) upon exposure to factor XII_a, X_a, IX_a or thrombin[30,31]. There is some evidence that both molecular forms possess serine protease activity, but conversion of the single-chain species to the two-chain form (VII_a) results in an increase in coagulant activity of more than hundredfold[32,33]. Other studies suggest, however, that only VII_a possesses proteolytic activity[34–36]. Either way, the procoagulant activity of factor VII in an in-vitro assay will be very sensitive to trace amounts of circulating VII_a. A raised factor VII coagulant activity may therefore serve as a marker of hypercoagulability in asymptomatic individuals, because it represents the result of exposure of factor VII to raised levels of factor XII_a, X_a and thrombin activity in vivo.

In the rabbit, Mitropoulos and Esnouf[37] have shown that injection of the fragment 1 region of $F_{1.2}$ (residues 1–156) is followed by a transient increase in the plasma concentrations of the vitamin K-dependent factors X and prothrombin. This raises the possibility that, when a hypercoagulable state is sustained, the increased turnover of $F_{1.2}$ will be associated with increased synthesis of all vitamin K-dependent clotting factors including factor VII. Thus, the high factor VII activity in men at high risk may consist in variable proportion of increased levels of both VII_a and single-chain native factor VII. More detailed study of this problem awaits a method of distinguishing between the two forms of factor VII in vivo. Of course, if a persistent hypercoagulable state is accompanied not only by increased concentrations of $F_{1.2}$, but also by an increased VII_c, then the expectation would be that these two variables are positively correlated. Studies are currently in progress to test this possibility.

FACTOR VII AND OTHER CORONARY RISK FACTORS

Plasma lipids

In the Northwick Park Heart Study, the association between coronary risk and VII_c was independent of serum cholesterol concentration[8]. Nevertheless, a highly significant positive association was found between VII_c and serum cholesterol levels[8]. A subsequent examination of 62 healthy men and women showed that VII_c was independently and positively associated with both serum cholesterol and non-fasting serum triglyceride concentrations[38], relations which persisted after allowance for factor

VII concentration. The strongest relations between VII_c and plasma lipids reside within the large triglyceride-rich lipoprotein classes, namely the chylomicrons and very-low density lipoproteins[39]. These associations, combined with in-vitro studies of the effects of large multi-lamellar liposomal vesicles and free fatty acids[40], prompted the suggestion that the in-vivo association arises because large lipoproteins provide a contact surface for activation of the intrinsic pathway of coagulation (specifically factor XII), with subsequent cleavage of some factor VII to VII_a by factor XII_a.

Many clinical conditions in which there is a hyperlipidaemia are associated with an increased factor VII_c, for example the primary hyperlipoproteinaemias[41,42], pregnancy[43] and uncontrolled diabetes mellitus[44]. Reduction of plasma lipid levels, particularly triglyceride, is associated with a decrease in factor VII_c[45]. When plasma lipid concentrations tend to be low, as in vegetarians, factor VII_c is also reduced[46].

Dietary fat intake

Dietary experimental studies in healthy adults have shown that a significant positive association exists between day-to-day variation in total fat intake and VII_c[47]. Indeed, the influence of fat consumption on VII_c is sufficiently rapid for an association to exist between the diurnal variation in plasma triglyceride concentration induced by the meal pattern, and the diurnal fluctuation in VII_c[48]. The diurnal rhythm in VII_c lags behind that in plasma triglyceride by approximately two or three hours. The link between total fat intake and subsequent VII_c is probably the postprandial chylomicronaemia, the large lipoprotein particles inducing a rise in factor VII coagulant activity. By contrast, no association appears to exist between diurnal fluctuation in factor VII antigen concentration and plasma triglyceride[48].

The association between factor VII_c and total dietary fat intake can be observed in the general community. The demonstration of such a relation is handicapped of course by the difficulty in measurement of fat intake in the habitual diet; a problem that has thwarted most attempts to show an association between fat intake and serum cholesterol concentration within communities. Nevertheless, a significant positive correlation has been demonstrated in middle-aged men when fat intake was expressed relative to body size, since it is overconsumption rather than absolute intake that is important for factor VII_c[49].

Two experimental studies, one of seven days duration[48] and one of 14 days[50], examined the effects of dietary fat composition on factor VII_c. Unlike total fat intake, the ratio of polyunsaturated fatty acid to saturated fatty acid in the diet (P/S ratio) had no demonstrable effect on VII_c.

Age and sex

Several cross-sectional studies have demonstrated an increase in factor VII_c with age been 20 and 60 years in both sexes[51,52]. When standardised for age, factor VII_c is significantly higher in women taking low-dose oestrogen contraceptives and in women after the menopause[51–53]. Scarabin and others[54] have shown that the rise with age in women is greater for factor VII_c than for factor VII antigen concentration, so that the ratio of VII_c/VII antigen (an index of factor VII activation) also increases significantly with age.

Other risk factors

Factor VII_c is unrelated to smoking habit[52,55]. The increases observed with obesity in some groups[52,55,56] and with increasing alcohol consumption[57] are probably reflections of the raised triglyceride concentrations in these conditions.

FIBRINOGEN AND THROMBOTIC RISK

Plasma fibrinogen concentration is strongly predictive of risk of coronary heart disease and stroke[8–14]. As such it is often considered to be an index of hypercoagulability. There is an evolving consensus, however, that the term hypercoagulability should be restricted to a state of increased flux within the coagulant pathway, with increased transformation of zymogen to enzyme at one or more stages in the system. Fibrinogen is a substrate rather than an enzyme; hence a raised concentration does not fit easily into this working definition. Rather, a high fibrinogen level is thought to increase the risk of an acute thrombotic event through its influence on platelet aggregability and blood viscosity and may, therefore, be more properly considered to be a determinant of the pre-thrombotic state through these mechanisms. Fibrinogen may also have an important role to play in the development of atheroma.

Viscosity effects

Increased blood viscosity reduces blood flow and increases platelet adhesion to damaged vascular surfaces. Its principal determinants are a raised haematocrit and an increased plasma viscosity. Fibrinogen, because of its size, structure and concentration, is the major determinant of plasma viscosity. The effect of fibrinogen on whole blood viscosity is particularly marked at low shear rates (low rates of flow), because the shear forces are no longer adequate to overcome the tendency of fibrinogen to aggregate red cells[58]. This increased resistance to flow will raise the likelihood of ischaemia and thrombus formation but, as argued above, should probably be thought of as separate from the phenomenon of hypercoagulability. Hyperviscosity effects associated with hyperfibrinogenaemia may play an important role in thrombus formation in areas of disturbed blood flow in the vicinity of artificial heart valves.

Platelet effects

Thrombus consists of fibrin polymer and aggregated platelets in various proportions. Grey thrombus consists mainly of aggregated platelets bound together by adhesive proteins, of which the most important is fibrinogen (see also Chapter 3.1). The fibrinogen receptor on the platelet surface (consisting of glycoproteins IIb and IIIa) is not expressed until the platelet is activated by exposure to agonists such as ADP (released from damaged cells), collagen, or thrombin. The responsiveness of platelets to low doses of ADP is increased[59,60] although the maximal rate of aggregation at higher ADP concentrations appears to be reduced by a high fibrinogen level[60]. It is by no means certain whether an increased aggregatory response in vitro on exposure to low doses of ADP reflects a hyperaggregable state in vivo. However, a contribution of hyperfibrinogenaemia to the risk of acute thrombosis through an influence on platelet aggregation cannot be discounted, particularly when platelets have been activated by contact with artificial surfaces or exposure to agonists such as ADP released from damaged endothelial cells, red cells and other platelets (see also Chapters 2.3, 3.1 and 3.4). Warfarin anticoagulation will not offset the viscosity or platelet aggregatory effects of a high plasma fibrinogen concentration.

FIBRINOGEN AND OTHER CORONARY AND STROKE RISK FACTORS

Smoking

High plasma fibrinogen concentration is strikingly associated with cigarette smoking. Current smokers of both sexes have higher levels than those who never smoked or gave up the habit and there is evidence for a dose-response relation among current smokers[13,52,61,62]. With discontinuation of smoking, fibrinogen levels tend to fall to those of age matched never-smokers within about 5 years[61]. In prospective data[61], cessation and resumption of smoking were accompanied by a reduction and an increase in plasma fibrinogen of about 0.15 g/l, respectively.

Plasma lipid concentrations

Patients with primary type II hyperlipoproteinaemia have a higher fibrinogen level than age matched control subjects[63]. Increased fibrinogen concentrations have also been reported in hypertriglyceridaemia, but unlike factor VII_c, fibrinogen levels did not fall significantly with reduction in plasma triglyceride[45]. Plasma fibrinogen and serum cholesterol also have a significant positive correlation in the general population, although the strength of this association is very weak[8] and its nature is unclear.

Dietary fat

Plasma fibrinogen concentration appears to be uninfluenced by acute changes in either total fat intake[47] or dietary fat composition (unpublished data). In a community study of asymptomatic middle-aged men, no association was observed between total dietary fat intake and plasma fibrinogen concentration[49]. With respect to dietary consumption of fish oil (n–3 very-long-chain polyunsaturated fatty acids), some studies have reported a reduction in fibrinogen with increased intake[64,65] whereas others have observed no significant effect[66–68].

Age and sex

Fibrinogen concentration increases with age in both sexes and is significantly higher in women[52,62,69], in whom the onset of the menopause is associated with an appreciable rise in plasma fibrinogen, more so when the former is natural rather than induced[53,62].

Other risk factors

In a study of British civil servants, Markowe and associates[70] noted a higher mean fibrinogen concentration in men belonging to lower grades of employment than in higher grades. This difference persisted when age and smoking habits had been taken into account and was thought to offer a possible explanation for the higher coronary heart disease mortality among men in lower grade employment, and possibly also for social class differences in coronary heart disease prevalance in Britain. A summary measure of job stress was also inversely related to fibrinogen concentration in these men[70]. A similar social class gradient has been reported in Scotland[62].

Fibrinogen concentration is inversely related to alcohol intake[62,69] and positively related to adiposity[52,62,69] in both sexes.

IDENTIFICATION AND CORRECTION OF INCREASED THROMBOEMBOLIC RISK

Whether preoperative hypercoagulability (as defined by high factor VII_c, $F_{1.2}$ or FPA levels) or hyperfibrinogenaemia increase the risk of prosthetic valve thrombosis and systemic embolism postoperatively is currently unknown. Prospective studies on this important aspect are long overdue. It is possible that patients in a prethrombotic state before valve replacement are at increased risk of such complications, especially in the early weeks and months after surgery (Chapter 3.4). Other patients may acquire a prethrombotic state in the late postoperative period as the result of a new disease process or change in lifestyle (Chapter 2.4) and experience an embolic event for the first time many years after operation.

Adequate anticoagulation with warfarin would be expected to convert a hypercoagulable state to a hypocoagulable state. However, because hypercoagulability is only one component of the prethrombotic state, anticoagulants cannot ensure freedom from valve thrombosis and embolism. Damaged or activated endothelial surfaces, high fibrinogen levels induced perhaps by cigarette smoking or acute infection, increased blood viscosity and local blood flow disturbances may combine with hyperaggregable platelets to generate platelet thrombi either in the vicinity of the prosthetic valve or at sites elsewhere. Thus measures which might reduce the risk of thrombotic and embolic complications include stopping cigarette smoking, prompt treatment of infection[71] and general steps to reduce the risk of atherosclerosis, such as correction of hyperlipidaemia and control of diabetes mellitus. Several lipid-lowering drugs reduce plasma fibrinogen concentration, including a number of fibrate[72] (but not gemfibrozil[73]) and nicotinic acid derivatives[74]. Whether such treatment in prosthetic heart valve patients with combined hyperlipidaemia and hyperfibrinogenaemia will reduce the risk of thromboembolism remains uncertain. The antiplatelet drug ticlopidine is reported to have a fibrinogen-lowering effect also[75–79], but as yet no clinical trials have been carried in patients with prosthetic valves.

CONCLUSIONS

Epidemiological studies since 1970 have provided strong evidence for the existence of a pre-thrombotic state in men at high risk of coronary heart disease. This appears to arise in part through a hypercoagulable state and in part through the effects of a high fibrinogen concentration on the viscosity and platelet aggregability components of thrombotic tendency. The former may be in response to exposure of blood to pro-coagulant surfaces. A high factor VII_c appears to serve as a marker of hypercoagulability. The associations of VII_c and fibrinogen with other coronary risk factors are consistent with the overall epidemiology of coronary heart disease.

The past decade has also witnessed the development of activation peptide assays as promising new measurements of hypercoagulability. The value of these peptides as markers of coronary heart disease risk, and their relations with other haemostatic, lipid and life-style risk factors are currently being explored, but results are not yet available. Current advice given for coronary heart disease prevention, for example consumption of a low fat diet, avoidance of smoking and obesity, will coincidentally reduce VII_c and fibrinogen concentration, and may be equally applicable to patients with prosthetic valves. Inclusion of these haemostatic indices with other major risk factors (plasma lipids, smoking habits, blood pressure) should significantly improve the assessment of individual risk for prosthetic heart valve patients also. Further research into these important aspects is urgently required.

REFERENCES

1. Grunkemeier GL, Rahimtoola SH. Artificial heart valves. Annu Rev Med 1990;41:251–263.
2. De Wood MA, Spores J, Notske R, et al. Prevalence of total coronary occlusion during the early hours of transmural myocardial infarction. N Engl J Med 1980;303:897–902.
3. Davies MJ. Thrombosis in acute myocardial infarction and sudden death. Cardiovasc Clin 1987;18:151–159.
4. Davies MJ, Thomas A. Thrombosis and acute coronary artery lesions in sudden cardiac ischaemic death. N Engl J Med 1984;310:1137–1140.
5. El Fawal MA, Berg GA, Wheatley DJ, Harland WA. Sudden coronary death in Glasgow: nature and frequency of acute coronary lesions. Br Heart J 1987;57:329–335.
6. Meade TW, Howarth DJ, Stirling Y, Welch TP, Crompton MR. Fibrinopeptide A and sudden coronary death. Lancet 1984;2:607–609.
7. Meade TW, North WRS, Chakrabarti R, et al. Haemostatic function and cardiovascular death: early results of a prospective study. Lancet 1980;1:1050–1054.
8. Meade TW, Mellows S, Brozovic M, et al. Haemostatic function and ischaemic heart disease: principal results of the Northwick Park Heart Study. Lancet 1986;2:533–537.
9. Wilhelmsen L, Svardsudd K, Korsan-Bengtsen K, Larsson B, Welin L, Tibblin G. Fibrinogen as a risk factor for stroke and myocardial infarction. N Engl J Med 1984;311:501–505.
10. Stone MC, Thorp JM. Plasma fibrinogen – a major coronary risk factor. In: Lenzi S and Descovitch GC (Eds). Atherosclerosis and Cardiovascular Diseases. Bologna, Editrice Compositori, 1984:3–10.
11. Kannel WB, Castelli WP, Meeks SL. Fibrinogen and cardiovascular disease. Abstract, 34th Annual Scientific Session of the American College of Cardiology, March 1985, Anaheim, California.
12. Kannel WB, D'Agostino RB, Belanger AJ. Fibrinogen, cigarette smoking, and risk of cardiovascular disease: insights from the Framingham Study. Am Heart J 1987;113:1006–1010.
13. Kannel WB, Wolf PA, Castelli WP, D'Agostino RB. Fibrinogen and risk of cardiovascular disease. J Am Med Assoc 1987;258:1183–1186.
14. Yarnell JWG, Baker IA, Sweetnam PM, et al. Fibrinogen, viscosity and white cell count are major risk factors for ischaemic heart disease. Circulation 1991;83:836–844.
15. Lau HK, Rosenberg JS, Beeler DL, Rosenberg RD. The isolation and characterisation of a specific antibody population directed against the prothrombin activation fragments F_2 and F_{1+2}. J Biol Chem 1979;254:8751–8761.
16. Tietel JM, Bauer KA, Lau HK, Rosenberg RD. Studies of the prothrombin activation pathway utilizing radioimmunoassays for the F_2/F_{1+2} fragment and thrombin-antithrombin III complex. Blood 1982;59:1086–1097.
17. Bauer KA, Kass BL, ten Cate H, Hawiger JJ, Rosenberg RD. Factor IX is activated in vivo by the tissue factor mechanism. Blood 1990;76:731–736.
18. Bauer KA, Kas BL, ten Cate H, Bednarek MA, Hawiger JJ, Rosenberg RD. Detection of factor X activation in humans. Blood 1990;74:2007–2015.
19. MacFarlane RG. An enzyme cascade in the blood clotting mechanism, and its function as a biochemical amplifier. Nature 1964;202:498–499.
20. Davie EW, Ratnoff OD. Waterfall sequence for intrinsic blood clotting. Science 1964;145:1310–1312.
21. Rosenberg RD, Rosenberg JS. Natural anticoagulant mechanisms. J Clin Invest 1984;74:1–6.
22. Nemerson Y, Silverberg SA, Jesty J. Self-damping mechanism in blood coagulation. Thromb Diath Haem 1974;32:57–64.
23. Bauer KA, Goodman TL, Kass BL, Rosenberg RD. Elevated factor X_a activity in the blood of asymptomatic patients with congenital antithrombin III deficiency. J Clin Invest 1985;76:826–836.
24. Bauer KA, Broekmans AW, Bertina RM, et al. Haemostatic enzyme generation in the blood of patients with hereditary protein C deficiency. Blood 1988;71:1418–1426.

25. Dittman WA, Majerus PW. Structure and function of thrombomodulin: a natural anticoagulant. Blood 1990;75:329–336.
26. Ishii H, Majerus PW. Thrombomodulin is present in human plasma and urine. J Clin Invest 1985;76:2178–2181.
27. Nawroth P, Stern D. Modulation of endothelial hemostatic properties by TNF. J Exp Med 1986;163:740–745.
28. Bevilacqua M, Pober J, Majeau G et al. Recombinant TNF induces procoagulant activity in endothelium. Proc Natl Acad Sci USA 1986;83:4533–4537.
29. Bauer KA, Weiss LM, Sparrow D, Vokonas PS, Rosenberg RD. Aging associated changes in indices of thrombin generation and protein C activation in humans. J Clin Invest 1987;80:1527–1534.
30. Radcliffe R, Nemerson Y. Activation and control of factor VII by activated factor X and thrombin. J Biol Chem 1975;250:388–395.
31. Kisiel W, Fujikawa K, Davies EW. Activation of bovine factor VII (proconvertin) by factor XII_a (activated Hageman factor). Biochemistry 1977;16:4189–4194.
32. Zur M, Radcliffe RD, Oberdick J, Nemerson Y. The dual role of factor VII in blood coagulation. J Biol Chem 1982;257:5623–5631.
33. Bach R, Oberdick J, Nemerson Y. Immunoaffinity purification of bovine factor VII. Blood 1984;63:393–398.
34. Rao LVM, Rapaport SI, Bajaj SP. Activation of human factor VII in the initiation of tissue factor-dependent coagulation. Blood 1986;68:685–691.
35. Williams EB, Krishnaswamy S, Mann KG. Zymogen/enzyme discrimination using peptide chloromethyl ketones. J Biol Chem 1989;264:7536–7545.
36. Wildgoose P, Berkner KL, Kisiel W. Synthesis, purification and characterization of an Arg 152-Glu site-directed mutant of recombinant human blood clotting factor VII. Biochemistry 1990;29:3413–3420.
37. Mitropoulos KA, Esnouf MP. The prothrombin activation peptide regulates synthesis of the vitamin K-dependent proteins in the rabbit. Thromb Res 1990;57:541–549.
38. Miller GJ, Walter SJ, Stirling Y, Thompson SG, Esnouf MP, Meade TW. Assay of factor VII activity by two techniques: evidence for increased conversion of VII to VII_a in hyperlipidaemia, with possible implications for ischaemic heart disease. Br J Haematol 1985;59:249–258.
39. Mitropoulos KA, Miller GJ, Reeves BEA, Wilkes HC, Cruickshank JK. Factor VII coagulant activity is strongly associated with the plasma concentration of large lipoprotein particles in middle-aged men. Atherosclerosis 1989;76:203–208.
40. Mitropoulos KA, Martin JC, Reeves BEA, Esnouf MP. The activation of the contact phase of coagulation by physiologic surfaces in plasma; the effect of negatively charged liposomal vesicles. Blood 1989;73:1525–1533.
41. Constantino M, Merskey C, Kudzma DJ, Zucker MB. Increased activity of vitamin K-dependent clotting factors in human hyperlipoproteinaemia – association with cholestrol and triglyceride levels. Thromb Haemost 1977;38:465–474.
42. Carvallo de Sousa J, Bruckert E, Giral P, et al. Plasma factor VII, triglyceride concentration and fibrin degradation products in primary hyperlipidaemia: a clinical and laboratory study. Haemostasis 1989;19:83–90.
43. Stirling Y, Woolf L, North WRS, Seghatchian MJ, Meade TW. Haemostasis in normal pregnancy. Thromb Haemost 1984;52:176–182.
44. Fuller JH, Keen H, Jarrett RJ, et al. Haemostatic variables associated with diabetes and its complications. Br Med J 1979;2:964–966.
45. Simpson HCR, Mann JI, Meade TW, Chakrabarti R, Stirling Y, Woolf L. Hypertriglyceridaemia and hypercoagulability. Lancet 1983;1:786–790.
46. Haines AP, Chakrabarti R, Fisher D, Meade TW, North WRS, Stirling Y. Haemostatic variables in vegetarians and non-vegetarians. Thromb Res 1980;19:139–148.
47. Miller GJ, Martin JC, Webster J, et al. Association between dietary fat intake and plasma factor VII coagulant activity – a predictor of cardiovascular mortality. Atherosclerosis 1986;60:269–277.
48. Miller GJ, Martin JC, Mitropoulos KA, et al. Plasma factor VII is activated by postprandial triglyceridaemia, irrespective of dietary fat composition. Atherosclerosis 1991;86:163–171.
49. Miller GJ, Cruickshank JK, Ellis LJ, et al. Fat consumption and factor VII coagulant activity in middle-aged men. An association between a dietary and thrombogenic coronary risk factor. Atherosclerosis 1989;78:19–24.
50. Marckmann P, Sandstrom B, Jespersen J. Effects of total fat content and fatty acid composition in diet on factor VII coagulant activity and blood lipids. Atherosclerosis 1990;80:227–233.
51. Brozovic M, Stirling Y, Harricks C, North WRS, Meade TW. Factor VII in an industrial population. Br J Haematol 1974;28:381–391.
52. Balleisen L, Bailey J, Epping P-H, Schulte H, van de Loo J. Epidemiological study on factor VII, factor

VIII and fibrinogen in an industrial population: 1. Baseline data on the relation to age, gender, body weight, smoking, alcohol, pill-using, and menopause. Thromb Haemost 1985;54:475–479.
53. Meade TW, Dyer S, Howarth DJ, Imeson JD, Stirling Y. Antithrombin III and procoagulant activity: sex differences and effects of the menopause. Br J Haematol 1990;74:77–81.
54. Scarabin PY, van Dreden P, Bonithon-Kop C, et al. Age-related changes in factor VII activation in healthy women. Clin Sci 1988;75:341–343.
55. Meade TW. Epidemiology of atheroma, thrombosis and ischaemic heart disease. In: Bloom AL, Thomas DP (Eds). Haemostasis and Thrombosis, 2nd edition, Edinburgh, Churchill Livingstone, 1987;697–720.
56. Iso H, Folsom AR, Wu KK, et al. Haemostatic variables in Japanese and Caucasian men. Am J Epidemiol 1989;130:925–934.
57. Meade TW, North WRS, Chakrabarti R, Haines AP, Stirling Y. Population-based distributions of haemostatic variables. Br Med Bull 1977;33:283–288.
58. Lowe GD, Forbes CD. Blood rheology and thrombosis. Clin Haematol 1981;10:343–367.
59. Bloom AL, Evans EP. Plasma fibrinogen and the aggregation of platelets by adenosine diphosphate. Lancet 1969;1:349–350.
60. Meade TW, Vickers MV, Thompson SG, Seghatchian MJ. The effect of physiological levels of fibrinogen on platelet aggregation. Thromb Res 1985;38:527–534.
61. Meade TW, Imeson J, Stirling Y. Effects of changes in smoking and other characteristics on clotting factors and the risk of ischaemic heart disease. Lancet 1987;2:986–988.
62. Lee AJ, Smith WCS, Lowe GDO, Tunstall-Pedoe H. Plasma fibrinogen and coronary risk factors: The Scottish Heart Health Study. J Clin Epidemiol 1990;43:913–919.
63. Lowe GDO, Drummond MM, Third JLHC, et al. Increased plasma fibrinogen and platelet aggregates in type II hyperlipoproteinaemia. Thromb Haemost 1979;42:1503–1507.
64. Saynor R, Gillott T. Fish oil and plasma fibrinogen. Br Med J 1988;297:1196.
65. Hostmark AT, Bjerkedal T, Kierulf P, Flaten H, Ulshagen K. Fish oil and plasma fibrinogen. Br Med J 1988;297:180–181.
66. Sanders TAB, Vickers M, Haines AP. Effect on blood lipids and haemostasis of a supplement of cod liver oil, rich in eicosapentaenoic acid and docosahexaenoic acids, in healthy young men. Clin Sci 1981;61:317–324.
67. Berg-Schmidt E, Ernst E, Varming K, Pederson JO, Dyerberg J. The effect of n–3 fatty acids on lipids and haemostasis in patients with type II_a and type IV hyperlipidaemia. Thromb Haemost 1989;62:797–801.
68. Hansen J-B, Olsen JO, Wilsgard L, Osterud B. Effects of dietary supplementation with cod liver oil on monocyte thromboplastin synthesis, coagulation and fibrinolysis. J Intern Med 1989;225 (Suppl 1):133–139.
69. Meade TW, Chakrabarti R, Haines AP, North WRS, Stirling Y. Characteristics affecting fibrinolytic activity and plasma fibrinogen concentrations. Br Med J 1979;1:153–156.
70. Markowe HLJ, Marmot MG, Shipley MJ, et al. Fibrinogen: a possible link between social class and coronary heart disease. Br Med J 1985;291:1312–1314.
71. Baumann H, Gauldie J. Regulation of hepatic acute phase plasma protein genes by hepatocyte stimulating factors and other mediators of inflammation. Mol Biol Med 1990;7:147–159.
72. O'Brien JR, Etherington MD, Jamieson S, Sussex J. The effect of ICI 55,897 and clofibrate on platelet function and other tests abnormal in atherosclerosis. Thromb Haemost 1978;40:75–82.
73. Anderson P, Smith P, Seljeflot I, Brataker S, Arnesen H. Effects of gemfibrozil on lipids and haemostasis after myocardial infarction. Thromb Haemost 1990;63:174–177.
74. Pickart L. Fat metabolism, the fibrinogen/fibrinolytic system and blood flow: new potentials for the pharmacological treatment of coronary heart disease. Pharmacology 1981;23:271–280.
75. Conard J, Lecrubier C, Scarabin PY, Horellou MH, Samama M, Bousser MG. Effects of long term administration of ticlopidine on platelet function and haemostatic variables. Thromb Res 1980;20:143–148.
76. Auckland A, Hurlow RA, George AJ, Stuart J. Platelet inhibition with ticlopidine in atherosclerotic intermittent claudication. J Clin Pathol 1982;35:740–743.
77. Randi ML, Fabris F, Crociani ME, Battocchio F, Girolami A. Effects of ticlopidine on blood fibrinogen and blood viscosity in peripheral atherosclerotic disease. Drug Res 1985;35:1847–1849.
78. Palareti G, Poggi M, Torricelli P, Balestra V, Coccheri S. Long-term effects of ticlopidine on fibrinogen and haemorheology in patients with peripheral arterial disease. Thromb Res 1988;52:621–629.
79. Finelli C, Palareti G, Poggi M et al. Ticlopidine lowers plasma fibrinogen in patients with polycythaemia rubra vera and additional thrombotic risk factors. A double blind controlled study. Acta Haematol 1991;85:113–118.

Chapter 1.6

The Influence of Surgery on Thromboembolic Risk: Timing of Operation and Technical Factors

Peter J. K. Starek

The timing of valve repair or replacement has traditionally depended on the severity of patient symptoms and/or the presence of certain indicators of depressed ventricular function that are predictive of further deterioration unless surgical intervention is instituted. Surgical intervention in patients with cardiac valve disease is often too late to prevent atrial fibrillation, which commonly occurs as a consequence of valve malfunction and is a strong risk factor for thromboembolic complications. Valve replacement or repair procedures are an independent source of thromboembolic complications. A discussion of timing in surgical intervention must try to balance the risk factors that are a consequence of the patient's disease and those that are introduced by the procedure itself. These latter risk factors are probably determined by the choice of procedure, substitute valve and suture materials and by technical factors.

RELATIONSHIP OF ATRIAL FIBRILLATION, THROMBOEMBOLIC COMPLICATIONS, AND HEART VALVE DISEASE

Incidence of atrial fibrillation

Any discussion of the timing of surgical treatment in relation to embolic risk must take into account the incidence of atrial fibrillation associated with particular types of heart valve disease. According to the Framingham Heart Study data, the overall incidence of atrial fibrillation in the adult population is about 0.4%. The frequency of atrial fibrillation seems to increase with age and is approximately 2–4% in patients over 60 years of age[1]. Patients with cardiac disease have a higher incidence of atrial fibrillation[2]. Patients with mitral stenosis requiring valve replacement have an incidence of atrial fibrillation of about 40%, while those with mitral regurgitation requiring surgical correction have an incidence of about 75%. Congestive cardiomyopathy, pericardial constriction, and hypertension carry a 25%, 35%, and 5–10% incidence of atrial fibrillation, respectively (Table 1.6–1). Ischaemic heart disease has been reported as a cause for atrial fibrillation in up to 40% of cases, as it often appears following a myocardial infarction or temporarily after coronary artery bypass surgery[3,4]. It is interesting that aortic valve disease has a very low 1% incidence of atrial fibrillation.

Mechanism of atrial fibrillation

Atrial biopsies in patients with atrial fibrillation due to rheumatic mitral valve

Table 1.6–1
Prevalance of Atrial Fibrillation (AF) Reported in Various Disease Populations*

Diagnosis of Population	Prevalence of AF (%)
Valvular heart disease	
Mitral stenosis (requiring valve replacement)	41
Mitral regurgitation (requiring valve replacement)	75
Aortic stenosis/aortic insufficiency	1
Coronary artery disease	
Angina	0.8
Immediately after myocardial infarction (transient)	7–16
Immediately after coronary artery bypass grafting (transient)	10
Cardiomyopathy	
Congestive cardiomyopathy	25
Primary hypertrophic cardiomyopathy	8–10
Idiopathic hypertrophic subaortic stenosis	8–10
Pericardial disease	
Acute pericarditis	5
Pericardial constriction	35
Miscellaneous	
Systemic arterial hypertension	5–10
Atrial septal defect (age, >50y)	53
Hyperthyroidism	12–18

*Reproduced, with permission , from Wipf JE, Lipsky BA: Atrial fibrillation: thromboembolic risk and indications for anticoagulation. Arch Intern Med 1990;150:1598–1603.

stenosis show varying amounts of fibrosis and muscular preservation or muscle atrophy. Bailey and associates graded these morphological changes, with Grade 1 being essentially normal myocardium, Grade 2 showing moderate to severe fibrosis in the muscle wall, although the muscle mass and architecture were essentially preserved, and Grade 3 showing extensive fibrosis with disruption of the architecture and considerable loss of muscle mass (Fig. 1.6–1). Grade 3 changes were associated with atrial fibrillation of more than 5 years' duration. In their experience, it was often possible to cardiovert patients with Grade 1 or 2 changes to normal sinus rhythm, whereas successful long term cardioversion was usually not possible in patients with Grade 3 changes[5]. This interesting study has clear implications for the timing of any surgical procedure that may improve the reversibility of atrial fibrillation.

The development of atrial fibrillation in patients with rheumatic mitral insufficiency can occur in the same way as in patients with rheumatic mitral stenosis. In other patients with chronic mitral insufficiency, left atrial size can increase and disrupt the normal architecture, thus predisposing these patients to the development of atrial fibrillation. This theory is supported by laboratory observations in a dog model of left atrial enlargement in arrhythmias[6]. Clinical studies in patients with atrial enlargement have suggested that arrhythmias are caused by the presence of fibres with low resting potentials and action potentials with slow upstrokes[7].

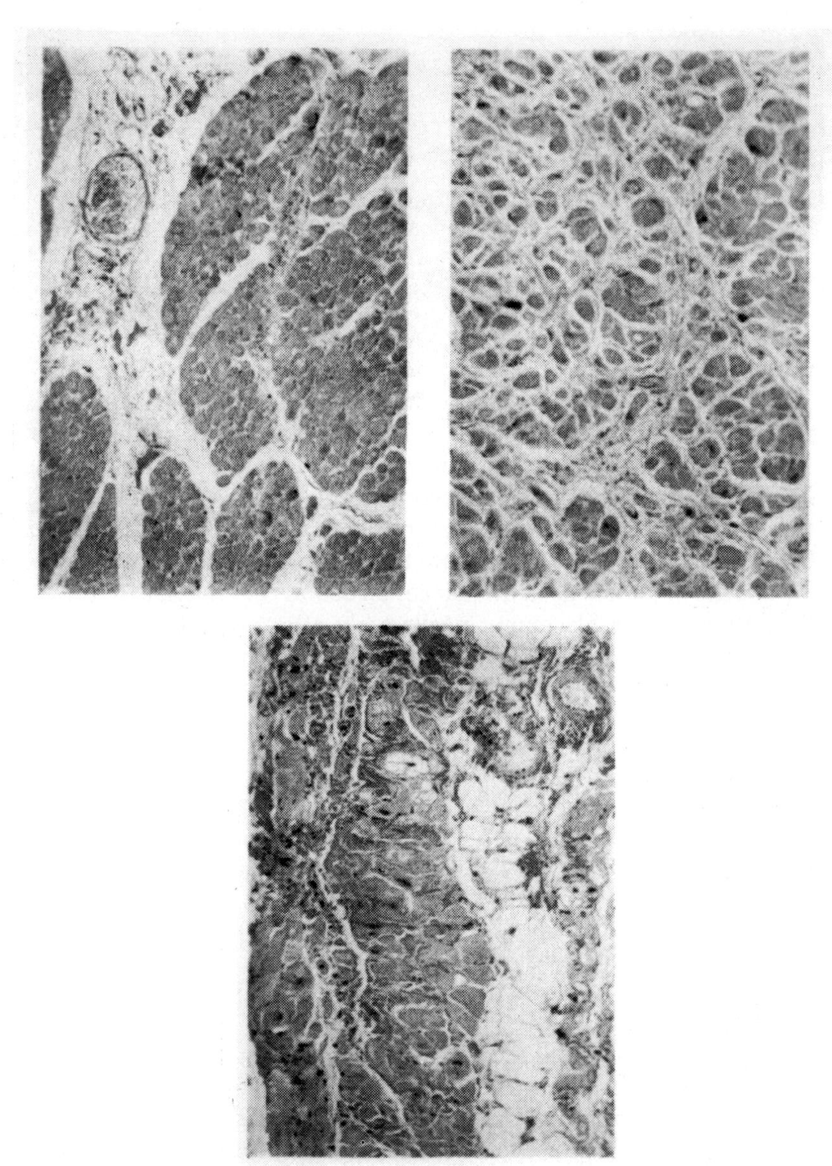

Figure 1.6–1: (Upper left) Normal posterior left atrial wall showing compact myocardium in bundles. (Verhoeff-Van Gieson stain, X 75.) (Upper right) Grade II biopsy showing diffuse net-like pattern of fibrosis. Muscle bundle architecture is preserved. (Verhoeff-Van Gieson stain, X 75.) (Lower left) Grade III biopsy showing severe fibrosis and obliteration of muscle bundle architecture. (Verhoeff-Van Gieson stain, X 75.) (Reproduced, with permission, from Bailey GWH et al.[5] © by The Lancet Ltd.)

Atrial fibrillation and thromboembolism

The risk of stroke in patients with non-rheumatic atrial fibrillation is 4–5% per annum, which is about a five-fold increase compared with controls in normal sinus rhythm[8] (see also Chapter 1.2). The risk of systemic embolism is greatly increased in atrial fibrillation of rheumatic aetiology[9,10]. Other factors which modify the risk of embolism in atrial fibrillation include the duration and stability of the rhythm[11–14], concomitant hypertension[14,15] and the presence of left atrial enlargement[16–20]. These factors are discussed in detail in Chapter 1.3. Because patients who have experienced preoperative embolism may not lose their embolic risk factors in the postoperative period, it is not surprising that one of the strongest independent predictors of embolism in the postoperative period is a history of embolism preoperatively[21].

THROMBOEMBOLISM AND PROSTHETIC VALVES

The normal mechanisms for preventing intravascular thrombus formation involve the equilibrium of the coagulation and fibrinolytic systems and the regulatory function of the endothelium[22–26]. When blood comes into contact with foreign surfaces, additional mechanisms come into play[27,28]. These are described in detail in Chapters 1.7 and 2.2. Of the available substitute valves, only free-hand inserted aortic homografts and pulmonary autografts contain no foreign surfaces. They are in consequence almost completely devoid of thrombotic and embolic complications[29] (see Chapter 2.4). All other prosthetic valves are thrombogenic to an extent determined by their design and the materials used in their construction[30]. The hazard function curve for embolism after valve replacement peaks early after operation, falling to a fairly stable constant hazard phase after the first 6 to 12 months[31,32] (see Fig 6.2–1a). It is probable that the embolic events in the early postoperative period are due to a com bination of factors, including alterations in coagulability (Chapter 3.4), low cardiac output and factors relating to materials and surgical technique.

Materials

The attachment of a prosthetic valve to the heart involves passing sutures through the annulus of the excised valve and the valve sewing ring. This can be accomplished with simple interrupted, continuous, horizontal mattress, or figure of eight sutures, or a combination of these. The desired result is apposition of the sewing ring to the endothelial surface of the annulus and the firm fixation of the valve in the appropriate position.

The sewing ring becomes covered with the patient's endothelium over a period of several months, and there is fibrous ingrowth into the sewing ring of the prosthetic valve (Fig. 1.6–2). The healing process begins with thrombus formation at the tissue fabric interface. This thrombus is eventually replaced by scar tissue. Two types of scar tissue are recognisable. One consists of simple fibrosis with an eventual covering of endothelial cells. If this type of scar tissue is fairly thin, it can survive by obtaining its nutrients directly from the bloodstream without the need of an intrinsic vascular blood supply. The second type of scar tissue is characterised by invasion of the sewing ring interstices by granulation tissue containing blood capillaries. The granulation tissue depends on its own capillary network and, should this be disrupted by any means (such as shrinkage of scar tissue and strangulation of the capillaries), necrosis and sloughing can take place, generating new thrombus and repetition of the healing process[33]. Surface thrombogenicity of sewing rings made out of different materials varies depending on the fabric covering. Pore size varies with the weave or knit, and this may have an effect on sewing ring healing. Expanded Teflon and Dacron velour are materials commonly used in sewing ring construction. Thrombogenicity tests on these

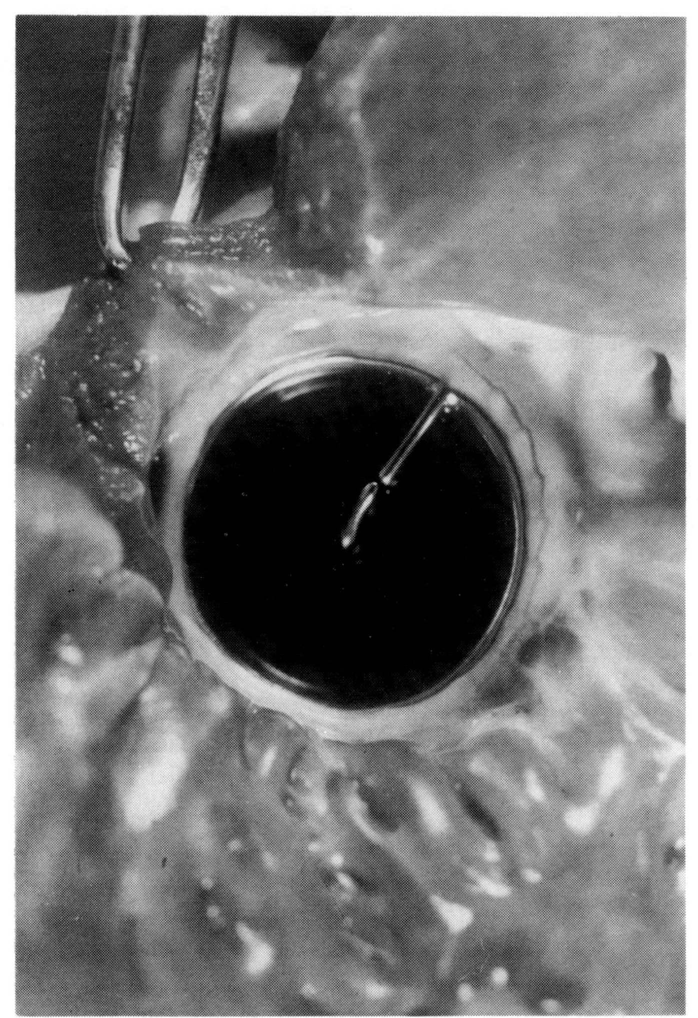

Figure 1.6–2: A thin layer of cardiac endothelium covers the valve sewing ring within two to three months of valve implantation and stops at the metal surface of the Medtronic Hall valve.

materials, used as vascular grafts, have shown that at three months after implant, expanded Teflon material has a better lining with cellular neointima; however, at six months the Dacron velour possesses the best neointima. The thrombogenicity of the two grafts is similar at six months, with slightly less thrombogenicity seen in the Teflon material at three months[34]. For further discussion of the embolic potential of the sewing ring and of the problem of tissue overgrowth, see Chapter 2.4.

The materials used for the construction of a prosthetic valve also have an important effect on its thrombogenicity[35–37]. These issues are explored in detail in Chapter 2.2.

IMPLANTATION TECHNIQUES AND THEIR INFLUENCE ON THROMBOGENICITY

When a prosthetic valve is implanted, it is the surgeon's responsibility to ensure 1) adequate fixation of the valve, 2) absence of paravalvular leaks, 3) free mobility of the occluder mechanism, 4) optimum orientation with regard to flow patterns, 5) absence of tissue distortion, insofar as possible, and 6) minimisation of endothelial injury in the implant site. These goals can be accomplished by careful attention to a series of steps.

Annulus preparation

Appropriate valve excision and annular preparation is a prerequisite to any satisfactory valve replacement. The diseased valve should be removed leaving an adequate annulus as a firm anchor for sutures. All calcium should be debrided, since a calcified annulus is not a satisfactory suture anchor and does not allow the flexibility required when the circular sewing ring of a valve prosthesis is sutured to a non-circular valve annulus. Excision of the valve beyond the annulus is occasionally necessary in difficult cases, particularly those involving endocarditis or heavy calcification. If this occurs, repair of the resulting defect with an appropriate material, such as pericardium or synthetic patch, should be accomplished to provide a satisfactory anchor for valve sutures.

Valve sizing

Appropriate sizing of the valve is very important. Both oversizing and undersizing are to be avoided. Oversizing invariably distorts and stretches the tissues once a rigid valve ring is implanted and can predispose the valve to tissue impingement of the occluder mechanism or create unnecessary stress in the suture line, thus predisposing to paravalvular leak. In addition, flow patterns may be distorted. All three of these undesirable effects increase the risk of thrombus formation and subsequent embolism.

Undersizing will compromise the haemodynamic performance of the valve and again may put unnecessary tension on the annulus, causing paravalvular leaks. In the author's experience of occasional bland paravalvular leaks, the sewing ring of the valve immediately adjacent to the paravalvular leak is often devoid of neointima. The turbulent blood flow through the paravalvular leak coming into contact with a raw Dacron surface may cause severe haemolysis[38] and, in addition, may provide a continuous stimulus towards thrombus formation. Chronic attempts at healing may generate emboli in a manner similar to freshly implanted valves.

Suture techniques

Suture techniques must ensure an even and equal distribution of sutures in the annulus and the matching portion of the prosthetic sewing ring. An uneven distribution of the sutures placed in the annulus and the sewing ring can cause unnecessary tension, resulting in paravalvular leaks or improper seating of the valve. A simple way of ensuring proper suture distribution is to slide the valve into position within the annulus once all of the annular sutures are in place, marking several key sutures and their appropriate corresponding location on the sewing ring. Once these sutures are passed through the sewing ring, the remaining sutures can then be evenly distributed between them.

A personal 20-year experience of suturing various types of prosthetic heart valves

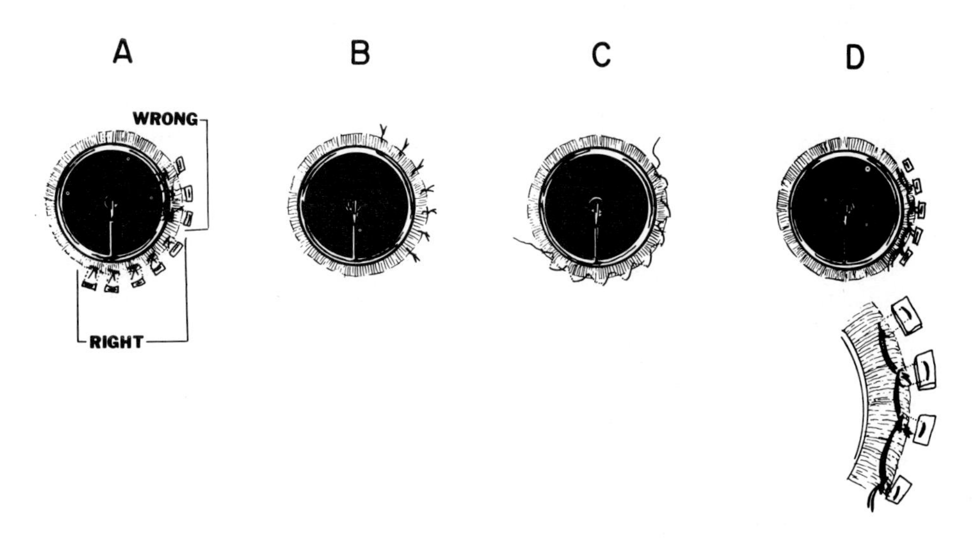

Figure 1.6–3: Suturing techniques and precautions suggested to avoid the possibility of prolapsing suture ends between the disc and valve ring. The surgeon can prevent potentially disastrous complications by adhering to the following principles: (A) do not suture through the sewing skirt close to the valve ring; (B) when using simple sutures, tie knots toward the tissue anulus; (C) use continuous suture whenever safe and convenient; (D) when using horizontal mattress sutures, either cut sutures short or tie down suture ends with adjacent sutures. (Reproduced from Starek[40].)

has shown that tissue valves are very 'forgiving' and can be safely sutured into place with virtually any suture technique, given the caveats mentioned above. In contrast, experience with suturing pivoting disc valves has taught the avoidance of horizontal mattress sutures incorporating reinforcing pledgets on the ventricular side of the mitral or aortic annulus, which may force the tissue annulus against the ventricular surface of the prosthesis. The author reported several cases of mitral valve thrombosis when this suture technique was used with Lillehei-Kaster pivoting disc valves[39]. In contrast, no cases of valve thrombosis were seen when the pledgets were placed on either the atrial or the aortic side of an annulus, thus seating the valve more or less within the annulus and somewhat protecting the occluder disc mechanism from impingement by tissue.

Disc valves are also vulnerable to impingement by sutures, and care must be taken to avoid tying knots too close to the disc occluder or cutting sutures too long, thus allowing the cut ends to prolapse between the ring housing and the disc occluder. The sutures can be cut by touching them with an ophthalmological cautery pencil, which simply melts the suture at point of contact and has the additional advantage of not allowing the two ends to unravel. Figure 1.6–3 shows several suggested ways of suturing pivoting disc valves without the risk of suture impingement[40].

The thrombogenicity of sutures varies with the different materials used. A study comparing the thrombogenicity of polypropylene, polyester, polygalactin, nylon and silk, using a scanning electron microscope to examine platelet deposition and thrombus formation, showed that polypropylene was the least thrombogenic material. Silk was the most thrombogenic, followed by nylon, polygalactin, and polyester[41]. In the author's experience in a non-randomised study of different suture materials, with and without pledgets, no difference in embolic incidence was noted between polypropylene and polyester sutures or between pledgets and no pledgets. The explanation of this probably lies in the fact that, within two months of implantation, most sutures and pledgets are covered with new endothelium, which probably decreases their thrombogenicity significantly.

Historically, some surgeons tried to reduce the thrombogenicity of the valve implantation procedure by using continuous sutures and tying the knots on the outside[42] or by covering the knots with a shield[43]. Hjelms and associates used a continuous suture technique in prosthetic aortic valve replacement, but reported a 26% incidence of paravalvular leaks and valve detachment in patients undergoing operation for aortic regurgitation, compared with a zero incidence of valve detachment in patients undergoing operation for aortic stenosis[44]. Messmer and associates reported a higher incidence of valve dehiscence using a continuous suture technique with the Bjørk-Shiley valve, particularly in patients operated on for mitral regurgitation[45]. Continuous suture with polypropylene is probably useful only in patients with a well preserved annulus and in patients where visualisation of the implantation site is good. Even then, this technique can be fairly cumbersome due to the length of suture and the need to pull up the suture loops with even tension while seating the valve before tying the knots. In the heavily calcified annulus where extensive decalcification is first necessary or in an annulus that is difficult to visualise, this technique is not as safe and efficient as the use of multiple interrupted sutures.

Although suture techniques and suture thrombogenicity vary, there are no randomised studies demonstrating the superiority of one technique or suture material over another. Rather, surgeons have learned to vary their technique and sutures depending on the condition of the annulus and the prosthesis being implanted.

Valve handling

Inasmuch as possible, valve implantation should be accomplished without handling the valve itself, except with the appropriate valve holder, a soft probe or a carefully gloved finger. Handling a valve leaflet, sewing ring, or struts with sharp instruments can bend or break struts and damage the finely polished surface of the mechanical valve, thus creating a nidus for thrombus formation. A tear in a glove when tying sutures can deposit skin oils and contaminants on the chemically clean surface of the valve, which then changes the interfacial potential of the valve surface and may predispose to thrombus formation[35].

Valve choice and orientation

The choice of an appropriate valve prosthesis and its orientation when implanted are both important in order to achieve optimal function. The caged ball valves, such as the Starr-Edwards and Smeloff-Cutter, can be easily implanted in a large heart with an adequate left ventricular cavity or in patients with a generous aortic annulus and ascending aorta. However, implanting a caged ball valve into the mitral position in a small left ventricular cavity is probably not wise; not only does the relatively bulky cage abut against the interventricular septum, partially obstructing the left ventricular outflow tract, but full ball travel may be prevented also, predisposing to thrombosis[46].

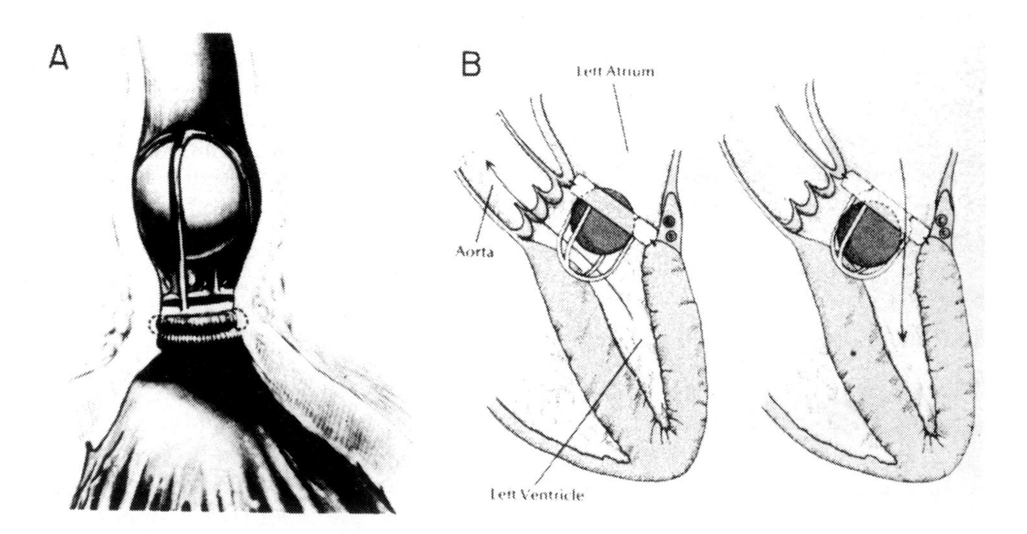

Figure 1.6–4: (A) Decreased secondary orifice between prosthetic valve ball and wall of ascending aorta. (B) Bulky cage and ball of mitral valve prosthesis partially obstructing left ventricular outflow tract in patient with a small left ventricle.

A caged ball valve in the small aortic root with a small ascending aorta provides a decreased secondary orifice be tween the ball in the open position and the aortic wall, producing relative obstruction to blood flow (Fig. 1.6–4).

In implanting stented bioprostheses, the surgeon must be aware of several potential complications related to valve orientation. In mitral valve implantation, placing a valve strut directly underneath the aortic valve should be avoided, since this obstructs the left ventricular outflow tract. In patients with a small left ventricular cavity, positioning a valve strut directly against the posterior wall, particularly in cases where the posterior leaflet has been removed, has been implicated as a potential cause of posterior left ventricular rupture due to strut perforation[47]. In implanting stented bioprostheses in the aortic position, one must avoid placing a strut directly in front of the right or left coronary orifice.

Opinions vary regarding the optimal orientation of the large opening when implanting pivoting disc valves such as the Bjørk-Shiley valve, the Medtronic Hall valve, or the Omniscience valve. The author's preference, based on 20 years' experience with pivoting disc valves, is to place the larger orifice anteriorly in the mitral position, providing that the disc moves freely in this orientation. De Wall and associates noted decreased thromboembolic complications with the mitral Omniscience valve in this orientation in comparison to a posterior orientation of the larger orifice[48]. However, many surgeons report satisfactory results with other pivoting disc valves using a posterior orientation of the larger orifice, and flow patterns within the left ventricle appear more physiological with this orientation (see Chapter 2.1). When implanting aortic pivoting disc valves, the larger orifice should be placed towards the non-coronary sinus, providing that the disc moves freely in this position. This orientation probably secures optimal blood flow around the outer curvature of the aorta.

There is a choice of orientation in both the aortic and mitral positions with bi-leaflet valves as well. In implanting a St. Jude mitral valve, Chaux and associates advocate orientating the pivoting axis of the two leaflets perpendicular to the interventricular septum in order to avoid asynchronous closure of the valve. In the aortic position, an orientation perpendicular to the interventricular septum is again recommended. Since the hinge guard protects the valve leaflets, Chaux and associates also recommend positioning the hinge guard towards any potential obstacle such as excessive bulging of a hypertrophied septum or an area of residual calcium, thus pushing this area away from the valve leaflets[49].

Left atrial appendage ligation

Patients who have a large left atrium, particularly those who also have atrial fibrillation in the presence of mitral valve disease, may have thrombus in the left atrium[50]. This has led some surgeons to routinely ligate the left atrial appendage on patients undergoing mitral valve surgery, in an attempt to reduce the incidence of thromboembolism[51,52]. Most cardiac surgeons have had the experience of operating on a patient with mitral valve disease and, on opening the left atrium, finding clot within the left atrium. In this circumstance, the left atrial appendage is almost always involved, and it is not unreasonable to exclude this source of potential thromboembolic complications by ligating or oversewing the entrance of the atrial appendage. Unfortunately there is no randomised clinical series reported in the literature clearly demonstrating that ligating the atrial appendage decreases the risk of thromboembolism, and this practice remains a personal choice for surgeons. For those who believe in obliterating the left atrial appendage, the use of an automatic surgical stapler may be a safe and expeditious way of accomplishing this procedure[53].

SUMMARY

Thromboembolism is a complex subject, influenced by many different patient-related factors, by prosthetic valve choice and surgical technique and by intensity of anticoagulation (Chapter 3.4). It is perhaps not surprising therefore that the literature offers no clear guidance on the timing of surgery in relation to the prevention of thromboembolism. Traditional indications for valve surgery are generally the progression of symptoms to NYHA Class 3, the development of ventricular failure, or deterioration of ventricular function. Unfortunately, these indications often postdate the development of atrial fibrillation or atrial and ventricular enlargement, all risk factors for thromboembolic complications even prior to valve replacement.

Ideally, one would like to operate on cardiac patients prior to the development of congestive heart failure, atrial fibrillation, or left atrial enlargement. If this ideal goal cannot be met, at least ventricular function and atrial fibrillation should be carefully anticipated and surgery of the diseased valve carried out before irreversible atrial and ventricular changes occur that preclude a return to sinus rhythm or an improvement in ventricular function. Appropriate valve repair techniques, where applicable, and careful accurate valve replacement should minimise the iatrogenic causes of thromboembolic complications.

REFERENCES

1. Kannel WB, Abbott RD, Savage DD, McNamara PM. Epidemiologic features of atrial fibrillation: the Framingham Study. N Engl J Med 1982;306:1018 1022.
2. Selzer A. Atrial fibrillation revisited. N Engl J Med 1982;306:1044 1045.
3. Davidson E, Weinberger I, Rotenberg Z, Fuchs J, Agmon J. Atrial fibrillation. Arch Intern Med 1989;149:457–459.
4. Cameron A, Schwartz MJ, Kronmal RA, Kosinski AS. Prevalence and significance of atrial fibrillation in coronary artery disease (CASS Registry). Am J Cardiol 1988;61:714–717.
5. Bailey GWH, Braniff BA, Hancock EW, Cohn KE. Relation of left atrial pathology to atrial fibrillation in mitral valvular disease. Ann Intern Med 1968;69:13–20.
6. Boyden PA, Tilley LP, Pham TD, Liu S-K, Fenoglio JJ Jr, Wit AL. Effects of left atrial enlargement on atrial transmembrane potentials and structure in dogs with mitral valve fibrosis. Am J Cardiol 1982;49:1896–1908.
7. Singer DH, Ten Eick RE, De Boar AA. Electrophysiologic correlates of human atrial tachyarrhythmias. In Dreifus L, Leikoff W, eds. Cardiac Arrhythmias. 25th Hahnemann Symposium. New York, Grune and Stratton, 1973:97 110.
8. Wolf PA, Dawber TR, Thomas HE, Kannel WB. Epidemiologic assessment of chronic atrial fibrillation and risk of stroke: The Framingham Study. Neurology 1978;28:973–977.
9. Szekely P. Systemic embolism and anticoagulant prophylaxis in rheumatic heart disease. Br Med J 1964;1:1209–1212.
10. Fleming HA, Bailey SM. Mitral valve disease, systemic embolism and anticoagulants. Postgrad Med J 1971;47:599–604.
11. Godtfredsen J. Atrial fibrillation, etiology, course and prognosis: a follow-up study of 1,212 cases. Copenhagen, Munksgaard, 1975.
12. Godtfredsen J, Petersen P. Thromboembolic complications in atrial fibrillation. In Refsum H, Sulg IA, Rasmussen K, eds. Heart and Brain, Brain and Heart. Heidelberg, Springer-Verlag, 1989:225–229.
13. Petersen P, Godtfredsen J. Embolic complications in paroxysmal atrial fibrillation. Stroke 1986;17:622–626.
14. Wolf PA, Kannel WB, McGee DL, Meeks SL, Bharucha NE, McNamara PM. Duration of atrial fibrillation and imminence of stroke: The Framingham Study. Stroke 1983;14:664–667.
15. Britton M, Gustafsson C. Non-rheumatic atrial fibrillation as a risk factor for stroke. Stroke 1985;16:182–188.
16. Petersen P, Kastrup J, Brinch K, Godtfredsen J, Boysen G. Relation between left atrial dimension and duration of atrial fibrillation. Am J Cardiol 1987;60:382–384.
17. Burchfiel CM, Hammermeister KE, Krause-Steinrauf H, et al. Left atrial dimension and risk of systemic embolism in patients with a prosthetic heart valve. J Am Coll Cardiol 1990;15:32–41.
18. Moss AJ. Atrial fibrillation and cerebral embolism (editorial). Arch Neurol 1984;41:707.
19. Caplan LR, D'Cruz I, Hier DB, Reddy H, Shah S. Atrial size, atrial fibrillation, and stroke. Ann Neurol 1986;19:158–161.
20. Sasaki W, Yanagisawa S, Maki K, Onodera A, Awaji T, Kanazawa T. High incidence of silent small cerebral infarction in the patients with atrial fibrillation (abstract). Circulation 1987;76(suppl IV):104.
21. Mitchell S, Miller G, Stinson E, et al. Significant patient-related determinants of prosthetic valve performance. J Thorac Cardiovasc Surg 1986;91:807–817.
22. Moncada S, Gryglewski R, Bunting S, Vane JR. An enzyme isolated from arteries transforms prostaglandin endoperoxides to an unstable substance that inhibits platelet aggregation. Nature 1976;263:663–665.
23. Weksler BB, Marcus AJ, Jaffe EA. Synthesis of prostaglandin I_1 (prostacyclin) by cultured human and bovine endothelial cells. Proc Natl Acad Sci (USA) 1977;74:3922–3926.
24. Esmon CT, Esmon NB, Harris KW. Complex formation between thrombin and thrombumudulin inhibits both thrombin-catalyzed fibrin formation and Factor V activation. J Biol Chem 1982;257:7944–7947.
25. Loskutoff DJ, Levin E. Properties of plasminogen activators produced by endothelial cells. In Jaffe EA, ed. Biology of Endothelial Cells. Boston, Martinus Nijhoff, 1984:200–208.
26. Collen D. On the regulation and control of fibrinolysis. Thromb Hemostat 1979;43:77–89.
27. Colman RW, Scott CF, Schmaier AH, Wachtfogel YT, Pixley RA, Edmunds LH Jr. Initiation of blood coagulation at artificial surfaces. Ann NY Acad Sci 1987;516:253–267.
28. Edmunds LH Jr. The Sangreal. J Thorac Cardiovasc Surg 1985;90:1–6.
29. Kirklin JW, Barratt-Boyes BG. Cardiac Surgery. New York, Wiley, 1986;414.
30. Edmunds LH Jr. Thrombotic and bleeding complications of prosthetic heart valves. Ann Thorac Surg 1987;44:430–445.
31. Miller DC, Stinson EB, Jamieson SW, Baumgartner WA, Shumway NE. Ten to fifteen year reassessment

of the performance characteristics of the Starr-Edwards Model 6120 mitral valve prosthesis. J Thorac Cardiovasc Surg 1983;85:1–20.
32. Kuntze CEE, Eijgelaar A, Ebels T, van der Heide JNH. Rates of thromboembolism with three different mechanical heart valve prostheses: randomized study. Lancet 1989;1:514–517.
33. Berger K, Sauvage LR, Wood SJ, Wesolowski SA. Sewing ring healing of cardiac valve prostheses. Surgery 1967;61:102–117.
34. Roon AJ, Moore WS, Goldstone J, Towan H, Campagna G. Comparative surface thrombogenicity of implanted vascular grafts. J Surg Res 1977;22:165–173.
35. Lee ME, Murakami T, Stanczewski B, Parmeggiani A, Srinivasan S, Sawyer PN. Etiology of thrombus formation on prosthetic metal heart valves. J Thorac Cardiovasc Surg 1972;63:809–819.
36. Bokrow JC, LaGrange LD, Schoen JF. Control of structure of carbon for use in bioengineering. In Walker PL, ed. Chemistry and Physics of Carbon. Vol. 9. New York, Dekker, 1972:117–154.
37. Salzman EW. Non-thrombogenic surfaces: a critical review. Blood 1971;38:509–523.
38. Okita Y, Miki S, Kusuhara K, et al. Intractable hemolysis caused by perivalvular leakage following mitral valve replacement with St. Jude Medical prosthesis. Ann Thorac Surg 1988;46:89–92.
39. Starek PJK, McLaurin LP, Wilcox BR, Murray GF. Clinical evaluation of the Lillehei-Kaster pivoting disc valve. Ann Thorac Surg 1976;22:362–368.
40. Starek PJK. Immobilization of disc heart valves by unraveled sutures. Ann Thorac Surg 1981;31:66–69.
41. Dahlke H, Dociu N, Thurau K. Thrombogenicity of different suture materials as revealed by scanning electron microscopy. J Biomed Mater Res 1980;14:251–268.
42. Wada J. The knotless suture method for prosthetic valve fixation. Int Surg 1966;46:317–320.
43. Lefrak EA, Starr A. The Starr Edwards ball valve. In: Cardiac Valve Prostheses. New York, Appleton Century Crofts, 1979:72.
44. Hjelms E, Vilhelmsen R, Rygg IH. Continuous suture technique in prosthetic aortic valve replacement. J Cardiovasc Surg 1982;23:145–148.
45. Messmer BJ, Okies JE, Hallman GL, Cooley DA. Mitral valve replacement with the Bjørk-Shiley tilting disc prosthesis. J Thorac Cardiovasc Surg 1971;62:938–946.
46. Roberts WC, Morrow AG. Mechanisms of acute left atrial thrombosis after mitral valve replacement: pathologic findings indicating obstruction to left atrial emptying. Am J Cardiol 1966;18:497–503.
47. Bortolotti U, Thiene G, Casarotto D, Mazzucco A, Gallucci V: Left ventricular rupture following mitral valve replacement with a Hancock bioprosthesis. Chest 1980;77:235–237.
48. De Wall RA. Thrombotic complications with the Omniscience valve: a current review. J Thorac Cardiovasc Surg 1989;98:298–299.
49. Chaux A, Blanche C. Technical aspects of valvular replacement with the St. Jude prosthesis. J Cardiovasc Surg 1987;28:363–368.
50. Bailey CP, Glover RP, O'Neill TJ. Surgery of mitral stenosis. J Thorac Cardiovasc Surg 1950;19:16–49.
51. Thomas TV. Left atrial appendage and valve replacement. Am Heart J 1972;84:838–839.
52. Matloff JM, Collins JJ, Sullivan JM, Gorlin R, Harker DE. Control of thromboembolism for prosthetic heart valves. Ann Thorac Surg 1969;8:133 145.
53. DiSesa VJ, Tamm S, Cohen LH. Ligation of left atrial appendage using an automatic surgical stapler. Ann Thorac Surg 1988;46:652–653.

Chapter 1.7

The Effects of Cardiopulmonary Bypass and its Pharmacological Management

Kenneth M Taylor

This chapter focuses on the subject of haemostasis during and after heart surgery. This subject has occupied the minds and the time of cardiac surgeons from the earliest days of cardiac surgery, principally because cardiac surgical patients have a propensity to bleed excessively and, until recently, there was no consistently effective therapeutic approach to this problem available. Interest in bleeding and haemostasis in cardiac surgery has, of course, been significantly increased in the past four years as a result of the major emphasis on blood conservation. Not only are homologous blood products a precious and relatively scarce resource, but more importantly there is concern among patients and their surgeons regarding the risks associated with blood and blood product transfusions - particularly the transmission of virus infections such as hepatitis and HIV infections[1] (Table 1.7–1). Gone are the days when blood transfusions were regarded as wholly therapeutic and completely safe. Today caution must be exercised in the approach to blood or blood product transfusion. It should be stressed that blood products (platelets, cryoprecipitate, fresh frozen plasma, etc.) constitute a quantitatively greater risk, since the patient is exposed to more donors; for example one unit of a blood product may be pooled from several donors.

Blood conservation is now mandatory in cardiac surgical practice and surgical techniques have been modified in order to facilitate this. Apart from the sine qua non of good surgical technique, there are two principal approaches, namely (a) blood salvage and autotransfusion and (b) the use of pharmacological agents to prevent and/or correct the haemostatic defect.

Autotransfusion techniques may be applied before, during and after surgery. Donation of the patient's own blood in the weeks prior to surgery has been reported in many centres[2], although geographical and logistical factors limit its applicability. Intraoperative retrieval of shed blood, and its subsequent processing by washing/concentrating systems, has been used successfully to provide autotransfusion blood of apparently acceptable quality, with consequent reduction in the need for homologous transfusions[3,4]. This concept has been extended into the postoperative period, using relatively inexpensive and simple chest drainage systems to collect, filter and reinfuse the blood which is lost through the chest drain in the early postoperative period[5].

Intra- and postoperative salvage techniques raise the question of the quality of the blood processed for reinfusion. Although the oxygen carrying capacity of the red cells appears to be satisfactory, other reports have suggested that vasoactive and blood cell activation agents (e.g. thromboxane) may be present in potentially harmful concentrations[6]. Although impressive results have been reported with autotransfusion techniques in patients having their first heart operation, patients exposed to the high

Table: 1.7–1

Hazard		*Incidence per Unit Transfusion*
Transmission of infective agent:	hepatitis	1:100
	HIV	1:40,000 – 10^6
	CMV	–
	HTLV I/II	–
Immunological reactions	fever, urticaria	1:100
	haemolysis	1:6,000
	fatal haemolysis	1:100,000

risk of bleeding associated with redo procedures or septic endocarditis still require considerable volumes of blood and blood product transfusions.

The emphasis of this chapter is on the use of pharmacological agents to reduce or even prevent the underlying haemostatic defects associated with cardiac surgery.

HAEMOSTATIC MECHANISMS DURING CARDIAC SURGERY

This is an area of considerable complexity. In order to perform open heart surgery, the use of cardiopulmonary bypass is mandatory. Extracorporeal circulation imposes the requirement of full systemic anticoagulation and also induces major changes in blood cells and their activity. The changes begin with the activation of circulating coagulation factor XII when blood contacts the artificial surfaces of the extracorporeal circuit. Activated factor XII (XIIa) stimulates a number of important cascade mechanisms, including coagulation, fibrinolysis, kallikrein release and complement activation[7,8] (Fig. 1.7–1). Platelet and white blood cell activation also occurs, resulting in a systemic inflammatory response. The latter is seen in most vital organs, but is particularly well demonstrated in the lungs[9–11], where neutrophil sequestration occurs in the pulmonary capillaries, with adherence and subsequent damage to the capillary endothelium (Fig. 1.7–2). The haemostatic mechanisms during cardiac surgery may be influenced by several factors, including (a) heparin anticoagulation, (b) fibrinolysis, kallikrein and complement pathways (via factor XIIa) and (c) disturbances of platelet function.

HEPARIN AND PROTAMINE

The pharmacology of heparin is described in detail in Chapter 3.2. Its mechanism of action is summarised briefly here to facilitate understanding of this chapter. Heparin is a negatively charged mucopolysaccharide, which itself has no direct effect on coagulation. However, once bound to circulating antithrombin III, also known as heparin co-factor, the heparin-antithrombin III complex exerts a powerful inhibitory effect on coagulation[12]. Although initially the effect was thought to be via thrombin and fibrinogen inhibition, it is now known that the complex inhibits many factors in the coagulation cascade, including factors XIIa, XIa and Xa, in addition to inhibitory effects

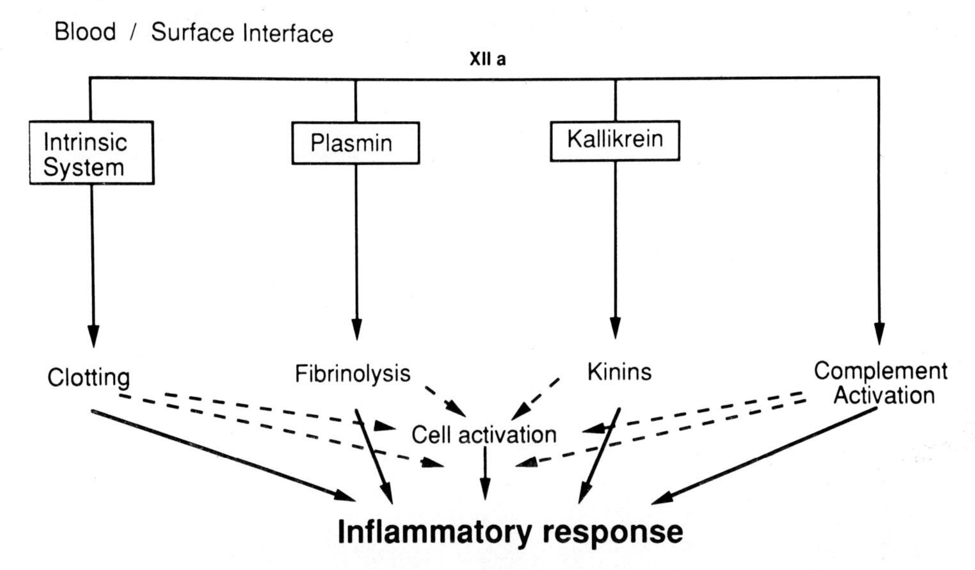

Figure 1.7–1: Contact activation pathways, including stimulation of coagulation, fibrinolysis and complement activation.

on plasmin and kallikrein[13]. It is recognised that there is a considerable variability in the anticoagulant activity of different heparin preparations and even of different batches. Comparative studies of beef lung heparin and pork mucosal heparin suggest that this variability in activity relates to the variations in heparin molecular weight fractions. Commercial heparin preparations have molecular weights ranging from 5,000 to over 25,000 daltons. Heparin with low molecular weight (including recently studied and specifically prepared preparations with molecular weights around 4-6,000 d) have been shown to exert low levels of thrombin inhibition, but high levels of factor Xa inhibition with consequent inhibition of both intrinsic and extrinsic coagulation systems[14].

Protamine is a positively charged peptide, derived from fish sperm, which binds to heparin, forming a heparin-protamine complex that prevents heparin from enhancing the anticoagulant effect of antithrombin III, and hence allows the coagulation cascade to proceed. Although heparin neutralisation with protamine is well tolerated in most patients, numerous protamine side effects have been described, including severe arterial hypotension and allergic reactions which may be life threatening.

Heparin and protamine dosage and administration

In view of the considerable variability in anticoagulant activity of heparin preparations, monitoring of anticoagulation levels during cardiac surgery is mandatory. Most cardiac units use either the accelerated or activated clotting time (ACT). The technique was introduced by Hattersley in 1966[15] and is based on a 10-fold acceleration of the whole blood clotting time. As with the whole blood clotting time[16], a dose response curve exists between heparin dosage and prolongation of the ACT. The normal range for ACT is quoted as 81-133 seconds (95% range)[15]. Although there is considerable individual variation in the ACT prolongation after a specified dose of

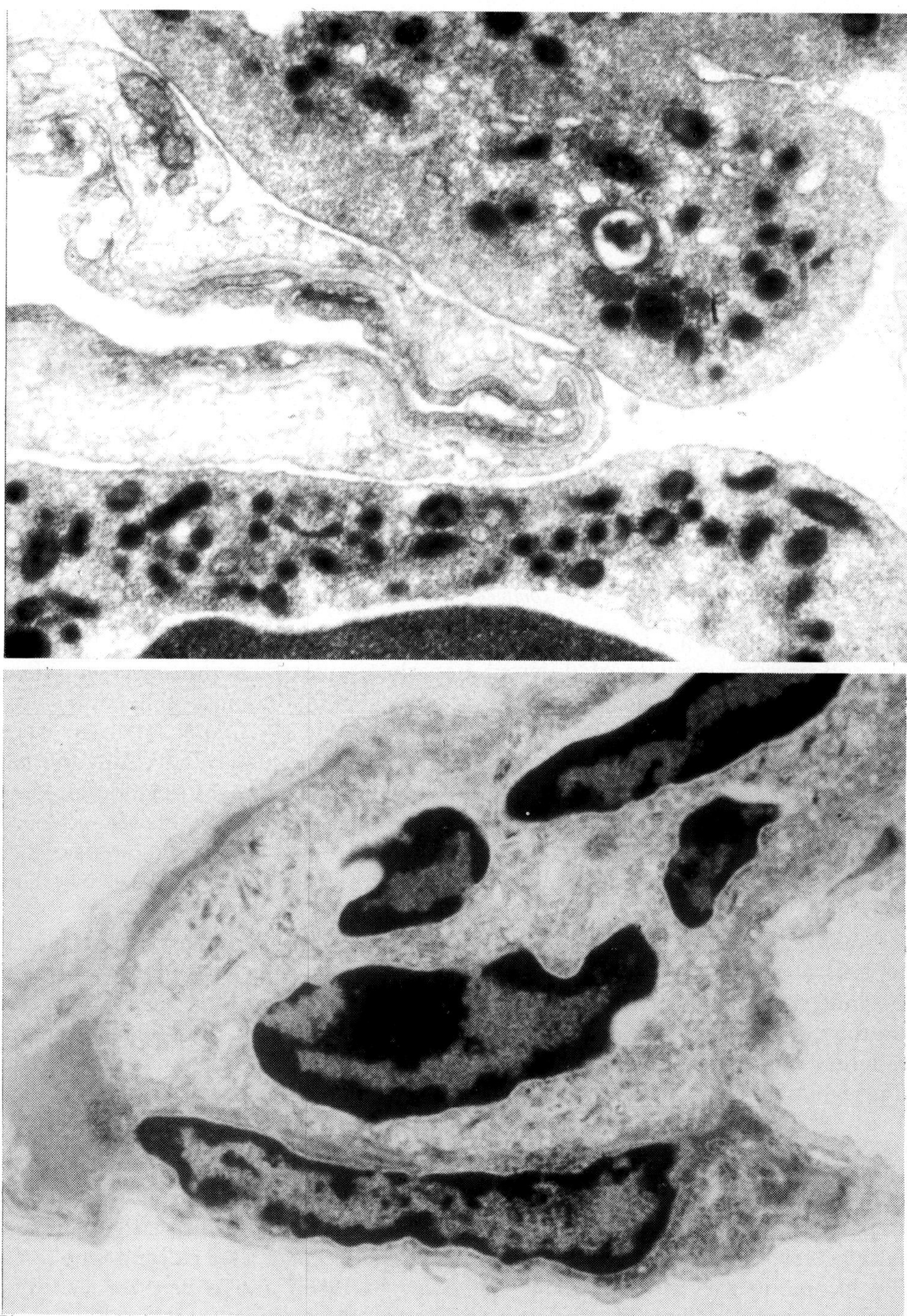

Figure 1.7–2 (a): Scanning electron microscope (SEM) picture of pre-CPB neutrophil circulating within pulmonary capillary. (x 16,000)

Figure 1.7–2 (b): SEM of post-cardiopulmonary bypass (30 min) period, showing neutrophil adherent to pulmonary capillary endothelium. (x 12,600)

heparin[17], the relationship for any one individual between heparin dose and ACT prolongation is approximately linear, up to an ACT of about 500 seconds[18,19].

Although the ACT is widely used, the test has some limitations. They include reduced accuracy at high heparin dosage levels and under conditions of systemic hypothermia. An alternative test is that which measures heparin activity based upon protamine neutralisation[20]. Although considered to be more accurate than the ACT system, this test is more complex and more expensive.

Currently, most units use a heparin/protamine dosage protocol similar to the following:

- Initial heparin dose: 300 units heparin/kg body weight
- Target ACT level: over 450–480 sec. throughout cardiopulmonary bypass
- Histamine reversal dose: 0.75–1.0 mg protamine/100 units of initial heparin dose.

Fibrinolysis, kallikrein and complement pathways

Contact activation of factor XII (Fig. 1.7–1) is considered to be the principal event in triggering host defence mechanisms when blood is exposed to any foreign surface. Activated factor XII (factor XIIa) itself initiates (a) intrinsic coagulation via factor XI, (b) kallikrein release via pre-kallikrein and (c) bradykinin release via factor XII binding to high molecular weight kininogen.

Kallikrein itself activates neutrophils and, together with bradykinin, activates the fibrinolytic system both via plasmin production (a kallikrein effect on pro-urokinase) and via release of tissue plasminogen activator (tPA) from endothelium (a bradykinin effect). Finally, contact activation is also directly involved in complement activation in a complex relationship involving factor XII, kallikrein and plasmin[21,22].

During cardiopulmonary bypass, contact activation inevitably occurs on a massive scale as the circulating blood passes over the foreign surfaces of the extracorporeal circuit. Such activation of host-defence mechanisms results in a systemic inflammatory reaction within which increased fibrinolysis and platelet activation are of particular concern in relation to haemostasis.

Fibrinolysis during cardiac surgery

The possibility of increased fibrinolysis during cardiac surgery has been addressed in a number of reports, some dating back many years[23–25]. Some reports suggested that increased fibrinolytic activity was evident before the onset of cardiopulmonary bypass and persisted for some hours afterwards, and that hypothermia and prolonged cardiopulmonary bypass times increased fibrinolytic activity even further[23]. The perception that increased fibrinolysis was a major adverse factor in cardiac surgery prompted the use of antifibrinolytic agents such as epsilon-amino-caproic-acid (EACA)[26] and aprotinin[23], in attempts to reduce bleeding.

In fact, the evidence for a hyperfibrinolytic state during routine cardiac surgery is unclear[27,28]. Certainly it has been shown by Tanaka and co-workers that tissue plasminogen activator (tPA) levels increase prior to the onset of cardiopulmonary bypass, and rise to maximal levels after 60 minutes on bypass[29]. Recent studies have, however, suggested that increased fibrinolysis is usually not the principal cause of increased bleeding, and that many of the changes in coagulation factors, fibrinogen, plasminogen and fibrin-degradation products are simply attributable to haemodilution[30].

Platelet function during cardiac surgery

Considerable evidence exists that platelet function is significantly disturbed during cardiac surgery. In addition to the anticipated fall in platelet count as a result of haemodilution, an increase in bleeding time and impaired aggregation have been described[31,32].

Although it is generally agreed that contact activation is of primary importance in inducing platelet dysfunction, the precise mechanisms are not defined. Some studies suggest that cardiopulmonary bypass induces a state of activation similar to that induced by adenosine diphosphate (ADP), as shown by increases in plasma levels of release factors including platelet factor 4, beta-thromboglobulin and thromboxane B_2[31,33,34]. In addition, the morphological shape changes in platelets, which have been demonstrated in cardiac surgical studies, are essentially identical to those seen during platelet activation.

Other studies have focused on the changes in platelet membrane receptor populations during cardiopulmonary bypass. In particular, significant reductions in the glycoprotein receptors, GpIb and GpIIb/IIIa complex have been reported[35,36]. Although it would be convenient to relate reduced platelet surface receptors to impaired haemostasis, the relationship appears complex, and may require major loss of surface receptors (particularly the GpIIb/IIIa complex which binds fibrinogen) before any haemostatic impairment could be anticipated.

DRUG THERAPY TO REDUCE BLOOD LOSS DURING CARDIAC SURGERY

Epsilon-amino-caproic acid (EACA)

EACA is a lysine analogue which exerts an antifibrinolytic effect by blocking the lysine binding sites by which plasminogen and plasmin bind to fibrin[37]. EACA has been used successfully to reduce blood loss in several clinical situations (for example transurethral prostatectomy[38]), but its efficacy in reducing blood loss in cardiac surgery is controversial[39,40]. Thrombotic complications have been reported in association with its use[41,42] and, despite 25 years' availability, its value in cardiac surgical practice remains dubious.

Tranexamic acid

This drug is also a lysine analogue with a reported increase in plasminogen binding 6 times that of EACA. Despite the anticipated increase in efficacy, studies have shown little increase in clinical benefit[43].

Desmopressin acetate (DDAVP)

Desmopressin is a synthetic vasopressin analogue which has reduced vasoconstrictor effects. Its mode of action in haemostasis is thought to be related to improved platelet adhesion, mediated through release of von Willebrand factor (vWF) from endothelial cells[44,45]. DDAVP is particularly effective in reducing bleeding times in patients with von Willebrand's disease and in haemophiliacs.

In recent studies using DDAVP therapy (0.3 μg/kg) in cardiac surgery, some authors reported significant reductions in blood loss, while others failed to demonstrate any real effect on bleeding[46,47]. In a randomised double-blind trial of patients undergoing heart valve surgery with or without coronary grafting, Salzman and associates showed a reduction in blood loss of almost 1 litre over 24 hours in the treated group[48]. Transfusion requirements in the first 24 hours were not, however, significantly different for treated and control groups.

Prostacyclin and other prostaglandin derivatives

Prostacyclin (PGI2) is a naturally occurring prostaglandin that inhibits platelet activation by increasing platelet cyclic adenosine monophosphate (AMP) levels, mediated by stimulation of adenyl cyclase[49]. PGI2 has a short duration of action, but is a relatively potent vasodilator. As a consequence, arterial hypotension has been a feature in several reported studies, limiting drug delivery and compromising its usefulness[50,51].

The potential role for prostacyclin in cardiac surgery, to preserve platelet numbers and function without impairing the coagulation process, led to its use in several clinical studies. Although several authors reported the expected effects of preserving circulating platelets, there was no consistent or convincing evidence that bleeding was reduced. Interpretation of the studies was complicated by great variability in the dose of prostacyclin administered, ranging from 10 to 100 mg/kg/min. The variability in dosage used may reflect the problem of excessive vasodilation and consequent hypotension at higher dose levels[50–54].

More recently, carbacyclin and oxycyclin derivatives of prostacyclin have been developed in an attempt to reduce the hypotensive side effects of the parent[55]. Reported experience with these analogues has, however, been disappointing[56].

Aprotinin

Aprotinin is a serine proteinase inhibitor (molecular weight = 6512) isolated from bovine lung. It inhibits several proteinases, including trypsin, plasmin and kallikrein. In view of its antiplasmin effect, it is also considered to be an antifibrinolytic agent. The drug must be given by intravenous injection, and its plasma half-life is around 2 hours.

Aprotinin has been used in the past in a number of clinical situations, including acute pancreatitis, septic and haemorrhagic shock and adult respiratory distress syndrome (ARDS). In 1964, Tice and co-authors reported its use in cardiac surgical patients as an antifibrinolytic agent[23]. Although subsequent use by others suggested that aprotinin might be effective in reducing bleeding after cardiac surgery[57,58], these results were not widely recognised and the drug's potential role in cardiac surgery was effectively ignored.

The recent resurgence of interest in aprotinin was prompted by reports from the Hammersmith group that high dose aprotinin therapy, used initially in an attempt to block complement and kallikrein induced lung damage, showed remarkable efficacy in reducing blood loss and blood transfusion requirements in cardiac surgical patients [59–61].

Initial clinical studies and dosage regime

An empirical dose regime was calculated prior to carrying out these initial studies, based on a 4μ molar plasma concentration of aprotinin, which would effectively block kallikrein. Aprotinin dosage or activity is hence expressed in kallikrein-inhibitory units (KIU). 100,000 KIU is equivalent to 14 mg protein. The actual regime used in the clinical studies was as follows:

- Loading dose of 2×10^6 KIU (280 mg)
- Pump prime dose of 2×10^6 KIU (280 mg)
- Maintenance infusion of 0.5×10^6 KIU per hour until the end of the operation (70 mg per hour).

Two distinct cohorts of patients were studied:-

Study 1: Primary coronary artery surgery. Placebo-controlled, randomised, double blind study in 80 patients (Table 1.7–2).

Study 2: Re-do cardiac surgery procedures. Prospective, randomised study in 22 patients (Table 1.7–3).

In the primary study[59], blood loss in the control group was 573 ml compared to 309 ml in the aprotinin group ($p < 0.01$). Haemoglobin loss was around 37 gm in the controls compared to 12 gm in the aprotinin group. Seventy-five units of blood were transfused in the control (n=40), compared to 13 units in the aprotinin patients (n=40) despite a strict, standard post-operative transfusion protocol for all. At the 7th postoperative day, plasma haemoglobin levels were normal and identical in both groups.

The results in the re-do study[60] were even more impressive, since patients having repeat median sternotomy procedures often bleed excessively and require substantial volumes of blood and blood product transfusions. Postoperative blood loss was 286 ml in the aprotinin group compared to 1,509 ml in controls ($p<0.001$). Haemoglobin losses were 8 gm and 78 gm, respectively ($p<0.001$). Five units of blood were transfused in the 11 aprotinin patients, compared to 41 units in the 11 control patients. Seven of the 11 patients receiving aprotinin did not require any intra- or postoperative blood or blood product transfusion.

Table 1.7–2
Aprotinin Study 1 Results: Primary Coronary Surgery[59]

	Aprotinin (n=40)	*Control (n=40)*
Post-op blood loss (ml)	309 ± 133	573 ± 166 (p<0.01)
Post-op haemoglobin loss (gm)	12 ± 12.6	37.1 ± 18.3
Total no of blood units transfused	13	75
% of patients transfused	20%	95%
Average no of graphts	3.88 ± 0.5	3.86 ± 0.8

(Results expressed as mean ± S.D.)

Table 1.7–3
Aprotinin Study 2 Results: Re-do Cardiac Surgery[60]

	Aprotinin (n=11)	*Control (n=11)*
Post-op blood loss (ml)	286 ± 48	1509 ± 388 (p<0.001)
Post-op haemoglobin loss (gm)	8.3 ± 2.4	78 ± 23 (p<0.001)
Total no of blood units transfused	5	41
% of patients transfused	36%	100%

(Results expressed as mean ± S.E.M.)

Confirmatory studies on efficacy and safety

Since the initial reports from the Hammersmith group, aprotinin has been used extensively in many cardiac surgical centres in Europe, with similar reported efficacy and safety. A five-centre study of aprotinin therapy in primary coronary artery surgery patients, recently reviewed by Royston[62], reported significant reductions in blood loss and blood transfusion requirements in each study centre (Fig. 1.7–3). Similar results have also been reported from other centres in both primary and reoperations[63,64]. The high levels of efficacy, particularly in higher risk reoperations, have encouraged many cardiac surgeons to use aprotinin therapy routinely in such cases.

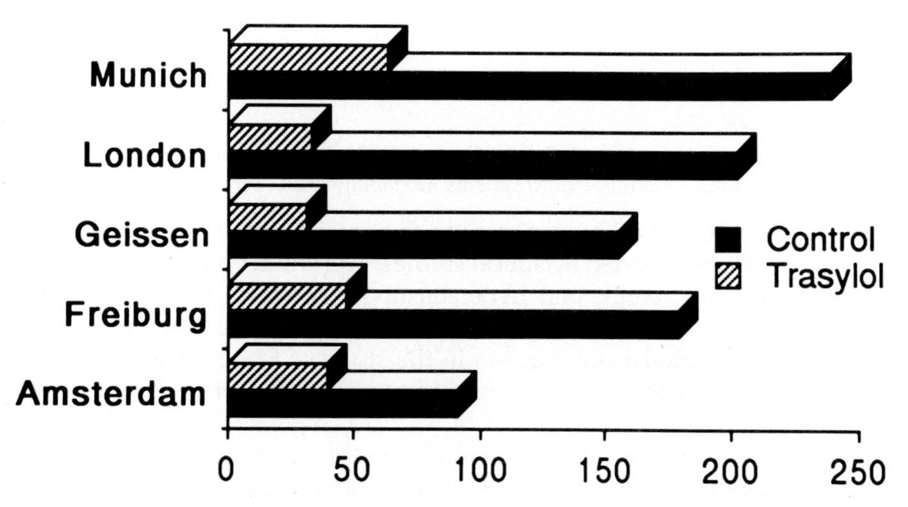

Figure 1.7–3: Donor blood transfusion units (per 100 cases) in five-centre study of aprotinin (Trasylol) therapy in primary coronary surgery patients. (Reproduced with permission from Royston D[68].)

Colloid required (ml/kg/24h)	73±40	49±32	NS

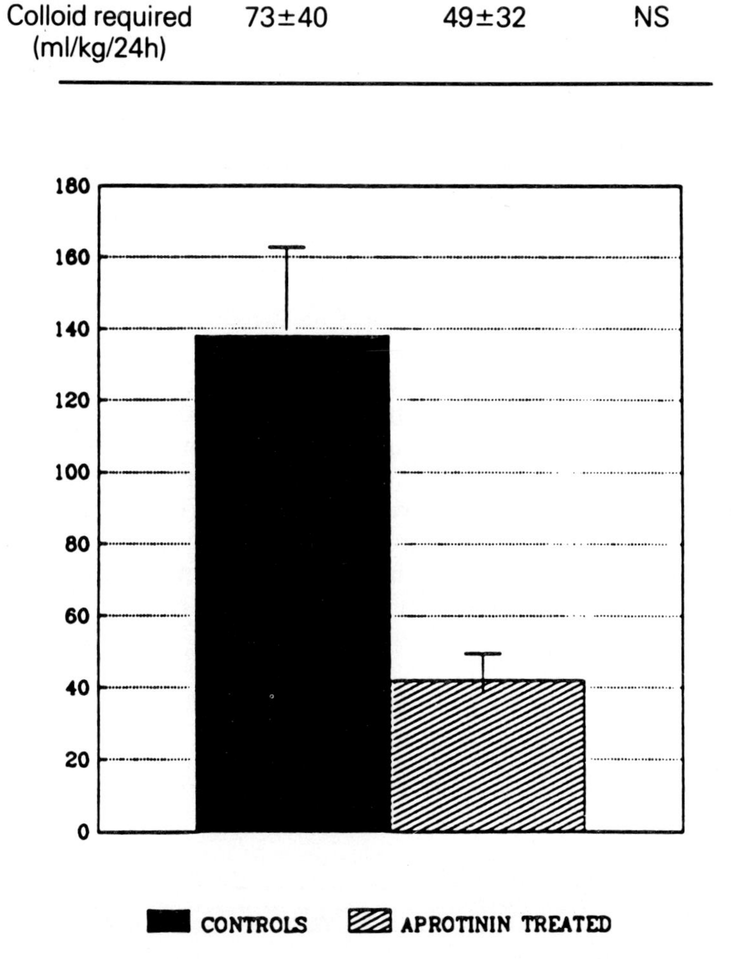

Figure 1.7–4: Chest closure times (minutes) and colloid requirements in paediatric cardiac surgical cases: placebo controls compared to aprotinin-treated patients. (Reproduced with permission from Elliott MJ[66].)

In addition to its proven efficacy, aprotinin therapy appears to be safe, with a low incidence of side effects reported in clinical studies. Aprotinin is a polypeptide derived from animal tissue and allergic and hypersensitivity reactions might be anticipated with its use. In fact, the incidence of allergic reactions appears to be extremely low, with only one report of anaphylactoid reaction in the study of Fraedrich and associates[63], and one severe allergic reaction in an open study of over 200 patients. There have been no clinical reports of renal or hepatic toxicity.

Although concerns have been raised that aprotinin therapy might be pro-thrombotic, with an increased incidence of myocardial Infarction and coronary vein graft occlusion, such fears have not been borne out in any of the studies reported to date. Prospective studies of coronary graft patency are in progress, although the multiple factors known

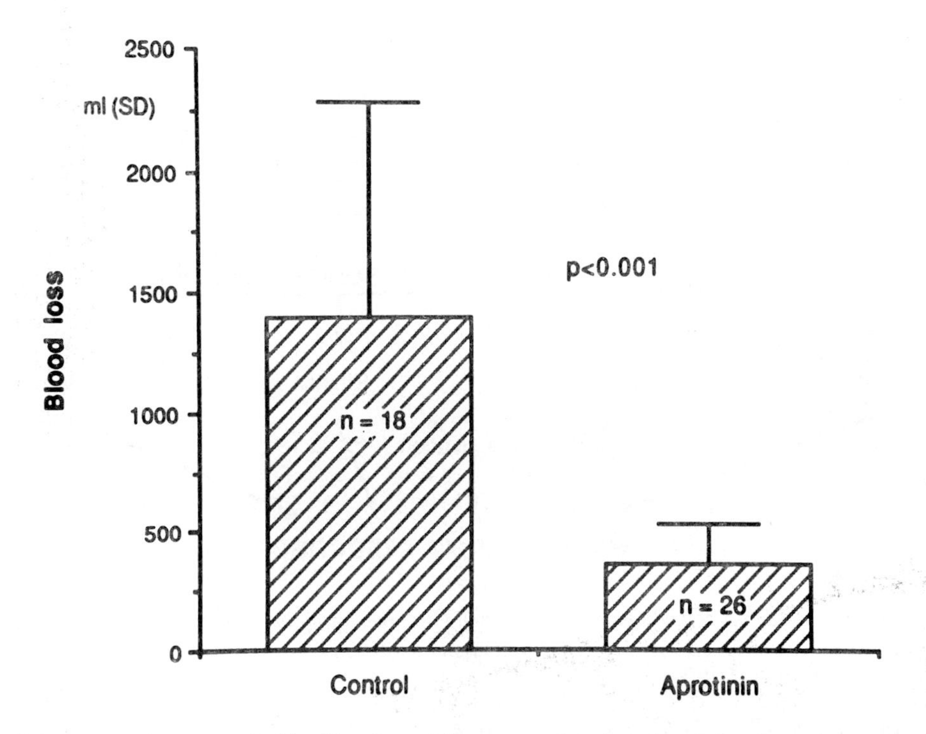

Figure 1.7–5: Post-operative blood loss in aspirin-pretreated patients (control and aprotinin groups). (Reproduced with permission from Bidstrup et al[67].)

to affect graft patency will make meaningful interpretation of results very difficult if not impossible. In fact, aprotinin is a mild anticoagulant (as evidenced by the increase in ACT levels seen in patients receiving the drug) and convincing evidence of pro-thrombotic tendency with aprotinin therapy is currently lacking.

Extended clinical use of aprotinin

In addition to the indications already described, aprotinin therapy appears to be effective in reducing blood loss in other cardiac and non-cardiac surgical procedures. Elliott[65] has recently reported beneficial effects in paediatric cardiac surgical cases (Fig. 1.7–4), with the time taken to achieve haemostasis and chest closure being reduced from 138 minutes in placebo controls to 42 minutes in treated cases ($p < 0.01$). Bidstup and others[66] have shown that patients maintained on aspirin therapy, who are known to bleed excessively during and after cardiac surgery, may successfully be treated with aprotinin (Fig. 1.7–5), reducing mean blood loss from 1,393 ml in controls to 352 ml in treated patients ($p < 0.001$).

Experience with the drug in heart and heart/lung transplantation, liver transplantation and major vascular surgery appears encouraging. There seems to be little doubt that aprotinin will prove useful in many other non-cardiac surgical procedures where blood loss and blood transfusion volumes are significant.

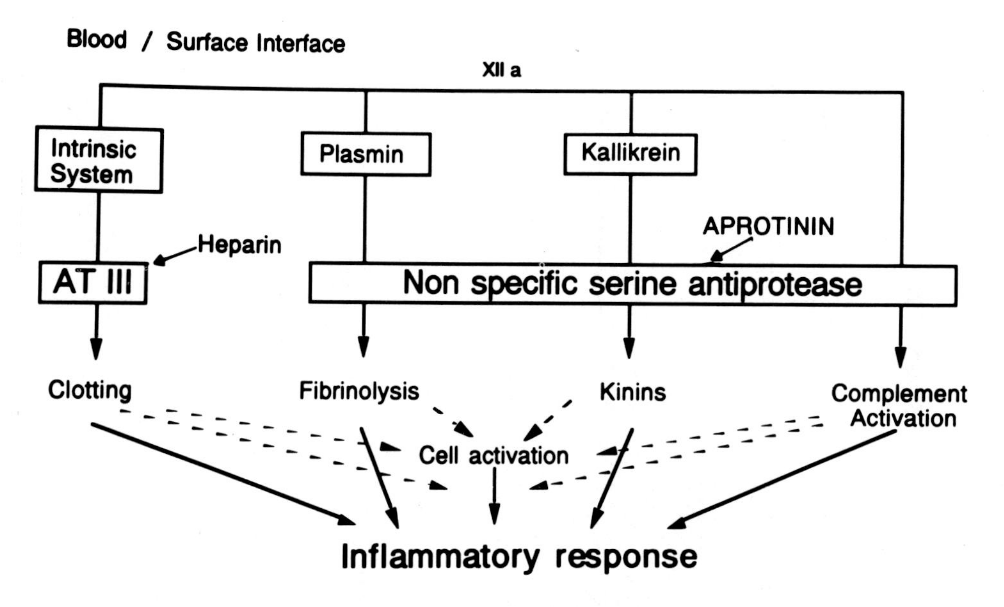

Figure 1.7–6: Contact activation pathways showing the broad range of inhibition induced by serine protease inhibition (aprotinin).

Mechanisms of action

The undoubted efficacy of aprotinin therapy in reducing bleeding in cardiac surgical patients raises intriguing questions as to its precise mode of action. Unfortunately, the broad range of antiprotease activity might indicate several, potentially interlinked mechanisms (Fig. 1.7–6). In addition, although most of the recent studies have been in cardiac cases, the fact that efficacy has been demonstrated in other forms of surgery (e.g. vascular and orthopaedic) might suggest that aprotinin acts via mechanisms that are not specific to the haemostatic disorders induced by cardiopulmonary bypass.

Certainly, aprotinin should act as an a antifibrinolytic agent by virtue of its antiplasmin effect. Although the arguments against a principal role for fibrinolysis in cardiac surgery have been reviewed previously in this chapter, a recent report has demonstrated elevated levels of fibrin degradation products during cardiopulmonary bypass, and significant suppression of this response by aprotinin[68]. Aprotinin has also been shown to be effective in preventing excessive bleeding in a patient requiring emergency coronary surgery 60 minutes after being given thrombolytic therapy[69].

Aprotinin may also exert a beneficial effect on platelets, specifically by preserving the glycoprotein surface receptor sites. van Oeveren and co-workers[70] have recently reported relative preservation of GpIb receptor sites in patients treated with aprotinin during cardiopulmonary bypass. Further studies on the effects of aprotinin on other receptor site populations are in progress. Finally, the antikallikrein effect of aprotinin may be important, particularly in relation to contact activation of factor XII and to plasmin release.

The numerous studies currently investigating the mechanisms of action of aprotinin may well lead to greater understanding of the complex and inter-related processes of coagulation, fibrinolysis, complement and blood cell activation, and of the inflammatory response in general. Until that time, aprotinin can be used 'empirically' to reduce blood loss in cardiac surgical practice, improving patient safety and making an unequalled contribution to blood conservation.

REFERENCES

1. NIH Consensus Conference: Perioperative red blood cell transfusion. JAMA 1988;60:2700–2703
2. Utely JR, Moores WY, Stephens DB. Blood conservation techniques. Ann Thorac Surg 1981;31:482–490
3. Noon GP. Intraoperative autotransfusion. Surgery 1978;84:719 -721
4. Schaff HV, Hauer JM, Brawley RK. Autotransfusion in cardiac surgical patients after operation. Surgery 1978;84:713–718
5. Cosgrove DM, Amiot DM, Meserko JJ. An improved technique for autotransfusion of shed mediastinal blood. Ann Thorac Surg 1985;40:519 -520
6. Moran S, Taylor KM. Prostaglandin concentrations in retrieved mediastinal blood. Perfusion (in press)
7. Kluft C, Dooijewaard G, Emeis JJ. Role of the contact system in fibrinolysis. Semin Thromb Hemost 1987;13:50–68
8. Kirklin JK, Westaby S, Blackstone EH et al. Complement and the damaging effects of cardiac surgery. J Thorac Cardiovasc Surg 1983;86:845–852
9. Ratliff NB, Young WG, Hacket DB et al. Pulmonary injury secondary to extracorporeal circulation. J Thorac Cardiovasc Surg 1973;65:425–431
10. Royston D, Fleming JS, Desai JB et al. Increased peroxide product generation associated with open heart surgery: Evidence for free radical generation. J Thorac Cardiovasc Surg 1986;91:759–766
11. Braude S, Nolop KB, Fleming JS et al. Increased pulmonary transvascular protien flux after canine cardiopulmonary bypass: Association with lung neutrophil sequestration and tissue peroxidation. Am Res Respir Dis 1986;134:867–872
12. Aren C. Heparin and Protamine Therapy. Seminars in Thorac and Cardiovasc Surg 1990;2:4, 364–372
13. Akkerman JWN, Bouma BN, Sixma JJ. Hemostasis. Ingelheim am Rhein, Boehringer Sohn, 1979; 100–121
14. Holmer E, Kurachi K, Soederstroem G. The molecular weight-dependance of the rate enhancing effect of heparin on the inhibition of thrombin, factor Xa, factor IXa, factor XIa, factor XIIa and kallikrein by antithrombin. Biochem J 1981;193:395–400
15. Hattersley PG. Activated coagulation time of whole blood. JAMA 1966; 196:150–154
16. Lee RI, White PD. A clinical study of the coagulation time of blood. Am J Med 1913;145:495–498
17. Bull BS, Korpman RA, Huse WM et al. Heparin therapy during extracorporeal circulation. I. Problems inherent in existing heparin protocols. J Thorac Cardiovasc Surg 1975;69:674–684
18. Bull BS, Huse WM, Brauer FS et al. Heparin therapy during extracorporeal circulation. II. The use of a dose-response curve to individualise heparin and protamine dosage. J Thorac Cardiovasc Surg 1975;69:685–689
19. Akl BF, Vargas GM, Neal J et al. Clinical experience with the activated clotting time for the control of heparin and protamine therapy during cardiopulmonary bypass. J Thorac Cardiovasc Surg 1980;79:97–102
20. Gundry SR, Drongowski RA, Coran AG et al. A comparison of methods to calculate the heparin reversal dose of protamine in cardiovascular surgery. Trans Am Soc Artif Intern Organs 1985;31:143–145
21. Wiggins RC, Ciclas PC, Henson PM. Chemotactic activity generated from the fifth component of complement by plasma kallikrein. J Exp Med 1981;153:1391–1404
22. Ward PA. A plasmin-split fragment of C3 as a new chemotactic factor. J Exp Med 1967;126:189–206
23. Tice DA, Reed GE, Clauss RH, Worth MH. Hemorrhage due to fibrinolysis occuring with open-heart operations. J Thorac Cardiovasc Surg 1963;46:673–676
24. Baier RE, Dutton RC. Initial events in interaction of blood with a foreign surface. J Biomed Mater 1969;3:191–206
25. Bentall HH, Allwork SP. Fibrinolysis and bleeding in open-heart surgery. Lancet 1968;1:4–6
26. Gans H, Krivit W, Runyeon A, McAuley M, Gans MA. Problems in hemostasis during open-heart surgery. III. Epsilon aminocaproic acid as an inhibitor of plasminogen activator activity. Ann Surgery 1962;155:268-271
27. Umlas J. Fibrinolysis and disseminated intravascular coagulation in open-heart surgery. Transfusion 1976;16:460–465

28. Griffith LD, Billman GF, Daily PO, Lane TA. Apparent coagulopathy caused by infusion of shed mediastinal blood and its prevention by washing of the infusate. Ann Thorac Surg 1989;47:400–405
29. Tanaka K, Takao M, Yada I et al. Alterations in coagulation and fibrinolysis associated with cardiopulmonary bypass. J Cardiothorac Anaesth 1989;3:181–188
30. Stibbe J, Kluft C, Brommer EJP, Gomes M, De Jong DS, Nauta J. Enhanced fibrinolytic activity during cardiopulmonary bypass in open-heart surgery in man is caused by extrinsic (tissue-type) plasminogen activator. Eur J Clin Invest 1984;14:357–379
31. Harker L, Malpass TW, Branson HE, Hessel II EA, Slichter SA. Mechanism of abnormal bleeding in patients undergoing cardiopulmonary bypass: Acquired transient platelet dysfunction associated with selective granule release. Blood 1980;56:824–834
32. Zilla P, Fasol R, Groscurth P, Kleptko W, Reichenspurner H, Wolner E. Blood platelets in cardiopulmonary bypass operations. Recovery occurs after initial stimulation, rather than continual activation. J Thorac Cardiovasc Surg 1989;97:379–383
33. Malpass TW, Hanson SR, Savage B, Hessel II EA, Harker LA. Prevention of acquired transient defect in platelet plug formation by infused prostacyclin. Blood 1981;57:736–741
34. Addonizio VP Jr, Strauss JF III, Colman RW, Edmunds LH Jr. Effects of prostaglandin E1 on platelet loss during in vivo and in vitro extracorporeal circulation with a bubble oxygenator. J Thorac Cardiovasc Surg 1979;77:119–123
35. George JN, Pickett EB, Saucerman S et al. Platelet surface glycoproteins. Studies on resting and activated platelets and platelet membrane microparticles in normal subjects, and observations in patients during adult respiratory distress syndrome and cardiac surgery. J Clin Invest 1986;78:340–348
36. Dechavanne M, French M, Pages J et al. Significant reduction in the binding of a monoclonal antibody (LYP 18) directed against the IIb/IIIa glycoprotein complex to platelets of patients having undergone extracorporeal circulation. Thromb Haemost 1987;57:106–109
37. Verstraete M. Clincal application of inhibitors of fibrinolysis, Drugs 1985;29:236–242
38. Madsen P, Stanch A. The effect of aminocaproic acid on bleeding following transurethral prostatectomy. J Urol 1974;96:255–256
39. DelRossi AJ, Cernaianu AC, Botros S, Lemole GM, Moore R. Prophylactic treatment of postperfusion bleeding using EACA. Chest 1989;96:27–32
40. Van der Salm TJ, Ansell JE, Okike ON et al. The role of epsilon-aminocaproic acid in reducing bleeding after cardiac operation:a double-blind randomized study. J Thorac Cardiovasc Surg 1988;95:538–540
41. Hoffman EP, Koo AH. Cerebral thrombosis associated with amicar therapy. Radiology 1979;131:667–672
42. Naeye RL. Thrombotic state after a hemorrhagic diathesis, a possible complication of therapy with epsilon-aminocaproic acid. Blood 1962;19:694–698
43. Horrow JC, Hlavacek J, Strong MD et al. Prophylactic tranexamic acid decreases bleeding after cardiac operations. J Thorac Cardiovasc Surg 1990;99:70–75
44. Manucci PM, Canciani MT, Rota L, Donovan BS. Response of factor VIII.von Willebrand factor to DDAVP in healthy subjects and patients with haemophilia A and von Willebrand's disease. Br J Haematolo 1981;47:283-93
45. Takeuchi M, Nagura H, Kaneda T. DDAVP and epinephrine induced changes in the localization of von Willebrand factor antigen in endothelial cells of human oral mucosa. Blood 1988;72:850–854
46. Hackmann T, Gascoyne RD, Naiman SC et al. A trial of desmopressin (1-desamino-8-d-argine vasopressin) to reduce blood loss in uncomplicated cardiac surgery. N Engl J Med 1989;321:1437–1439
47. Rocha E, Llorens R, Paramo JA, Arcas R, Cuesta B, Trenor AM. Does desmopressin acetate reduce blood loss after surgery in patients on cardiopulmonary bypass? Circulation 1988;77:1319
48. Salzman EW, Weinstein MJ, Weintraub RM et al. Treatment with desmopressin acetate to reduce blood loss after cardiac surgery. N Engl J Med 1986;314:1402–1406
49. Weskler BB. Platelet interactions with the blood vessel wall. In: Coleman RW, Hirsh J, Marder VJ, Salzman EW (eds): Hemostatis and Thrombosis (ed2) Philadelphia, PA, Lippincott 1987; 793–812
50. Walker ID, Davidson JF, Faichney A, Wheatley DJ, Davidson KG. A double blind study of prostacyclin in cardiopulmonary bypass surgery. Br J Hematol 1981;49:415–419
51. Aren C, Feddersen K, Raedegran K. Effects of prostacyclin infusion on platelet activation and postoperative blood loss in coronary bypass. Ann Thorac Surg 1983;36:49–53
52. Longmore DB, Guerrara D, Bennett G et al. Prostacyclin: A solution to some problems of extracorporeal circulation: Experiments in greyhounds. Lancet 1979;1:1002–1004
53. Disesa VJ, Huval W, Lelcuk S et al. Disadvantages of prostacyclin infusion during cardiopulmonary bypass: A double-blind study of 50 patients having coronary revascularization. Ann Thorac Surg 1984;38:514–520
54. Fish KJ, Sarnquist FH, van Steennis C et al. A prospective, randomised study of the effects of prostacyclin on patelets and blood loss during coronary bypass operations. J Thorac Surg 1986;91:436–441

55. Addonizio VP Jr, Fisher CA, Jenkin BK, Strauss JF III, Musial JF, Edmunds LH Jr. Iloprost (ZK36374), a stable analogue of prostacyclin, preserves platelets during stimulated extracorporeal circulation. J Thorac Cardiovasc Surg 1985;89:926–930
56. Blauth C, Brady A, Arnold J, Brannan JJ, Taylor KM. A double blind trial of Iloprost during cardiopulmonary bypass. Perfusion 1987;2:271-276
57. Mammen EF. Natural protease inhibitors in extracorporeal circulation. Ann NY Acad Sci 1968;146:754–762
58. Ambrus JL, Schimert G, Lajos TZ et al. Effect of antifibrinolytic agents and estrogens on blood loss and blood coagulation factors during open heart surgery. J Med 1971;2:65–81
59. Bistrup BP, Royston D, Sapsford RN, Taylor KM. Reduction in blood loss and blood use after cardiopulmonary bypass with high dose aprotinin (Trasylol). J Thorac Cardiovasc Surg 1989;97:364–372
60. Royston D, Bidstrup BP, Taylor KM, Sapsford RN. Effect of aprotinin on need for bleed transfusions after repeat open heart surgery. Lancet 1987;ii:1289–1291
61. Bidstrup BP, Royston D, Taylor KM, Spasford RN. Effect of aprotinin on need for blood transfusion in patients with septic endocarditis having open heart surgery. Lancet 1988;i:366–367
62. Royston D. The serine anti-protease aprotinin: a novel approach to reducing post-operative bleeding. Blood Coagulation and Fibrinolysis 1990;1:55–69
63. Fraedrich G, Weber C, Bernard A, Hettwer A, Schlosser V. Reduction of blood transfusion requirement in open heart surgery by administration of high dose aprotinin – preliminary results. Thorac Cardiovasc Surg 1989;37:89–91
64. Dietrich W, Barankay A, Dilthey G et al. Reduction in homologous blood requirement in cardiac surgery by intraoperative aprotinin application – clinical experience in 152 cardiac surgical patients. Thorac Cardiovasc Surg 1989;37;92–98
65. Elliott MJ, Allen A. Aprotinin in paediatric cardiac surgery. Perfusion 1990;5(suppl):73–76
66. Bidstrup BP, Royston D, McGuinness C, Sapsford RN. Aprotinin in aspirin pretreated patients. Perfusion 1990;5 [suppl]:77–81
67. Royston D. Aprotinin in open heart surgery. Perfusion 1990; 5 [suppl]:63–72
68. van Oeveren W, Jansen NJ, Bidstrup BP et al. Effects of aprotinin on haemostatic mechanisms during cardiopulmonary bypass. Ann Thorac Surg 1987;44:640–645
69. Efstratiadis T, Munsch C, Crossman D, Taylor KM. Aprotinin therapy after thrombolytic treatment. Ann Thorac Surg 1991;52: 1320–1321.
70. van Oeveren W, Eijsman L, Roozendaal KJ, Wildevuur Ch RH. Platelet preservation by Aprotinin during cardiopulmonary bypass. Lancet 1988;i:644

Part 2

Prosthesis-related factors

Chapter 2.1

Influence of Flow Characteristics of Prosthetic Valves on Thrombus Formation

Ajit P. Yoganathan, Timothy M. Wick and Helmut Reul

As stated by Roberts, the 1960s will probably be remembered most in the annals of cardiology as the decade during which cardiac valve replacement became a successful reality[1]. However, even after 30 years of experience, problems associated with heart valve prostheses have not been eliminated. The most serious problems and complications are: (i) thrombosis and thromboembolism, (ii) tissue overgrowth, (iii) infection, (iv) paravalvar regurgitation, (v) haemolysis, (vi) valve failure due to material fatigue or chemical change, (vii) damage to endothelium adjacent to the valve, and (viii) regurgitation caused by failure of the valve to close properly. Problems (i), (ii), (v), and (vii) are *directly* related to the velocity and turbulence fields created by the various valve designs, and have been addressed in detail during the past decade by investigators studying cardiovascular fluid mechanics[2–14].

It has been established that shear stresses in the order of 1500–4000 dynes/cm^2 can cause lethal damage to red cells[15,16]. However, in the presence of foreign surfaces red cells can be destroyed by shear stresses on the order of 10–100 dynes/cm^2[17,18]. Sutera and Mehrjardi[19] have observed that sub-lethal damage to red cells can occur at turbulent shear stress levels of 500 dynes/cm^2 (see also Chapter 2.2). Platelets appear to be more sensitive to shear, and can be damaged by shear stresses on the order of 100–500 dynes/cm^2[20–24]. Evidence that platelet activation, aggregation, and thrombosis is induced by fluid shear forces have been predominantly generated by viscometric studies performed under well defined fluid mechanical conditions[25,26]. In viscometers, the extent and reversibility of shear-induced platelet aggregation are a function of both the magnitude and duration of the applied shear stress. For example, at 150 dynes/cm^2, platelet aggregation is not observed until shear is applied for 300 seconds[27]. But, as the intensity of the applied shear stress increases, platelet activation and aggregation occur more rapidly. For example, at a shear stress of 600 dynes/cm^2, platelet aggregation occurs within 30 seconds[28,29] and at 6500 dynes/cm^2, platelet activation occurs in less than 5 milliseconds[29]. As the magnitude of the applied shear increases, formed platelet aggregates tend not to separate when the shear forces are discontinued[20,27,28,30]. Furthermore, platelet damage increases linearly with time of exposure to constant shear stress[27], indicating that shear-induced platelet damage is cumulative.

Even with anticoagulant compliance, the risk of valve-induced thromboembolic events has not been eliminated. The frequency of these events has been monitored for more than 20 years and data indicate that thromboembolic complications vary with the anatomical site of implantation, mitral valve replacement carrying a slightly higher risk of thromboembolism than aortic valve replacements[31]. This difference in risk may be associated with haemodynamics, since mitral valve disease leads to conditions, including an enlarged left atrium, chronic atrial fibrillation, and low cardiac output, which may contribute to stagnation regions behind the prosthetic valve[32]. As compared to mechanical valves, bioprosthetic valves have more favourable haemodynamics than mechanical valves[33] and patients are generally subject to fewer thromboembolic complications[34–39]. To further decrease or minimise the risk of shear-induced platelet activation, thrombosis and embolism, additional studies are required to better characterise the fluid dynamics of each valve design under conditions expected in vivo and to propose new design criteria to reduce and/or eliminate regions of high turbulent shear stresses, flow stagnation and flow separation.

In order to assess the fluid dynamic characteristics of a prosthetic heart valve design, the following in vitro studies can be conducted: (i) pressure drop or gradient; (ii) regurgitant volume; (iii) flow visualisation; (iv) velocity mapping; and (v) turbulence mapping. This chapter will describe in vitro velocity and turbulence mapping studies conducted with a variety of size 27 mm prosthetic valve designs, both mechanical and tissue, that have been used clinically during the last three decades. The studies were conducted under simulated physiological pulsatile flow conditions in the aortic position of the Georgia Tech left heart simulator. The velocity and turbulence measurements were performed with a two dimensional laser Doppler velocimeter system[3].

During the past two years an additional *potential* source of blood cell damage has been identified in mechanical valves: the appearance of cavitation bubbles at valve closure. One of the authors of this chapter (HR) initiated a study to detect cavitation in several clinically used mechanical heart valves in vitro, in a simulated mitral position, using distilled water as the model fluid. The study was designed to determine the threshold value of artificially created 'left ventricular' dp/dt required to produce cavitation, and to assess the influence of valve size and design parameters on this threshold value.

VELOCITY AND TURBULENT SHEAR STRESS STUDIES

The figures of the in vitro flow field studies are presented as schematic diagrams, and represent velocity and turbulence profiles obtained at peak systole, at a cardiac output of 6.0 l/min and a heart rate of 70 beats/min. All downstream distances are measured from the valve sewing rings. Table 2.1–1 lists the maximum and cross-sectionally averaged mean turbulent shear stresses measured downstream of the valves at different times during systole. More detailed descriptions of the in vitro experimental conditions and methodology have already been published[2–7,14].

(i) Starr-Edwards caged-ball valve (Model 1260)

The flow emerging from the valve formed a circumferential jet that separated from the ball, hit the wall of the flow chamber and then flowed along the wall. It had very high velocities in the annular region. The maximum velocity, measured 12 mm downstream of the valve, was 220 cm/s at peak systole. Even during the acceleration phase, the jet had already developed in this region with a peak velocity of 180 cm/s, then gradually diverged as it flowed downstream. The peak systolic velocity, measured 30 mm downstream of the valve, was 180 cm/s, as shown in Figure 2.1–1A. High

Table 2.1–1.
Peak and Mean Turbulent Shear Stresses
Measured Downstream of the Different Valve Designs

Valve	*Location (mm)*	*Acceleration Phase*		*Peak Systole*		*Deceleration Phase*	
		Peak (dynes/cm²)	*Mean (dynes/cm²)*	*Peak (dynes/cm²)*	*Mean (dynes/cm²)*	*Peak (dynes/cm²)*	*Mean (dynes/cm²)*
S-E	26, centerline	750	450	1800	1000	1400	700
(1260)	30, centerline	600	200	1850	1100	1300	750
B-S	7, centerline	2400	900	3400	1600	1100	600
(C-C)	7, major orifice	900	450	1800	600	400	200
	7, minor orifice	1500	650	1800	900	900	600
	11, centerline	1050	550	1500	650	550	250
	11, major orifice	700	400	1100	400	750	450
	11, minor orifice	400	250	1800	900	1050	500
	14, 90 degree rotated (Fig. 2.1–2C)	600	300	1200	600	1000	450
M-H	7, major orifice	450	250	1200	450	600	300
	7, minor orifice	950	400	1000	350	850	450
	13, centerline	1200	600	1000	550	800	400
	13, major orifice	400	320	1500	370	700	300
	13, minor orifice	1250	550	1450	700	700	450
	16, centerline	300	100	2000	1000	850	450
	15, 90 degree rotated (Fig. 2.1–3C)	300	170	1450	700	900	450
O-C	8mm, major orifice	300	80	1400	250	900	600
	8mm, minor orifice	730	110	850	200	770	250
	8mm, centerline	400	60	1250	190	600	220
	14mm, major orifice	800	250	2000	220	800	200
	14mm, minor orifice	650	120	1200	320	1050	450
	14mm, centerline	530	190	1700	320	650	270
	17mm, 90° rotated	800	210	1800	470	1100	380
SJM	8, centerline	820	450	1150	500	600	320
	8, 6.25mm lateral to centerline	1600	1050	2000	1000	1000	650
	13, centerline	950	470	1500	750	1400	900
	13, 6.25mm lateral to centerline	1400	800	2000	1050	1000	700
	11, 90 degree rotated (Fig. 2.1–5D)	950	550	1700	1200	1000	700
DU	13mm, centerline	1120	300	1500	750	1000	460
	13mm, 6.25mm lateral to centerline	650	380	2300	1250	1000	550
	13mm, 90° rotated (Fig. 2.1–6D)	800	260	1700	680	780	420
C-E	10, centerline	900	400	2750	1200	1750	1000
(2625)	15, centerline	1400	700	4500	2000	1700	900
HC MO	10, centerline	1000	400	2900	1100	1150	550
(250)	15, centerline	1750	950	2450	1900	2100	1400

Table 2.1–1 (Continued)
Peak and Mean Turbulent Shear Stresses
Measured Downstream of the Different Valve Designs

Valve	*Location (mm)*	*Acceleration Phase*		*Peak Systole*		*Deceleration Phase*	
		Peak (dynes/cm²)	*Mean (dynes/cm²)*	*Peak (dynes/cm²)*	*Mean (dynes/cm²)*	*Peak (dynes/cm²)*	*Mean (dynes/cm²)*
HC II	18, centerline	1000	400	2500	900	1100	450
(410)	33, centerline	1100	350	2200	950	1300	750
C-E	15, centerline	1100	200	2000	350	1900	350
(2650)	20, centerline	700	200	1750	500	1050	300
I-S	21, centerline	1100	150	2100	450	950	250
(Peri-cardial)	27, centerline	600	350	2500	450	800	400
C-E	17, centerline	500	100	850	200	1000	350
(Peri-cardial)	33, centerline	850	200	1130	450	900	370

HC MO: Hancock modified orifice, HC II: Hancock II, C-E: Carpentier-Edwards IS: Ionescu-Shiley

velocity gradients were observed at the edges of the jet. The maximum velocity gradient (1700 cm s^{-1}/cm) was observed in the annular region adjacent to the surface of the ball during peak systole. A large velocity defect was observed in the central part of the flow chamber as a wake developed distal to the ball. A region of low velocity reverse flow was observed at peak systole and during the deceleration phase, with a diameter of about 8mm immediately distal to the apex of the cage. The maximum reverse velocity measured was –25 cm/s; it occurred at peak systole 30 mm downstream of the valve (Fig. 2.1–1A). The intensity of the reverse flow during the deceleration phase was not as high as that observed at peak systole. The maximum reverse velocity (–20 cm/s) was measured 26 mm downstream of the valve during this phase of the cardiac cycle. The maximum reverse velocity measured 30 mm downstream of the valve was –10 cm/s, since the flow field had started to recover from separation. No reverse flow was observed during the acceleration phase. However, the velocity in the central part of the flow channel was low.

High turbulent shear stresses were observed at the edges of the jet. The maximum turbulent shear stress measured was 1850 dynes/cm², which occurred at the location of the highest velocity gradient (Fig. 2.1–1B). The intensity of turbulence during peak systole did not decay very rapidly downstream of the valve (Table 2.1–1). Elevated turbulent shear stresses occurred during most of systole. Turbulent shear stresses as high as 3500 dynes/cm² were estimated in the annular region between the flow channel wall and the ball.

(ii) Bjørk-Shiley Convexo-Concave valve

This valve produced two high-velocity-jet type flow fields. The larger corresponded in location to the major, the smaller to the minor orifice outflow region. The region between the two jets appeared to be stagnant at all three cardiac cycle times at which

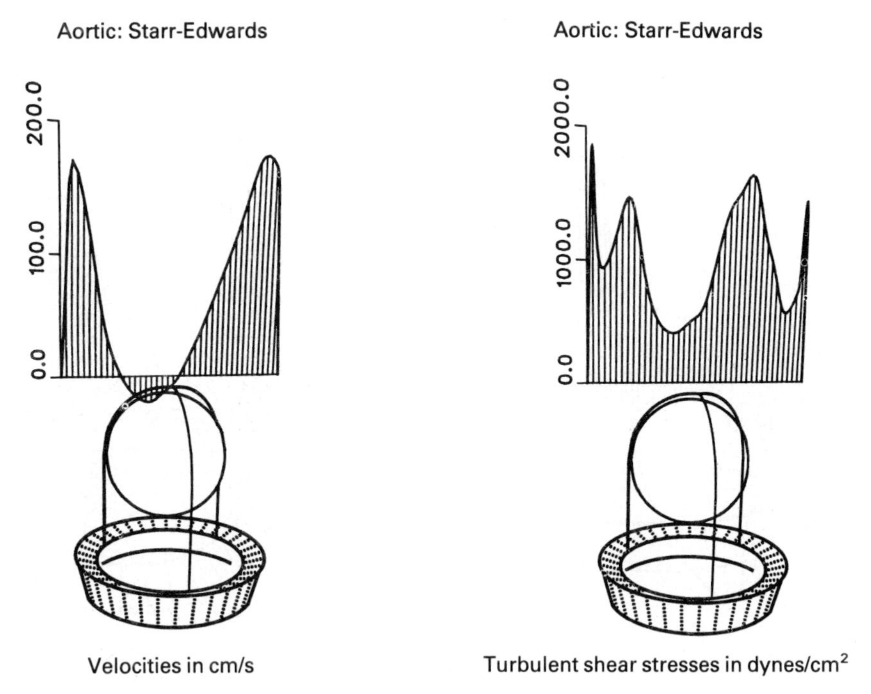

Figure 2.1–1A; Velocity profile 30 mm downstream on the centerline for the Starr-Edwards ball valve, at peak systole.
Figure 2.1–1B: Turbulent shear stress profile 30 mm downstream on the centerline for the Starr-Edwards ball valve, at peak systole.

velocity measurements were conducted. This region of stagnation and/or flow separation extended as far downstream as 15 mm from the valve sewing ring. During the acceleration and deceleration phases, a region of stagnation about 2 mm wide was still present 14 mm downstream of the valve.

The major orifice jet developed more rapidly than the minor, as indicated by the velocity profile obtained during the acceleration phase. However, both jets reached about the same maximum velocity (200cm/s) at peak systole (Figs. 2.1–2A and 2.1–2B). A small region of flow separation and reversal was observed between the major orifice jet and the wall of the flow chamber, with a maximum reverse velocity of –10 cm/s. A much larger region of flow separation and reversal was observed below the minor orifice jet (Fig. 2.1–2A), since the jet was directed laterally by the occluder. This region of flow separation was not observed during the acceleration phase, since the jet was not fully developed and the flow field recovered from separation rapidly. At peak systole, a region of reverse flow was observed which extended 7 mm from the wall (Figs. 2.1–2A and 2.1–2B). The effect of the struts on the flow field could be clearly seen in the velocity profile obtained across the minor orifice as shown in Figure 2.1–2B.

The flow in the minor orifice region was very disturbed with a maximum turbulent shear stress at peak systole of 1800 dynes/cm^2 (Figs. 2.1–2C and 2.1–2D). Elevated turbulent shear stresses were also observed during the acceleration and the deceleration phases (Table 2.1–1). The flow was more disturbed in the minor orifice region (Figs. 2.1–2C and 2.1–2D). High turbulent shear stresses were observed at the edges of

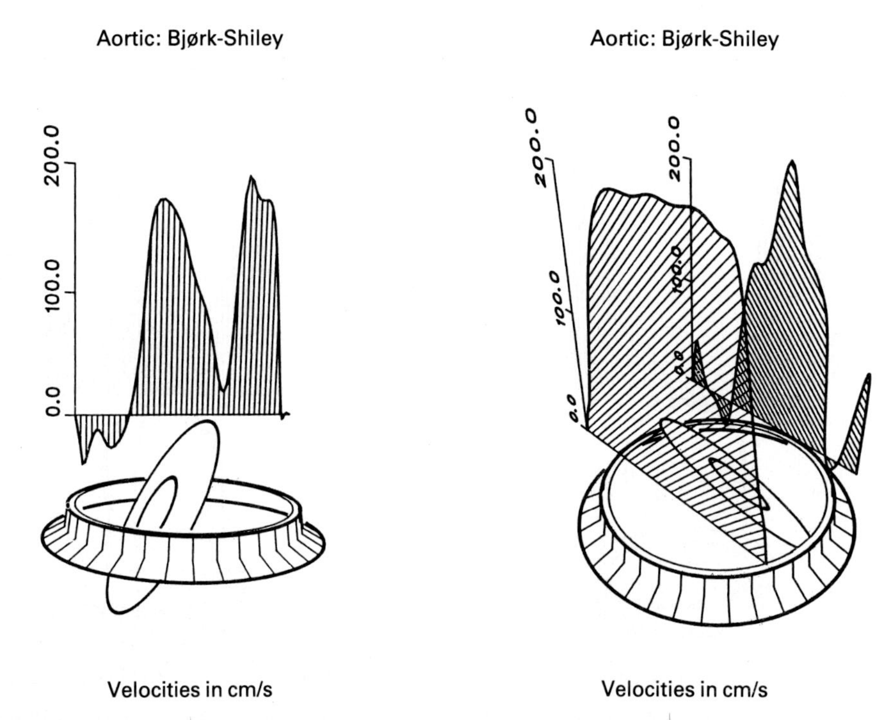

Figure 2.1–2A: Velocity profile 14 mm downstream on the centerline across the major and minor orifices of the Bjørk-Shiley tilting disc valve (major orifice to the right), at peak systole.
Figure 2.1–2B: Velocity profiles 11 mm downstream in the major and minor orifices of the Bjørk-Shiley tilting disc valve, at peak systole.

the jet, which corresponded to the locations of high velocity gradients. These high turbulent shear stresses were confined to narrow regions and decayed rapidly.

(iii) Medtronic Hall valve

High velocity jet like flows were observed from both the major and the minor orifice outflow regions. The orientation of the jets with respect to the axial direction changed as the valve opened and closed. The major orifice jet was larger in size than the minor orifice jet and had a slightly higher velocity. The peak velocities measured 7 mm downstream of the valve were 210 cm/s and 200 cm/s in the major and the minor orifice regions, respectively. The velocity of the major orifice jet did not decrease much as the flow travelled from 7 to 15 mm downstream of the valve. The peak velocity of the major orifice jet measured 15 mm downstream of the valve was 200cm/s (Figs. 2.1–3A and 2.1–3B). The peak velocity in the minor orifice was lower than that in the major orifice (Figs. 2.1–3A and 2.1–3B), especially during the acceleration phase. A region of reverse flow was observed adjacent to the wall in the minor orifice region at peak systole, which extended 2 mm from the wall with a maximum reverse velocity of –25 cm/s. The size of this region increased during the deceleration phase to 8 mm from the wall. No area of stagnation was observed in the region between the major and minor orifice jets, in contrast to findings with the Bjørk-Shiley valve. A small region of flow separation was observed adjacent to the wall in the major orifice region as illustrated by Figure

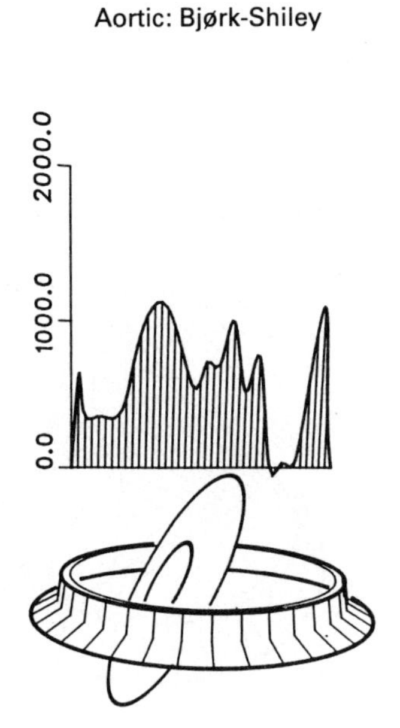

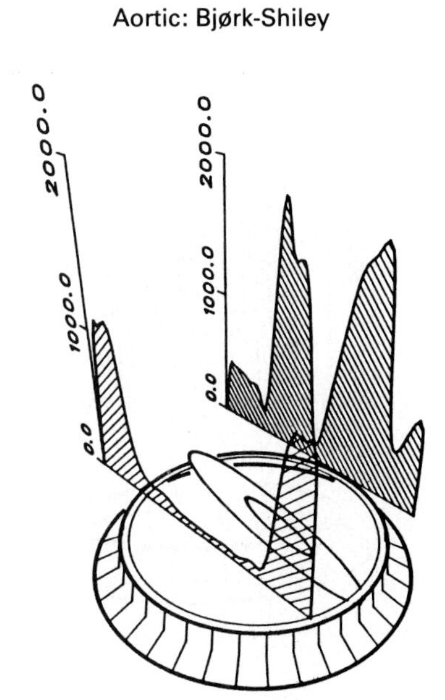

Figure 2.1–2C: Turbulent shear stress profile 14 mm downstream on the centerline across the major and minor orifices of the Bjork-Shiley tilting disc valve (major orifice to the right), at peak systole.
Figure 2.1–2D: Turbulent shear stress profiles 11 mm downstream in the major and minor orifices of the Bjørk-Shiley tilting disc valve, at peak systole.

2.1–3B. In the minor orifice region, a profound velocity defect was observed 7 and 11 mm distal to the minor orifice strut (Fig. 2.1–3B). Furthermore, the region adjacent to the wall immediately downstream from the minor orifice was stagnant during the acceleration and deceleration phases, and had very low velocities (< 15 cm/s) during peak systole.

In the major orifice region, high turbulent shear stresses were confined to narrow regions at the edges of the major orifice jet (Figs. 2.1–3C and 2.1–3D). The peak turbulent shear stresses measured at peak systole were 1200 and 1500 dynes/cm^2, 7 and 13 mm downstream of the valve, respectively. During the acceleration and deceleration phases the turbulent shear stresses were relatively low. High turbulent shear stresses were more dispersed in the minor than those in the major orifice region as shown by Figures 2.1–3C and 2.1–3D. The turbulent shear stresses during the acceleration and deceleration phases were also high (Table 2.1–1). The turbulent shear stress profiles across the major and the minor orifices 15 mm downstream of the valve (Fig. 2.1–3C), showed a maximum turbulent shear stress of 1450 dynes/cm^2 at the lower edge of the minor orifice jet. Since these high turbulent shear stresses in the minor orifice region were observed 15 mm downstream of the valve, it is probable that even higher turbulent shear stresses occurred in the minor orifice region closer to the valve, where they could not be measured because of the obstruction of the laser beams by the occluder.

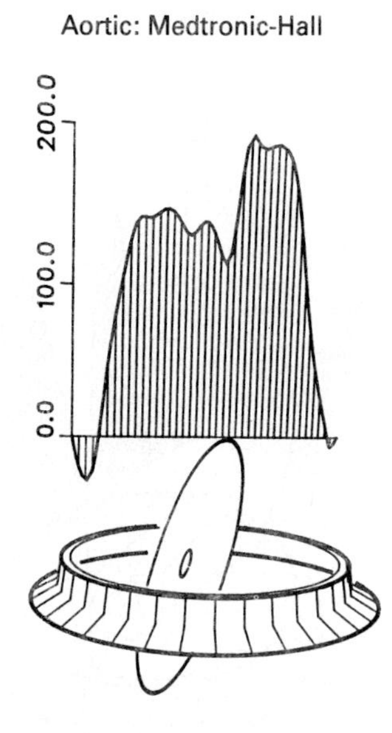

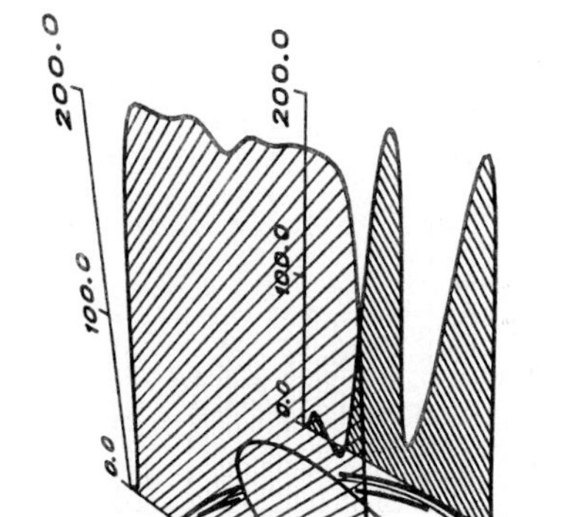

Figure 2.1–3A: Velocity profile 15 mm downstream on the centerline across the major and minor orifices of the Medtronic-Hall tilting disc valve (major orifice to the right), at peak systole.
Figure 2.1–3B: Velocity profiles 13 mm downstream in the major and minor orifices of the Medtronic-Hall tilting disc valve, at peak systole.

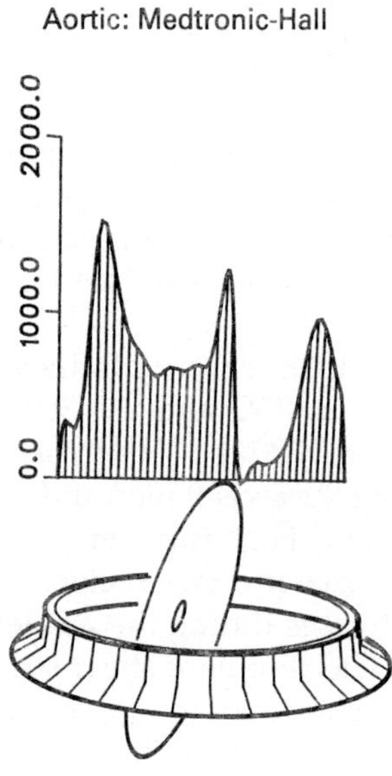

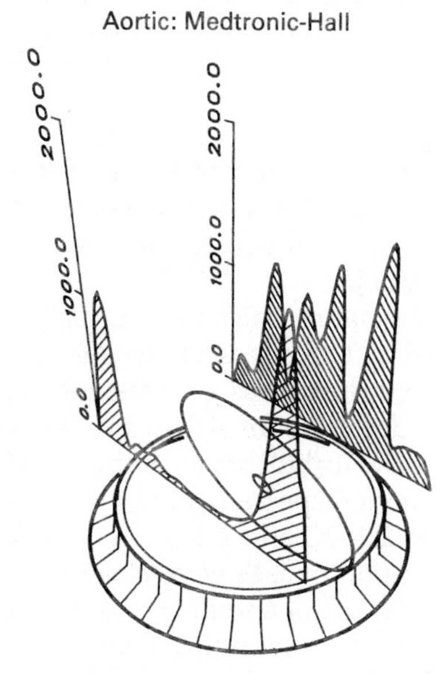

Figure 2.1–3C: Turbulent shear stress profile 15 mm downstream on the centerline across the major and minor orifices of the Medtronic-Hall tilting disc valve (major orifice to the right), at peak systole.
Figure 2.1–3D: Turbulent shear stress profiles 13 mm downstream in the major and minor orifices of the Medtronic-Hall tilting disc valve, at peak systole.

(iv) Omnicarbon valve

Velocity profiles taken in the major orifice region, 8 mm downstream of the valve, showed a blunt jet type flow during the acceleration phase and at peak systole. The maximum velocities measured were 130 and 225 cm/s, respectively. In the major orifice region, 14 mm downstream, a blunt jet type flow field was observed at all three phases at which measurements were made (Fig. 2.1–4A). The velocity profile taken along the centreline plane 8 mm downstream of the valve showed that the region adjacent to the pivot guards was relatively stagnant during the acceleration and the deceleration phases. At peak systole, forward flow was observed adjacent to the pivot guards with a velocity of 35 cm/s. Measurements along the centreline plane 14 mm downstream of the valve showed that the flow field had increased in magnitude, especially during the deceleration phase. The maximum velocities measured were 130, 225, and 125 cm/s, during the acceleration peak systole and deceleration phases, respectively.

In the minor orifice region, the forward flow occurred in the centre part of the flow channel. The maximum velocity measured 8 mm downstream of the valve at peak systole was 225 cm/s. The region adjacent to the wall appeared to be relatively stagnant during the acceleration phase. At peak systole and the deceleration phase, a small amount of forward flow was observed in this region. The velocities in the minor orifice jet did not appear to change significantly as the flow travelled from 8 to 14 mm downstream from the valve sewing ring (Fig. 2.1–4A). The velocity profiles taken 17 mm downstream of the valve across the major and minor orifices (Fig. 2.1–4B), showed

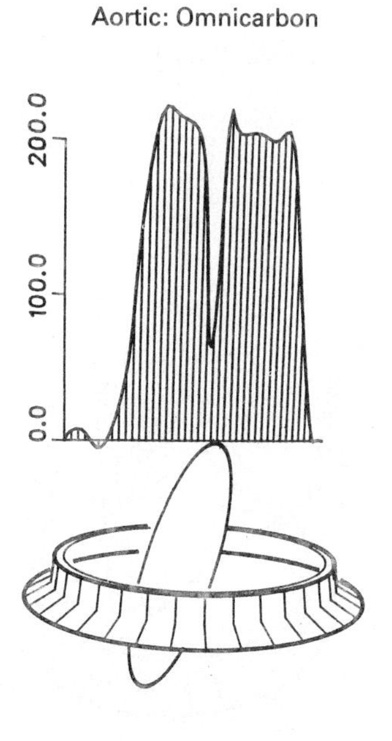

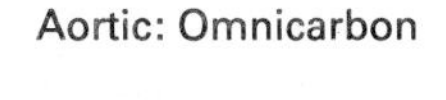

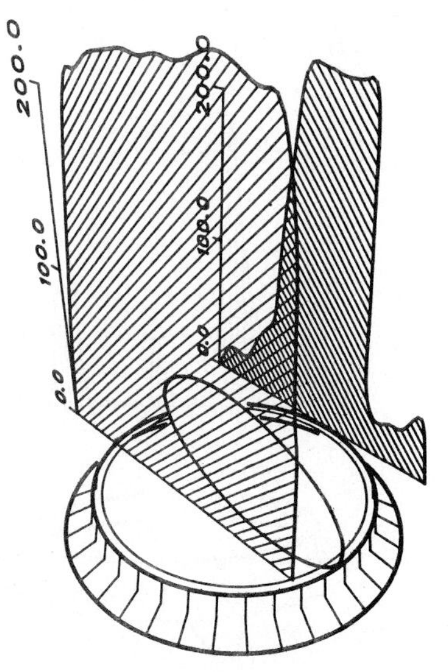

Figure 2.1–4A: Velocity profiles 14mm downstream in the major and minor orifices of the Omnicarbon tilting disc valve, at peak systole.

Figure 2.1–4B: Velocity profile 14mm downstream on the centreline across the major and minor orifices of the Omnicarbon tilting disc valve (major orifice to the right), at peak systole.

that the minor orifice jet had a slightly higher maximum velocity than the major orifice jet, especially during the acceleration phase and at peak systole. An area of flow separation was observed in the minor orifice region adjacent to the flow channel wall at peak systole and during the deceleration phase. The velocity profiles across the major orifices also showed that the forward flow emerging from the minor orifice was sharply reduced during the deceleration phase.

Turbulent shear stress measurements obtained in the major orifice 14 mm downstream of the valve, showed elevated turbulent shear stresses only at the edges of the jet during all three phases. Along the centreline plane, high turbulent shear stresses were also confined to a narrow region. The maximum measured turbulent shear stress increased from 1250 to 1700 dynes/cm^2 as the flow travelled from 8 to 14 mm downstream of the valve, as shown in Figure 2.1–4C. In the minor orifice region, high turbulent shear stresses occurred in a small region during the acceleration phase and at peak systole, but were spread over a larger region during the deceleration phase (Table 2.1–1). The turbulent shear stress measurements across the major and minor orifices, shown in Figure 2.1–4D, indicated that the flow field in the minor orifice region was more disturbed. The maximum turbulent shear stress measured (1800 dynes/cm^2) occurred at the central edge of the minor orifice jet.

(v) St. Jude Medical valve

The St. Jude valve has two semicircular leaflets which divide the area available for forward flow into three regions, two lateral orifices and a central orifice. The major part

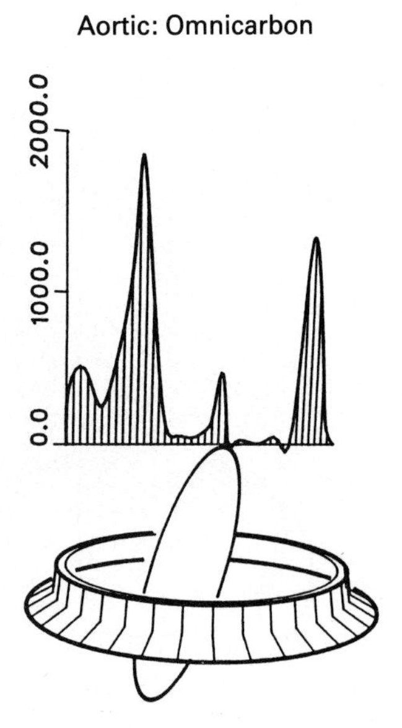

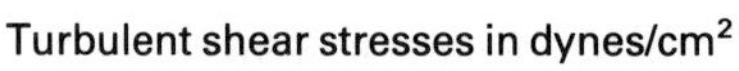

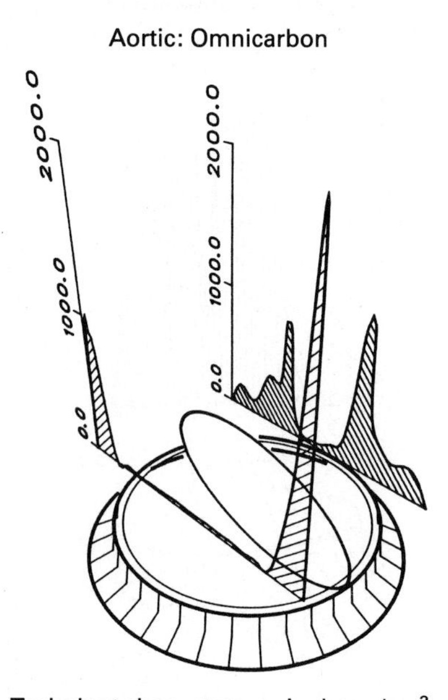

Figure 2.1–4C: Turbulent shear stress profiles 14mm downstream on the major and minor orifices of the Omnicarbon tilting disc valve, at peak systole.

Figure 2.1–4D: Turbulent shear stress profile 14mm downstream on the centreline across the major and minor orifices of the Omnicarbon tilting disc valve (major orifice to the right), at peak systole.

of the forward flow emerged from the two lateral orifices. The measurements along the centreline plane 8 mm downstream of the valve showed at peak systole a maximum velocity of 220 cm/s and 200 cm/s for the lateral and central orifice jets, respectively. The velocity of the jets remained about the same as the flow travelled from 8 to 13 mm downstream (Fig. 2.1–5A). The velocity profiles showed two defects which corresponded to the locations of the two leaflets. The velocity measurements conducted during the acceleration and deceleration phases showed that the flow was more evenly distributed across the flow chamber during the deceleration than during the acceleration phase. Regions of flow separation were observed around the jets adjacent to the flow channel wall as the flow separated from the orifice ring. The measurements across the central orifice illustrated in Figure 2.1–5B show that the maximum velocity in the central orifice was 220 cm/s. Small regions of low velocity reverse flow were observed adjacent to the pivot/hinge mechanism of the valve (Figure 2.1–5B). The maximum velocities measured during the acceleration and deceleration phase were 110 and 115 cm/s, respectively. More flow emerged from the central orifice during the deceleration phase than during the acceleration phase.

High turbulent shear stresses occurred at locations of high velocity gradients and at locations immediately distal to the valve leaflets (Fig. 2.1–5C). The flow along the centreline plane became more disturbed as the flow travelled from 8 to 13 mm downstream of the valve. The peak turbulent shear stresses measured along the centreline plane at peak systole were 1150 and 1500 dynes/cm^2 at 8 and 13 mm downstream of the valve, respectively. The profiles across the central orifice showed

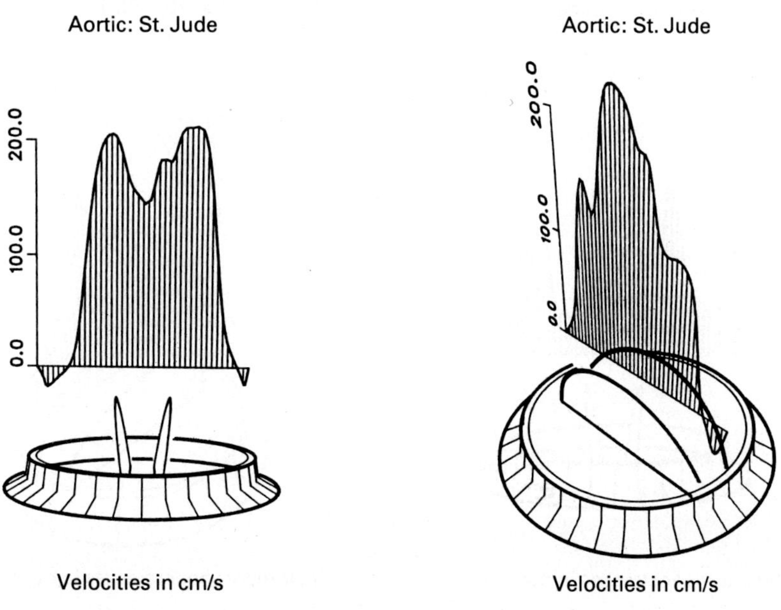

Figure 2.1–5A: Velocity profile 13 mm downstream on the centerline for the St. Jude Medical bileaflet valve, at peak systole.

Figure 2.1–5B: Velocity profile 13 mm downstream across the central orifice for the St. Jude Medical bileaflet valve, at peak systole.

that the flow was very disturbed in this region. The maximum turbulent shear stress measured in the central orifice as shown in Figure 2.1–5D (1700 dynes/cm^2) occurred at peak systole. Since these high turbulent shear stresses across the central orifice were measured 11 mm downstream, it is probable that even higher turbulent shear stresses occurred closer to the valve.

(vi) Edwards-Duromedics valve

This valve has two curved semi-circular leaflets which divide the area available for flow into three regions, two lateral orifices and a central orifice. Experiments with this valve design were conducted 13 mm downstream of the valve along the centreline plane, and 6.25 mm lateral to the centreline. Measurements across the central orifice (with the two leaflets opening and closing in the horizontal plane), were also made at the same downstream location. The results of the velocity measurement studies showed that the major part of the forward flow occurred through the two lateral orifices. The velocity profiles obtained along the centreline plane showed that the three jet like flow fields which emerged from three orifices had about the same maximum velocity, 210 cm/s (Fig. 2.1–6A). The profile obtained during the acceleration phase showed that the jet emerging from the central orifice was located in the central part of the aortic flow channel. The velocity profiles obtained at peak systole and during the deceleration phase, however, showed that the jet like flow from the central orifice was located more towards one side of the flow channel, rather than being centrally located. In addition, the two velocity defects which separated the three jets were not of the same

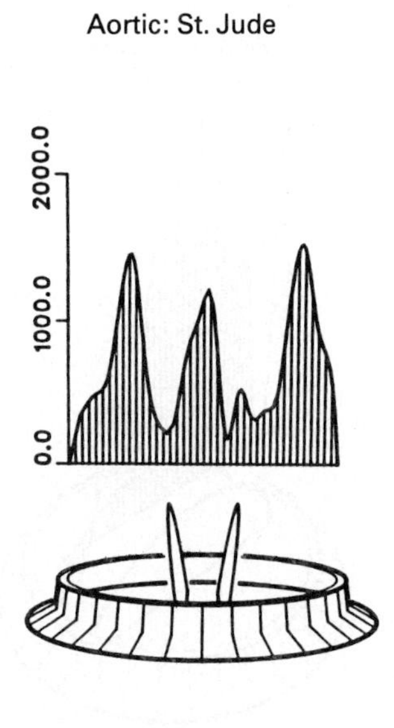

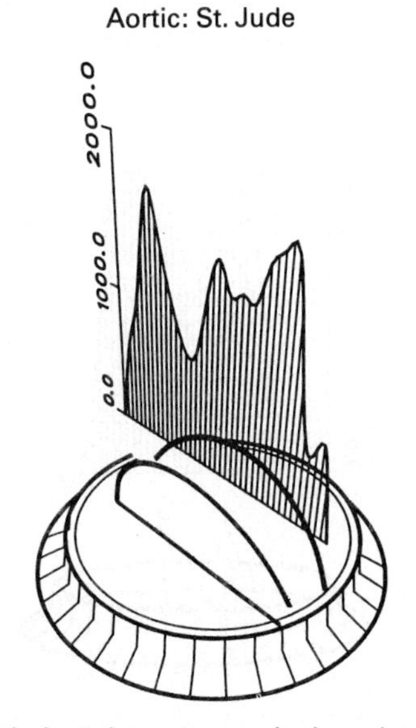

Figure 2.1–5C: Turbulent shear stress profile 13 mm downstream of the centerline orifice for the St. Jude Medical bileaflet valve, at peak systole.

Figure 2.1–5D: Turbulent shear stress profile 13 mm downstream across the central orifice for the St. Jude Medical bileaflet valve, at peak systole.

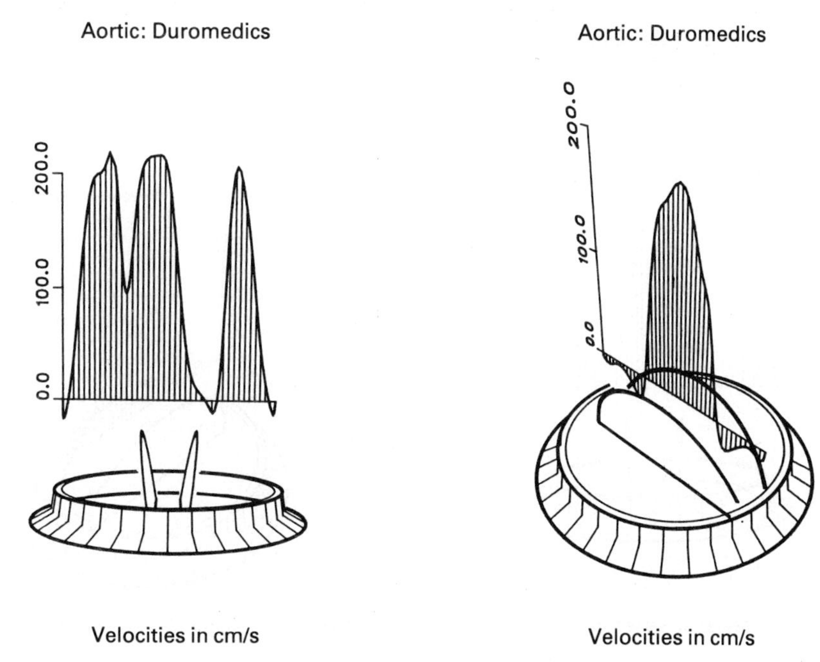

Figure 2.1–6A: Velocity profile 13 mm downstream on the centerline for the Duromedics bileaflet valve, at peak systole.

Figure 2.1–6B: Velocity profile 13 mm downstream across the central orifice for the Duromedics bileaflet valve, at peak systole.

size, with one being larger than the other (Fig. 2.1–6A). The velocity profiles obtained across the central orifice clearly indicated that the forward flow mainly occurred in the central part of the aorta, with large regions of flow separation on either side of the jet (i.e., adjacent to the pivot/hinge mechanism of the valve), as shown schematically in Figure 2.1–6B.

High turbulent shear stresses were generally observed at locations corresponding to regions of high velocity gradients. The maximum turbulent shear stress measured across the centreplane was 1500 dynes/cm^2 (Fig. 2.1–6C), with a mean value of 750 dynes/cm^2. The off-centreline turbulent shear stress measurements showed a maximum of 2300 dynes/cm^2, with a mean value of 1250 dynes/cm^2. The maximum turbulent shear stress measured across the central orifice, as shown in Figure 2.1–6D, was 1700 dynes/cm^2.

(vii) Carpentier-Edwards porcine valve (Model 2625)

The velocity profiles taken 10 mm downstream of the valve, along the centreline plane, showed that the peak velocity of the jet like flow emerging from the valve was as high as 330 cm/s at peak systole. The peak velocities measured during the acceleration and deceleration phases were about the same, 175 and 170 cm/s, respectively. However, the flow was much more evenly distributed during the acceleration than during the deceleration phase. No regions of flow separation were observed throughout the systolic period in this plane of measurement. However, the annular region between the outflow surfaces of the leaflets and the flow chamber wall was

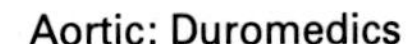

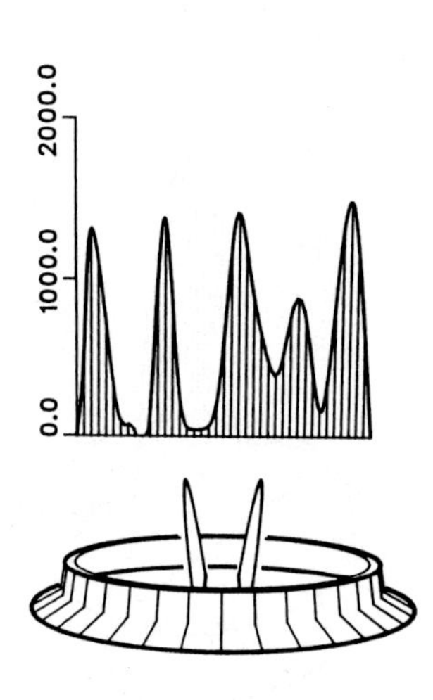

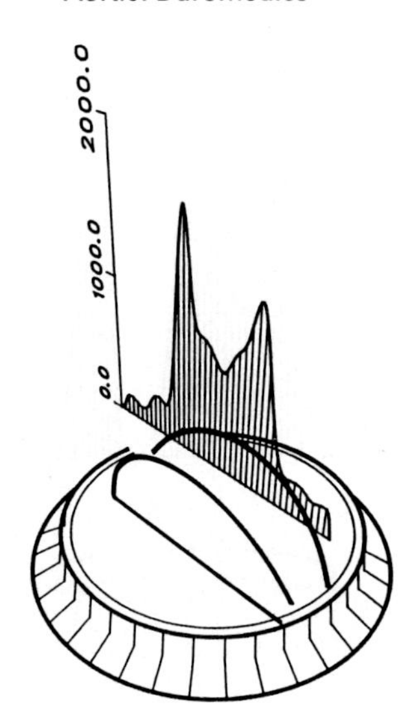

Figure 2.1–6C: Turbulent shear stress profile 13 mm downstream on the centerline across the major and minor orifices for the Duromedics bileaflet valve, at peak systole.
Figure 2.1–6D: Turbulent shear stress profile 13 mm downstream across the central orifice for the Duromedics bileaflet valve, at peak systole.

relatively stagnant throughout systole. The velocity of the jet increased to about 370 cm/s at peak systole, as the flow travelled from 10 to 15 mm downstream of the valve. This indicated that the flow tended to accelerate toward the centre of the flow channel. Velocity profiles measured 15 mm downstream of the valve (Fig. 2.1–7A) showed a small velocity defect in the centre of the flow channel during the acceleration phase and at peak systole.

High turbulent shear stresses occurred at the edge of the jet (Fig. 2.1–7B). The maximum turbulent shear stress measured 10 mm downstream of the valve along the centreline plane at peak systole was 2,750 dynes/cm^2. The turbulent shear stresses at the edge of the jet increased as the flow travelled from 10 to 15 mm downstream of the valve. The maximum and mean turbulent shear stress measured at peak systole increased to 4,500 and 2,000 dynes/ cm^2, respectively (Table 2.1–1).

(viii) Hancock Modified Orifice porcine valve (Model 250)

In this design, a size 25 mm valve was studied, since a size 27 mm valve is not manufactured. The velocity measurements showed that this valve design also produced a very high velocity jet like flow field. The jet had a maximum velocity of 330 cm/sec, which was measured along the centreline plane, 10 mm downstream of the valve. The jet, however, started to dissipate very rapidly as it flowed downstream. The maximum velocity measured 15 cm downstream of the valve was 180 cm/sec, as shown in Figure 2.1–8A. A velocity defect was observed 15 mm downstream in the central part of the flow channel at peak systole and during the deceleration phase, but was not observed along the centreline plane 10 mm downstream of the valve. Once again, the annular region between the outflow surfaces of the leaflets and the flow chamber wall was relatively stagnant during systole.

Turbulent shear stress measurements showed that the high turbulent shear stresses measured 10 mm downstream of the valve were confined to a narrow region at the edge of the jet, with a peak value of 2,900 dynes/cm^2 (Table 2.1–1). This peak turbulent shear stress decreased to 2,400 dynes/cm^2 as the flow travelled from 10 to 15 mm downstream of the valve (Fig. 2.1–8B). The region of high turbulence, however, became more diffuse as a result of energy dissipation.

(ix) Hancock II porcine valve (Model 410)

The velocity profiles obtained along the centreline plane 18 mm downstream of this valve showed that the maximum velocity of the forward flow was 260 cm/s during peak systole. A relatively stagnant region was observed adjacent to the wall of the flow channel, which extended about 3 mm from the wall. The jet was still present 33 mm downstream of the valve as indicated by the velocity profiles obtained along the centreline plane at this downstream location (Fig. 2.1–9A). Regions of flow separation were observed adjacent to one side of the flow chamber wall during peak systole and the deceleration phase.

Turbulent shear stress measurements along the centreline plane 18 mm downstream of the valve (Table 2.1–2) showed that this valve produced turbulent shear stresses as high as 2,500 dynes/cm^2. The maximum turbulent shear stress measured along the

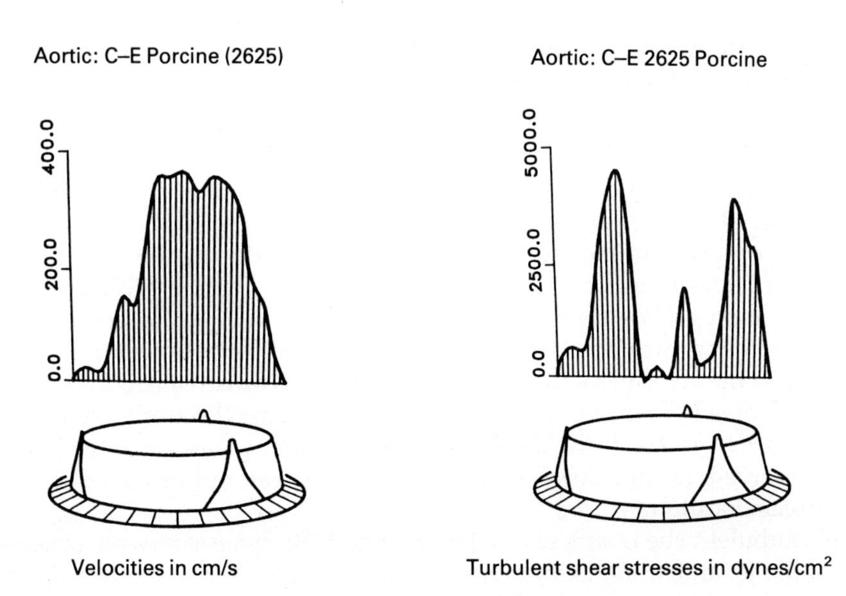

Figure 2.1–7A: Velocity profile 15 mm downstream on the centerline for the Carpentier-Edwards 2625 porcine valve, at peak systole.

Figure 2.1–7B: Turbulent shear stress profile 15 mm downstream on the centerline for the Carpentier-Edwards 2625 porcine valve, at peak systole.

Aortic: Hancock Porcine (MO)

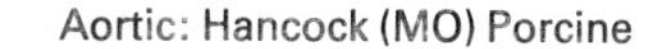

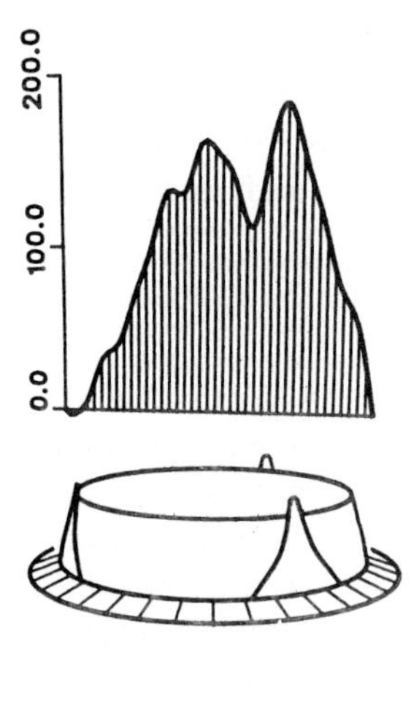

0.0 1000.0 2000.0 3000.0

Velocities in cm/s

Turbulent shear stresses in dynes/cm^2

Figure 2.1–8A: Velocity profile 15 mm downstream on the center for the Hancock modified orifice porcine valve, at peak systole.
Figure 2.1–8B: Turbulent shear stress profile 15 mm downstream on the centerline for the Hancock modified orifice porcine valve, at peak systole.

centreline plane 33 mm downstream of the valve during peak systole (2,200 dynes/cm^2) was slightly lower than that measured 18 mm downstream of the valve.

(x) Carpentier-Edwards porcine valve (Model 2650)

The forward flow emerging from the valve had a maximum velocity of 200 cm/s at peak systole along the centreline plane, 15 mm downstream of the valve. A velocity defect was observed in the centre of the flow channel during the deceleration phase. The forward flow occupied a major portion of the flow channel with a small region of flow separation and/or stagnation, adjacent to the wall of the flow chamber. The velocity profiles measured along the centreline plane 20 mm downstream of the valve showed that the velocities and the flow fields at this downstream location were similar to those observed 15 mm downstream of the valve during the acceleration phase and at peak systole (Fig. 2.1–10A). During the deceleration phase, however, the velocity defect observed 15 mm downstream of the valve was not observed at this farther downstream location.

High turbulent shear stresses of the order of 1750 dynes/cm^2 were observed at the edge of the jet and at the location of the velocity defect (Fig. 2.1–10B). The maximum turbulent shear stress measured along the centreline plane 15 mm downstream of the valve was 2,000 dynes/cm^2, which occurred at the edge of the jet during peak systole (Table 2.1–1). The maximum turbulent shear stress appeared to decay as the flow travelled downstream.

Aortic: Hancock II Porcine

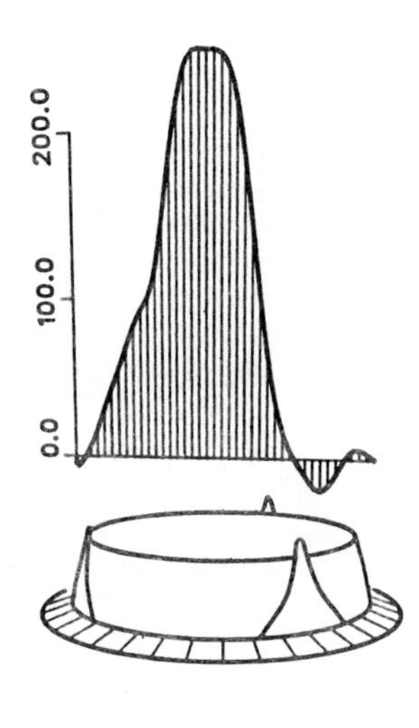

Velocities in cm/s

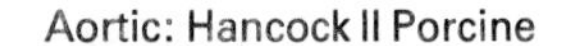

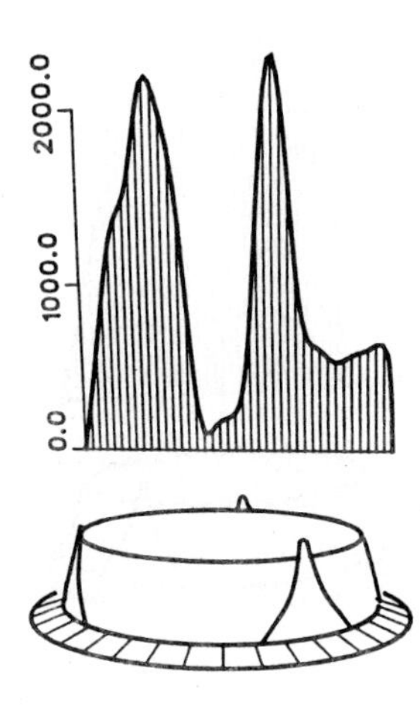

Turbulent shear stresses in dynes/cm^2

Figure 2.1–9A: Velocity profile 33 mm downstream on the centerline for the Hancock II porcine valve, at peak systole.

Figure 2.1–9B: Turbulent shear stress profile 33 mm downstream on the centerline for the Hancock II porcine valve, at peak systole.

(xi) Ionescu-Shiley Standard pericardial valve

This valve produced a jet like flow field with very high velocity gradients at the edges of the jet. Regions of flow separation and/or stagnation were observed around the periphery of the jet. The maximum velocity of the jet measured 21 mm downstream of the valve at peak systole was 200 cm/s. The flow lateral to the centreline plane accelerated toward the centreline plane as the flow travelled from 21 to 27 mm downstream of the valve. As a result, the maximum velocity of the jet at peak systole increased to 230 cm/s, 27 mm downstream of the valve (Fig. 2.1–11A). This acceleration phenomenon was also observed during late systole, but it was not obvious during early systole.

High turbulent shear stresses were confined to a narrow region around the jet (Fig. 2.1–11B). The maximum turbulent shear stress measured 21 mm downstream of the valve was 2,100 dynes/cm^2 and increased to 2,500 dynes/cm^2 as the flow travelled to 27 mm downstream of the valve (Table 2.1–1). This higher turbulent shear stress could be a result of the acceleration of the flow towards the centreline plane.

(xii) Carpentier-Edwards pericardial valve (Model 2900)

The velocity profiles obtained along the centreline plane 17 mm downstream of the

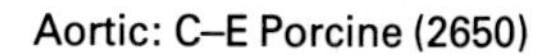

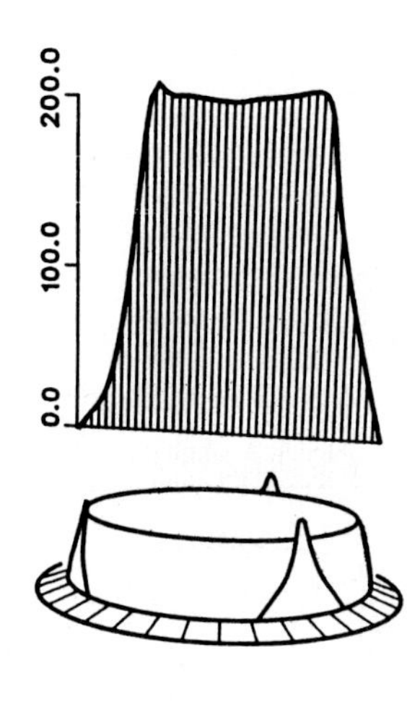

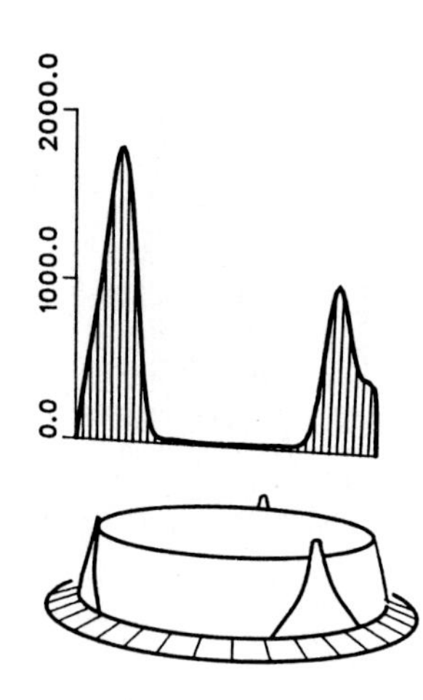

Figure 2.1–10A: Velocity profile 15 mm downstream on the centerline for the Carpentier-Edwards 2650 porcine valve, at peak systole.
Figure 2.1–10B: Turbulent shear stress profile 15 mm downstream on the centerline for the Carpentier-Edwards 2650 porcine valve, at peak systole.

valve at peak systole showed a maximum velocity of 180 cm/s. The maximum velocities measured during the acceleration and deceleration phases were 120 and 80 cm/s, respectively. A velocity defect was observed during the deceleration phase in the central part of the flow channel. A region of flow separation which extended about 6 mm from the wall was observed at peak systole and during the deceleration phase. This region was relatively stagnant during the acceleration phase. The maximum velocity of the jet at peak systole did not change as the flow travelled from 17 to 33mm downstream of the valve (Fig. 2.1–12A). However, the size of the region of flow separation decreased and extended only 1 mm from the wall. No regions of flow separation or stagnation were observed during the acceleration phase.

Turbulent shear stress measurements taken along the centreline plane 17 mm downstream of the valve showed that, during the deceleration phase, elevated turbulent shear stresses were spread out over a wide region (with a maximum value of 1,000 dynes/cm^2). At peak systole, the high turbulent shear stresses were confined to a narrow region, with a maximum value of 850 dynes/cm^2 (Fig. 2.1–12B). The intensity of turbulence at peak systole increased as the flow travelled from 17 to 33 mm downstream of the valve.

IMPLICATIONS FOR THROMBUS DEPOSITION

In the vicinity of mechanical heart valves, where peak shear stresses can easily exceed 1500 dynes/cm^2 and mean shear stresses are frequently in the range of 200–600

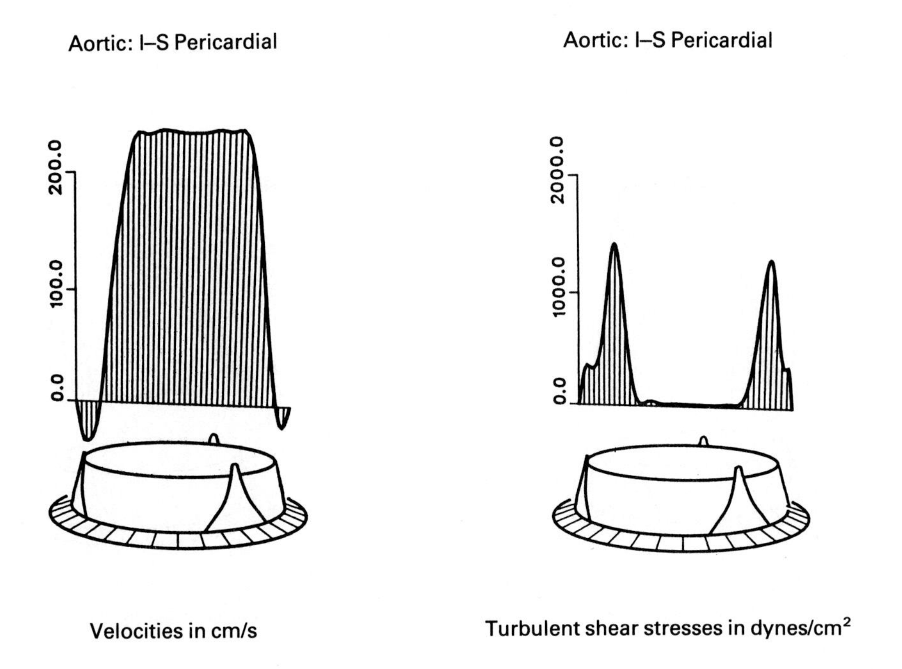

Figure 2.1–11A: Velocity profile 27 mm downstream on the centerline for the Ionescu-Shiley pericardial valve, at peak systole.

Figure 2.1–11B: Turbulent shear stress profile 27 mm downstream on the centerline for the Ionescu-Shiley pericardial valve, at peak systole.

dynes/cm^2 (Table 2.1–1), platelet activation and aggregation can readily occur. Data indicating that shear-induced platelet damage is cumulative[27] are particularly relevant to heart valves. During an individual excursion through the replacement valve, the combination of shear magnitude and exposure time may not induce platelet aggregation. However, as a result of multiple journeys through the artificial valve, shear-induced damage may accumulate to a degree sufficient to promote thrombosis and subsequent embolisation.

All of the aortic valve designs (mechanical and tissue) studied create mean turbulent shear stress in excess of 200 dynes/cm^2 during the major portion of systole (Table 2.1–1), which could lead to damage to blood elements. In the case of mechanical prostheses, due to the presence of foreign surfaces, the chances for blood cell damage are increased. Furthermore, the regions of flow stagnation and/or flow separation that occur adjacent to the superstructures of these valve designs, could promote the deposition of damaged blood elements, leading to thrombus formation on the prosthesis.

Starr-Edwards caged-ball valve (Model 1260)

The large wall shear stresses (1940 dynes/cm^2), created by the Starr-Edwards valve could cause lethal damage to the endothelial lining of the aortic wall adjacent to the valve and allow thrombus deposition and subsequent intimal thickening (see Chapter 2.4). The bulk turbulent shear stresses measured are large enough to cause damage to the red cells and platelets. The turbulent shear stresses in the annular region are also

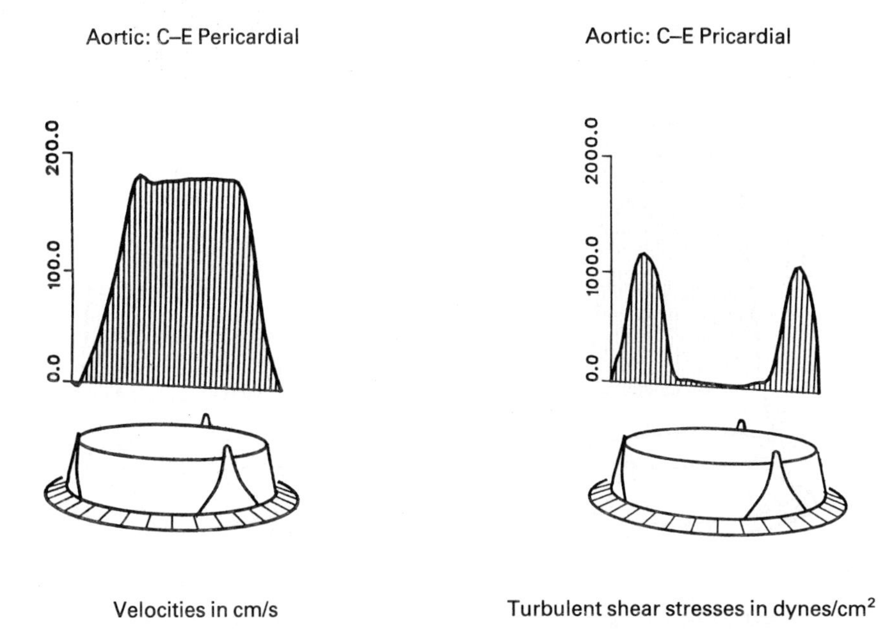

Figure 2.1–12A: Velocity profile 17 mm downstream on the centerline for the Carpentier-Edwards pericardial valve, at peak systole.
Figure 2.1–12B: Turbulent shear stress profile 17 mm downstream on the centerline for the Carpentier-Edwards pericardial valve, at peak systole.

large enough to lethally damage blood elements, which may then adhere to the valve cage or poppet. The region of stasis at the cage apex and the flow separation distal to the ball set the scene for thrombus formation on the apex of the cage (see Figure 2.4–3 in Chapter 2.4). The region of flow separation adjacent to the sewing ring could lead to tissue overgrowth. Both thrombus formation and tissue overgrowth occurring on various parts of the superstructure of this valve design are well documented in the clinical literature.

Bjørk-Shiley convexo-concave valve

As with the preceeding valve, the wall shear stresses (1380 dynes/cm^2) created by this valve are probably high enough to cause damage to the endothelial lining of the aortic wall. The turbulent shear stresses (3300 dynes/cm^2) are large enough to damage red cells and platelets. The in vitro studies have indicated that the valve creates two unequal regions of flow. There is a region of stasis below the outflow face of the disc and low flow through the minor orifice. Therefore, thrombus formation could occur on the aortic face of the disc and along the struts in the minor orifice region. A region especially vulnerable to thrombus formation would be the edge of the disc, near the centre-line plane. The high-velocity, jet-like flow adjacent to the flow channel wall leads to high turbulent shear stresses. Blood elements, damaged as a result, could easily be trapped in the region of stagnant flow below the edge of the disc and then become adherent to the disc. This part of the disc does not move much when the valve opens and closes and the damaged blood elements adhering to it are not likely to be washed away, hence increasing the risk of thrombus formation. The large region of flow separation adjacent to the sewing ring in the minor orifice region would encourage the growth of excess fibrous tissue along the sewing ring.

Medtronic Hall valve

The wall shear stress created by this valve also (700 dynes/cm^2) could cause sublethal damage to the endothelial lining of the aortic wall and the measured turbulent shear stresses (1900 dynes/cm^2) could damage red cells and platelets. The leakage backflow occurring through the small clearance of the central pivot hole (when the valve is closed) created turbulent shear stresses of the order of 700 dynes/cm^2. These turbulent shear stresses, although not very great in comparison to the turbulent shear stresses measured in the bulk flow downstream of the valve, could lead to damage to the blood elements, due to surface effects. The region of flow separation in the minor orifice could lead to excess tissue overgrowth along the sewing ring. The wake observed downstream from the strut in the minor orifice region could theoretically make this strut a possible location for thrombus formation. In addition, fibrous tissue growing along the sewing ring adjacent to this location might encapsulate this metal surface. If thrombus formation and/or tissue overgrowth started at these locations, the region of the wake could become larger and worsen the obstruction to flow. The region of stagnant flow observed at the edge of the occluder, adjacent to the stops, could trap damaged blood elements which might subsequently adhere to the occluder and lead to thrombus formation.

Omnicarbon valve

This valve produced turbulent shear stresses as high as 2000 dynes/cm^2, which are large enough to cause damage to the blood elements. The occluder of the Omnicarbon valve opens to a 79 degree angle and has a low pivot axis, allowing for more flow through the major orifice region compared with the minor orifice region. The region adjacent to the pivot guards was relatively stagnant during the acceleration and deceleration phases, and thus could be vulnerable to thrombus formation. The flow field produced by this valve during the deceleration phase was very unstable and disturbed, which could be a result of the large opening angle and the low pivoting point of the occluder. Furthermore, hydrodynamic instability of the occluder was occasionally observed during the deceleration phase.

St. Jude Medical valve

The wall shear stresses were relatively low (630 dynes/cm^2), but could still cause damage to the endothelial lining of the aortic wall. The high turbulent shear stresses (2000 dynes/cm^2) could cause damage to blood elements. Furthermore, the leakage backflow through the pivot area leads to turbulent shear stresses in the order of 500 dynes/cm^2. Such turbulent shear stresses could cause damage to red cells and platelets due to surface effects, and lead to haemolysis. The region of flow separation observed adjacent to the downstream sewing ring could lead to tissue overgrowth and/or thrombus formation in this region. The region adjacent to the pivot mechanism is especially vulnerable to thrombus formation, because of the combination of high turbulent shear stresses and flow separation observed in this region.

Edwards-Duromedics valve

This bileaflet valve design also created elevated turbulent shear stresses high enough to damage blood elements. The region of flow separation adjacent to the sewing ring could lead to tissue overgrowth. The velocity profiles taken across the central orifice of the Edwards-Duromedics valve showed a large region of flow separation and/or stagnation on either side of the central orifice, adjacent to the pivot mechanism of the valve (Fig. 2.1–7A). The elevated turbulent shear stresses (as high as 1700 dynes/cm^2) measured adjacent to these regions of flow separation and/or stagnation could damage blood elements, which would tend to become trapped within the regions of flow separation and/or stagnation and adhere to the surface of the valve adjacent to the pivot mechanism. Since the regions of the pivot mechanism of the Duromedics valve design are never fully washed during the cardiac cycle, as is the case in the St. Jude Medical valve design, thrombus formation may occur in these regions.

Bioprosthetic valves

All tissue valves, porcine and pericardial, create jet type central flow fields, although the newer generation bioprostheses tend to create somewhat flatter velocity profiles, producing more evenly distributed downstream flow fields and lower levels of turbulent shear stresses. The turbulent shear stresses are, however, large enough to damage the formed elements of blood. Furthermore, the annular region between the outflow surfaces of the valve leaflets and the flow channel wall is relatively stagnant during most of systole. All tissue valves studied have demonstrated this phenomenon, although the size of the stagnant region is smaller with the newer valve designs. The effect of these regions of stagnation is magnified by low cardiac output, during which one of the three leaflets may fail to open. Stagnation can lead to the deposition of thrombus on the outflow surfaces of the leaflets (see Figure 2.4–2 in Chapter 2.4).

CAVITATION STUDIES

With the exception of the Bicer and Sorin valves, all mechanical valve designs studied in distilled water showed cavitation at valve closure in a simulated mitral position when the artificially created 'left ventricular' dp/dt reached 5500 mm Hg/s and some showed cavitation within the range 1800 to 2000 mm Hg/s (equivalent to the physiological range under resting conditions).

Using the same valve size (27 mm), a comparison of the threshold values of dp/dt which produced cavitation showed that the Omnicarbon (875 mmHg/s), Medtronic Hall (1375 mmHg/s) and the Bjørk-Shiley Convexo-Concave (1500 mmHg/s) had the lowest values, cavitation occurring within the physiological dp/dt range. From the group of bileaflet valves, the Duromedics had the lowest threshold with 2250 mmHg/s, but this and the value for the St. Jude valve (2875 mmHg/s) were above the physiological level at rest (Table 2.1–2). It should be stressed that although all valves were of clinical quality, in most cases only one valve per size was investigated, so that the comparative results must be regarded as preliminary at this stage.

Table 2.1–2
Threshold values of 'left ventricular' dp/dt required to produce cavitation in 27mm mitral prostheses in vitro

Prosthesis	*dp/dt (mmHg/s)*
Sorin-Medical	5,500
Bicer	5,100
Bjørk-Shiley Spherical	4,250
Carbomedics	3,000
St. Jude Medical	2,875
Bjørk-Shiley Monostrut	2,450
Duromedics-Edwards	2,250
Bjørk-Shiley Concavo-convex	1,500
Medtronic-Hall	1,375
Omnicarbon	875

Note. In most cases, only one example of each prosthesis was tested.

The cavitation threshold was found to increase with valve size in some prostheses (Omnicarbon, Medtronic Hall and Bjørk-Shiley Monostrut). Conversely, for the same dp/dt value the bubble field increased with decreasing valve size, suggesting that the tendency to cavitation is greater in the smaller valve sizes[52].

Cavitation in a simulated mitral position can be observed with nearly all mechanical heart valves during in vitro testing. The 'left ventricular' dp/dt values associated with the onset of cavitation under these artificial conditions are equivalent to values of true left ventricular dp/dt within the physiological range at resting conditions. Therefore, it is possible that cavitation also occurs in vivo. Because no appropriate in vivo measurement techniques exist, this has yet to be confirmed.

Among single and bileaflet valves, the designs with the lowest leakage rates[53] seem to have the lowest cavitation thresholds, indicating that tight sealing at valve closure promotes the generation of high negative pressure downstream of the sealing area, at least under in vitro conditions.

Despite these interesting results, it is impossible to simulate in vitro true in vivo conditions in terms of the damping properties of adjacent tissues on high negative pressures. Nevertheless the present results suggest that measurements of cavitation should be included in any assessment of mechanical heart valve function and longevity. With respect to haemolysis and thromboembolism, cavitation may have to be added to the list of potential sources of blood cell damage following heart valve replacement.

CONCLUSIONS

The quantitative in vitro flow studies clearly indicate an improvement in both mechanical and tissue valve designs during the past decade. The mechanical valve designs, however, have less than ideal regurgitation characteristics which must be improved. The prosthetic valves designed after 1975 have superior pressure drop characteristics, and tend to create more centralised flow fields with lower levels of turbulence. However, the lower levels of turbulent shear stresses created by the newer valve designs, both mechanical and tissue, are still large enough to cause damage to the formed elements of the blood. Such damage to red cells and platelets may lead in some cases to significant haemolytic anaemia or, when combined with regions of stagnation and/or low velocity reverse flow, to the deposition of thrombus on the valve mechanism. There remains ample scope for further improvement in valve design to optimise haemodynamic characteristics, and thus reduce thrombus formation and thromboembolic complications.

ACKNOWLEDGEMENTS

This work was supported by research contracts from the Food and Drug Administration, and grants from the American Heart Association – Georgia Affiliate, various prosthetic heart valve manufacturers, and NIH (HL#45485). The help of Susan Elliott in preparing and typing this chapter is greatly appreciated.

REFERENCES

1. Roberts WC. Choosing a substitute cardiac valve: type, size, surgeon. Am J Cardiol 1976;38:633–644.
2. Woo Y-R. *In Vitro* Velocity and Shear Stress Measurements in the Vicinity of Prosthetic Heart Valves, PhD Thesis, Georgia Institute of Technology, 1984.
3. Woo Y-R, Yoganathan AP. An instrument for the measurement of in vitro velocity and turbulent shear stress in the immediate vicinity of prosthetic heart valves. Life Support Syst 1986;4:47–62.
4. Woo Y-R, Yoganathan AP. *In vitro* pulsatile flow velocity and turbulent shear stress measurements in the vicinity of mechanical aortic heart valve prostheses. Life Support Syst 1985;3:283–312.
5. Woo Y-R, Yoganathan AP. *In vitro* pulsatie flow velocity and shear stress measurements in the vicinity of mechanical mitral heart valve prostheses. J Biomech 1986;19:39–51.
6. Yoganathan AP, Woo Y-R, Sung H-W, Williams FP, Franch RH, Jones M. *In vitro* haemodynamic characteristics of tissue bioprostheses in the aortic position. J Thorac Cardiovasc Surg 1986;92:198–209.
7. Yoganathan AP, Woo Y-R, Sung H-W. Turbulent shear stress measurements in the vicinity of aortic heart valve prostheses. J Biomech 1986;19;433–442.
8. Yoganathan AP, Corcoran WH, Harrison EC. *In vitro* velocity measurements in the near vicinity of aortic valve prostheses. J Biomech 1979;12:135–152.
9. Yoganathan AP, Corcoran WH, Harrison EC, Carl JR. The Bjørk-Shiley aortic prosthesis: flow characteristics thrombus formation and tissue overgrowth. Circulation 1978;58:70–76.
10. Bruss K-H. Reul H, van Gilse J, Knott E. Pressure drop and velocity fields at four mechanical heart valve prostheses: Bjørk-Shiley Standard, Bjørk-Shiley Concave-Convex, Hall-Kaster and St. Jude Medical. Life Support Syst 1983;1:3–15.
11. Chandran KG, Cabell GN, Khalighi B, Chen C-J. Laser anemometry measurements of pulsatile flow past aortic valve prostheses. J Biomech 1983;16:865–873.
12. Chandran KB, Cabell GN, Khalighi B, Chen C-J: Pulsatile flow past aortic valve bioprosthesis in a model human aorta. J Biomech 1984;17:609–619.
13. Jones M, McMillan ST, Eidbo EE, Woo Y-R, Yoganathan AP. Evaluation of prosthetic heart valves by Doppler flow imaging. Echocardiography 1986;3:513–525.
14. Yoganathan AP, Sung H-W, Woo Y-R, Jones M. *In vitro* velocity and turbulence measurements in the vicinity of three new mechanical aortic heart valve prostheses. J Thorac Cardiovasc Surg 1988;95:929–939.
15. Nevaril C, Hellums J, Alfrey C Jr. Lynch E. Physical effects in red blood cell trauma. J Am Inst Chem Engr 1969;15:707–711.
16. Sallam A, Hwang NHC. Red blood cell hemolysis in a turbulent jet. Presented at ASME Biomechanics Symposium, Houston, TX, USA. New York, American Society of Mechanical Engineers, 1983;83–86.
17. Blackshear PL. Haemolysis at prosthetic surfaces. Chemistry of Biosurfaces 1972;2:523–561.
18. Mohandas H, Hochmuth RM, Spaeth EE. Adhesion of red cells to foreign surfaces in the presence of flow. J Biomed Mater Res 1974;8:119–136.
19. Sutera SP, Merjhardi MH. Deformation and fragmentation of human red cells in turbulent shear flow. Biophys J 1975;15:1–15.
20. Hung TC, Hochmuth RM, Joist JH, Sutera SP. Shear induced aggregation and lysis of platelets. Trans Am Soc Artif Int Organs 1976;22:285–290.

21. Ramstack JM, Zuckerman L, Mockros LF. Shear induced activation of platelets. J Biomech 1979;12:113–125.
22. Hellums JD, Brown CH, III. Blood cell damage by mechanical forces. In Hwang NHC, Norman NA (Eds.). Cardiovascular Fluid Dynamics and Measures. Baltimore, University Park Press, 1977;1–42.
23. Wurzinger LJ, Schmid-Schonbein H. Species difference in platelet aggregation and the influence of citrate and heparin anticoagulation thereon. Am Soc Artif Intern Organs J 1981;4:149–156.
24. Wurzinger LJ, Opitz R, Blasberg P, Echweiler H, Schmid-Schonbein H. The role of hydrodynamic factors in platelet activation and thrombotic events. In Schettler G (Ed.). The Effects of Shear Stress of Short Duration, Fluid Dynamics as a Localizing Factor for Atherosclerosis. Berlin, Springer, 1983;91–102.
25. Stein PD, Walburn FJ, Sabbah NH. Turbulent stresses in the region of aortic and pulmonary valves. J Biomech Eng 1982;104:238–244.
26. Hanle DD. Fluid dynamics of prosthetic aortic heart valves in steady and pulsatile flow. PhD Thesis, Calfornia Institute of Technology, CA, 1984.
27. Brown CH, III, Lemuth RF, Hellums JD, Leverett LB, Alfrey CP. Response of human platelets to shear stress. Trans ASAIO 1977;21:35–39.
28. Anderson GH, Hellums JD. Platelet lysis and aggregation in shear fields. Blood Cells 1978;4:499–507.
29. Colantuoni G, Hellums JD, Moake JL, Alfrey CP Jr. The response of human platelets to shear stress at short exposure times. Trans ASAIO 1977;23:626–631.
30. Moritz MW, Reimers RC, Baker RK, Sutera SP, Joist JH. Role of cytoplasmic and releasable ADP in platelet aggregation induced by laminar shear stress. J Lab Clin Med 1983;101:537–544.
31. Clagett GP. Artificial devices in clinical practice. In Colman RW, Hirsh J, Marder VJ, Salzman EW (Eds.). Hemostasis and Thrombosis. Basic Principles and Clinical Practice. Second edition. Philadelphia, JB Lippincott Co., 1987:1348–1365.
32. Cohn, LH. Thromboembolism in different anatomical positions:Aortic, mitral, and multiple valves. In Rábago G, Cooley DA (Eds.). Heart Valve Replacement: Current Status and Future Trends. Mount Kisco, NY, Futura Publishing, 1987:259–270.
33. Becker RM, Strom J, Frishman W, Oka Y, Lin YT, Yellin EL, Frater RWM. Performance of the Ionescu-Shiley valve prosthesis. J Thorac Cardiovasc Surg 1980;80:613–620.
34. Grunkemeier GL. Stastitical analysis of prosthetic valve series. In Rábago G, Cooley DA (Eds.). Heart Valve Replacement: Current Status and Future Trends. Mount Kisco, NY, Futura Publishing, 1987:11–26.
35. Dale J. Arterial thromboembolic complications in patients with Starr-Edwards aortic ball valve prostheses. Am Heart J 1976;91:653–659.
36. Fuster V, Pumphrey CW, McGoon MD, Chesbro JH, Pluth JR, McGoon DC. Systemic thromboembolism in mitral and aortic Starr-Edwards prostheses: A 10–19 year follow-up. Circulation 1982;66 (suppl I):157–161.
37. Starr A. The Starr-Edwards valve. J Am Coll Cardiol 1985;6:899–903.
38. Moore CH, Martelli V, Al-Janabi N, Ross DN. Analysis of homograft valve failure in 311 patients followed up to 10 years. Ann Thorac Surg 1975;20:274–281.
39. Barratt-Boyes B. Aortic valve disease. In Kirklin JW, Barratt-Boyes BG, (Eds.). Cardiac Surgery. New York, Wiley, 1986;373–429.
40. Horstkotte D, Körfer R, Siepel L, Bircks W, Loogen F. Late complications in patients with Bjørk-Shiley and St. Jude Medical heart valve replacement. Circulation 1983;68 (suppl II):175–184.
41. Jacobs ML, Buckley MJ, Austen WG, Swinski LA, Daggett WM, Akins CW. Mechanical valves: Ten year follow-up of Starr-Edwards and Bjørk-Shiley prostheses. Circulation 1985;72 (suppl III):208.
42. Czer LSC, Matloff J, Chaux A, DeRobertis M, Yoganathan Y, Gray RJ. A 6 year experience with the St. Jude medical valve: Haemodynamic performance, surgical results, biocompatibility and followup. J Am Coll Cardiol 1985;6:904–912.
43. Arom KV, Nicoloff DM, Kersten TE, Northrop WF III, Lindsay WG. Six years of experience with the St. Jude Medical valvular prosthesis. Circulation 1985;72 (suppl II):153–158.
44. Baudet EM, Oca CC, Roques XF, Laborde MN, Hafez AS, Collot MA, Ghidoni IM. A 5½ year experience with the St. Jude Medical cardiac valve prosthesis. J Thorac Cardiovasc Surg 1985;90:137–144.
45. Hall KV, Nitter-Hauge S, Abdelnoor M. Seven and one-half years' experience with the Medtronic-Hall valve. J Am Coll Cardiol 1985;6:1417–1421.
46. Callaghan JC, Teijeira J, Bonneau D, Gelfand ET, Casey P, Drutz J. A five year study of the incidence of valve-related complications with the Omniscience cardiac prosthesis. J Cardiovasc Surg 1986;27:500–502.
47. Martinell J, Fraile J, Artiz V, Morena J, Rábago G. Long-term comparative analysis of the Bjørk-Shiley and Hancock valves implanted in 1975. J Thorac Cardiovasc Surg 1985;90:741–749.

48. Jamieson WRE, Pelletier LC, Janusz MT, Chaitman BR, Tyers GFO, Miyagishima M. Five year evaluation of the Carpentier-Edwards porcine bioprosthesis. J Thorac Cardiovasc Surg 1984;88:324–333.
49. Pelletier C, Chaitman BR, Baillot R, Val PG, Bonan R, Dyrda I. Clinical and haemodynamic results with the Carpentier-Edwards porcine bioprosthesis. Ann Thorac Surg 1982;34:612–624.
50. Brais MP, Bédard JP, Goldstein W, Korshal A, Keon WJ. Ionescu-Shiley pericardial xenografts: Follow-up of up to 6 years. Ann Thorac Surg 1985;39:105–111.
51. Borovetz HS, Kormos RL, Griffith, Hung T-C. Clinical utilization of the artificial heart. Crit Rev Biomed Eng 1989;17:179–201.
52. Knott E, Reul H, Knoch M, Steinseifer G, Rau G. *In vitro* comparision of aortic heart valve protheses. J Thorac Cardiovasc Surg 1988;96:952–961.
53. Graf T, Fischer H, Reul H, Rau G. Cavitation potential of mechanical heart valve protheses. Int J Artif Organs 1991;14:169–171.

Chapter 2.2

Haematological Effects of Turbulent Blood Flow

S. P. Sutera and J. H. Joist

THE NATURE OF TURBULENT SHEAR FLOW.

The word turbulent is derived from the Latin adjective *turbulentus,* which means disturbed, confused, stormy or boisterous. The related Latin noun *turba* means a tumult, uproar, disturbance or commotion, especially one caused by a crowd of people. It is easy to understand therefore how the word turbulent when applied to blood flow has come to be used by many as a description for any type of violently disturbed flow pattern. However, in the terminology of fluid dynamics, turbulence has a much more specific and restricted definition.

In 1883, Osborne Reynolds, while studying the flow of pure liquids in tubes, discovered that two basic flow regimes were possible: *laminar,* in which the fluid appears to move smoothly in concentric layers or *laminae,* and *turbulent,* wherein dye streaks would curl up, break up and spread out rapidly until they were no longer recognisable as streaks. Turbulent flow is characterised by an unsteady and irregular eddying motion, which is superimposed on the mean flow. At a fixed point in a turbulent flow, velocity and pressure fluctuate rapidly about their mean values (Fig.

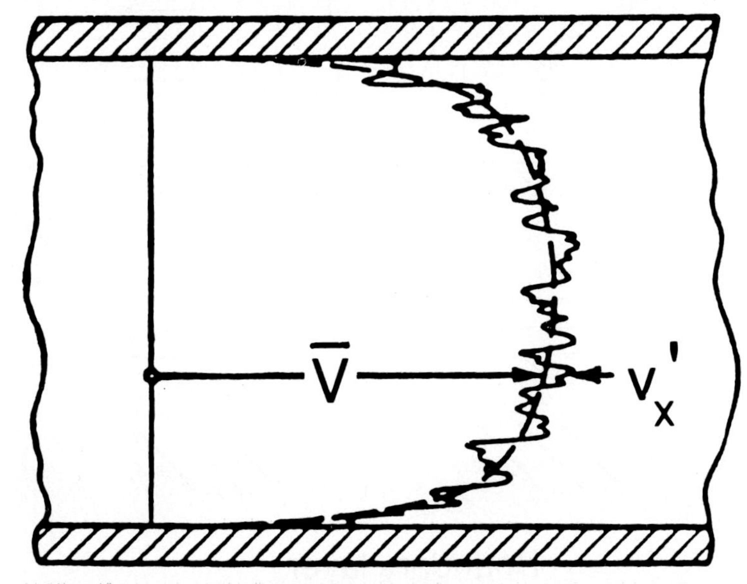

Figure 2.2–1: Representation of an instantaneous velocity profile in turbulent tube flow. At any point in the flow (except within a thin layer next to the tube wall) the velocity consists of a time-averaged or mean component and a randomly fluctuating component.

2.2–1). These fluctuations appear random in space and time and possess a continuous spectrum of length scales and frequencies. They can only be described in statistical terms.

Reynolds learned that the transition from laminar to turbulent flow in pipes was governed by a combination of the fluid density and viscosity, the average flow velocity and the tube diameter. This dimensionless combination is known as the Reynolds number; it is expressed mathematically as

$$Re \equiv \frac{\rho V D}{\mu}, \tag{1}$$

where

ρ = liquid density (g/cm^3),
μ = dynamic viscosity ($dyn.sec./cm^2$ = poise),
V = cross-sectional average velocity (cm/sec),

and

D = pipe diameter (cm).

Experiments showed that laminar flow in pipes becomes unstable when Re exceeds approximately 2000. As shown in Figure 2.2–2, steady turbulent flow in a tube is characterised by a mean velocity profile, which is more blunt than the parabolic laminar profile; hence a steeper velocity gradient or shear rate at the wall. Note that, in either flow regime, the fluid in contact with the solid boundary does not slip past the

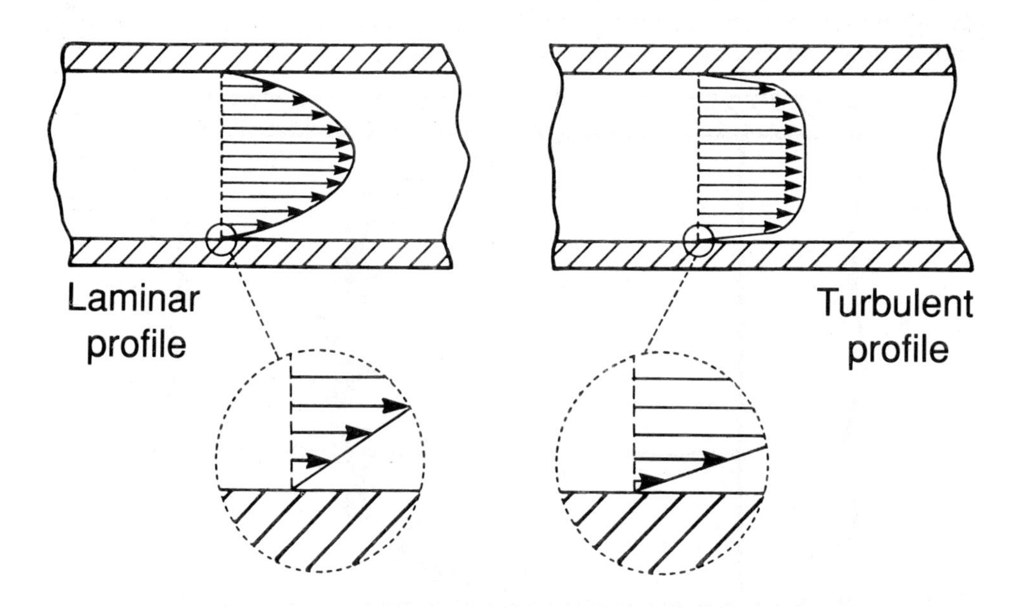

Figure 2.2–2: Laminar versus turbulent mean flow velocity profiles in tube flow. The latter is more blunt and has a steeper slope (i.e., shear rate) at the tube wall.

surface and so has zero velocity there. Turbulent fluctuations are damped out very close to a solid boundary resulting in a thin laminar region (the viscous sublayer) adjacent to the boundary.

Since Reynolds' discovery we have learned that this dichotomous nature of fluid flow occurs everywhere in nature. With each particular flow geometry there is a critical Reynolds number beyond which a *steady* laminar flow becomes unstable and will degenerate into turbulent flow. For example, jet flows issuing from a relatively small orifice, like a stenotic valve or a paravalvular leak into a relatively quiescent body of fluid entrain some of the latter into a "free" shear layer, that is one which is unassociated with a solid boundary (Fig. 2.2–3). This shear layer becomes turbulent when the jet Reynolds number surpasses a critical value. Flows past bluff or unstreamlined bodies such as the ball of a caged ball prosthetic valve or the disc of a tilting disc valve at high angle of attack (Fig. 2.2–4) typically separate from the body surface and form turbulent wakes bounded by free shear layers.

Turbulent versus 'disturbed' flow

Published values of critical Reynolds numbers, that is values of *Re* at which transition from laminar to turbulent flow will occur somewhere in the flow field, generally pertain to steady, non-pulsatile flows. In the circulation, of course, the geometry of the heart and large arteries is constantly changing in a periodic fashion, and blood flow is consequently pulsatile. In the normal aorta, the peak Reynolds number can surpass the critical value of 2000, but the systolic pulse, lasting only tenths of a second, is too brief to permit the full development of turbulent flow with a complete spectrum of eddy sizes, especially those of microscopic scale comparable to

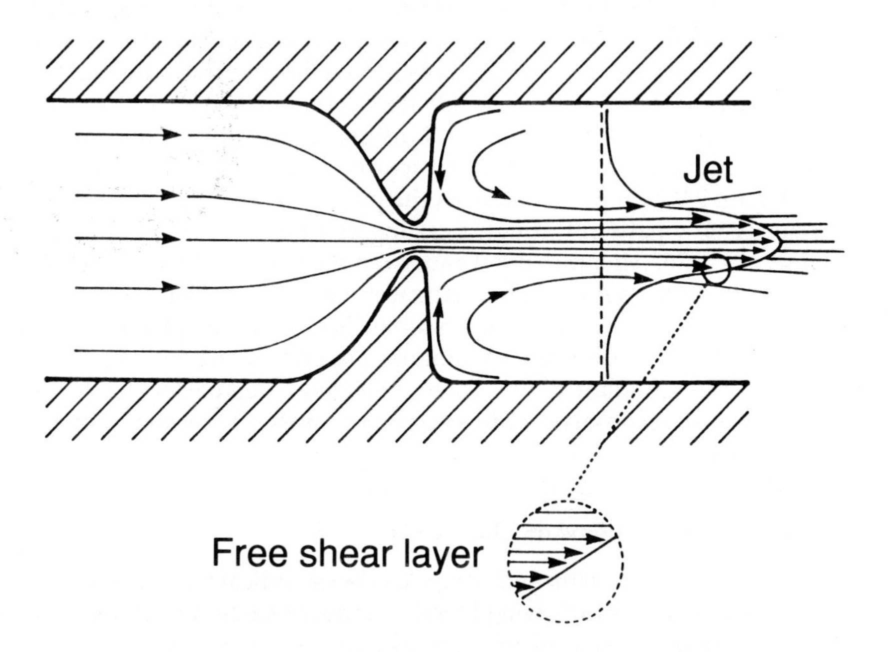

Figure 2.2–3: Free shear layer generated by jet flow emerging from an orifice.

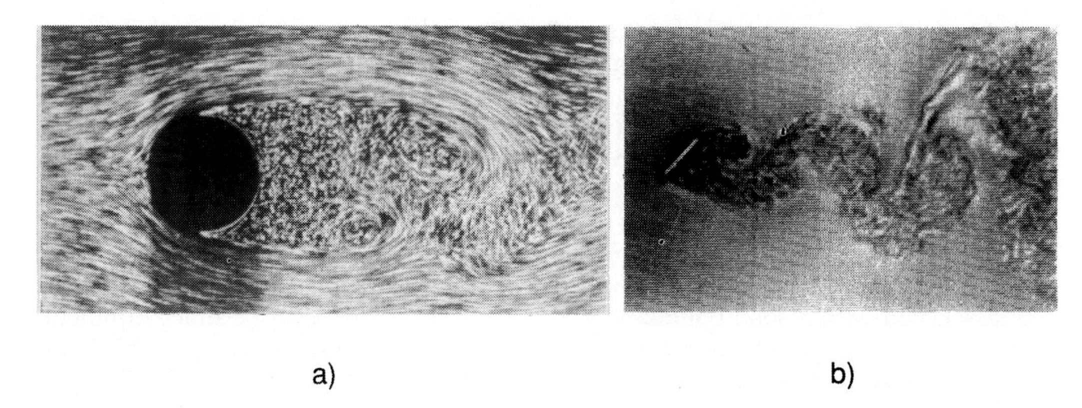

Figure 2.2–4: Photographs of turbulent wakes generated in steady flows normal to bluff bodies. (a) Flow past a sphere. (b) Flow past a tilted disk. The flow patterns are made visible by fine aluminium particles carried by the flow.

blood cells. Periodic, turbulence-like fluctuations or 'turbulence bursts' have been measured in the aortic flows of man, dog and horse. However, the application of hot-film anemometry to surveys of blood flow in the normal aorta and large arteries of humans, dogs and horses has excluded the presence of turbulence in these areas[1–3]. Furthermore, these anemometric measurements usually give no indication of the length scale or 'eddy-size' of the fluctuations. Special configurations of two or more hot-film probes are necessary to determine the size spectrum of the eddies. Further along the descending aorta, measurements have indicated either undisturbed or, at worst, 'disturbed flow', but not true turbulence.

Disturbed flow is a descriptive term which generally implies that, relative to a stationary sensor, the flow is unsteady (time-varying) and also has a complex structure, including separated regions and large vortices. Given the pulsatile nature of blood flow and the compliance of the vessels, unsteady flow is the normal condition. The careful flow visualisation work done by Karino and his group at McGill University has given considerable insight to the complex flow structures that occur in the vicinity of vessel branchings. Figure 2.2–5, reproduced from the publication of Motomiya and Karino[4], shows the steady flow pattern through a casting of a human carotid bifurcation. The flow is laminar (Re = 762, entering flow) and, even though it is steady, it separates and forms a large vortex in the sinus. Individual tracer particles are deflected at the divider, then travel laterally along the daughter vessel walls describing spiral orbits about the mainstream. These so-called secondary motions superimposed on the primarily axial mainstream give the resultant flow a three-dimensional character. Such flows look disturbed to the eye of an observer or to a stationary sensor. However, they are clearly not turbulent flows.

In vitro effects of turbulent flow on blood cells

There is a large body of *in vitro* and *in vivo* evidence indicating that shear affects (a) the interaction of blood cells in flowing blood, (b) the interaction of platelets and other cells with the injured vessel wall or artificial surface, (c) the surface properties of platelets, resulting in the expression of receptors for biologically important agonists

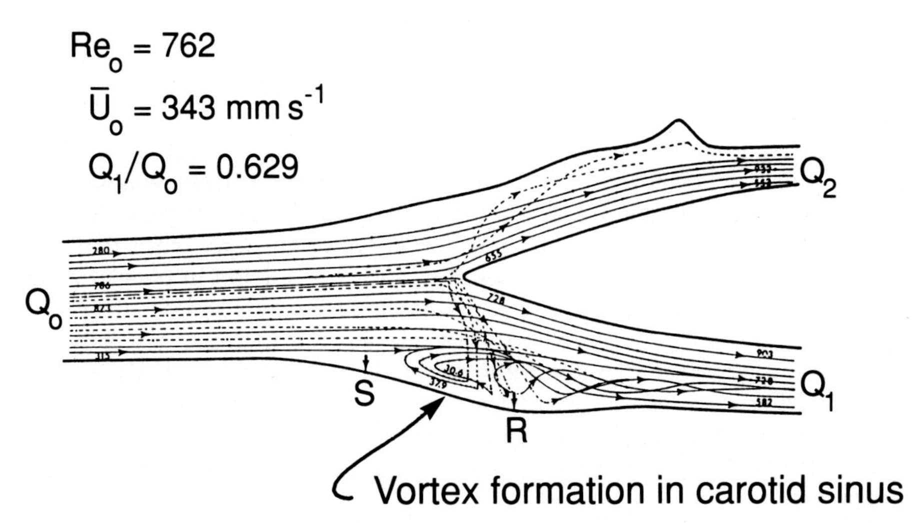

Figure 2.2–5: Steady flow pattern in a human common carotid bifurcation, constructed from tracer particle trajectories. The Reynolds number is representative of physiological flow rates. A large vortex has formed in the carotid sinus. S and R denote the respective separation and reattachment points. (From Motomiya and Karino[4] with permission).

(leading to release and aggregation) or adhesive glycoproteins, and (d) cell membrane integrity, resulting in sublethal or lethal cell injury.

The effects of prolonged exposure (in the order of several minutes) to controlled turbulent shear flow on erythrocytes and platelets have been studied *in vitro*. These showed a stress threshold for haemolysis of 1500 to 2500 dynes/cm^2[5,6], a range which is roughly ten times the maximum shear stress possible in the *normal* human circulation. It is important to note that this same threshold was found in independent *in vitro* studies performed in *laminar* shear flow[7]. In contrast to erythrocytes, platelets have a substantially lower tolerance to injury by shear stress when the period of exposure is in the order of five minutes. Major platelet damage evidenced by loss from platelets of large molecules such as lactic dehydrogenase (LDH) may be induced in human, platelet-rich plasma by shear stresses in the range of 100–150 dynes/cm^2, but this threshold appears to be similar in laminar[8–11] and turbulent shear flows[12]. At sustained (5 minutes) shear stresses as low as 25 dynes/cm^2, human platelets *in vitro* release serotonin and adenine nucleotides[9] and aggregate. The key point to bear in mind, however, is the sustained exposure (minutes) of the blood cells to shear stresses in most of these *in vitro* experiments.

In experiments in which platelets were exposed to viscometric shear stresses *in vitro* for shorter periods of time, extensive aggregation of human platelets was observed in citrated platelet-rich plasma exposed to pulsatile shear stress of one second duration at 25 dyn/cm^2. Aggregation was associated with small amounts of serotonin release and generation of platelet procoagulant activity[13]. However, *in vivo*, the exposure of blood cells passing through a region of high shear stress, turbulent or not, would be measured in milliseconds. Under such circumstances the stress thresholds for cellular damage would probably be enormously increased[14]. Indeed, Wurzinger and Schmid-Schönbein[15] have reported the induction of platelet aggregation and platelet damage with exposure of human platelets to shear stresses of 2550 dyn/cm^2 for only seven milliseconds.

The difficulties encountered in both *in vitro* and *in vivo* attempts to evaluate the effects of turbulent flow are demonstrated in Figure 2.2–6. Human citrated platelet-rich plasma (platelets, 300,000/μl) was exposed to continuous (5 min) shear stresses of different intensity in a computerised cone-plate viscometer[16]. There was a progressive increase in platelet aggregation and serotonin release as the flow regime changed from strictly laminar (up to 40 dyn/cm^2) to transitional. To test the hypothesis that reduction in the Reynolds number would be associated with a reduction in platelet activation, aliquots of platelet-rich plasma were exposed to the same shear stress in the presence of 40% (vol/vol) of normal red blood cells ghosts, to increase viscosity without introducing the potentially confounding effects of red cell-derived ADP[17]). Interestingly, the addition of red cell ghosts potentiated platelet aggregation probably via increased platelet diffusivity[17]. However, there was little if any decrease in serotonin release or platelet damage (LDH loss) as a result of the attenuation of transitional flow disturbances.

Turbulent flow associated with prosthetic valves and its haematological consequences

While it is safe to say that fully developed turbulent flow is unlikely to occur in the normal human vascular tree, flow even in the normal heart and aorta during the systolic pulse is rapid and comprises intense, localised shear layers which can generate

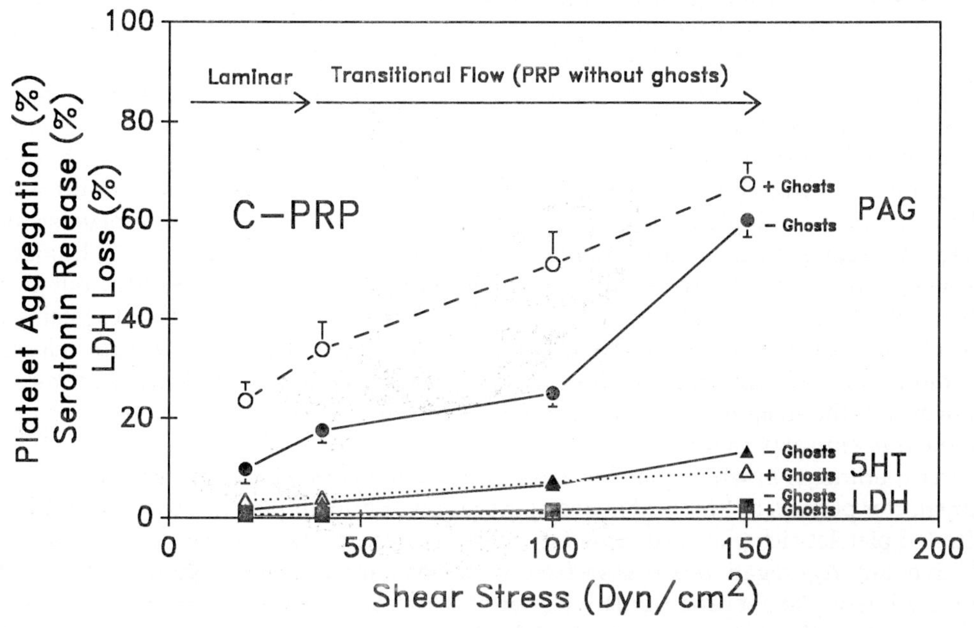

Figure 2.2–6: Platelet aggregation, serotonin release and LDH loss induced by shear in citrated, human platelet rich plasma (C-PRP) in a cone-plate viscometer; laminar and transitional flow in the presence and absence of red blood cell (RBC) ghosts. PAG: platelet aggregation, 5HT: serotonin, LDH: lactic dehydrogenate. For details see text.

brief bursts of turbulent flow fluctuations. Stein and Sabbah demonstrated the occurrence of disturbed flow and turbulent fluctuations near the normal aortic valve during and after peak systolic flow[18]. Turbulence intensity was magnified markedly in patients with severe aortic stenosis or aortic regurgitation, but in both normal and pathological situations the flow disturbances did not endure past the aortic arch. Using *in vitro* simulation techniques Yoganathan and co-workers[19] have measured turbulent shear stresses in flows distal to a variety of prosthetic valves. Localised shear stresses as high as 1000–2000 dynes/cm^2 were frequently observed. The possibility of extraordinary levels of shear stress is enhanced under the abnormal conditions imposed by a severely stenosed valve or certain prosthetic valve designs[20] (see Chapter 2.1). An extreme condition can arise in the event of a paravalvular leak; the resulting regurgitant jet can generate supraphysiological shear stresses sufficient to cause haemolysis, platelet activation and platelet damage. An important question then follows. When such shear-induced cellular damage occurs, to what extent does the presence of turbulent flow, however transient, contribute to that damage? To answer this we must examine the mechanisms underlying shear stress in a turbulent shear flow.

In laminar flow, the shear stress at any point in the flow is the product of the fluid viscosity and the velocity gradient or shear rate at that point. In turbulent flow, an additional mechanism arising from the eddy motion increases the effective viscosity and, thereby, the shear stress. This mechanism is described empirically in terms of an 'eddy viscosity' and the corresponding shear stress transmitted between adjacent layers of the flow is called the 'Reynolds stress'. Figure 2.2–7 shows schematically the physical mechanism of this turbulent component of shear stress. A slow moving fluid 'particle' (a small but macroscopical packet of fluid) from below the imaginary dashed line 'jumps' into the faster moving fluid above and causes the fluid around it to decelerate. In other words, it exerts a negative force on the fluid in its new surroundings. In like manner, a particle from the faster moving fluid jumps into the slow moving fluid below the line (there is no net exchange of mass across the imaginary line) and causes that fluid to accelerate. This exchange of momentum (per unit area) is interpretable as a virtual shear stress (the Reynolds stress). In mathematical terms the Reynolds shear stress is expressible as

$$\tau_T = -\overline{\rho \upsilon^1 v^1}, \qquad (2)$$

where

ρ = mass density of the fluid,
υ^1 = velocity fluctuation in the X (horizontal) direction,
v^1 = velocity fluctuation in the y (vertical) direction.

The overbar signifies the time average of the product. It is important to understand that, in the normal circulation, the Reynolds stress does not operate at a solid boundary because the velocity fluctuations are damped out in the vicinity of the boundary. For this reason there will always exist a laminar boundary layer (the sublayer) between a smooth boundary and a turbulent core flow. Flow conditions in the vicinity of a prosthetic valve are, however, very different from those in the vascular tree and

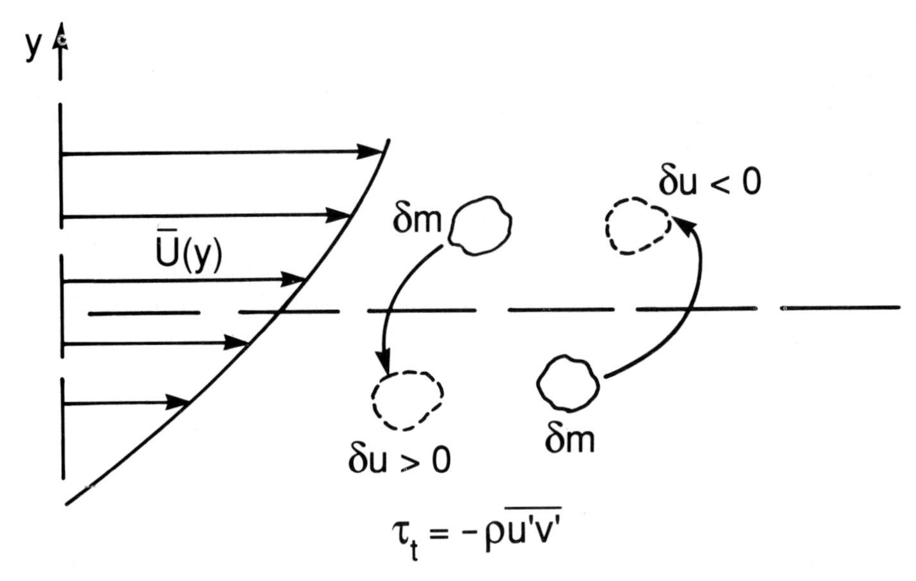

Figure 2.2–7: Diagram illustrating the physical mechanism of the turbulent component of shear stress, also known as the Reynold stress, i.e., transverse movement of fluid particles. At a solid boundary the Reynolds stress does not operate and the tangential stress exerted on the boundary is purely viscous.

endothelial damage caused by localised high shear stresses has been described (see Chapter 2.1).

If one visualises a red cell embedded in a turbulent flow as sketched in Figure 2.2–8, one can think of two extremes. First, if the turbulent eddies are large with respect to the suspended cells (Fig. 2.2–8a), the cells could probably be transported inside the eddies and experience a basically viscous, laminar flow around them. Shear stress in the mean flow is still transmitted through the eddies and would generate distortional surface forces on the cells. Second, if the eddies are small compared with the cells, then, in addition to the shear stress exerted by the mean flow, a cell would experience additional distortional shear due to 'micro-gusts' which buffet different regions of the cell at different times. The effect of clear air turbulence causing 'wind shear' on an airliner is an analogous phenomenon. In reality, turbulent flows generally contain a multiplicity of eddy sizes. The largest have the same scale as the flow itself and by the action of viscosity these break down into smaller and smaller eddies until the very smallest are dissipated to thermal energy. This cascading process of eddy development takes time, however, and in the millisecond existence of the turbulent bursts generated by a normal aortic valve, it is extremely unlikely that eddies of a size smaller than a red cell or a platelet will develop. Hence, the most probable situation is the first one, that eddies much larger than the blood cells will be generated.

This conclusion is supported by studies on turbulent shear flows bearing red cells and platelets[6,12], the results of which suggested that turbulent fluctuations did not aggravate the effects of shear on the suspended cells. To pursue this point further, glutaraldehyde was used to fix human red cells while they were subjected to intense, but well defined turbulent shear flows *in vitro*[21]. The fixed post-shear cell shapes thus observed were remarkable for their regularity and uniformity. Virtually all of the cells

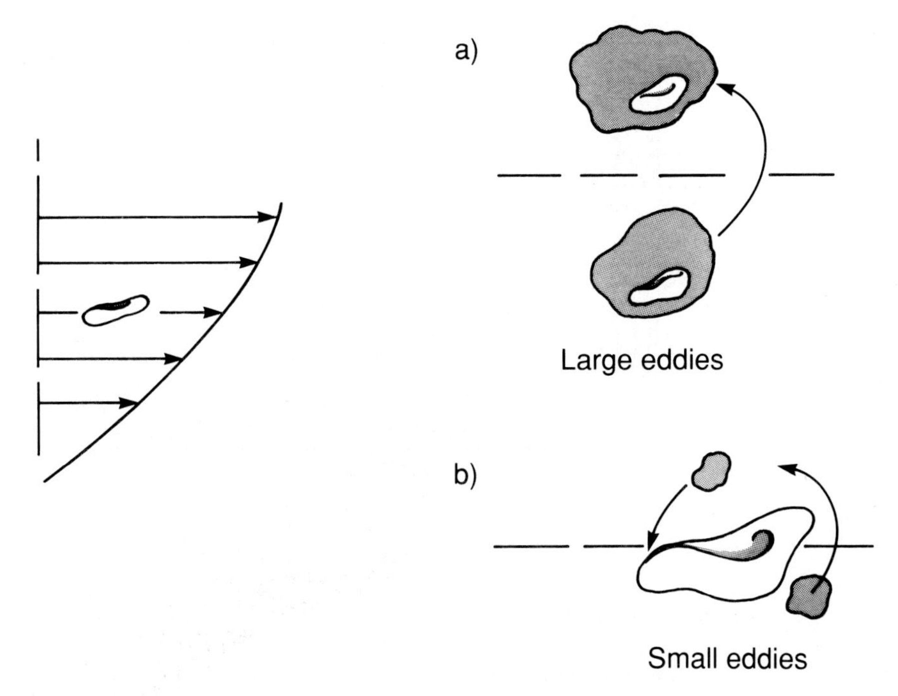

Figure 2.2–8: Illustration of the effect of eddy (dark) motion on red blood cells (light) in a turbulent shear flow (a) when eddies are larger than the cells and (b) when eddies are smaller than the cells.

were stretched into smooth, ellipsoidal forms well known from rheoscopic observations in uniform laminar shear flows[22]. The lack of any morphological reflection of the randomness or chaos of turbulence could be interpreted to indicate that the scale of the turbulent fluctuations was not small enough to cause distortion of the red cells. Subsequently, it was estimated that the dominant, energy-bearing eddies present in the flow were about 200μm in diameter, which is an order of magnitude greater than the disc diameter of the human red cell. Sustained (4 min) exposure of human red cells to higher, haemolytic levels of shear stress, again in the turbulent regime, revealed the same type of shear-induced fragmentation produced in laminar shear flows of comparable stress[6].

CONCLUSIONS

Damage to circulating blood cells is determined primarily by the magnitude of shear stress encountered and by the duration of exposure. Immediately distal to a prosthetic aortic valve, zones of turbulent shear flow can occur during systole. The same may be true for a severely stenosed natural valve. Paravalvular leaks can also generate extremely high shear stresses. In all of these situations the short duration (tenths of a second) of high shear rates makes it unlikely that normal erythrocytes will lyse. Conceivably, some fragile members of the cell population, perhaps the senescent ones, may not be able to resist fragmentation. On the other hand, the combination of stress intensity and duration seem quite sufficient to activate or damage platelets that are transported through the high shear regions. However, any activation or damage so

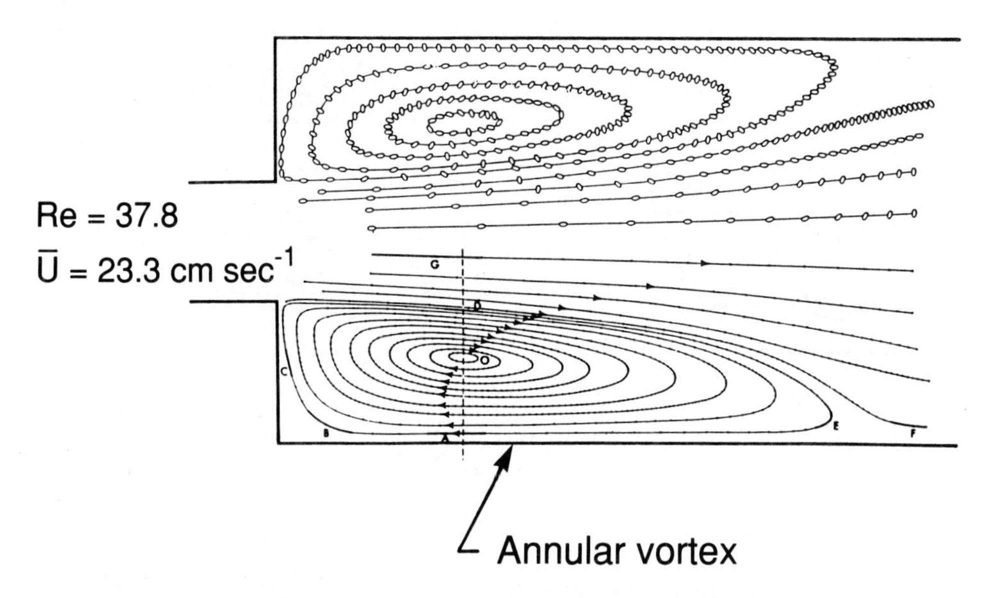

Figure 2.2–9: Visualisation of flow through a sudden expansion from a 150μm tube. The flow is steady and laminar. A large annular vortex is formed in which glutaraldehyde-hardened human red cells circulate in closed orbits. (From Karino et al.[24], *with permission).*

produced is probably not attributable to the presence of turbulence, in the strict scientific sense of the word, because the dominant turbulent eddies will be much larger than either the red cells or the platelets.

Thus turbulent flow, as strictly defined, does not appear to be a serious factor in either blood cell activation or damage associated with prosthetic valves. However, one fluid-mechanical factor which certainly can be implicated is the potential for flow separation and stable recirculation zones provoked by geometrical discontinuities in the flow boundaries. Figure 2.2–9 (taken from reference 23) exemplifies the danger. Laminar flow through a sudden expansion from a 150μm diameter tube to 500μm (a step height of 175 μm) generates a stable annular vortex, in which platelets could be entrained and held for long periods of time. Since the mural boundary layer of the entering flow is likely to be richer in platelets than the mainstream, the vortex will provide conditions conducive to platelet collisions and aggregation and also interaction with the wall, processes which are involved in thrombus formation.

REFERENCES

1. Stein PD, Sabbah HN, Anbe DT, Walburn FJ. Blood velocitiy in the abdominal aorta and common iliac artery of man. Biorheology 1979;16:249–255.
2. Nerem RM, Rumberger JA Jr, Cross DR, Hamlin RL, Geiger GL. Hot-film anemometer velocity measurements of arterial blood flow in horses. Circ Res 1974;34:193–203.
3. Nerem RM, Seed WA. An *in vivo* study of aortic flow disturbances. Cardiovasc Res 1972;6:1–14.
4. Motomiya M, Karino T. Flow patterns in the human carotid artery bifurcation. Stroke 1984;15:50–56.
5. Sutera SP, Croce PA, Mehrjardi MH. Haemolysis and sub-haemolytic alterations of human RBC induced by turbulent shear flow. Trans Am Soc Artif Intern Organs 1972;18:335–341.
6. Sutera SP, Mehrjardi HM. Deformation and fragmentation of human RBC in turbulent shear flow. Biophys J 1975;15:1–10.

7. Leverett LB, Hellums JD, Alfrey CP, Lynch EC. Red blood cell damage by shear stress. Biophys J 1972;12:257–273.
8. Brown CH, Lemuth RF, Hellums JD, Leverett LB, Alfrey CP. Response of human platelets to shear stress. Trans Am Soc Artif Intern Organs 1975;21:35–38.
9. Brown CH, Leverett LB, Lewis CN, Alfrey CP, Hellums JD. Morphological, biochemical and functional changes in human platelets subjected to shear stress. J Lab Clin Med 1975;86:462–471.
10. Moritz MW, Sutera SP, Joist JH. Factors influencing shear-induced platelet alterations: Platelet lysis is independent of platelet aggregation and release. Thromb Res 1981;22:445–455.
11. Moritz MW, Reimers RC, Baker RK, Sutera SP, Joist JH. Role of cytoplasmic and releasable ADP in platelet aggregation induced by laminar shear stress. J Lab Clin Med 1983;101:537–544.
12. Hung TC, Hochmuth RM, Joist JH, Sutera SP. Shear-induced aggregation and lysis of platelets. Trans Am Soc Artif Intern Organs 1976;22:265–290.
13. Joist JH, Bauman JE, Sutera SP. Platelet alterations in response to repetitive, short duration laminar shear stress. Thromb Haemost 1987;58:12(Abstract).
14. Hellums JD, Peterson DM, Stathopoulos NA, Moake JL, Georgio TD. Studies on the mechanisms of shear-induced platelet activation, in *Cerebral Ischemia and Hemorheology*. Hartmann A, Kuschinsky W, Eds. Berlin, Springer Verlag, 1987:80–89.
15. Wurzinger LJ, Schmid-Schönbein H. Surface abnormalities and conduit characteristics as a cause of blood trauma in artificial internal organs: The interaction of fluid-dynamic, physicochemical and cell-biological reactions in thrombus formation. Ann NY Acad Sci 1987;516:316–332.
16. Sutera SP, Nowak MD, Joist JH, Zeffren DJ, Baumann JE. A programmable computer-controlled cone-plate viscometer for the application of pulsatile shear stress to platelet suspensions. Biorheology 1988;25:449–459.
17. Reimers RC, Sutera SP, Joist JH. Potentiation by red blood cells of shear-induced platelet aggregation: Relative importance of chemical and physical mechanisms. Blood 1984;64:1200–1206.
18. Stein PD, Sabbah HN. Turbulent blood flow in the ascending aorta of humans with normal and diseased aortic valves. Circ Res 1976;39:58–65.
19. Yoganathan AP, Woo Y-R, Sung H-W. Turbulent shear stress measurements in the vicinity of aortic valve prostheses. J Biomech 1986;19:433–42.
20. Giersiepen M, Wurzinger LJ, Opitz R, Reul H. Estimation of shear stress-related blood damage in heart-valve prostheses – *in vitro* comparison of 25 aortic valves. Int J Artif Organs 1990;13:300–306.
21. Sutera S, Mehrjardi M, Mohandas M. Deformation of erythrocytes under shear. Blood Cells 1975;1:369–374.
22. Schmid-Schönbein H, Wells R. Fluid drop-like transition of erythrocytes under shear. Science 1972;165:288–291.
23. Karino T, Motomiya M. Goldsmith HL. Flow patterns in model and natural vessels. In Stanley JC, Ed. Biologic and Synthetic Vascular Protheses. New York, Grune and Stratton, 1982:Chapter 10.

Chapter 2.3

Interactions of Blood with Artificial Surfaces

James M. Anderson and Frederick J. Schoen

The major causes of prosthetic valve failure can frequently be linked to inappropriate or adverse blood/material interactions leading to thrombosis or thromboembolism, organisation and healing of thrombus, or haemolysis[1–3]. Despite extensive experimental efforts over the past three decades, an artificial surface suitable for prosthetic valve application, that is as non-thrombogenic as the natural circulatory endothelial lining, has not been realised. This is not surprising if one considers the complexity of the issues important in the design of a non-thrombogenic surface. From the biological perspective, these issues and their complexity may be best viewed as perturbations of Virchow's triad of factors that potentiate thrombosis and predict the extent and location of thrombus formation in the cardiovascular system[4].

In this context, Virchow's triad may be viewed as surface thrombogenicity, alterations in blood homeostasis towards coagulation and thrombosis, and haemorrheological factors. Clinically, these factors interact in largely unknown ways to compromise the function of blood-contacting prostheses. For example, an artificial surface may be relatively non-thrombogenic in a laminar, moderate flow and shear stress state, whereas the same surface under conditions of turbulent flow and high shear stress or low flow with stasis may lead to thrombosis. In this regard, prosthetic valves have regions of both high flow with shear stress and possibly turbulence and low flow with shear stress and stasis.

In considering the interactions of blood with artificial surfaces, the unique biological and design characteristics of each type of prosthesis must be considered in the context of Virchow's triad. A specific material may display variable degrees of thrombogenic and non-thrombogenic behaviour depending on its applications. For example, blood interactions with the same artificial surface in an arterial catheter, pacemaker lead, prosthetic valve, vascular graft or ventricular assist device would be expected to yield different thrombogenic potentials. In many respects, prosthetic valves offer the greatest challenge for the development of a non-thrombogenic cardiovascular prosthesis. The enormity of this challenge is due to our incomplete knowledge of initial events and determinants of blood/materials interactions, platelet interactions with artificial surfaces and lack of appropriate materials for appropriate prosthetic valve design and development[5–10]. The following discussion confronts these issues, their complex interactions and the present and future strategies for the development of new non-thrombogenic materials.

The consequences of thrombi on prosthetic heart valves are: (1) interference with function by partial or complete immobilisation of the occluder or obstruction of the valve orifice, or (2) generation of thromboemboli to distal arterial beds[1,11] (Fig. 2.3–1). Design-specific flow abnormalities largely determine the propensity to and location of valve thrombi on prosthetic heart valves (Chapter 2.1). Indeed, flow abnormalities

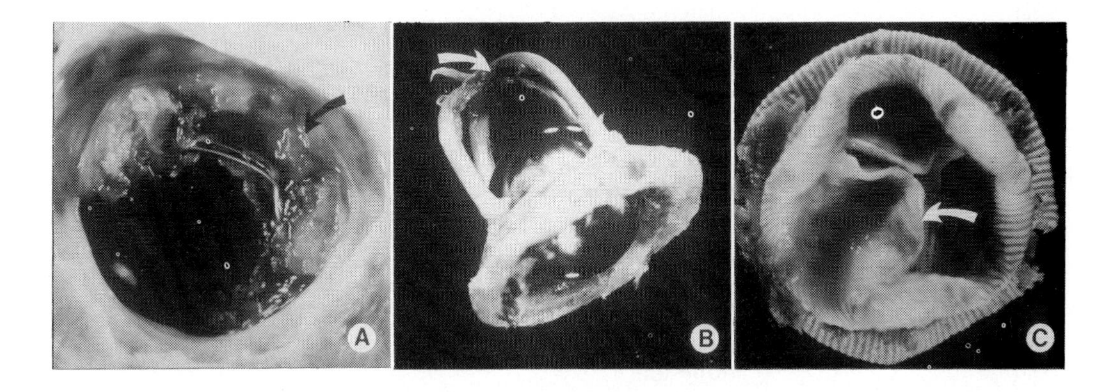

Figure 2.3–1: Prosthetic heart valve thrombosis. (A) Fatal thrombosis of a Bjork-Shiley tilting disk valve. Thrombus formation is initiated in the minor orifice as viewed from the outflow aspect (arrow); (B) thrombus formation at the apex of the cage of a caged-ball valve (arrow). This thrombus did not interfere with poppet motion but resultant emboli necessitated removal; (C) porcine bioprosthetic valve thrombosis, involving the outflow portion of a single cusp (arrow).

probably contribute more to the thromboembolic problems of prosthetic heart valves than those associated with other cardiovascular prosthetic devices[12–15]. In most clinical series, thromboembolic complications are much less frequent with aortic than mitral replacements, and with bioprosthetic than mechanical valves[2,3,16–18]. Unstented aortic homografts have a very low risk of thromboembolism[19,20](see Chapter 2.4).

Platelet (white) or fibrin (red) thrombi that form on bioprosthetic or mechanical valves undergo histological organisation extremely slowly, if at all, because of the absence of adjacent vascularised tissue[1]. Microscopic determination of the age of such thrombi is thus imprecise, and such thrombi can be friable for long periods of time, prolonging the embolic risk. Normally functioning endothelium is highly thromboresistant. Endothelium resists local thrombus formation despite circulating activated platelets or components of the coagulation system by active processes[1,21,22]. Endothelial cell thromboresistance largely derives from synthesis by normal vascular endothelial cells of prostacyclin (PGI_2, a potent inhibitor of platelet aggregation), thrombomodulin (a surface receptor that inhibits thrombin and contributes to activation of the inhibitor protein C), heparin sulphate (which activates antithrombin III) and plasminogen activator (which induces fibrinolysis). Nevertheless, the thromboresistance of endothelial cells can be impaired in certain pathological conditions[23,24]. Platelet adhesion to artificial surfaces is largely analogous to adhesion of platelets to the vascular subendothelium following endothelial denudation.

Turbulent flow and blood material surface interactions contribute to the destruction of red blood cells by prosthetic heart valves (haemolysis). In patients receiving earlier generation heart valve prostheses, haemolysis was common; long-term survivors often had renal tubular haemosiderosis or cholelithiasis, indicative of chronic haemolysis[25–27]. However, contemporary valves generally yield slight and well-compensated haemolysis. Thus, haemolytic anaemia is presently unusual and its onset should suggest paravalvular leak or valvular dysfunction due to materials degeneration or thrombosis.

Table 2.3–1
Initial events in blood/material interactions

Protein Adsorption and Activation
Intrinsic and Extrinsic Coagulation
Fibrinolysis
Complement
Adhesion Molecules
Others
Platelet Interactions
Adhesion
Activation
Release
Aggregation
White Cell Adhesion and Activation

INITIAL BLOOD/MATERIALS INTERACTIONS

The exposure of blood to artificial surfaces initiates a complex series of interrelated reactions that involve protein adsorption, adhesion and activation of platelets and white blood cells, the blood coagulation/fibrinolytic system, and the complement system[7,8]. Table 2.3–1 presents initial events which have been considered to be important in blood interactions with artificial surfaces. It has been hypothesised that the extent or degree of these interrelated interactions may lead to thrombogenic or non-thrombogenic conditions.

Artificial materials exposed to blood initially and spontaneously adsorb a film of plasma components, primarily protein[7,8,28]. The composition and conformational changes of proteins in this layer have been considered to dictate the further interaction of blood with the surface. However, little is known regarding the development, composition and changes that may occur within this protein layer. Recent studies utilising anticoagulated whole human blood have shown that significant protein adsorption occurs within one minute of blood contact. While fibronogen, IgG and albumin predominate on the surface, other significant proteins such as factor XII (Hageman factor), factor VII, fibronectin, haemoglobin, factor V3.vWF and complement are also present in the protein layer at the blood contacting surface. These studies were carried out with clinically used materials such as Dacron fabric, ePTFE, polyethylene, and silicone rubber[29–31]. It is generally considered that the dynamic process of protein adsorption and desorption and protein/protein interaction lead to progressive passivation of the artificial surfaces. Albumin has been implicated as a significant passivating protein whereas fibrinogen and gamma globulin have been suggested to promote platelet adhesion and activation[7].

In regard to initial blood/material interactions, little is known about the role which coagulation factors play in the formation of a localised stable thrombus which subsequently undergoes dissolution by fibrinolysis or organisation[7,8]. Furthermore, virtually no studies have been carried out in whole human blood under steady or

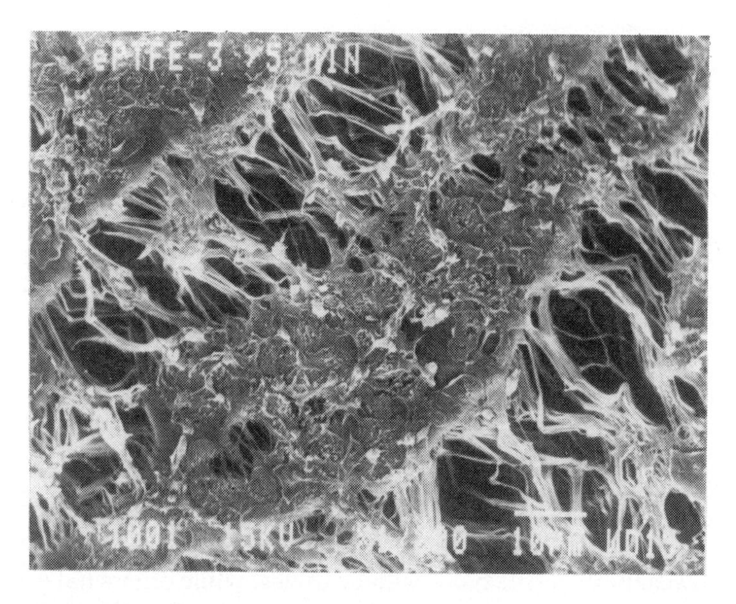

Figure 2.3–2: Platelet adhesion to expanded polytetrafluoroethylene from anticoagulated (citrate) whole human blood after 5 minutes in an in vitro *recirculation system. Original magnification:1,200X.*

pulsatile flow conditions to investigate the artificial surface activation of the intrinsic and/or extrinsic coagulation systems. Studies such as these would be important to better understand initial blood/material interactions and the role of the material in dictating thrombogenic/non-thrombogenic behaviour.

PLATELET INTERACTIONS WITH ARTIFICIAL SURFACES

Initial blood-surface interactions with prosthetic valves and other cardiovascular material devices are dominated by platelet-surface interactions (Fig. 2.3–2). Platelet activation by exposure of blood to artificial surfaces, particularly in complex flow systems such as the prosthetic valve, may lead to local thrombus formation, thromboembolic complications, consumption coagulopathy, and excessive local or generalised bleeding. As described earlier, the blood compatibility of prosthetic valves is not merely a function of blood/materials interactions but mechanical and rheological factors play a large role. In this respect, it is difficult to separate and identify the significance or contribution of each of these major factors to thrombosis and thromboembolism. Excessive shear and vortical flow with a valve prosthesis can cause haemolysis and platelet damage[32]. Excessive shear alone can cause platelet degranulation, activation, and haemolysis[33].

There is a strong relationship between prosthetic valve thromboembolism and altered platelet function. Numerous studies have examined platelet function in prosthetic heart valve recipients to detect persons at risk for thrombosis and thromboembolism and drug regimens capable of decreasing the risk (see Chapter 3.1). Systemic anticoagulation with warfarin reduces the incidence of thromboembolism in heart valve recipients and has become a mainstay in the management of prosthetic valve recipients[34](see Chapter 3.4). The clinical use of antiplatelet agents, such as sulfinpyrazone, suloctidyl and a combination of dipyridamole and acetylsalicylic acid, has been shown to decrease the incidence of thrombosis and thromboembolism with some prosthetic heart valves[35–41]. Moreover, these studies have indicated that platelets are a major contributing factor in valve thrombus formation.

The primary role of platelet function abnormalities in thrombosis after valve replacement is supported by the studies presented in Table 2.3–2. Platelet interactions have been evaluated by platelet counts, platelet adhesion, platelet release, platelet aggregation, and platelet kinetics. It is noteworthy that rarely has a comprehensive evaluation of platelet function been undertaken in the clinical studies. Partial or incomplete studies of platelet function have inhibited the development of a more comprehensive view of the role of platelet interactions with prosthetic valves.

Platelet counts are known to decrease during and immediately after valve implantation, presumably due to the thrombocytopenic effect of cardiopulmonary bypass during surgery[41]. The thrombocytopenia reverses within a week following surgery and may even reach levels above normal[37,41,47]. Long-term platelet counts generally have been found to be lower than normal controls, although some studies have found platelet counts not significantly different from normals[35,39,44–46]. Some studies have suggested that there is no significant difference in platelet counts in patients with mechanical versus bioprosthetic valves, while others have indicated that platelet counts are lower in patients with mechanical valves[44,45,48]. However both bioprosthetic and mechanical valves vary in their thrombogenicity (see Chapter 2.4) and this may explain these apparently contradictory findings.

Platelet adhesion to prosthetic valve surfaces in vivo have been measured by direct imaging with ^{111}In-labelled platelets[49,50]. Using this technique, platelet deposition on various parts of Bjørk-Shiley valves was quantified. The largest percentage of valve associated platelets was adherent to the Teflon sewing ring or involved in sewing ring thrombi. The percentage of platelets adhering to the disc and valve housing was about 1% of those adhering to the sewing ring. In vitro platelet retention studies assessed by the glass bead column method have shown that platelet retention increases immediately after surgery and subsequently decreases below normal[37,41,46]. The decreased platelet retention is suggestive of either consumption of adhesive platelets or circulation of inactive or exhausted platelets. Aspirin and dipyridamole were not able to increase this depressed platelet adhesion behaviour[39].

Stimulated or damaged platelets in prosthetic valve recipients produce elevated plasma levels of platelet release products. High levels of the platelet release products platelet factor 4 (PF4) and beta-thromboglobulin (bTG) have been found in prosthetic valve patients (Table 2.3–2). Furthermore, the bTG content of circulating platelets has been found to be decreased in patients with valve prostheses, indicating that degranulated platelets continue to circulate[45]. Studies of the platelet release product bTG *in vivo* have suggested that there is no difference in bTG levels between any of the valve types[44,45,48]. Platelet factor 4 levels were found to be significantly elevated in patients with double versus single valve replacement[44]. Use of antiplatelet drugs such as suloctidil and sulfinpyrazone has been shown to decrease bTG and PF4 levels slightly in valve recipients[33,37]. Platelet release can also be assessed by the measurement of products of arachidonic acid metabolism, namely thromboxane B_2 (TxB_2) and malondialdehyde. Both thromboxane B_2 and malondialdehyde have been found to be elevated in valve recipients and malondialdehyde levels have correlated well with increased levels of PF4 and bTG[42].

Table 2.3–2
Human platelet function studies with prosthetic valves

			Platelet studies				
Heart Valve Type	*Test system*	*Anticoagulant*	*Platelet count*	*Platelet adhesion*	*Platelet release*	*Platelet aggregation*	*Platelet kinetics*
1. Aortic and mitral valves[23]	Implanted valves and tested at various times post-surgery	Variable	Yes		Malondial-dehyde production		
2. Aortic and mitral valves[16, 24]	Implanted valves and tested antiplatelet drug	Warfarin	Yes		ßTG, PG4		^{51}Cr-platelet
3. Starr Edwards, Bjørk Shiley[18]	Drug trial 2 wks after valve implantation	Acenocoumarine	Yes	Glass bead column	PF4	ADP, epinephrine- and collagen-induced	^{51}Cr-platelet
4. Disc valves & heterograft valves[25]	Implanted mitral and aortic valves	Warfarin	Yes		ßTG, PF4 TxB_2 production		
5. Mechanical and biological valves[26]	Implanted valves and tested at various times post-surgery	NS	Yes		ßTG and Plt ßTG content		
6. Starr Edwards[20, 27]	Implanted valves and tested at various times post-surgery	Variable	Yes	Glass bead column		ADP- and epinephrine-induced	^{51}Cr-platelet
7. Starr Edwards[22]	Implanted valves in children and tested antiplatelet drugs	NS	No	Glass bead column			^{51}Cr-platelet
8. Beall, Starr Edwards, Bjørk Shiley[17]	Tested antiplatelet drugs 2–6 mo. after implantation	Warfarin	No				^{51}Cr-platelet
9. Starr Edwards, Bjork Shiley[28]	Studied platelet function before and after valve implantation	NS	Yes				^{51}Cr-platelet
10. Ball valves and porcine valves[29]	Implanted valves and tested at various times post-surgery	Phen-procoumon	Yes		PF4, ßTG		

Platelet aggregation has been evaluated in patients with prosthetic valves. In general, the aggregating ability of platelets to stimulation by ADP, epinephrine, and collagen remains normal after valve replacement[37,39]. There is some suggestion that certain prostheses may affect collagen-induced aggregation. Aspirin therapy has been shown to reduce the aggregating response of platelets to collagen[39,46].

The most frequently studied platelet function parameter in clinical prosthetic valve series is platelet kinetics. Platelet kinetic studies suggest a correlation between shortened platelet survival times and increased frequency of thromboembolic complications[51]. Abnormal platelet kinetics following valve replacement have been characterised by decreased platelet survival, shortened half-life and increased platelet consumption[35–39,46]. Some studies have suggested that patients with replacement valves have a higher consumption of platelets and are at greater risk of thromboembolism. Antiplatelet drugs have been shown to increase platelet survival in valve recipients[35–39](see Chapter 3.1).

MODIFICATION OF BLOOD/MATERIAL INTERACTIONS: PRESENT AND FUTURE STRATEGIES

New materials for application in prosthetic valves must be both durable and non-thrombogenic. To realise these properties, investigators have directed their efforts toward preparing surface modified materials, where appropriate surface properties are introduced into the materials for non-thrombogenic behaviour, while maintaining adequate and appropriate mechanical properties for prosthetic valve function.

Virtually every physical and chemical property of materials has been suggested as being important in blood coagulation and thrombosis. Some of the more well known and widely investigated hypotheses are presented in Table 2.3–3. The hypotheses dealing with surface charges and energetics were extensively studied in the 1960's and

Table 2.3–3
Hypotheses for surfaces and blood compatibility

Property	*Biological Response*	*Reference*
Negative surface charge	Decreased protein and cell adsorption	5, 52–55
Minimal surface energy	Decreased protein and cell adsorption	5, 52–55
Minimal interfacial free energy	Decreased protein	5, 52–55
Albumin surfaces	Passivated surface, decreased thrombosis	56–61
Plasma polymerised surfaces	Decreased protein and platelet interactions	61–64
Hydrated, dynamic surfaces	Decreased protein adsorption	65–68
Microphase separated surfaces	Decreased protein and platelet interactions	69–74
Pharmacologically active surfaces	Direct coagulation and platelet interactions	74–80

1970's. Results from these studies were not promising for several reasons. First, the experimental models and methods of assessment were naive and crude. For example, protein adsorption was mainly studied utilising single proteins in buffer solution and plasma or whole blood was rarely used. Secondly, the experiments were most commonly carried out under static conditions and the importance of flow and shear stress was not taken into consideration. As methods of assessment such as radioimmunoassay, ELISA and material surface characterisation techniques such as ESCA and SIMS became available, our understanding of surfaces and blood/material interactions increased. In part, this was related to the explosion of techniques and methods in cell and molecular biology. In addition, our understanding of the function and interactions within the coagulation system and other related systems as well as the function of platelets permitted a more in-depth appreciation of blood/material interactions and led to the development of new hypotheses. Current concepts under active investigation include albuminated surfaces, hydrated dynamic surfaces, microphase separated surfaces, and pharmacologically active surfaces.

The development of albuminated surfaces came from early observations that materials precoated with albumin appeared to produce less thrombus in contact with blood when compared to the base artificial material. These observations led to numerous and extensive studies by a large number of groups in the area of protein adsorption. The albumin concept is based on the fact that albumin itself is a blood component which does not interact adversely with other blood components. Albumin does not contain peptide sequences known to interact with either adhesion receptors on cell membranes or enzymes in the coagulation and complement cascades. Several surface modification methods have been developed to enhance the surface binding of albumin[56–60]. Plasma gas discharge techniques have been developed to immobilise albumin onto various polymers[61]. Direct surface alkylation or acetylation of suitable polymers such as polyurethanes, polyamides, and cellulosics with 16 or 18 carbon chains create a more hydrophobic surface which efficiently binds albumin.

Plasma gas discharge techniques have been used to modify surfaces, producing variable hydrophobic/hydrophilic and ionic/non-ionic characteristics[62,63]. This technique offers promise for the future in that it only provides a surface modification and does not alter the bulk physical and mechanical properties of the material being modified. Thus, materials with apparent thrombogenic surfaces such as tough engineering plastics, metals, ceramics, and composites can be chemically modified to produce surfaces which exhibit decreased thrombogenic behaviour. Moreover, this technique permits the introduction of chemical groups capable of subsequent reaction for the attachment of anticoagulants such as heparin and hirudin, hydrophilic molecules such as polyethylene oxide, and other pharmacologically active agents known to inhibit blood coagulation and platelet activation.

Plasma gas discharge polymers, also known as plasma polymerisation polymers, when prepared using fluorinated hydrocarbons, have been shown to markedly reduce platelet consumption when tested in an *in vivo* baboon shunt model. Similar experiments utilising ePTFE vascular grafts modified with a plasma polymer based on hexafluroethane/H_2 showed a reduction by 87% in *in vivo* platelet deposition when measured by ^{111}In-platelets[61].

Polymer surfaces modified with polyethylene oxide chains, with molecular weights up to 2000, provide hydrated dynamic surfaces[65–67]. These materials are based on the concepts of hydrophilicity and steric exclusion through molecular mobility at the surface. These molecules may be chemically coupled to surface active groups on a wide variety of materials. As previously mentioned, surface active groups can be produced by the plasma gas discharge or plasma polymerisation technique. Plasma protein adsorption and platelet adhesion onto these materials have been found to be significantly decreased when compared to appropriate controls.

The study of protein adsorption and cellular adhesion to segmented polyurethane block copolymers coupled with sophisticated characterisation of the polymer surface morphology have revealed that two-phase or microdomain surface morphologies result in decreased protein adsorption and cellular adhesion[69–74]. Studies have indicated that microdomain sizes on the same scale as proteins, platelets and white cells, can effectively alter the adsorption and adhesion phenomenon. Studies on a HEMA (2-hydroxy ethyl methacrylate) and styrene block copolymer have indicated that albumin selectively adsorbs to the hydrophilic (HEMA) domains and gamma globulin selectively adsorbs to the hydrophobic (styrene) domains. Platelet interactions with these materials have indicated that while platelet adhesion was increased, platelet activation was decreased[72]. The development and exploitation of this concept to produce polymers with decreased thrombogenic behaviour were the result of sophisticated biological assay systems as well as surface and bulk polymer characterisation techniques. These efforts illustrate the necessary coupling of biomedical science and materials science to produce hypotheses for the development of new blood-contacting materials.

Attempts to develop pharmacologically active surfaces which inhibit blood coagulation and thrombosis have been carried out over the past three decades[75–80]. Early attempts utilised heparin in various forms as coatings which leached or were released from the blood-contacting surfaces. Early attempts to prepare these types of non-thrombogenic surfaces were hampered by the lack of knowledge of biological interactions which lead to thrombosis on surfaces. As our knowledge of blood coagulation and platelet interactions with surfaces has increased, approaches to the development of pharmacologically active surfaces have become more sophisticated.

Activity in this area has mainly focused on the covalent attachment of heparin, prostaglandins and fibrinolytic enzymes to surfaces without loss of biological activity. Heparin immobilised polymer surfaces are currently being used clinically in catheter applications. Heparin grafted onto surfaces interacts with circulating antithrombin III in such a manner as to increase the interaction of antithrombin III with thrombin and other activated clotting factors. The use of hydrophilic spacer groups to extend the heparin molecule away from the surface is believed to decrease the steric hindrance on the binding and interactions of heparin and antithrombin III[78]. Thus, spacer groups may increase the efficiency of the anticoagulant effect of heparin. While extensive work is already in progress to exploit these techniques, long-term efforts are needed in the study of blood-surface interactions before the clinical efficacy of such systems can be determined.

Efforts to develop new materials for prosthetic valve application must be interdisciplinary. The development of new materials will permit new prosthetic valve designs based on material/property relationships. However, our knowledge of the effects of blood flow and artificial material surfaces on thrombosis in the setting of prosthetic valves is markedly incomplete. A full understanding of these blood/material interactions must be developed. Experimental model systems which appropriately mimic the prosthetic valve clinical situation are necessary, possibly involving animal models. Surface modification techniques to produce tough, durable, and possibly flexible materials which are non-thrombogenic are distinct possibilities. Extensive efforts are necessary to fully exploit these techniques for use in new prosthetic valves.

REFERENCES

1. Schoen FJ. Interventional and surgical cardiovascular pathology. Clinical correlations and basic principles. 1989; WB Saunders Co, Philadelphia.
2. Edmunds LH. Thrombotic and bleeding complications of prosthetic heart valves. Ann Thorac Surg 1987;44:430–445.
3. Bloomfield P, Wheatley DJ, Prescott RJ, Miller HC. Twelve-year comparison of a Bjork-Shiley mechanical heart valve with porcine bioprostheses. N Engl J Med 1991;324:573–579.
4. Wessler S, Thye Yin E. On the mechanism of thrombosis. Prog Hematol 1969;6:201–232.
5. Guidelines for blood-materials interactions Report of the National Heart, Lung, and Blood Institute Working Group. US Deapartment of Health and Human Services. 1985;NIH Pub 85–2185.
6. Andrade JD, Coleman DL, Didisheim P, et al. Blood-materials interactions – 20 years of frustration. Trans Am Soc Artif Intern Org 1981;27:659–662.
7. Salzman EW, Merrill EW. Interaction of blood with artificial surfaces. In Colman RW, Hirsh J, Marder VJ, Salzman EW, ed. Haemostasis and thrombosis. Basic principles and clinical practice. 2nd ed. Philadelphia:JB Lippincott, 1987:1335–1347.
8. Vroman L. The importance of surfaces in contact phase reactions. Sem Thromb Haemost 1987;13:79–85.
9. Anderson JM, Kottke-Marchant K. Platelet interactions with biomaterials and artificial devices. CRC Crit Rev Biocompat 1985;1:111–203.
10. Joist JH, Pennington DG. Platelet reactions with artificial surfaces. Trans Am Soc Artif Intern Org 1987;33:341–344.
11. Chesebro JH, Fuster V. Thromboembolism in heart valve replacement. In Kwaan HC, Bowie EJW, ed. Thrombosis. Philadelphia:WB Saunders, 1982;146.
12. Schoen FJ. Cardiac valve prostheses. Pathological and bioengineering considerations. J Cardiac Surg 1987;2:65–108.
13. Schoen FJ, Hobson CE. Anatomic analysis of removed prosthetic heart valves: causes of failure of 33 mechanical valves and 58 bioprostheses, 1980 to 1983. Hum Pathol 1985;16:549–559.
14. Yoganathan AP, Corcoran WH, Harrison EC, Carl JR. The Bjork-Shiley aortic prosthesis: flow characteristics, thrombus formation and tissue overgrowth. Circulation 1978;58:70–76.
15. Yoganathan AP, Reamer HH, Corcoran WH, et al. The Starr-Edwards aortic ball valve: flow characteristics thrombus formation, and tissue overgrowth. Artif Org 1981;5:6–17.
16. Edmunds LH. Thrombotic and bleeding complications of prosthetic heart valves. Ann Thorac Surg 1987;44:430–445.
17. Cohn LH, Allred EN, DiSesa VJ, et al. Early and late risk of aortic valve replacement. A 12-year concomitant comparison of the porcine bioprosthetic and tilting disc prosthetic aortic valves. J Thorac Cardiovasc Surg 1984;88:695–705.
18. Cohn LH, Allred EN, Cohn LA, et al. Early and late risk of mitral valve replacement. A 12-year concomitant comparison of the porcine bioprosthetic and prosthetic disc mitral valves. J Thorac Cardiovasc Surg 1985;90:872–881.
19. Barratt-Boyes BG, Roche AHG, Subramanyan R, et al. Long-term follow-up of patients with the antibiotic sterilised aortic homograft valve inserted freehand into the aortic position. Circulation 1987;75:768–777.
20. O'Brien MF, Stafford EG, Gardner MAH, et al. Comparison of aortic valve replacement with viable cryopreserved and fresh allograft valves, with a note on chromosomal studies. J Thorac Cardiovasc Surg 1987;94:812–823.
21. Stern DM, Carpenter B, Nawroth PP. Endothelium and the regulation of coagulation. Pathol Immunopathol Res 1986;5:29–36.
22. Rodgers GM. Haemostatic properties of normal and perturbed vascular cells. FASEB J 1988;2:116–123.
23. Nawroth PP, Stern DM. Endothelial cell procoagulant properties and the host response. Sem Thromb Hemost 1987;13:391–397.
24. Bevilacqua MP, Gimbrone MA. Inducible endothelial functions in inflammation and coagulation. Sem Thromb Hemost 1987;13:425–433.

25. Bernstein EF. Certain aspects of blood interfacial phenomena. Red blood cells. Fed Proc 1971;30:1510–1515.
26. Roberts WC, Morrow AG. Renal haemosiderosis in patients with prosthetic aortic valves. Circulation 1966;33:390–398.
27. Harrison EC. Roschke EJ, Meyers HI, et al. Cholelithiasis: A frequent complication of artificial heart valve replacement. Am Heart J 1978;95:483–488.
28. Andrade JD, Hlady V. Protein adsorption and materials biocompatibility: a tutorial review and suggested hyopotheses. Adv Polymer Sci 1986;79:1.
29. Pankowsky DA, Ziats NP, Topham NS, Ratnoff OD, Anderson JM. Morphologic characteristics of adsorbed human plasma proteins on vascular grafts and biomaterials. J Vasc Surg 1990;11:599–606.
30. Ziats NP, Pankowsky DA, Tierney BP, Ratnoff OD, Anderson JM. Adsorption of Hageman factor (factor XII) and other human plasma proteins to biomedical polymers. J Lab Clin Med 1990;116:687–696.
31. Ziats NP, Topham NS, Pankowsky DA, Anderson JM. Analysis of protein adsorption on retrieved human vascular grafts using immunogold labelling with silver enhancement. Cells & Materials 1991;1:73–82.
32. Brown CH III, Leverett LB, Lewis CW, Alfrey CP Jr, Hellums JD. Morphological, biochemical and functional changes in human platelets subjected to shear stress. J Lab Clin Med 1975;86:462–471.
33. Bernstein EF, Marzec U, Johnston GG. Structural correlates of platelet functional damage by physical forces. Trans Am Soc Artif Intern Organs 1977;23:617–625.
34. Gadboys HL, Litwak RS, Niemetz J, Wisch N. Role of anticoagulants in preventing embolisation from prosthetic heart valves. J Am Med Assoc 1967;202:282–286.
35. Ludlam CA, Allan N, Blandford RB, Dowdle R, Bentley NJ, Bloom AL. Platelet and coagulation function in patients with abnormal cardiac valves with sulphinpyrazone. Thromb Haemost 1981;46:743–746.
36. Steele P, Rainwater J, Vogel R. Platelet suppressant therapy in patients with prosthetic cardiac valves. Relationship of clinical effectiveness to alteration of platelet survival time. Circulation 1979;60:910–913.
37. Col-de Beys C, Ferrant A, Moriau M. Effects of suloctidil on platelet survival time following cardiac valve replacement. Thromb Haemost 1981;46:550–553.
38. Turpie AGG, deBoer AC, Giroux M, et al. Platelet survival and betathromboglobulin after heterograft mitral valve replacement: Effect of suloctidil. Thromb Haemost 1983;50:63–68.
39. Dale J, Myhre E, Rootwell K. Effects of dipyridamole and acetylsalicylic acid on platelet functions in patients with aortic ball valve prostheses. Am Heart J 1975;89:613–618.
40. Brott WH, Zajtchuk R, Bowen TE, Davia J, Green DC. Dipyridamole-aspirin as thromboembolic prophylaxis in patients with aortic valve prostheses. J Thorac Cardiovas Surg 1981;81:632–635.
41. Wyss M. Diez C, Balavoine JF, Martin D, Bouvier CA. Prevention of thromboembolic complications of valve prostheses by agents affecting platelet function. Eur J Cardiol 1978;813:336–347.
42. Sullivan JM, Taylor JC, Samaha JK. Platelet malondialdehyde in cardiovascular disease: effect of prosthetic heart valves and cardioactive drugs on production. Thromb Haemost 1981;46:76–80.
43. Ludlam CA, Allan N. Blandford RB, Dowdle R, Bentley N. Bloom AL. BTG and platelet survival in patients with rheumatic heart disease and prosthetic cardiac valves and their treatment with sulphinpyrazone. Thromb Haemost 1979;42:329–334.
44. Cella G, Schivazappa L, Casonato A, et al. In vivo platelet release reaction in patients with heart valve prostheses. Haemostasis 1980;9:263–275.
45. Pumphrey CW, Dawes J. Platelet alpha granule depletion: findings in patients with prosthetic heart valves and following cardiopulmonary bypass surgery. Thromb Res 1983;30:257–264.
46. Dale J, Myhre E. Platelet functions in patients with aortic ball valves. Am Heart J 1977;94:359–366.
47. Dumoulin M. Tirmarche M. Horellou MA, Acar J, Samama M. Study of platelet diameter distribution in patients with valvular heart disease and with prosthetic heart valve replacement. Haemostasis 1981;10:28–36.
48. Dudczak R, Neissner H. Thaler E, et al. Plasma concentration of platelet-specific proteins and fibrinopeptide A in patients with artificial heart valves. Haemostasis 1981;10:186–194.
49. Dewanjee M, Trastek V, Tago M, Torianni M, Kaye M, Didisheim P. Noninvasive radioisotopic technique for detection of platelet deposition in bovine pericardial mitral valve prosthesis (BPMVP) and in vitro quantification of visceral microembolism in dogs. Trans Am Soc Artif Intern Organs 1983;29:188–193.
50. Dewanjee MK, Kaye MP, Fuster V, Rao SA. Noninvasive radioisotopic technique for detection of platelet deposition in mitral valve prosthesis and renal microembolism in dogs. Trans Am Soc Artif Inter Organs 1980;26:475–480.
51. Steele P, Weily H, Davies H, Pappas G, Genton E. Platelet survival time following aortic valve replacement. Circulation 1975;51:358–362.
52. Leininger RI. Polymers as surgical implants. CRC Crit Rev Bioeng 1972;1:333–381.

53. Andrade JD. Interfacial phenomena and biomaterials. J Assoc Adv Med Inst 1973;7:110–119.
54. Vroman L, et al. Reactions of formed elements of blood with plasma proteins at interfaces. Ann NY Acad Sci 1977;283:65–76.
55. Sawyer PN. Surface charge and thrombosis. Ann NY Acad Sci 1983;416:561–584.
56. Tsai C-C, Huo H-H, Kulkarni P, Eberhart RC. Biocompatible coatings with high albumin affinity. ASAIO Trans 1990;36:M307-M310.
57. Tsai CC, Frautschi JR, Eberhart RC. Enhanced albumin affinity of silicone rubber. Trans Am Soc Artif Intern Organs 1988;34:559–563.
58. Eberhart RC, Munro MS, Frautschi JR, et al. Influence of endogenous albumin binding on blood-material interactions. Ann NY Acad Sci 1987;516:78–95.
59. Pitt WG, Cooper SL. Albumin adsorption on alkyl chain derivatised polyurethanes: The effect of C–18 alkylation. J Biomed Mater Res 1988;22:359–382.
60. Grasel TG, Pierce JA, Cooper SL. Effects of alkyl grafting on surface properties and blood compatibility of polyurethane block copolymers. J Biomed Mater Res 1987;21:815–842.
61. Ishikawa Y, Sasakawa S, Takase M, Osada Y. Effect of albumin immobilisation by plasma polymerisation on platelet reactivity. Thromb Res 1984;35:193–202.
62. Hoffman AS. Biomedical applications of plasma gas discharge processes. J Appl Polym Sci:Appl Polym Symp 1988;42:251–267.
63. Gombotz WR, Hoffman AS. Gas discharge techniques for modification of biomaterials. In Williams D (Ed): Critical reviews in biocompatibility. 4th ed. Boca Raton:CRC Press, 1987;1–42.
64. Yeh Y-S, Iriyama Y, Matsuzawa Y, Hanson SR, Yasuda H. Blood compatibility of surfaces modified by plasma polymerization. J Biomed Mater Res 1988;22:795–818.
65. Merrill EW, Salzman EW. Polyethylene oxide as a biomaterial. ASAIO J 1983;6:60–64.
66. Mori Y, Nagaoka S. A new antithrombogenic material with long polyethylene oxide chains. Trans Am Soc Artif Intern Organs 1982;28:459–463.
67. Hoffman AS, Horbnett TA, Ratner BD. Interaction of blood and blood components at hydrogel interfaces. Ann NY Acad Sci 1977;283:372–382.
68. Nagaoka S, Mori Y. Takiuchi H, Yokota K, Tanzawa H, Nishiumi S. A new antithrombogenic material with long polyethylene oxide chains. Trans Am Soc Artif Intern Organs 1982;28:459–463.
69. Okano T, Nishiyama S, Shinohara I, et al. Effect of hydrophilic and hydrophobic microdomains on mode of interaction between block polymer and blood platelets. J Biomed Mater Res 1981;15:393–402.
70. Okano T, Kataoka I, Sakurai Y, Shimada M, Akaika T, Shinohara I. Molecular design of block and graft copolymers having the ability to suppress platelet adhesion. Artif Organs 1981;5:468–470.
71. Okano T, Shimada M. Aoyagi T, et al. The hydrophilic-hydrophobic microdomain surface having the ability to suppress platelet aggregation and their in vivo antithrombogenicity. J Biomed Mater Res 1986;20:919–928.
72. Nojiri C, Okano T, Jacobs HA, et al. Blood compatibility of PEO grafted polyurethane and HEMA/styrene block copolymer surfaces. J Biomed Mater Res 1990;24:1151–1171.
73. Goodman SL, Simmons SR, Cooper SL, Albrecht RM. Preferential adsorption of plasma proteins onto apolar polyurethane microdomains. J Coll Inter Sci 1990;139:561–570.
74. Okkema AZ, Grasel TG, Zdrahala RJ, Solomon DD, Cooper SL. Bulk, surface, and blood-contacting properties of polyetherurethanes modified with polyethylene oxide. J Biomater Sci Polymer Edn 1989;1:43–62.
75. Nojiri C, Park KD, Grainger DW, et al. *In vivo* nonthrombogenicity of heparin immobilised polymer surfaces. ASAIO Trans 1990;36:M168-M172.
76. Heyman P, Cho CS, McRea JC, Olsen POB, Kim SW. Heparinised polyurethane in vitro and in vivo studies. J Biomed Mater Res 1985;19:419–436.
77. Kim SW, Feijen J. Surface modification of polymers for improved blood compatibility in biocompatibility. CRC Crit Rev Biocompat 1985;1:229–260.
78. Park KD, Okano T, Nojiri C, Kim SK. Heparin immobilisation onto segmented polyurethaneurea surfaces – effect of hydrophilic spacers. J Biomed Mater Res 1988;22:977–992.
79. Jacobs HA, Okano T, Kim SW. Antithrombogenic surfaces: Characterisation and bioactivity of surface immobilised PGE_1-heparin conjugate. J Biomed Mater Res 1989;23:611–630.
80. Ohshiro T, Kosaki G. Urokinase immobilised on medical polymeric materials: Fundamental and clinical studies. Artif Org 1980;4:58–64.

Chapter 2.4

Thrombogenicity, Thrombosis and Embolism

Eric G. Butchart

In health, the normal heart valves are regarded as non-thrombogenic structures. However, systemic illnesses such as malignant disease[1,2], autoimmune disease[3,4], and septicaemia (Chapter 1.4) may lead to the deposition of thrombus on previously normal valves. Valves whose structure or surface has been modified by disease processes may also attract thrombus deposition and the subsequent thrombus organisation and fibrous tissue formation can lead to further thickening of valve leaflets[4–7].

It can be seen that defining thrombogenicity, even as it applies to natural heart valves, is fraught with difficulties. Whilst a natural valve under physiological conditions could be said to possess zero thrombogenicity, the same valve under abnormal flow conditions[7] or the influence of a systemic illness may become thrombogenic[4–7]. The difficulties are magnified when discussing the thrombogenicity of artificial heart valves. It has to be acknowledged that all such devices are thrombogenic to a greater or lesser degree[8], no matter how close to the original human 'design' they may be. To the extent that, in most patients, all currently available mechanical valves require life-long anticoagulation to prevent gross thrombus accumulation of their working surfaces, whereas biological valves do not, mechanical valves as a group must be regarded as more thrombogenic than biological valves. However, there are considerable differences among the various prostheses; some mechanical valves are more thrombogenic than others and even bioprostheses are not immune from gross thrombus deposition, showing a gradation from the least thrombogenic homografts and pulmonary autografts through pericardial valves to the relatively more thrombogenic porcine valves (vide infra).

All replacement heart valves represent a foreign body within the circulation, initiating a pathophysiological response which endeavours to encapsulate the foreign body with thrombus and exclude it[9]. The extent to which thrombus adheres to the various components of a prosthesis is proportional to the thrombogenicity of the component and can be modified on some components by anticoagulation (see also Chapter 3.4). The propensity of adherent thrombus for embolism also varies with its site of attachment to the prosthesis, the type of tissue or artificial surface to which it is attached and with the level of anticoagulation (vide infra). In general terms however, it appears to be more difficult for the body to immobilise thrombus and prevent embolism on an artificial or foreign surface than on a natural valve surface.

The thrombogenicity of an artificial heart valve can be defined in terms of its capacity to induce, anywhere in the circulation, thrombus formation which would not have occurred without its presence. Two distinct types of thrombogenicity can be identified: primary and secondary. Primary thrombogenicity relates to the tendency of thrombus to form on the prosthesis itself, either accumulating to cause functional impairment or breaking off and embolising. Secondary thrombogenicity refers to thrombus which is *initiated* at a site remote from the prosthesis as the result of the presence of the prosthesis in the circulation.

PRIMARY THROMBOGENICITY

In discussing thrombogenicity, it is important to distinguish between microthrombus formation and gross (visible) thrombosis. Microthrombus formation occurs on natural human heart valves in autoimmune disease[4], rheumatic disease[5,6] and congenital valve abnormalities[7] and by organisation and fibrosis contributes to progressive thickening of valve cusps. It rarely gives rise to embolism. A similar process of microthrombus formation occurs as part of the 'incorporation' of any substitute heart valve and is described in detail below. It occurs to a variable extent on the sewing rings of both mounted biological valves and mechanical valves, on the Dacron-covered stents of bioprostheses and on the cusps of homografts and heterografts. Its propensity for embolism varies with the nature of the surface to which it is attached. It has been traditional to describe the thrombogenicity of substitute heart valves in terms of gross thrombus deposition only. However, 'microthrombogenicity', or the tendency for excessive microthrombus formation on part of an artificial valve is also important since its consequences, particularly in biological valves, can contribute to valve failure (vide infra).

The mechanisms of thrombosis and embolism, both microscopic and gross, are better understood by first examining the different pathological reactions which occur on each of the three main valve components; sewing rings, biological cusps and the artificial surfaces of mechanical valves.

Sewing rings

The fibrous tissue which ultimately results in the incorporation of the sewing ring of a prosthesis is of two types. Both follow the initial deposition of a layer of thrombus. One results from organisation of thrombus to become avascular fibrous tissue and is the type more frequently seen *covering* the sewing ring[9]. The other evolves through granulation tissue and the growth of capillaries to form vascular fibrous tissue. This latter type extends into the spaces in the sewing ring between the material fibres and under some circumstances (vide infra) is involved in covering the surface of the sewing ring also[9]. Eventually there is a covering of endothelium of variable completeness and uncertain functional ability[10]. Endothelium in such an 'adverse' and non-physiological environment may not exhibit anticoagulant properties and indeed may show procoagulant activity[11–13].

The extent and thickness of the 'normal' tissue which covers the sewing ring is affected by several factors (excessive pathological thickness is discussed later):

1. *Interspecies variability.* In comparison to the animal species commonly used for experimental heart valve implantation (calf, pig and dog), man's ability to incorporate fabrics placed in the circulation appears limited[14]. These interspecies differences probably relate at least in part to age (calf v middle-aged man for example), presence or absence of disease in the annulus and coagulation differences[14,15]. In man, complete tissue coverage in the aortic position seems limited to a maximum inward growth of about 7 mm whereas the calf is capable of

20 mm of inward growth over fabric[14]. Thus the results of animal experiments on sewing ring healing cannot be extrapolated directly to man.

2. *Anatomical location*. The local flow conditions to which the sewing ring is exposed govern the degree of initial thrombus formation and the local pressure to which it is exposed controls the type of fibrous tissue formed and its extent[14,16]. Sewing rings exposed to arterial pressure (both aortic and ventricular sides of aortic prostheses and ventricular sides of mitral prostheses) become covered by avascular fibrous tissue of limited extent[14,16]. In the mitral position, about twice as much tissue usually grows on the atrial side of the sewing ring as on the ventricular[14]. A similar situation is seen in the tricuspid position, except that sewing ring tissue thickness is even greater in the right atrium and the fibrous tissue more commonly contains capillaries, as the result of the lower pressures to which it is exposed[9].
3. *Anticoagulation*. The ultimate thickness of the tissue covering the sewing ring is probably at least partly determined by the amount of thrombus to be organised. Animal experiments have shown that anticoagulation commenced early in the post operative period can minimise the degree of thrombosis of the sewing ring and hence reduce the thickness of the fibrous covering[17,18]. If this is also true in man, it is a further indication for commencing anticoagulation as early as possible (see also Chapter 3.4).

Radioactive labelled platelet studies in animals have shown that large numbers of platelets adhere to the sewing ring soon after operation and that as its incorporation proceeds over several weeks fewer and fewer platelets become adherent[19]. In this period before endothelialisation takes place, microembolism from the sewing ring occurs frequently and can be detected in other organs using labelled platelets[19]. It is likely therefore that some larger symptomatic emboli in the early post operative weeks also originate from this site.

Tissue ingrowth

If satisfactory incorporation of the sewing ring has taken place with a thin fibrous tissue and endothelial covering, a relatively non-thrombogenic surface should eventually be created, unless suture knots protrude above the endothelium. Under some circumstances however, the fibrous tissue covering the sewing may become excessively thickened and overgrow the margin of the sewing ring. The pathogenesis of this exuberant tissue ingrowth or pannus formation is not fully understood but is probably multifactorial with fabric damage[16], local flow conditions[20], inadequate anticoagulation[17,18], degree of fibrous tissue vascularity[9] and degree of foreign body reaction and fibroblast activity[21] all playing a part. The type of implantation technique used may also have an effect[22].

Severe fabric wear can result in unrolling of the fabric which, when covered by tissue ingrowth, leads to the formation of a stiff subvalvar membrane in the aortic position or an atrial shelf in the mitral position, each producing narrowing of the valve orifice[16]. Some have theorised that a minimum shear stress is required throughout the circumference of the annulus to prevent extension of tissue onto the mechanism of the prosthesis and that local areas of sluggish flow will predispose to its development[20].

Tissue ingrowth appears commoner in excessively sedentary patients, suggesting that low cardiac output may be a factor.

Tissue ingrowth is widely regarded as a late phenomenon, occurring after several years of implantation and accounting for a gradual decrease in valve performance even before acute signs and symptoms develop[23]. However, it has been observed as early as one month after implantation[24]. In one large series of obstructed mechanical valves reported from South Africa, tissue ingrowth contributed to obstruction in 46% and was seen as early as six weeks after operation[25]. In another series from South Africa, valve thrombosis was only seen in association with tissue ingrowth (Chapter 4.4). Many of the patients in these series were from 'third world' communities receiving inadequate anticoagulation. Bearing in mind the experimental work referred to above[17,18] it is possible that lack of anticoagulation is a major factor in early tissue ingrowth in Africans. The higher fibrinogen levels of rural African communities as a consequence of the high incidence of parasitic infestation[26] may also be relevant in this respect, since the effects of raised fibrinogen levels on coagulability are enhanced in abnormal blood flow situations such as those seen in proximity to prosthetic valves (Chapters 1.5 and 2.1). However, the lower factor VII levels, lower platelet counts and greater fibrinolytic activity of these population groups[26,27] may counteract the hypercoagulable potential of raised fibrinogen levels to some extent. Ethnic differences in fibroblast activity[21] offer an alternative or additional explanation for tissue ingrowth in Africans (vide infra).

The intriguing question is whether intermittently inadequate anticoagulation over many years also contributes to *late* tissue ingrowth. Is it possible for repeated episodes of thrombus deposition and subsequent organisation to build up layers of increasing thickness similar to that seen on rheumatic mitral valves[5,6]? Unfortunately, there are currently no data to directly answer this question, although infrequent reports of excessive tissue ingrowth in non-anticoagulated bioprostheses suggest that this is not the most likely explanation unless the phenomenon goes unnoticed at reoperation or autopsy because it is not the primary cause of valve failure or death.

In some patients, the explanation for excessive tissue ingrowth appears to lie in an unusually exuberant foreign body reaction with active granulation tissue adjacent to the sewing ring laying down successive layers of fibrous tissue which gradually increase in thickness, becoming less and less cellular (Fig. 2.4–1). This basket-weave collagen is similar to that seen in pleural plaques which can attain a thickness in excess of 1 cm despite being devoid of capillaries[28]. Excessive granulation tissue, especially if it contains large histiocytes with prominent PAS-positive, diastase resistant inclusions, raises the possibility of a starch-induced reaction secondary to contamination of the sewing ring by surgical glove powder[29] (nowadays made from maize starch). Interestingly, unidentified filterable substances from glove powder particles have been shown to be cytotoxic to human vascular endothelial cells grown in tissue culture[30], underlying the importance of minimising glove contact with endocardium and aortic endothelium during valve replacement.

Exuberant tissue ingrowth in Africans may be related to inappropriately excessive production of collagen by fibroblasts in responses to injury or foreign material, since several diseases involving excess production of collagen are commoner in blacks than whites both in Africa and the USA[21]. These include keloid, scleroderma, systemic lupus erythematosus, uterine fibroids, neurofibromas, fibrosarcomas and endomyocardial fibrosis[21]. The comparison to endomyocardial fibrosis is perhaps

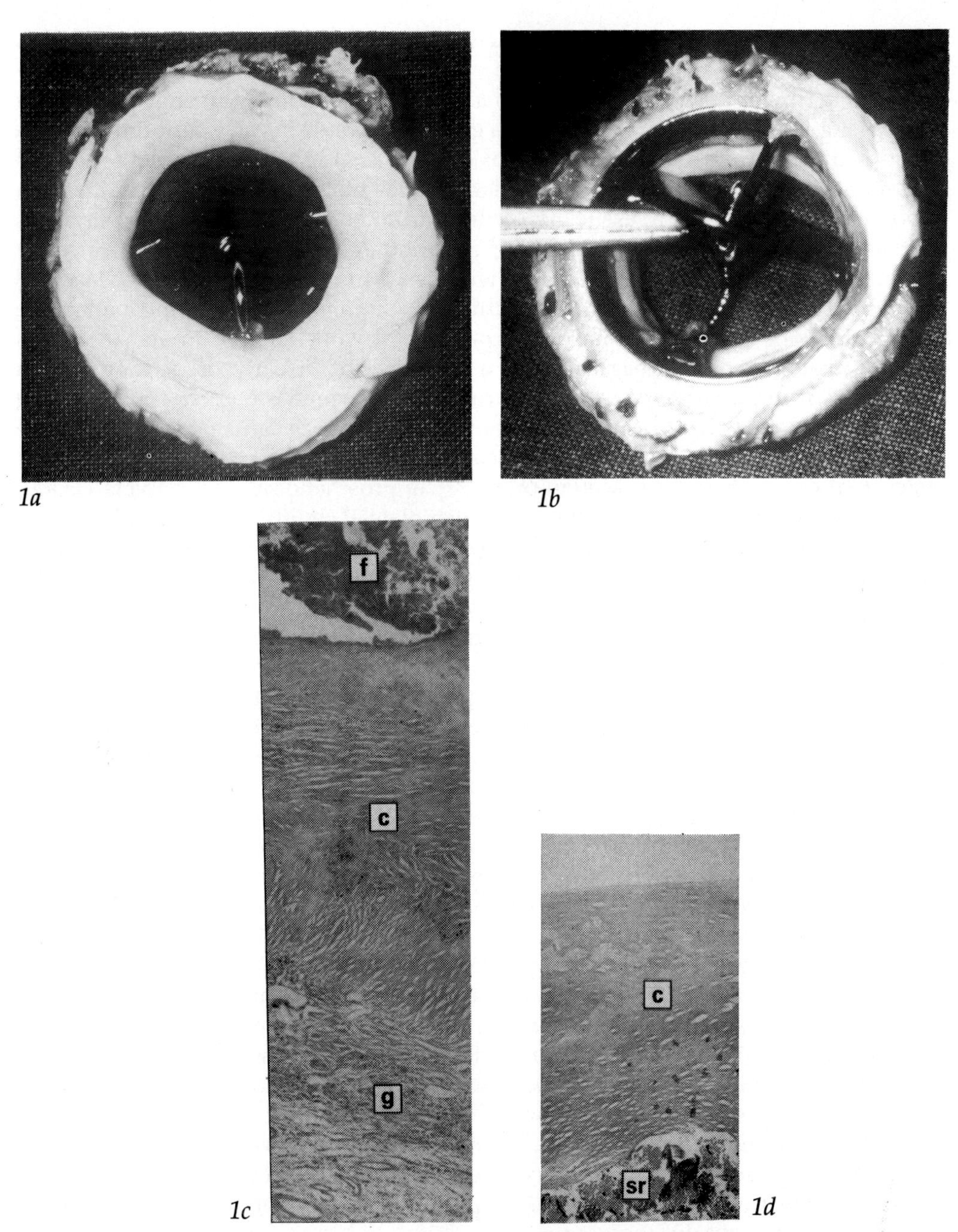

Figure 2.4–1: Excessive tissue ingrowth on a Medtronic Hall mitral valve, resulting from an exuberant foreign body reaction. a) Inflow (atrial) aspect of prosthesis. b) Outflow (ventricular) aspect of prosthesis showing the concentric narrowing of the orifice caused by the tissue ingrowth. c) Photomicrograph (x80) showing unusually thick, active granulation tissue and successive layers of fibrous tissue with diminishing cellularity. NOTE: Sewing ring not shown to limit size of illustration. d) Photomicrograph (x80) of 'normal' sewing ring healing for comparison showing much thinner fibrous tissue and no granulation tissue. Key f=fibrin c=collagen g=granulation tissue sr=sewing ring material

particularly relevant since this condition is relatively common in tropical Africa[31] and microscopically bears a striking resemblance to the excessive tissue ingrowth seen on sewing rings[31]. The aetiology of endomyocardial fibrosis remains uncertain with opinion divided between dietary influences[32] and cardiotoxic hypereosinophilia secondary to parasite infestation[33]. Alternatively, the condition may simply represent the end stage of a common response to injury initiated by different agents[32] and characterised by excessive fibrous tissue production[21]. Whether any of these agents may also be involved in initiating excessive tissue ingrowth on sewing rings remains speculative.

Sewing ring tissue ingrowth, whatever its aetiology, has several deleterious effects. In bioprostheses, excessive overgrowth onto the cusps causes progressive stiffening with eventual stenosis[22,34–36] or cusp retraction[37]. Prostheses in the tricuspid position are particularly prone to this problem[9,34,35,37] probably because low right atrial pressures allow the development of thicker fibrous tissue fuelled by neovascularity[9,37] (vide infra). In mechanical valves, extension of fibrous tissue onto the mechanism of the prosthesis can narrow the orifice, interfere with occluder movement and act as a site from which emboli may be discharged when the occluder strikes thrombus on its leading edge[25]. It also sets the scene for gross valve thrombosis by further reducing flow in areas of relative stagnation[20] (See also Chapter 2.1).

Homograft and heterograft valve cusps

Both homograft and heterograft valve cusps consist of foreign biological material that is either of dubious initial viability in homografts or completely dead in heterografts, having been treated with one of a number of chemical fixatives[38]. Unmounted homografts in the aortic position have the advantages of normal anatomical configuration, physiological flow patterns and the absence of a sewing ring and stents to attract thrombus formation[39]. Yet, like heterograft valves, they are not biologically inert and share the same surface reactions at least qualitatively if not quantitatively[38].

Unimplanted heterograft bioprostheses usually show widespread loss of endothelium or mesothelium (in the case of pericardial valves) as the result of harvesting, preparation and preservation techniques, exposing either basement membrane or collagen[40–42]. Although information on unimplanted homografts is lacking in the literature, a certain amount of endothelial loss is to be expected in these valves also prior to implantation. In both homografts and heterografts, any remaining endothelial or mesothelial cells on the cusps are probably lost soon after implantation[40,43–46]. The underlying basement membrane or exposed collagen attracts a thin layer of fibrin and platelets within hours of implantation[38,40]. In the case of bioprostheses, tanning with glutaraldehyde is thought to diminish the ability of exposed collagen to aggregate platelets[47]. It should be stressed that this early thrombus deposition is mainly at microscopic level only, although small flecks of thrombus visible to the naked eye have been seen on both homografts and heterografts recovered within a few weeks of implantation[34,44]. Fibrin deposits and large thrombi occur to a greater extent on the outflow surface of cusps than on the inflow surfaces[34] probably because the outflow surfaces are exposed to lower shear stresses[40,43]. After the initial healing of the sewing ring, the leaflets become the most thrombogenic parts of bioprostheses in terms of platelet deposition[19].

The organisation of microthrombus on the surface of the cusp leads to the formation of a fibrous sheath which varies in extent and thickness according to the duration of implantation and several other factors[38]. In some cases it extends only a few millimetres onto the base of the cusp[48], in others it covers almost the whole cusp[45]. In homografts, the extent of the fibrous sheath varies with the mode of preparation, being least in chemically treated valves, of moderate extent in antibiotic treated valves and greatest in fresh homografts where it can lead to cusp shrinkage[44,45]. In heterografts, the different forms of preimplantation treatment do not appear to influence the extent of the fibrin sheath[40], which is more dependent on valve site, being least extensive in the aortic position and most extensive in the tricuspid position[37,43], almost certainly as the result of local pressures and shear stresses, as discussed above. In general, fibrous sheathing occurs to a greater extent in homografts than in heterografts[43].

Host endothelialisation of biological valve cusps is variable in extent and usually incomplete[43], if not absent altogether[43,46]. Even when present, its functional ability is uncertain[10–13]. When endothelialisation does take place, it only occurs over previously deposited fibrin or fibrous sheath, never over exposed donor collagen[13]. Thus in homografts, the degree of endothelialisation varies with the extent of the fibrous sheath, which in turn depends on how the valve has been processed (vide supra). However a fibrous sheath does not guarantee endothelialisation. Freeze-dried and gamma irradiated homografts are reported to be almost devoid of endothelium up to 4 years and one and a half years respectively despite extensive fibrous sheathing in the latter[46]. Antibiotic treated and fresh homografts appear to have a greater covering of endothelium[44,45]. On porcine heterografts, endothelialisation increases with time but is never complete. No endothelial cells are seen in the first year of implantation, but after 5 years, up to 70% of valves show some degree of endothelialisation[43]. Endothelium is more likely to remain in place in areas of lower shear stresses and is therefore seen more on outflow surfaces of cusps than inflow surfaces and is more frequent on tricuspid prostheses than mitral prostheses and more frequent on mitral prostheses than aortic prostheses[43].

Because both homograft and heterograft cusps have either very incomplete or absent endothelial covering for most or all of their implantation lifespan it is inevitable that the non-endothelialised surfaces will have some degree of microthrombus covering[40,46]. There are four possible fates for this microthrombus: organisation to fibrous tissue, increase in size, lysis or embolism. Fibrin deposition and evidence of organisation is greater on outflow surfaces than on inflow surfaces due to the difference in shear stresses[40]. In most bioprostheses this microscopic fibrin deposition is not progressive and therefore probably undergoes continuous cycles of lysis or microembolism without giving rise to any symptoms[40,48]. This may account for increased platelet activation and turnover in some patients with bioprostheses[48–52]. Long-term aspirin has been recommended to minimise platelet adhesion[53] but in vitro studies have shown no significant decrease in platelet adherence to bioprosthetic cusps in media containing therapeutic levels of aspirin[47]. It is possible therefore that the therapeutic benefit of aspirin is mediated through its effect on associated non-prosthetic risk factors[54,55] (see also Chapters 3.1 and 3.4).

Symptoms attributable to cusp thrombus formation and its consequences arise under three circumstances:

1. Increase in size of thrombus. Small deposits of thrombus visible to the naked eye

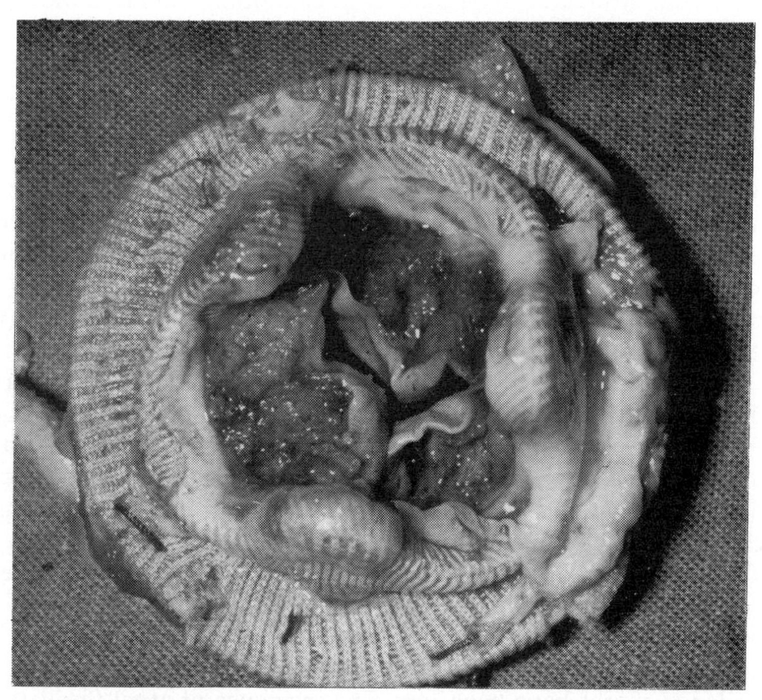

Figure 2.4–2: Thrombosed aortic porcine bioprosthesis, with thrombus filling each of the cusp sinuses (by kind permission of Prof. F.J. Schoen).

are occasionally seen on both homograft and heterograft cusps removed at operation or autopsy[34,44]. These thrombi have in most instances been asymptomatic and are 'incidental findings'. Symptoms occur when the thrombus becomes large enough to fill one or more of the three cusp sinuses (Fig. 2.4–2), limiting cusp mobility and causing stenosis[35]. This type of valve thrombosis has never been reported in homografts and is generally regarded as a rare occurrence in heterografts. Yet many reports of porcine valve thrombosis have appeared in the literature[35,56–64] with incidences between 0.4%[63] and 2.2%[57]. Bioprostheses in the mitral position have been shown experimentally to exhibit asynchronous opening of the cusps and to create areas of relative stagnation in the cusp sinuses during systole[65]. These adverse features when combined with a low cardiac output syndrome in the post operative period probably account for most of the early mitral valve thromboses[34,35,57]. Some late valve thromboses in both aortic and mitral positions are related to structural deterioration and associated cusp stiffness[48] or cusp tears[34]. However, in many patients no obvious structural abnormality or low output state precedes the valve thrombosis[35,57,61,63,64]. In these cases, primary tissue thrombogenicity[35], abnormal flow conditions[57,65] or a hypercoagulable state (Chapter 1.5) seem the only explanations. Gross cusp thrombosis has not been reported in bovine pericardial valves, possibly as the result of their superior haemodynamic performance in comparison to porcine valves[66].

2. Embolism. Despite the occasional finding of visible thrombus on homograft cusps following removal[44,45,67], symptomatic embolism from unstented homografts in the aortic position is widely regarded as a rare occurrence[39] although it has been reported in association with structural deterioration in chemically sterilised valves[67]. In fact, linearised rates of embolism reported after homograft aortic valve replacement vary from 0.034%[68] to 1.2% per year[69], a 35-fold difference. The series from Stanford reporting 1.2% per year included a small number of stented homografts also but no analysis of embolism according to implantation technique was reported[69]. Physiological flow patterns probably discourage thrombus deposition on the unstented homograft cusp and any micro-thrombus that does form probably has a secure attachment because of its adherence to the microscopically rough surface of collagen fibrils. For this reason, embolism from the cusp itself probably is indeed a rare occurrence. As in reported series of other types of prosthetic valve, it should be remembered that some, if not most, emboli arise from non-prosthetic sites (vide infra), as part of the 'background incidence' of stroke and TIA (Chapters 1.1 and 6.4) which is higher in the presence of atrial fibrillation (Chapter 1.2) and left atrial enlargement (Chapter 1.3). Barratt-Boyes is so convinced that homograft cusps do not give rise to emboli[70] that he does not report strokes, TIAs and peripheral emboli as valve-related events[71], recording valve-related thromboembolism as zero[70,72]. However, in most instances it is impossible to determine the site of origin of an embolus and it is a huge assumption that none whatsoever originate from the valve.

In the 20-year experience from the National Heart Hospital in London, reporting an incidence of 0.034% per year[68] (one embolus in one patient), the mean age of the patients was lower than the average valve series in Western countries and lower than other homograft series reporting higher embolic incidence[69,73,74] so that the 'background incidence' might have been low. The incidence of atrial fibrillation was not stated. However, a third of the 555 patients had additional procedures of which almost half (78) were mitral valvotomies. Bearing in mind that the incidence of embolism following mitral valvotomy averages 2.1% per year[75], it is rather surprising that a few embolic events did not occur in this subgroup at least, especially since none of the patients were anticoagulated[76]. In contrast, an 11-year experience of 200 aortic homografts in Southampton demonstrated a probable effect of concomitant mitral valve surgery on embolic incidence, even though only 15 patients (7.5%) underwent double valve surgery[73]. Three of the four embolic events in the series occurred in these 15 patients who were also in atrial fibrillation. Overall the embolic incidence was 0.36% per year but in 179 patients undergoing isolated aortic homograft replacement with no additional procedure, the incidence was 0.1% per year.

Another series of isolated aortic homografts also reported exceptionally low embolic risk[77]; thromboembolism was reported as zero but 18.6% of patients were excluded from analysis either because they underwent emergency valve replacement (5%) or because of insufficient follow-up information (13.6%). Pulmonary autografts can be considered very similar or even superior to unstented homografts in terms of their embolic potential since they are not 'foreign' tissue. When used in predominantly young patients, embolism is reported to be zero[78].

The true, *valve-related* embolic incidence after unstented homograft aortic valve replacement is difficult to determine. As with prosthetic valves, the reported incidences will depend on age, heart rhythm, stroke risk factors and other valve pathology[69,73,74]. For this reason, the embolic rate is probably a poor guide to the thrombogenicity of the homograft, as Barratt-Boyes has pointed out[70]. However one should enter the caveat that the degenerating, calcified homograft may be prone to

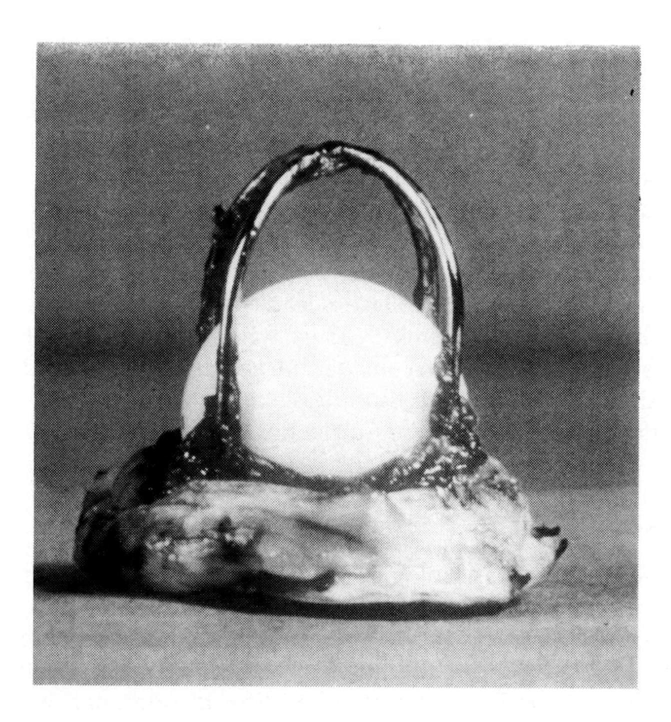

Figure 2.4–3: Thrombosis of Starr-Edwards mitral prosthesis, showing thrombus accumulation around the orifice, on the struts and on the apex of the cage, from which emboli may be dislodged by repetitive ball impact.

accumulate small thrombi and to embolise[67]. Further studies on his important aspect are required. Although now only of historical interest since their use has been discontinued, both stented[79,80] and unstented[81] homografts used in the mitral position yielded embolic incidences similar to those reported for heterografts.

The frequency of embolism from heterograft *cusps* is also difficult to establish. Although small fibrin thrombi on the outflow surfaces of the cusps are relatively common, the incidence of embolism from these thrombi appears to be low[34]. The risk of embolism is probably higher from thrombi on inflow surfaces[82], but most early emboli of valve origin in patients with heterograft valves probably arise from the sewing ring[19,35,57] or stent[83]. If gross bioprosthetic thrombosis develops, embolism is a frequent accompaniment, occurring in 50% of cases in one series[57]. Late bioprosthetic embolism is sometimes associated with degenerating cusps, when some emboli may be calcific[84,85]. Platelet studies suggest that bioprostheses may become more thrombogenic when they degenerate[86], although none of the bioprosthetic series in the literature report a late rise in embolic rate, coincident with degeneration. However, most of these series give insufficient information about embolism to determine whether a temporal effect exists or not. Furthermore if the overall embolic rate is low, a small late rise in incidence may be difficult to detect except in very large series or multicentre studies. More epidemiological and laboratory investigations are required on this fundamental aspect.

3. Organisation of thrombus. A thin sheath of fibrous tissue over the cusp allows ingrowth of endothelium and therefore probably has a protective effect, although it is rarely complete (vide supra). Thicker fibrous tissue however can be detrimental and interfere with valve function either by causing cusp shrinkage and incompetence[37,45] or by causing progressive stiffening of cusps leading to functional stenosis[22,34–36]. This latter complication occurs most frequently in the tricuspid position[9,34–37]. Calcium laid down in organised thrombus is also one of the mechanisms involved in the calcification of both homografts[67,87,88] and heterografts[89–91]. The growth in size of calcium deposits can lead to further thrombus formation and repeated cycles of thrombosis and calcification lead to a laminated appearance[89]. Calcification of thrombotic material superimposed on calcification of collagen leads to progressive stiffening[89–91] and increases the risk of calcific embolism[84,85]. Thus, when assessing the 'thrombogenicity' of biological valves it is important to consider the effects of thrombus deposition in the widest sense. Although gross valve thrombosis and embolism from valve cusps are unusual, the effects of microthrombus formation can lead to valve failure in other ways.

Mechanical valves

Mechanical valves differ from biological valves in four fundamental respects, each of which has an important bearing on the mechanisms of thrombosis and embolism. Firstly, the patterns of blood flow are non-physiological (although bioprostheses also show non-physiological flow patterns)[65], creating areas of relative stagnation, turbulent flow, flow separation and regurgitant flow through narrow gaps with high shear stresses (Chapter 2.1 and 2.2). Secondly, the surfaces presented to the blood

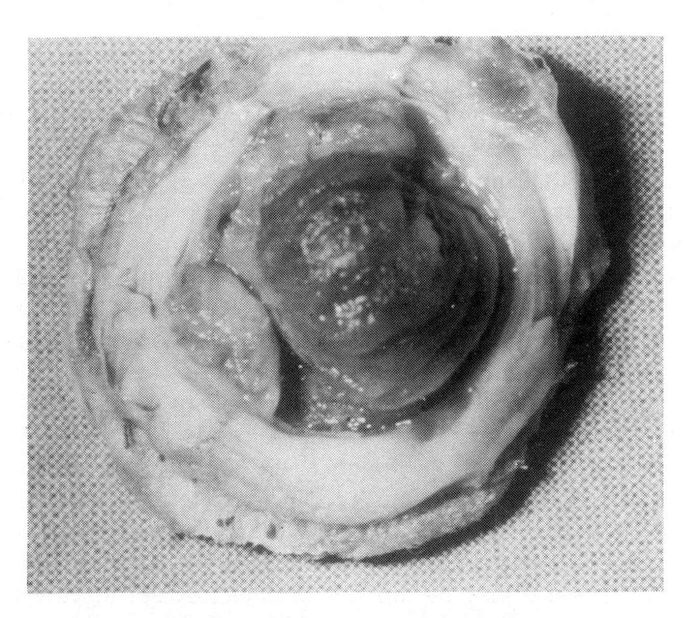

Figure 2.4–4: Thrombosis of Bjørk-Shiley Standard mitral prosthesis, seen from the ventricular aspect, showing almost complete immobilisation of the disc by firm thrombus. The laminated appearance, representing successive layers of thrombus deposition is readily seen. Length of history prior to diagnosis: 4 weeks.

stream are inorganic and highly polished with less secure attachment for any thrombus which does form (Chapter 2.3). Thirdly, the damage to erythrocytes and platelets which results from occluder impact and high shear stresses releases ADP which stimulates platelet aggregation (Chapter 2.2). Fourthly, in many mechanical valves, cavitation occurs on closure, generating microbubbles which, although they only last for a few milliseconds, may have important consequences (Chapter 2.1). The mechanisms whereby these factors lead to thrombus deposition on the working surfaces of mechanical valves has already been described in the foregoing three chapters. Embolism in patients with mechanical valves may originate from one of three sources: the highly polished working surfaces, the sewing ring or extra-valvar sites. The sewing ring as a source of emboli has already been discussed and extra-valvar sites are discussed later.

Embolism from the working surfaces is probably associated with one of four mechanisms:

1. Occluder impact. The risk of emboli being liberated by the occluder striking thrombus on some part of the valve housing varies according to the design of the prosthesis and the pattern of thrombus deposition (Figs 2.4–3,4 and 5). However in any mechanical valve, thrombus which extends from the sewing ring onto the annulus of the prosthesis is likely to be dislodged by the occluder before it becomes large enough to be detected clinically[92,93]. This is one reason why many prosthetic valves investigated following an embolic episode show no abnormality (Chapter 2.6). Similarly, thrombus which forms on the leading edge of tissue ingrowth (qv) is likely to be dislodged by occluder impact (Fig. 2.4–1a).

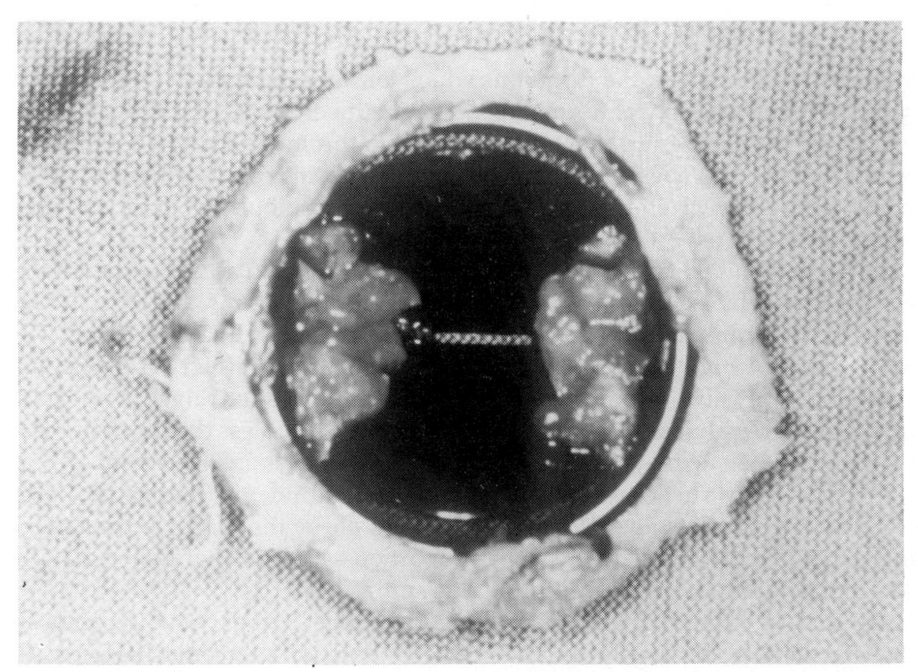

Figure 2.4–5: Thrombosis of St. Jude Medical mitral valve, showing almost complete immobilisation of both leaflets by a relatively small volume of thrombus (by kind permission of Dr P. Sareli).

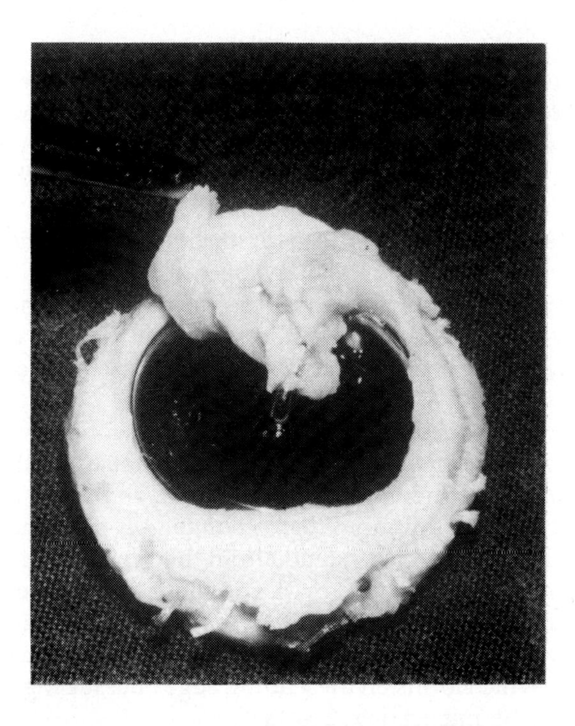

Figure 2.4–6: Thrombosis of Medtronic Hall mitral prosthesis, seen from the ventricular aspect. Thrombus can be seen gaining access to the central strut from the sewing ring and spiralling around it to spread out as a thin sheet resting on the surface of the disc but not adherent to it. This thrombus was flexible and rubbery in consistency, moving with the disc on opening and not limiting its movements.

In the ball valve design, the thrombus which forms preferentially on the apex of the cage because of local flow abnormalities[94] is repetitively struck by the ball with each cardiac cycle. In this design therefore gross valve thrombosis is often announced by repeated embolic episodes[95–98]. Following mitral ball valve replacement up to 35% of patients with *recurrent* emboli are found to have thrombosis of their prosthesis at reoperation or autopsy[98].

In tilting disc and bileaflet valves, thrombus is able to gain access to the mechanism of the prosthesis by extending along struts or over hinge points. In these situations it escapes occluder impact and is able to increase in size, initially moving with the occluder (Fig. 2.4–6) but eventually gradually immobilising it (Fig. 2.4–4). Because the typical pattern of valve thrombosis in tilting disc and bileaflet valves is not subject to occluder impact, embolism is a rare accompaniment[99–113] unless the thrombus is friable (vide infra). The somewhat higher incidence of embolism as an antecedent symptom in prosthetic valve obstruction among third world communities in South Africa receiving tilting disc and bileaflet valves[25] is probably explicable by the lack of anticoagulation in many patients and the relatively high proportion of tissue ingrowth as a cause of obstruction and thrombus deposition[25] (vide supra).

Thus in most patients with tilting disc and bileaflet valves valve thrombosis and embolism seem to be largely unrelated events with different mechanisms. Consequently, design changes among tilting disc valves in particular may have profound effects on the incidence of valve thrombosis but little effect on the incidence of

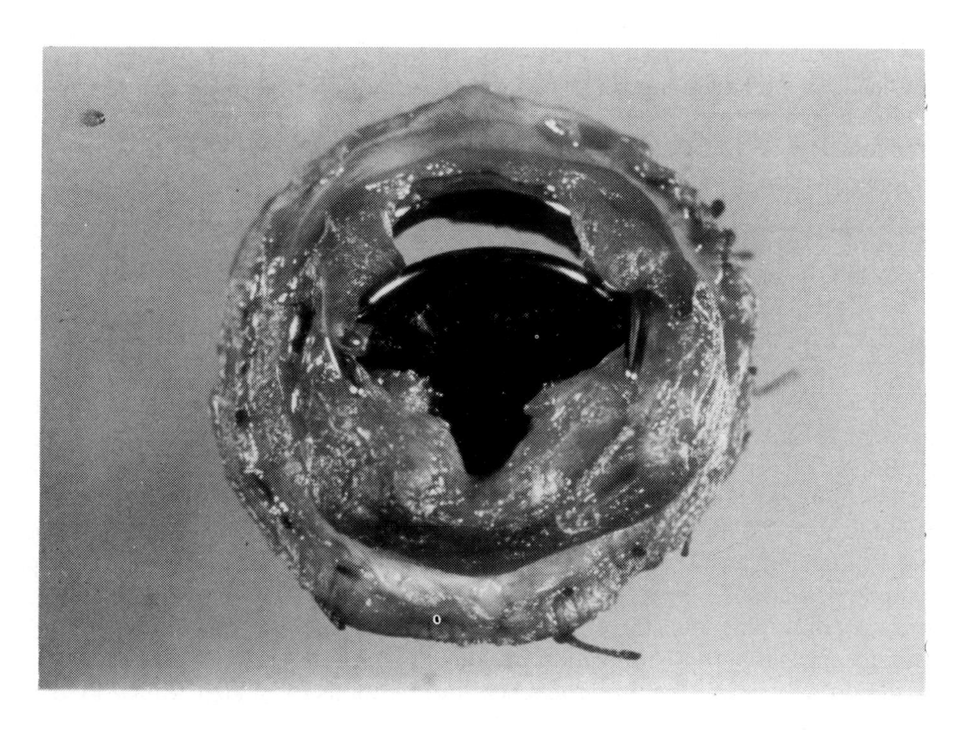

Figure 2.4–7: Acute thrombosis of a Lillehei-Kaster mitral prosthesis, seen from the ventricular aspect. The thrombus is dark red and friable, typical of thrombus developing in conditions of sluggish flow (see text). This type of thrombus may be more susceptible to embolism.

embolism[114–116]. For this reason the incidence of valve thrombosis (with certain caveats) is probably a better guide to thrombogenicity than embolic incidence. This aspect is discussed more fully in the section of this chapter on measurement of thrombogenicity.

2. Friability of thrombus. The thrombus seen adhering to thrombosed prosthetic valves is of two types: firm, pale, rubbery and flexible (Fig. 2.4–4 and 6) or soft, dark red and friable (Fig. 2.4–7). The texture of a thrombus is governed by a number of factors: blood flow conditions[117], the speed of its growth [117], the effect of the stabilising proteins factor XIII[118], fibronectin[119] and thrombospondin[120] and the degree of organisation (if any). Thrombus forming in fast-flowing 'arterial' conditions contains a high proportion of platelets and fibrin with relatively few enmeshed red cells[117,121]. It tends to form slowly and the effect of factor XIII in binding fibrin molecules together by catalysing cross-linkages takes place rapidly in fast-flowing blood[122]. The result of factor XIII activity under such conditions is to produce a firm, elastic, insoluble clot relatively resistant to fibrinolysis[118]. Conversely, thrombus forming under conditions of sluggish flow, such as exist in the left atrium in low cardiac output, contains much less fibrin (approximately the same proportion as the concentration of fibrinogen in liquid blood, ie 0.3%), is mainly composed of red cells and may grow rapidly[117], although its speed of growth will be determined to some extent by the intensity of anticoagulation[123]. The effect of factor XIII on the more widely spaced fibrin molecules in this red, friable thrombus is probably much reduced. This type of thrombus is likely to be more mobile, to show evidence of lysis and to be susceptible to embolism[124].

3. Change in anticoagulation level. Although firm, elastic 'arterial' thrombus is little influenced by anticoagulation[117], the adherence of thrombus to artificial surfaces is reduced when anticoagulation intensity is increased from subtherapeutic to therapeutic levels[123], increasing the risk of embolism. Therefore the large fluctuations in anticoagulation level, with troughs dipping below the therapeutic threshold, which are seen in many patients[125] may be an important factor in the pathogenesis of embolism[8]. Other factors which may have a bearing on the balance of the patient's coagulation system and therefore on embolism are discussed later.

4. Cavitation effect. This mechanism of embolism generation remains speculative at present. Cavitation results when sudden negative pressure is briefly generated during valve closure causing gases to come out of solution in the blood to form microbubbles[126]. When these bubbles collapse small pressure waves and fluid jets occur which can damage adjacent surfaces, causing pitting erosion. The effects of cavitation are seen more frequently in the mitral position due to higher closing velocities and are found in some prostheses more than others[126].

Bubbles up to 1.8 mm in diameter have been seen in the region of prosthetic valves tested in distilled water under simulated physiological flow conditions[126]. In water these bubbles last less than 0.1 millisecond. Whether they last longer in blood is speculative but platelets are known to adhere to bubble surfaces[127–129] and the possibility exists that this could either prolong the life of the bubble or enhance platelet aggregation when the bubble collapses. Air embolism is also know to damage endothelium and to predispose it to fibrin deposition[127].

Recent reports of asymptomatic microemboli detected by transcranial Doppler in some patients with prosthetic aortic valves[130,131] might at first sight appear to support a hypothesis of cavitation-generated microemboli. However, there was no correlation between the presence of microemboli and valve type or duration of implantation. Furthermore microemboli were detected in at least one patient with a porcine bioprosthesis. It is more likely therefore that an alternative explanation for this phenomenon exists (vide infra).

Embolism from extra-valvar sites is of course not unique to mechanical valves, although for convenience it is discussed here. It may occur as the result of disease processes present before valve replacement which remain unaltered postoperatively, for example atrial fibrillation and left atrial enlargement (see Chapters 1.1, 1.2 and 1.3). However, some thrombus formation at sites remote from the prostheses may occur solely or predominantly as the result of its presence in the circulation. This effect is termed secondary thrombogenicity and is described below. This thrombus also may result in embolism.

SECONDARY THROMBOGENICITY

Secondary thrombogenicity has two underlying mechanisms: obstruction and abnormal flow patterns. Obstructive thrombogenicity can be most readily identified in the mitral position, where prostheses with poor haemodynamics may produce significant 'stenosis'[132,133] with an incidence of left atrial thrombus formation and embolism typical of native valve stenosis[75,76,134–137]. Examples include oversized caged ball valves in small left ventricles where full ball travel is prevented by contact with the ventricular wall[138] and late stenosis in bioprostheses[35]. Abnormal flow patterns, by creating increased shear stresses which damage red cells and platelets, liberating ADP (see Chapter 2.2), can increase local coagulability[139]. This may induce thrombus deposition downstream from the prosthesis when activated platelets are transported onto pre-existing abnormal surfaces. Abnormal flow patterns generated by a mitral prosthesis could thus increase the possibility of thrombus formation on an abnormal native aortic valve[7] or on an aortic prosthesis in double valve replacement. This mechanism is almost certainly the explanation for the increased susceptibility to valve thrombosis of the St. Jude Medical valve in the aortic position when combined with a porcine bioprosthesis in the mitral position[112]. It has been shown that an area of stagnation and abnormal flow exists behind each cusp of a mitral porcine bioprosthesis[65]. It is thus possible that the resulting locally induced hypercoagulability predisposes an adjacent aortic mechanical valve to thrombosis. If this is indeed the explanation it represents an example of secondary thrombogenicity attributable to the porcine bioprosthesis. Abnormal flow and high shear stresses downstream from an aortic prosthesis could lead to endothelial damage[11,140,141] on the aortic wall. The combination of this damage with platelet activation associated with high shear stresses[139] could then result in thrombus deposition or even atheroma on the aortic wall[7] with subsequent embolism[142]. The same process probably also involves the proximal coronary arteries, since organisation of thrombus producing aortic and coronary intimal thickening and osteal coronary stenosis has been reported after aortic valve replacement with the Starr-Edwards valve[192]. Thus the possibility exists that some of the coronary embolism seen after aortic valve replacement[143,144] is related to aortic wall and coronary osteal thrombosis rather than thrombosis on the prosthesis itself.

Up to 38% of patients with primary coronary artery disease also have atheromatous plaques in the ascending aorta[145]. The combination of a pre-existing plaque with the adverse effects of abnormal prosthetic flow patterns could increase the possibility of thrombus deposition and may partly explain the increased incidence of embolism when coronary artery surgery is combined with valve replacement[8], although pre-existing ischaemic heart disease alone increases the risk of stroke between two- and fourfold[146]. It is possible that continuous cycles of microthrombus deposition on aortic atheromatous plaques as the result of prosthetic shear-induced platelet activation provide the source of the microemboli detected by transcranial Doppler in some patients with prosthetic aortic valves[130,131]. Further investigation is required to see if any correlation exists between these microemboli and the presence of aortic atheroma.

OTHER FACTORS INFLUENCING THROMBOGENICITY

The thrombogenicity of a prosthetic heart valve is not a constant phenomenon. From the foregoing discussion, it can be seen that such factors as cardiac output, degree of endothelialisation of the sewing ring and cusps (in the case of bioprostheses), structural deterioration (including the local flow changes this may cause), progression of disease in another valve, and anticoagulation intensity all have an impact on thrombogenicity.

In addition to these factors, any factor which increases coagulability has the potential to increase the risk of thrombus formation either on the prosthesis or on another intracardiac structure. These factors can be broadly divided into disease processes and lifestyle or environmental influences.

Disease processes

Several chronic diseases increase coagulability by a variety of mechanisms[147] (see also Chapter 1.5). Diabetes is associated with raised levels of fibrinogen[117,148,149] and von Willebrand factor[117] and reduced endothelial prostacyclin production[117]. Platelet function is also abnormal in diabetics[148] with increased thromboxane synthesis and greater sensitivity to aggregating stimuli[117]. Patients with nephrotic syndrome develop platelet dysfunction, hyperfibrinogenaemia and elevated levels of some coagulation factors[147,150]. Levels of the clot stabilising and bonding proteins, factor XIII and fibronectin are also raised[151] and levels of the natural anticoagulant, antithrombin III are reduced[152]. Malignant disease has a variety of effects on the coagulation system depending on the type of tumour, its pathological stage and the treatment employed[1,147]. Common abnormalities in many cancers include elevation of fibrinogen and some coagulation factors, thrombocytosis and increased platelet aggregability[1]. Some tumour cells also produce procoagulants that act either as tissue factor or as direct factor X activators[1]. Recent research work suggests that anti-endothelial cell antibodies may contribute to the endothelial damage of many autoimmune diseases[153] and that oxygen free radicals may damage endothelium in a number of pathological situations[154]. Both mechanisms may increase the procoagulant activity of endothelium. Whether they increase the risk of thrombus formation on endocardium or on the endothelium of 'healed' sewing rings requires further investigation.

Of the acute disease processes which increase coagulability, infection is by far the most important. In the author's experience, careful history taking in patients reporting embolic episodes or presenting with prosthetic valve thrombosis will often elicit an antecedent infective episode, even in the absence of endocarditis. Several mechanisms may be responsible for the hypercoagulability associated with infection. Fibrinogen levels are elevated[155,156], the inflammatory mediators, interleukin–1 and tumour necrosis factor, can induce endothelial procoagulant activity[12,13,157] and diminish its fibrinolytic activity[157], while endotoxins and other bacterial products can damage endothelium, directly activate the coagulation system and cause platelet aggregation[117]. Some viruses also damage endothelial cells and modify platelet function[117]. Severe infections associated with significant fluid loss, especially gastrointestinal infections, may lead to dehydration, further increasing the blood viscosity already raised by hyperfibrinogenaemia[158].

A seasonal variation in fibrinogen level occurs among elderly people. Higher levels are seen in the winter months[159], correlating with the higher mortality from coronary artery disease and stroke[160,161] at this time of year[162]. Higher fibrinogen levels are almost certainly explained by the winter rise in infection incidence. Although a seasonal fluctuation in white cell count does not occur[159], fibrinogen levels have been shown to be a more sensitive indicator of infection than white cell count in many mammalian species[155]. So far, there have been no studies undertaken to search for a seasonal fluctuation in embolic incidence after heart valve replacement in any age group. If such a seasonal fluctuation exists, it would provide indirect evidence for infection as an initiating factor in many emboli.

Lifestyle and environmental influences

Ethnic differences in coagulability[26,27,163–165] have already been briefly discussed earlier in this chapter. Whether these differences are genetically determined or due to differences in diet[166–168], tobacco[168–171] and alcohol consumption[168,172,173], exercise patterns[174,175] and the prevalence of chronic disease[26,176,177] has been the subject of much research work. Whatever their pathogenesis, differences in coagulability are almost certainly partly responsible for ethnic differences in stroke incidence[168,176,177] and probably affect the incidence of intracardiac thrombosis and embolism among different population groups after heart valve replacement also[25,112,178].

The predominant lifestyle influences on coagulability are diet and cigarette smoking. These are discussed in detail in Chapter 1.5. However, it is worth adding here that experimental work in animals suggests that a high fat, high carbohydrate, low protein diet can specifically induce *atrial* endothelial damage, predisposing to gross atrial thrombus formation[179]. Obesity and a sedentary lifestyle are associated with increased blood viscosity[164], elevated levels of factor VII and plasminogen activator inhibitor (PAI)[175] and reduced levels of antithrombin III[180]. Regular exercise in contrast can restore elevated factor VII and PAI levels to normal[175] and weight reduction can raise antithrombin III levels to normal[180]. The influence of social class is probably mediated through its effects on fibrinogen levels (see Chapter 1.5). Many drugs increase coagulability[181]. In particular, oral contraceptives enhance platelet sensitivity to ADP, increase some clotting factors[181] and decrease levels of antithrombin III[152,181]. They are known to increase the risk of stroke[182,183] and their use in patients with prosthetic valves should be discouraged. Oestrogen therapy in prostatic cancer has similar effects on coagulation[152].

DIFFERENTIATION BETWEEN EMBOLISM OF PROSTHETIC AND NON-PROSTHETIC ORIGIN

It has been traditional for many years to attribute all embolism in patients with replacement valves to the prosthesis itself[8]. However, there is no logic in this approach because many, if not most, emboli are likely to be patient-related rather than prosthesis-related, emanating from non-prosthetic sites as the result of pre-existing disease processes (Chapters 1.1, 1.2 and 1.3) and in response to variation in coagulability (vide supra). Because there is a 'background incidence' of stroke and TIA in the general population, gradually rising with age to around 2% per year by the age of 75 (Chapter 1.1), one should be very suspicious about any large series of replacement valves of whatever type which reports a zero or near-zero incidence of embolism. An exception might be a series composed entirely of young patients in sinus rhythm. Atrial fibrillation, even in the absence of valve disease, is associated with a fivefold increase in the incidence of *stroke* alone (Chapter 1.2). If TIAs are included also, the increased incidence is probably even greater. Therefore one can expect the presence of atrial fibrillation to have a major impact on the incidence of embolism after valve replacement also.

In the individual patient it is usually impossible to determine whether a particular embolus has arisen from the replacement valve or from another site, unless (on rare occasions) residual thrombus can be visualised on the prosthesis or on the left atrial wall, for example (Chapter 2.6). However, the embolic experience of a large series of patients with the same type of replacement valve may provide indirect evidence of embolic origin when the following aspects are examined:

Relation of embolism to atrial fibrillation (AF)

In the absence of valve disease, AF increases the incidence of embolism more than 5-fold (Chapter 1.2), while in rheumatic heart disease it increases the incidence almost 8-fold[76]. Although likely to be modified somewhat by anticoagulation (Chapter 1.2), a demonstrable effect of AF on embolic incidence postoperatively would be anticipated if most emboli were still originating from the left atrium. Conversely, the lack of such an effect *in a large series containing many patients in AF* would be very suggestive that the increased proportion of emboli occurring in sinus rhythm were actually originating from the prosthesis. The inability to demonstrate a difference in embolic incidence between AF and sinus rhythm in the large series of Starr-Edwards valves in which it was sought[184–189] could thus be considered tentative indirect evidence of the prosthetic origin of many emboli after valve replacement with this prosthesis, although some of the earlier series did not express their results in a time-related fashon. A prosthetic origin of many emboli is in keeping with the pattern of thrombus deposition on the apex of the cage and dislodgement by repetitive ball impact[94].

In contrast, in series of some tilting disc[190–192], bileaflet[193,194] and bioprosthetic[53,66,191,195–198] valves, the typical relationship between embolism and AF seems to persist postoperatively, suggesting that with these prostheses most emboli continue to originate from the left atrium. Interestingly, the positive relationship between embolism and AF noted in the Bjørk-Shiley Standard[190,191] and Concavo-Convex[191] models has not so far been seen in the later Monostrut model[199], although only short-term results are presently available for this prosthesis.

Relation of embolism to known stroke risk factors.

If all embolic events in a prosthetic valve series occur in patients with one or more known stroke risk factors, for example AF, systemic hypertension, diabetes, cigarette smoking or age greater than 70, the corollary is that patients without risk factors remain free of emboli and therefore that most, if not all, emboli are non-prosthetic in origin[192].

Relation of embolism to valve thrombosis.

As discussed earlier in this chapter, the relationship between valve thrombosis and embolism varies according to the design of the prosthesis, with repetitive emboli more likely to occur with thrombosed ball valves[95–98] than with thrombosed tilting disc or bileaflet valves[99–112].

Relation of embolism to change of prosthesis

If the embolic incidence falls significantly in a group of patients when one type of prosthesis is replaced by another of different type, this could be regarded as suggestive evidence of prosthetic origin of emboli from the first type of prosthesis[95]. However, an alternative explanation could be that the higher incidence with the first prosthesis was due to secondary thrombogenicity (qv) of obstructive type increasing the possibility of embolism from the left atrium.

Relation between pre-operative and postoperative embolism

Even successful closed mitral valvotomy does not significantly reduce the incidence of embolism in patients with rheumatic mitral valve disease[75,76]. Therefore it is probably unreasonable to expect any prosthetic mitral valve to lower the pre-operative embolic incidence overall, although some subgroups, for example those in sinus rhythm with small left atria and no other stroke risk factors, may escape embolism altogether[53,66,192]. If the embolic rate *rises* postoperatively however, as reported with some prostheses[200], this does not necessarily signify prosthetic origin of the additional emboli, because the risk factors for embolism may change after operation and with the passage of time as the patient becomes older. For example, a patient in sinus rhythm preoperatively may develop AF postoperatively, the left atrium may enlarge progressively[201] and left ventricular function may deteriorate[202–204] (see also Chapter 1.3). Advancing age per se also increases the risk of stroke and TIA (Chapter 1.1). Nevertheless a carefully controlled, prospective randomised study of different prostheses taking into account preoperative and postoperative embolism in the form of a 'progress proportion' could perhaps yield useful comparative information (see Chapter 6.4).

The ratio between major and minor emboli

The natural history of rheumatic heart disease is associated with a distribution of embolic size in which approximately 60% are minor or cause transient symptoms only[76]. Unfortunately, most prosthetic valve series in the literature do not stratify embolic events according to severity. In those that do, the percentage of minor or transient events varies from 25%[114] to 75%[192]. Does this wide disparity have any significance or is it simply due to variation in definitions and methods of data collection[77], since minor events are easily overlooked? The latter is probably the most likely explanation. However, there are alternative explanations. A prosthesis of low primary thrombogenicity with good haemodynamic performance will also have low secondary thrombogenicity, so that large thrombi are less likely to form in the left atrium. Alternatively the size of emboli may be determined more by patient-related factors such as left atrial size, cardiac output (Chapter 1.3) and the efficiency of anticoagulant control[8,123,192]. Variation between series may thus simply reflect the different patient populations. More studies on these fundamental aspects of embolism are long overdue.

MEASUREMENT OF THROMBOGENICITY

The assessment of thrombogenicity is an important component of the evaluation of any heart valve prosthesis. However, it is important to define the conditions under which thrombogenicity is assessed because there are many variables which can influence thrombus deposition. Applying Virchow's triad[205] of factors affecting thrombus formation (surface, blood flow, blood constituents), it can be seen that all three components may vary during the life of the prosthesis. The prosthesis is likely to be most thrombogenic immediately after implantation before endothelialisation of the sewing ring and (in the case of bioprostheses) other components has taken place (vide supra) and when cardiac output may be low. Thereafter, local flow conditions and variation in the coagulability of the blood will continue to exert a major influence on thrombus deposition. In the case of mechanical prostheses, wear of the components can lead to increased local blood trauma or altered flow patterns which may modify thrombogenicity[206]. In biological valves, tissue degeneration and calcification with advancing age of the prosthesis may theoretically increase the risk of thrombus deposition[67,86], although this effect remains unproven by currently available clinical studies.

Given the intrusion into clinical assessment of the many biological variables already discussed in this chapter, the in vitro laboratory testing of artificial heart valves appears superficially attractive. Each prosthesis can be tested under carefully controlled standardised conditions and various aspects of flow known to have an influence on thrombogenicity can be investigated[207]. Unfortunately there is no single measurement, or even a derived index from multiple measurements, which will accurately predict thrombogenicity in the clinical situation in every type of prosthesis or allow direct comparison of one prosthesis with another. Numerous studies exist comparing prostheses in terms of one or more hydrodynamic parameters (see Chapter 2.1). Whilst limited qualitative inferences can be made, each measurement has to be considered in the context of the particular design features of individual prostheses.

Recently an in vitro test model has been described which permits an evaluation of prosthesis thrombogenicity in a recirculating blood system[208]. It has also been suggested that conducting pulse duplicator tests on prostheses in a coagulable mixture of milk and rennet gives some indication of where clots will form in the clinical situation[209]. These types of artificial testing are mainly qualitative rather than quantitative, although they may allow limited comparison of one prosthesis with another under standardised conditions.

Animal implantation studies of prosthesis thrombogenicity have very limited value because coagulability and frequency of bacteraemia vary considerably from one animal species to another. Bacteraemia is a frequent occurrence in the dog for example[210,211] and gross bacteraemia from the bowel during cardiopulmonary bypass often leads to early massive valve thrombosis[212]. The dog is also hypercoagulable relative to man[15]. Hence, a prosthesis which appears prone to thrombosis in the dog[213] may not be prone to thrombosis in the clinical situation[115].

Clinical assessment of prosthesis thrombogenicity

Following implantation, prosthesis thrombogenicity assessment depends on the detection of thrombus formation, embolism or a milieu of altered coagulability using clinical observation and various laboratory investigations. In order to ascribe these pathological states to the prosthesis itself and thereby draw conclusions about its thrombogenicity, it is essential to have preoperative baselines for comparison, because some clinical observations and laboratory tests characterise the coagulability of the patient rather than the prosthesis and may have been present preoperatively.

Hypercoagulability is discussed in full in Chapter 1.5 and the various laboratory tests which can be employed to detect thrombosis, embolism or a prothrombotic state are described in detail in Chapter 2.5 and 2.6. Implanting a large foreign body into the circulation could be regarded as a rather extreme test of the coagulability of the patient. Those few percent of patients who suffer thrombotic or embolic complications may simply be those who were already hypercoagulable preoperatively or became hypercoagulable, either temporarily or permanently, postoperatively. Hazard function curves showing an early peak in the incidence of valve thrombosis are in keeping with this hypothesis[114,214,215], although not all prosthetic valve series demonstrate this effect.

Embolic rates

The incidence of systemic embolism following implantation of prosthetic valves of different design and manufacture is a superficially attractive means of attempting to distinguish between them[8,216]. However, it is dependent on so many variables that an *unqualified* embolic rate is meaningless. The large number of factors which can influence embolic rates are listed in Table 2.4–1 but by far the most important factors are anticoagulation level[8,192] (see also Chapter 3.4) and heart rhythm (Chapters 1.2 and 1.3). Associated cardiac pathology[217], age, ethnicity[163] and the presence of chronic disease[147] play important contributory roles and intercurrent illness, especially infection, may have a significant effect[117].

For embolic rates to have any meaning they must be stratified by patient risk factors and anticoagulation levels *achieved*. To take an extreme example, it would be ludicrous to compare an overweight, sedentary, diabetic, hypertensive, cigarette smoking patient of 75 in atrial fibrillation and congestive heart failure to a slim, athletic, normotensive non-smoker of 35 in sinus rhythm when the only factor they have in common is an artificial heart valve of the same make. If the 75 year-old also has low and poorly controlled anticoagulation and the 35 year-old has good control, the absurdity is increased to the point of farce. Yet the literature contains abundant examples of relatively small series of heterogeneous patients whose only common factor is a prosthetic heart valve of the same type. If the thrombogenicity of the replacement valve is low, as in homografts, most bioprostheses and some modern mechanical valves, embolism is probably much more dependent on established stroke risk factors and, in the case of mechanical valves, on anticoagulation level than on the prosthesis itself[192]. For this reason, there is as much variability in embolic rates between reported series of the same prosthesis as between different prostheses (Chapter 6.3).

In general, therefore, embolic rates as currently expressed in the literature must be regarded as an unreliable guide to the thrombogenicity of prostheses. Only by stratifying embolic rates according to categories of risk and anticoagulation and standardising definitions and methods of data collection will any useful results emerge in the future (see Chapter 6.4).

Thrombosis rates

The rates quoted in the prosthetic valve literature for valve thrombosis are subject to many of the limitations already discussed for embolic rates, in that there are variables other than the prosthesis which may affect thrombosis rates also (Table 2.4–2),

Table 2.4–1
Variables apart from the prosthesis influencing embolic rate after valve replacement

Methodology (Chapters 6.1 – 6.4)

Definition of embolism
Source of data
- clinical only
- clinical and investigation
- necropsy

Method of clinical data collection
- regular patient interview
- once only retrospective interview
- questionnaire
- review of patient records only

Specific questions asked
Percentage of patients lost to follow up
Exclusion criteria employed
Method of analysis of sudden death
Reporting methods and statistical analysis

Temporal effects (Chapters 6.2 and 6.4)

[Risk of embolism not constant]

Patient-related factors (Chapters 1.1 – 1.6)

Ethnic group
Known stroke risk factors
- age
- atrial fibrillation
- hypertension
- diabetes
- ischaemic heart disease
- hyperlipidaemia
- hyperfibrinogenaemia
- cigarette smoking
- alcohol consumption

Local cardiac factors
- valve position (mitral or aortic)
- aetiology of valve disease
- left atrial size
- left atrial appendage size
- previous left atrial thrombus
- other valve abnormalities and additional cardiac procedures
- impaired left ventricular function
- congestive cardiac failure
- endocarditis

Arterial factors
- carotid stenosis
- aortic atheroma
- aortic surgery

Surgical technique (Chapter 1.6)

Postoperative management (Chapter 3.4)

Immediate postoperative use of heparin or dextran
Level of anticoagulation *actually achieved*
Use of antiplatelet agents
Electrical cardioversion

Patient compliance (Chapters 2.4 and 3.4)

Anticoagulation compliance
Lifestyle influences
- diet
- cigarette smoking and alcohol
- exercise

Concomitant drug therapy

---

although these are fewer in number. The most important of these variables are anticoagulation level (vide infra) and cardiac output[34,35,57,218]. Low cardiac output, with or without the hypercoagulability discussed earlier, may contribute to the early peak in the hazard function curve for valve thrombosis in the series in which it is observed[114,214,215].

Although there are some limitations to their usefulness as an index of prosthesis thrombogenicity (notably the definition of valve thrombosis and the number of unexplained deaths in the series) valve thrombosis rates are probably more representative of thrombogenicity than embolic rates[115,219], providing that the intensity of anticoagulation is taken into account. As judged by valve thrombosis rates, unstented homografts in the aortic position have extremely low thrombogenicity[39], although pericardial heterografts appear almost as good in this respect since no case of gross cusp thrombosis has been reported with this prosthesis either[66]. Porcine heterografts in

Table 2.4–2
Variables apart from the prosthesis influencing prosthetic valve thrombosis rate

Methodology (Chapters 5.1 and 6.1 – 6.4)	*Surgical technique* (Chapter 1.6)
Definition of valve thrombosis	Orientation
Method of diagnosis	Sizing
. clinical only	Suture technique
. echocardiography	
. nuclear studies	*Postoperative management* (Chapters 2.4 and 3.4)
. operation	
. necropsy	Level of anticoagulation achieved
Percentage of patients lost to follow up	Use of antiplatelet agents
Exclusion criteria employed	
Method of analysis of unexplained death	*Patient compliance* (Chapter 3.4)
Temporal effects (Chapters 2.4 and 6.2)	Anticoagulation compliance
	Lifestyle influences (as for embolic rate)
Patient-related factors (Chapter 2.4)	
Low cardiac output	
Hypercoagulability	
. Pregnancy	

contrast have a measurable incidence of gross valve thrombosis[61,63] which, without anticoagulation, is about the same as the least thrombogenic mechanical valves with anticoagulation[115,219]. Mechanical valves vary greatly in their valve thrombosis rates. Figure 6.3–3 in Chapter 6.3 shows a comparison of valve thrombosis rates, taken from the literature, in four commonly used mechanical prostheses. The scatter of results for each prosthesis is almost certainly at least partly related to different anticoagulation levels used in the various series. An example of the effect of anticoagulation on the incidence of valve thrombosis can be seen in another similar compilation from the literature reported by Butchart and Grunkemeier[115], in which a striking difference in valve thrombosis rate was apparent between series of Omniscience valves in North America[220,221] and the UK[222]. Although the UK experience[222] when it was first reported triggered a number of acrimonious letters in the literature, the explanation for the difference in valve thrombosis rate was almost certainly the very different anticoagulation levels used on the two sides of the Atlantic at that time. The UK series was maintained at an INR between 2.0 and 3.0[223], whilst the North American series were maintained at prothrombin times equivalent to INRs between 5.0 and 10.0 (see chapter 3.3).

Hence, if valve thrombosis rates are to be useful as an index of thrombogenicity in the future, it is essential that full information is given about anticoagulation levels *actually achieved* in the patients under investigation, preferably expressed in the standardised internationally accepted terminology, the International Normalised Ratio or INR.

PROSTHESIS THROMBOGENICITY AND PATIENT SAFETY

It is probably fair to say that embolism can never be totally eliminated from any large series of replacement valves of whatever type given the 'background incidence' of stroke and TIA and the various patient risk factors that have been discussed. Although never mentioned in series of homografts and non-anticoagulated heterografts, there is also a 'background incidence' of bleeding which, because it is clearly not 'anticoagulant-related', is presumably dismissed as being irrelevant and unworthy of reporting. However, it is important to compare like with like and to acknowledge that a proportion of cases of 'anticoagulant-related bleeding' are in reality simply part of the 'background incidence' and due to underlying pathology. The unmasking effect of anticoagulation in revealing underlying pathology is almost certainly the explanation for the early peak in the hazard function curve for bleeding after commencing anticoagulation[189,224,225].

One could thus argue that in order to achieve fair comparison between prostheses, one should discount the first six months' or perhaps even the first year's experience of bleeding, valve thrombosis and embolism on the grounds that many instances will be primarily patient- rather than prosthesis-related. One would then be left with a long term comparison of all bleeding events (whether the patient is on anticoagulants or not), all events of valve thrombosis, all events of embolism (if not related to known stroke risk factors) and all events in which microthrombogenicity of valve cusps (in the case of homografts and heterografts) had led to valve failure.

Since the incidence of bleeding will be higher in the patients on anticoagulants, the homografts and heterografts are likely to score best on this assessment in the early years. However, the incidence of anticoagulant-related bleeding is very closely related to anticoagulation intensity[226]. If it is possible to maintain this at a very low level in a mechanical valve of low thrombogenicity without increasing the risk of valve thrombosis[115,192], the long-term safety of such a combination should compare well to that of biological valves, especially as the latter will eventually degenerate, possibly becoming more thrombogenic in the process, and ultimately fail altogether necessitating the increased risk of reoperation. Clearly, there will be a difference in patient safety between mechanical prostheses which require high levels of anticoagulation to reduce the risk of valve thrombosis and those which do not, since the risk of both valve thrombosis and bleeding will be higher in the former.

Lastly, the different mechanisms of valve thrombosis and their consequences vary between prostheses and have implications for patient safety. Gross thrombosis of porcine heterografts is associated with embolism in up to 50% of cases[57]. One of the advantages claimed for the ball valve is that it is thromboses gradually allowing time for recognition and elective reoperation[98]. However recognition can be difficult[227] and mortality following reoperation has been high in some series[188,189]. A further disadvantage is that thrombosis is often heralded by recurrent embolism[97,98] so that survivors of reoperation may be left with a neurological deficit.

Tilting disc and bileaflet valves are widely believed to thrombose rapidly or even suddenly[96]. However, examination of reports in the literature shows this to be a misconception[25,99–103,105–111,218,228–231]. Most patients have symptoms lasting several days or even weeks, although delay in diagnosis may lead to an acute presentation. Antecedent embolism is unusual (vide supra). A large series of thrombosed tilting disc and bileaflet valves in a predominantly third world population in South Africa detected no difference in presentation between the two types of valve[25]. However in many instances tissue ingrowth was the major component of the obstruction. Examination of

Table 2.4–3
Duration of symptoms prior to diagnosis of valve thrombosis
Comparison of tilting disc and bileaflet valves

	Tilting disc (Bjork-Shiley)	*Bileaflet (St Jude Medical)*
Case reports	45	10
Mean duration (days)	24.3 (range 1–180)	7.3 (range 1–21)
Duration ≥14 days	40%	20%

Data taken from all reports in the literature giving details of individual cases of mitral or aortic valve thrombosis in these two prostheses. See references 99–103, 105–111, 218, 228–230. Insufficient case report data was available in the literature on other tilting disc and bileaflet valves to include them in a comparative analysis.

many reports in the literature in contrast suggests that presentation is rather slower in tilting disc valves[99–103,218,228–231] than bileaflet valves[105–111] offering an extra margin of safety (Table 2.4–3). The explanation for this difference almost certainly lies in the lightweight construction and delicate hinge mechanism of the bileaflet valve which allows the leaflets to be immobilised by a smaller volume of thrombus[105] than that which would immobilise a tilting disc valve.

All replacement heart valves of whatever type have some degree of thrombogenicity, manifested in different ways and of varying impact on patient safety. Whilst much research continues in an endeavour to improve replacement devices, it is unlikely that the 'perfect' heart valve, not subject to wear or degeneration and totally non-thrombogenic, will ever be produced. Indeed, even the 'normal' heart valve is not immune from thrombus deposition in some systemic diseases. Improved patient safety therefore is more likely to result from choosing the most appropriate and least thrombogenic replacement valve for each patient, minimising anticoagulation levels so that they are no higher than necessary to prevent thrombosis and serious embolism (Chapter 3.4) and following patients carefully for any symptoms or signs of impending thrombosis or degeneration (Chapter 5.1), especially following major intercurrent illness or any non-cardiac surgery associated with anticoagulation interruption (see also chapter 4.5). Echocardiographic and other techniques are now becoming so sophisticated that there is no excuse for allowing any patient to deteriorate for several weeks and present in extremis before a diagnosis of valve thrombosis is made.

REFERENCES

1. Dvorak HF. Thrombosis and cancer. Hum Pathol 1987;18:275–284.
2. Deppisch LM, Fayemi AO. Non-bacterial thrombotic endocarditis: clinicopathologic correlations. Am Heart J 1976;92:723–729.
3. Straaton KV, Chatham WW, Reveille JD, Koopman WJ, Smith SH. Clinically significant valvular heart disease in systemic lupus erythematosus. Am J Med 1988;85:645–650.

4. Ford SE, Lillicrap D. Brunet D, Ford P. Thrombotic endocarditis and lupus anticoagulant. Arch Pathol Lab Med 1989;113:350–353.
5. Magarey FR. Pathogenesis of mitral stenosis. Br Med J 1951;1:856–857.
6. Tweedy PS. The pathogenesis of valvular thickening in rheumatic heart disease. Br Heart J 1956;18:173–185.
7. Stein PD, Sabbah HN, Pitha JV. Continuing disease process of calcific aortic stenosis: role of microthrombi and turbulent flow. Am J Cardiol 1977;30:159–163.
8. Edmunds LH Jr. Thrombotic and bleeding complications of prosthetic heart valves. Ann Thorac Surg 1987;44:430–445.
9. Berger K, Sauvage LF, Wood SJ, Wesolowski SA. Sewing ring healing of cardiac valve prostheses. Surgery 1967;61:102–117.
10. Schoen FJ. Biomaterials science, medical devices and artificial organs: Synergistic interactions for the 1990s. Trans Am Soc Artif Intern Organs 1991;37:44–48.
11. Dewey CF Jr, Bussolari SR, Gimbrone MA Jr, Davies PF. The dynamic response of vascular endothelial cells to fluid shear stress. J Biomech Eng 1981;103:177–185.
12. Nawroth PP, Stern DM. Endothelial cell procoagulant properties and the host response. Sem Thromb Hemost 1987;13:391–397.
13. Rodgers GM. Haemostatic properties of normal and perturbed vascular cells. FASEB J 1988;2:116–123.
14. Sauvage LR, Berger K, Wood SJ. The clinical significance of healing data obtained from study of prosthetic valves in animals. Adv Cardiol 1972;7:25–33.
15. Hawkey CM. The relationship between blood coagulation and thrombosis and atherosclerosis in man, monkeys and carnivores. Thromb Diathes Haemorrh 1974;31:103–118.
16. Marbarger JP, Clark RE. The clinical life history of explanted prosthetic heart valves. Ann Thorac Surg 1982;34:22–23.
17. Bonchek LI, Braunwald NS. Modification of thrombus formation on prosthetic heart valves by the administration of low molecular weight dextran. Ann Surg 1967;165:200–205.
18. Hannah H, Bull B, Braunwald NS. Development of an autogenous tissue covering on prosthetic heart valves: effect of warfarin and dextran. Ann Surg 1968;168:1075–1078.
19. Dewanjee MK, Trastek VF, Tago M, Torianni M, Kaye MP. Noninvasive radioisotopic technique for detection of platelet deposition on bovine pericardial mitral valve prostheses and in vitro quantification of visceral microembolism in dogs. Trans Am Soc Artif Intern Organs 1983;298:188–193.
20. Yoganathan AP, Corcoran WH, Harrison EC, Carl JR. The Bjørk-Shiley aortic prosthesis: flow characteristics, thrombus formation and tissue overgrowth. Circulation 1978;58:70–76.
21. Polednak AP. Connective tissue responses in negroes in relation to disease. Am J Phys Anthropol 1974;41:49–58.
22. Bortolotti U, Galluci V, Casarotto D, Thiene G. Fibrous tissue overgrowth on Hancock mitral xenograft: a cause of late prosthetic stenosis. Thorac Cardiovasc Surgeon 1979;27:316–318.
23. Planinc D, Jeric M, Mihatov S, Omcikus M, Pagon L, Rudar M. Doppler evaluation of prosthetic mitral valves. Acta Cardiol 1991;46:79–83.
24. Cleveland JC, Lebenson IM, Dague JR. Early postoperative development of aortic regurgitation related to pannus ingrowth causing incomplete disc seating of a Bjørk-Shiley prosthesis. Ann Thorac Surg 1982;33:496–498.
25. Deviri E. Sareli P, Wisenbaugh T, Cronje SL. Obstruction of mechanical heart valve prostheses: clinical aspects and surgical management. J Am Coll Cardiol 1991;17:646–650.
26. Meade TW, Stirling Y, Thompson SG et al. An international and interregional comparison of haemostatic variables in the study of ischaemic heart disease. Int J Epidemiol 1986;15:331–336.
27. Merskey C, Gordon H, Lackner H. Blood coagulation and fibrinolysis in relation to coronary heart disease: a comparative study of normal white men, white men with overt coronary heart disease and normal Bantu men. Br Med J 1960;1:219–227.
28. Gibbs AR, Seal RME. Atlas of Pulmonary Pathology. Lancaster, MTP Press, 1982.
29. Peters E, Gardner DG, Altini M, Crooks J. Granular cell reaction to surgical glove powder. J Oral Pathol 1986;15:454–458.
30. Sharefkin JB, Fairchild KD, Albus RA, Cruess DF, Rich NM. The cytotoxic effect of surgical glove powder particles on adult human vascular endothelial cell cultures: implications for clinical uses of tissue culture techniques. J Surg Res 1986;41:463–472.
31. Davies JNP. The heart of Africa: cardiac pathology in the population of Uganda. Lab Invest 1961;10:205–215.
32. Davies H. Endomyocardial fibrosis and the tuberous diet. Int J Cardiol 1990;29:3–8.
33. Spry CJF. The pathogenesis of endomyocardial fibrosis: the role of the eosinophil. Springer Semin Immunopathol 1989;11:471–477.
34. Spray TL. Roberts WC. Structural changes in porcine xenografts used as substitute cardiac valves. Am J Cardiol 1977;40:319–330.

35. Thiene G, Bortolotti U, Panizzon G, Milano A, Gallucci V. Pathological substrates of thrombus formation after heart valve replacement with the Hancock bioprosthesis. J Thorac Cardiovasc Surg 1980;80:414–423.
36. Hassoulas J, Rose AG. Experimental evaluation of the Mitroflow pericardial heart valve prosthesis. Part II: pathologic examination. Angiology 1988;39:733–741.
37. Murphy SK, Rogler WC, Fleming WH, McManus BM. Retraction of bioprosthetic heart valve cusps: a cause of wide-open regurgitation in right-sided heart valves. Hum Pathol 1988;19:140–147.
38. Ferrans VJ, Tomita Y, Hilbert SL, Jones M, Roberts WC. Pathology of bioprosthetic cardiac valves. Hum Pathol 1987;18:586–595.
39. Bodnar E, Ross DN. Valvular homografts. In Bodnar E, Frater RWM (Eds): Replacement Cardiac Valves. New York, Pergamon Press, 1991;287–306.
40. Ferrans VJ, Spray TL, Billingham ME, Roberts WC. Structural changes in glutaraldehyde-treated porcine heterografts used as substitute cardiac valves. Am J Cardiol 1978;41:1159–1184.
41. Riddle JM, Magilligan DJ, Stein PD. Surface morphology of degenerated porcine bioprosthetic valves four to seven years following implantation. J Thorac Cardiovasc Surg 1981;81:279–287.
42. Ishihara T, Ferrans VJ, Jones M, Boyce SW, Roberts WC. Structure of bovine pericardium and of unimplanted Ionescu-Shiley pericardial valvular bioprostheses. J Thorac Cardiovasc Surg 1981;81:747–757.
43. Ishihara T, Ferrans VJ, Jones M. Boyce SW, Roberts WC. Occurrence and significance of endothelial cells in implanted porcine bioprosthetic valves. Am J Cardiol 1981;48:443–454.
44. Gavin JB, Herdson PB, Monro JL, Barratt-Boyes BG. Pathology of antibiotic-treated human heart valve allografts. Thorax 1973;28:473–481.
45. Gavin JB, Barratt-Boyes BG, Hitchcock GC, Herdson PB. Histopathology of 'fresh' human aortic valve allografts. Thorax 1973;28:482–487.
46. Aparicio SR, Donnelly RJ, Dexter F, Watson DA. Light and electron microscopy studies on homograft and heterograft heart valves. J Pathol 1975;115:147–162.
47. Magilligan DJ, Oyama C, Klein S, Riddle JM, Smith D. Platelet adherence to bioprosthetic cardiac valves. Am J Cardiol 1984;53:945–949.
48. Angell WW, Angell JD. Porcine valves. Prog Cardiovasc Dis 1980:23:141–166.
49. Lee G, Joye JA, Rose A, DeNardo S, Kozina JA, Mason DT. Evaluation of platelet kinetics following porcine and mechanical valve replacement. Clin Cardiol 1981;4:11–14.
50. Dudczak R, Niessner H. Thaler E, Lechner K, Kletter K, Frischauf H, Domanig E, Aicher H. Plasma concentration of platelet-specific proteins and fibrinopeptide A in patients with artificial heart valves. Haemostasis 1981; 10:186–194.
51. Turpie AGG, de Boer AC, Giroux M et al. Platelet survival and betathromboglobulin after heterograft mitral valve replacement: effect of suloctidil (Abstract). Thromb Haemost 1983;50:63.
52. Koppensteiner R, Moritz A, Schlick W et al. Blood rheology after cardiac valve replacement with mechanical prostheses or bioprostheses. Am J Cardiol 1991;67:79–83.
53. Nunez L, Aguado GM, Larrea JL, Celemin D, Oliver J. Prevention of thromboembolism using aspirin after mitral valve replacement with porcine bioprostheses. Ann Thorac Surg 1984;37:84–87.
54. David TE, Ho WIC, Christakis GT. Thromboembolism in patients with aortic porcine bioprostheses. Ann Thorac Surg 1985;40:229–233.
55. Barnett HJM. Aspirin in stroke prevention: an overview. Stroke 1990; 21 (Suppl IV):IV–40-IV–43.
56. Fishbein MC, Gissen SA, Collins JJJr, Barsamian EM, Cohn LH. Pathologic findings after cardiac valve replacement with glutaraldehyde-fixed porcine valves. Am J Cardiol 1977;40:331–337.
57. Hetzer R, Hill DJ, Kerth WJ, Wilson AJ, Adappa MG, Gerbode F. Thrombosis and degeneration of Hancock valves: clinical and pathological findings. Ann Thorac Surg 1978; 26:317–322.
58. Franken P. Taeymans Y, Henuzet C, Rutsaert J, Primo G. Fatal thrombosis of a porcine aortic valve graft. N Engl J Med 1979; 300:197–198.
59. Craver JM, Jones EL, McKeown P, Bone DK, Hatcher CR, Kandrach M. Porcine cardiac xenograft valves: analysis of survival, valve failure and explantation. Ann Thorac Surg 1982;34:16–21.
60. Phillips HR, Spray TL, Lowe JE, Morris KG, Wechsler AS. Subvalvular thrombotic obstruction of an aortic porcine heterograft. Chest 1982;81:756–758.
61. Cohen DJ, Likoff M, Kishel J, Harken AH. Risk of prosthetic thrombosis with a porcine heterograft valve in the aortic position: case reports. Milit Med 1982;147:1056–1058.
62. Schoen FJ, Hobson CE. Anatomic analysis of removed prosthetic heart valves: causes of failure of 33 mechanical valves and 58 bioprostheses, 1980 to 1983. Hum Pathol 1985;16:549–559.
63. Croft CH. Buja LM, Floresca MZ, Nicod P, Estrera A. Late thrombotic obstruction of aortic porcine bioprostheses. Am J Cardiol 1986;57:355–356.
64. Baciewicz PA, de Rio C, Goncalves MA, Lattouf OM, Guyton RA, Morris DC. Catastrophic thrombosis of porcine aortic bioprostheses. Ann Thorac Surg 1990;50:817–819.

65. Jones M, Eidbo EE. Doppler colour flow evaluation of prosthetic mitral vales: experimental epicardial studies. J Am Coll Cardiol 1989;13:234–240.
66. Gonzalez-Lavin L, Tandon AP, Chi S et al. The risk of thromboembolism and haemorrhage following mitral valve replacement. A comparative analysis between the porcine xenograft valve and Ionescu-Shiley bovine pericardial valve. J Thorac Cardiovasc Surg 1984;87:340–251.
67. Davies H, Missen GAK, Blandford G, Robets CI, Lessof MH, Ross DN. Homogaft replcement of the arotic valve. A clinical and pathologic study. Am J Cardiol 1968;22:195–217.
68. Matsuki O, Robles A, Gibbs S, Bodnar E, Ross DN. Long-term performance of 555 aortic homografts in the aortic position. Ann Thorac Surg 1988;46:187–191.
69. Anderson ET, Hancock EW. Long-term follow-up of aortic valve replacement with the fresh aortic homograft. J Thorac Cardiovasc Surg 1976;72:150–156.
70. Barratt-Boyes BG. In discussion of Nashef SAM, Stewart M, Bain WH. Heart valve replacement, thromboembolism or thrombosis and embolism? In Bodnar E. Surgery for Heart Valve Disease. London, ICR Publishers, 1990;159–170.
71. Barratt-Boyes BG, Roche AHG, Brandt PWT, Smith JC, Lowe JB. Aortic homograft valve replacement; a long-term follow-up of an initial series of 101 patients. Circulation 1969;40:763–775.
72. Barratt-Boyes BG. Long-term follow-up of patients receiving a freehand antibiotic sterilised homograft aortic valve. In Rabago G, Cooley DA. Heart Valve Replacement and Future Trends in Cardiac Surgery. New York, Futura Publishing. 1987;167–179.
73. Virdi IS, Munro JL, Ross JK. Aortic valve replacement with antibiotic-sterilised homograft valves: 11 year experience at Southampton. In Bodnar E, Yacoub M (Eds): Biologic and Bioprosthetic Valves. Yorke Medical, 1986;29–37.
74. O'Brien MF, Stafford EG, Gardner MAH, Pohlner PG, McGiffin DC. A comparison of aortic valve replacement with viable cryopreserved and fresh allograft valves, with a note on chromosomal studies. J Thorac Cardiovasc Surg 1987;94:812–823.
75. Deverall PB, Olley PM, Smith DR, Watson DA, Whitaker W. Incidence of systemic embolism before and after mitral valvotomy. Thorax 1968;23:530–536.
76. Szekely P. Systemic embolism and anticoagulant prophylaxis in rheumatic heart disease. Br Med J 1964;1:1209–1212.
77. Khagani A, Dhalla N, Penta A et al. Patient status 10 years or more after aortic valve replacement using antibiotic sterilised homografts. In Bodnar E, Yacoub M (Eds): Biologic and Bioprosthetic Valves. Yorke Medical, 1986;38–57.
78. Abrams S, Somerville J, Ross DN. Pulmonary autograft for aortic valve disease: twenty two years experience. Eur Heart J 1991;12(Suppl):211(abstract).
79. Stinson EB, Griepp RB. Bieber CP, Shumway NE. Aortic valve allografts for mitral valve replacement. Surgery 1975;77:861–867.
80. Heng MK, Barratt-Boyes BG, Agnew TM, Brandt PWT, Kerr AR, Graham KJ. Isolated mitral replacement with stent-mounted antibiotic-treated aortic allograft valves. J Thorac Cardiovasc Surg 1977;74:230–237.
81. Qureshi SA. Halim MA, Campalani G, Coe YJ, Towers MK, Yacoub MH. Late results of mitral valve replacement using unstented antibiotic sterilised aortic homografts. Br Heart J 1983;50:564–569.
82. Bennett EV, Grover FL, Trinkel JK. Porcine valve bioprosthesis: early thrombosis with systemic emboli. Ann Thorac Surg 1982;33:197–199.
83. Stahmann F, Knott HW, Doty DB. Transient cerebral ischaemic attacks associated with worn porcine heterograft prosthesis. J Thorac Cardiovasc Surg 1979;77:872–874.
84. Bortolotti U, Milano A. Thiene G. Valente M, Mazzucco A, Galluci V. Evidence of impending embolisation of a calcific cusp fragment from a mitral porcine xenograft. Thorac Cardiovasc Surgeon 1982;30:405–406.
85. Johnson D, Gonzalez-Lavin L. Myocardial infarction secondary to calcific embolisation: an unusual complication of bioprosthetic valve degeneration. Ann Thorac Surg 1986;42:102–103.
86. Prandoni P. Pengo V; Boetto P, Zambon G, Menozzi L. Do malfunctioning bioprosthetic heart valves represent a potential thrombogenic focus? Haemostasis 1985;15:337–344.
87. Mohri H, Reichenbach DD, Barnes RW, Merendino KA. A biologic study of the homologous aortic valve in dogs. J Thorac Cardiovasc Surg 1967;54:622–629.
88. Jonas RA, Ziemer G, Britton L, Armiger LC. Cryopreserved and fresh antibiotic-sterilised valved aortic homograft conduits in a long-term sheep model. J Thorac Cardiovasc Surg 1988;96:746–755.
89. Ferrans VJ, Boyce SW, Billingham, ME, Jones M, Ishihara T, Roberts WC. Calcific deposits in porcine bioprostheses; structure and pathogenesis. Am J Cardiol 1980;46:721–734.
90. Dunn JM, Marmon LM. Mechanisms of calcification of tissue valves. Clin Cardiol 1985;3:385–396.
91. Schoen FS, Harasaki H, Kim KM, Anderson HC, Levy RJ. Biomateial-associated calcification: pathology, mechanisms and strategies for prevention. J Biomed Mater Res 1988;22:11–36.

92. Roberts WC, Morrow AG. Late postoperative pathological findings after cardiac valve replacement. Circulation 1967;35/36(Suppl I):I–48-I–62.
93. Bjørk VO, Wilson GJ, Sternlieb JJ, Kaminsky DB. The porous metal-surfaced heart valve. Long-term study without long-term anticoagulation in mitral position in goats. J Thorac Cardiovasc Surg 1988;95:1067–1082.
94. Yoganathan AP, Raemar HH, Corcoran WH, Harrison EC, Shulman IA, Parnassus W. The Starr-Edwards aortic ball valve: flow characteristics, thrombus formation and tissue overgrowth. Artif Organs 1981;5:6–17.
95. Reitz BA, Stinson EB, Griepp RB, Shumway NE. Tissue valve replacement of prosthetic heart valves for thromboembolism. Am J Cardiol 1978;41:512–515.
96. Metzdorff MT, Grunkemeier GL, Pinson PW, Starr A. Thrombosis of mechanical cardiac valves: a qualitative comparison of the silastic ball valve and the tilting disc valve. J Am Coll Cardiol 1984;4:50–53.
97. Acar J, Enriquez-Sarano M. Farah E, Kassab R, Tubiana P, Roger V. Recurrence systemic embolic events with valve prosthesis. Eur Heart J 1984;5(Suppl D):33–38.
98. Acar J, Vahanian A, Dorent R et al. Detection of prosthetic valve thrombosis using ^{111}indium platelet imaging. Eur Heart J 1990;11:389–398.
99. Fernandez J, Samuel A, Yang SS et al. Late thrombosis of the aortic Bjørk-Shiley prosthesis; its clinical recognition and management. Chest 1976;70:12–16.
100. Moreno-Cabrol RJ, McNamara JJ, Mamiya RT, Brainard SC, Chung GKT. Acute thrombotic obstruction with Bjørk-Shiley valves. J Thorac Cardiovasc Surg 1978;75:321–330.
101. Copans H, Lakier JB, Kinsley RH, Colsen PR, Fritz VU, Barlow JB. Thrombosed Bjørk-Shiley mitral prostheses. Circulation 1980;61:169–174.
102. Balram A, Kaul U, Rao BVR et al. Thrombotic obstruction of Bjørk-Shiley valves; diagnostic and surgical considerations. Int J Cardiol 1984;6:61–69.
103. Massad M, Fahl M, Slim M et al. Thrombosed Bjørk-Shiley standard disc mitral valve prostheses. J Cardiovasc Surg 1989;30:976–980.
104. Nashef SAM, Stewart M, Bain WH. Heart valve replacement, thromboembolism or thrombosis and embolism? In Bodnar E. (Ed) Surgery for Heart Valve Disease. London, ICR Publishers, 1990;159–170.
105. Nunez L. Iglesias A, Sotillo J. Entrapment of leaflet of St Jude Medical cardiac valve prostheses by miniscule thrombus: report of two cases. Ann Thorac Surg 1980;29:567–569.
106. Commerford PJ, Lloyd EA. DeNobrega JA. Thrombosis of St Jude Medical cardiac valve in the mitral position. Chest 1981;80:326–327.
107. Moulton AL, Singleton RT, Oster WF et al. Fatal thrombosis of a St Jude Medical valve despite 'adequate' anticoagulation: anatomic and technical considerations. J Thorac Cardiovasc Surg 1982;83:472–473.
108. Sharma A, Johnson DC, Cartmill TB. Entrapment of both leaflets of St Jude Medical aortic valve prosthesis in a child. J Thorac Cardiovac Surg 1983;86:453–456.
109. Turinetto B, Cahsai G, Dozza F, Marinelli G, Pierangeli A. Early thrombosis of an aortic St Jude valve in spite of effective anticoagulant treatment. J Cardiovasc Surg 1984;35:182–184.
110. Prabhu S, Friday KJ, Reynolds D, Elkins R, Lazzara R. Thrombosis of aortic St Jude valve. Ann Thorac Surg 1986;41:332–333.
111. Deuvaert FE, LeClerc JL, Primo G et al. Thrombosis of the St Jude Medical valve prosthesis in the aortic positon: a diagnostic and surgical emergency. J Cardiovasc Surg 1986;27:622–624.
112. Ribeiro PA, Al Zaibag M, Idris M et al. Antiplatelet drugs and the incidence of thromboembolic complications of the St Jude Medial aortic prosthesis in patients with rheumatic heart disease. J Thorac Cardiovasc Surg 1986;91:92–98.
113. Kinsley RH, Antunes MJ. Colsen PR. St Jude Medical valve replacement; an evaluation of valve performance. J Thorac Cardiovasc Surg 1986;92:349–360.
114. Lindblom D. Long-term clinical results after mitral valve replacement with the Bjørk-Shiley prosthesis. J Thorac Cardiovasc Surg 1988;95:321–333.
115. Butchart EG, Lewis PA, Grunkemeier GL, Kulatilake N, Breckenridge IM. Low risk of thrombosis and serious embolic events despite low intensity anticoagulation; experience with 1,004 Medtronic Hall valves. Circulation 1988;78(Suppl I):I–66-I–77.
116. Thevenet A. In discussion of Dewall RA, Raggio JMC, Dittrich H, Guilmet D, Morea M, Thevenet A. The Omni design; evolution of a valve. J Thorac Cardiovasc Surg 1989;98:999–1007.
117. Mustard JF, Packham MA, Kinlough-Rathbone RL. Mechanisms in thrombosis. In Bloom AL, Thomas DP (Eds): Haemostasis and Thrombosis. Edinburgh, Churchill Livingstone, 1987;618–650.
118. McDonagh J. Structure and function of factor XIII. In Colman RW, Hirsh J, Marder VJ, Salzman EW (Eds): Haemostasis and thrombosis. Philadelphia, JB Lippincott, 1987;289–300.
119. Mosher DF. Fibronectin, relevance to haemostasis and thrombosis. In Colman RW, Hirsh J, Marder VJ, Salzman EW. Haemostasis and Thrombosis. Philadelphia, JB Lippincott, 1987;210–218.

120. Lawler J. The structural and functional properties of thrombospondin. Blood 1986;67:1197–1209.
121. Vermylen J, Verstraete M, Fuster V. Role of platelet activation and fibrin formation in thrombogenesis. J Am Coll Cardiol 1986;8:2B–9B.
122. Francis JL: The detection and measurement of factor XIII activity: a review. Med Lab Sci 1980;37:137–147.
123. Madras PN, Thomsof01rLCJohnson WR. The effect of coumadin upon thrombus forming on foreign surfaces. Artif Organs 1980;4:192–198.
124. Yasaka M. Miyatake K, Mitano M, Beppu S, Nagata S, Yamaguchi T, Omae T. Intracardiac mobile thrombus and D-dimer fragment of fibrin in patients with mitral stenosis. Br Heart J 1991;66:22–25.
125. Butchart EG, Lewis PA, Kulatilake ENP, Breckenridge IM. Anticoagulation variability between centres: implications for comparative prosthetic valve assessment. Eur J Cardiothorac Surg 1988;2:72–81.
126. Graf T, Reul H, Rau G. Cavitation potential of mechanical heart valve prostheses. Int J Artif Organs 1991;14:221–226.
127. Warren BA, Philp RB, Inwood MJ. The ultrastructural morphology of air embolism: platelet adhesion to the interface and endothelial damage. Br J Exp Pathol 1973;54:163–172.
128. Thorsen T, Dalen H, Bjerkvig R, Holmsen H. Transmission and scanning electron microscopy of N_2-microbubble-activated human platelets in vitro. Undersea Biomed Res 1987;14:45–59.
129. Malmgren R, Thorsen T, Lie RT, Holmsen H. Microbubble-induced serotin secretion in human platelets. Thromb Haemost 1991;65:399–402.
130. Berger M, Davis D, Lolley DM, Rams JJ, Spencer M. Detection of subclinical microemboli in patients with prosthetic aortic valves. J Cardiovasc Technol 1991;9:282–283.
131. Berger M, Davis D, Rams JJ, Spencer M. Personal communication.
132. Westaby S, Karp RB, Blackstone EH, Bishop SP. Adult human valve dimensions and their surgical significance. Am J Cardiol 1984;53:552–556.
133. Rahimtoola SH. The problem of valve prosthesis-patient mismatch. Circulation 1978;58:20–24.
134. Coulshed N, Epstein EJ, McKendrick CS, Galloway RW, Walker E. Systemic embolism and mitral stenosis. Br Heart J 1970;32:26–34.
135. Fukuda Y, Kuroiwa Y, Okumiya K et al. Hypercoagulability in patients with mitral stenosis. Jpn Circulation J 1980;44:867–874.
136. Beppu S, Nimura Y, Sakakibara H et al. Smoke-like echo in the left atrial cavity in mitral valve disease: its features and significance. J Am Coll Cardiol 1985;6:744–749.
137. Chen YT, Kan MN, Chen JS et al. Contributing factors to formation of left atrial spontaneous echo contrast in mitral valvular disease. J Ultrasound Med 1990;9:151–155.
138. Roberts WC, Morrow AG. Mechanisms of acute left atrial thrombosis after mitral valve replacement. Am J Cardiol 1966;18:497–503.
139. Stein PD, Sabbah HN. Haemorheology of turbulence. Biorheology 1980;17:301–319.
140. Fry DL. Acute vascular endothelial changes associated with increased blood velocity gradients. Circulation Res 1968;22:165–197.
141. Fry DL. Certain histological and chemical responses of the vascular interface to acutely induced mechanical stress in the aorta of the dog. Circulation Res 1969;24:93–108.
142. Karalis DG, Chandrasekaran K, Victor MF, Ross JJJr, Mintz GS. Recognition and embolic potential of intra-aortic atherosclerotic debris. J Am Coll Cardiol 1991;17:73–78.
143. Prizel KR, Hutchins GM, Bulkley BH. Coronary artery embolism and myocardial infarction: a clinico-pathologic study of 55 patients. Ann Intern Med 1978;88:155–161.
144. Charles RG, Epstein EJ, Holt S, Coulshed N. Coronary embolism in valvular heart disease. Quart J Med 1982;202:147–161.
145. Tobler HG, Edward JE. Frequency and location of atherosclerotic plaques in the ascending aorta. J Thorac Cardiovasc Surg 1988;96:304–306.
146. Shaper AG, Phillips AN, Pocock SJ, Walker M, Macfarlane PW. Risk factors for stroke in middle aged British men. Br Med J 1991;302:1111–1115.
147. Schafer AI. The hypercoagulable states. Ann Intern Med 1985;102:814–828.
148. Mayne EE, Bridges JM, Weaver JA. Platelet adhesiveness, plasma fibronogen and factor VIII levels in diabetes mellitus. Diabetologia 1970;6:436–440.
149. Prentice CRM, Lowe GDO. Blood viscosity and the complications of diabetes. Adv Exp Med Biol 1984;164:99–103.
150. Kendall AG, Lohmann RC. Nephrotic syndrome, a hypercoagulable state. Arch Intern Med 1971;127:1021–1027.
151. Vaziri ND, Gonzales E, Barton CH, Chen HT, Nguyen Q, Arquilla M. Factor XIII and its substrates, fibronectin, fibronogen and alpha 2-antiplasmin in plasma and urine of patient with nephrosis. J Lab Clin Med 1990;117:152–156.
152. Buller HR, ten Cate JW. Acquired antithrombin III deficiency: laboratory diagnosis, incidence, clinical implications and treatment with antithrombin III concentrate. Am J Med 1989; 87(Suppl) 3B):44S–48S.

153. Editorial: Antibodies to endothelial cells. Lancet 1991;337:649–650.
154. Shatos MA, Dohety JM, Hoak JC. Alterations in human vascular endothelial cell function by oxygen free radicals: platelet adherence and prostacyclin release. Arteriosclerosis Thromb 1991;11:594–601.
155. Hawkey CM, Hart MG. Fibronogen levels in mammals suffering from bacterial infections. Vet Rec 1987;121:519–521.
156. DiMinno G, Ceebone AM. Fibrinogen: a coagulation protein in the cardiovascular risk factor profile. In Crepaldi G, Gotto AM, Manzato E, Baggio G (Eds): Atherosclerosis VIII. Amsterdam, Elsevier, 1989;469–474.
157. Bevilacqua MP, Gimbrone MA. Inducible endothelial functions in inflammation and coagulation. Sem Thromb Hemost 1987;13:425–433.
158. Wells RE, Gawronski TH, Cox PJ, Perera RD. Influence of fibronogen on flow properties of erythrocyte suspensions. Am J Physiol 1964;207:1035–1040.
159. Stout RW, Crawford V. Seasonal variations in fibrinogen concentrations among elderly people. Lancet 1991;338:9–13.
160. Wilhelmsen L, Svarsudd K, Bengsten KK, Larsson B, Welin L, Tibblin G. Fibrinogen as a risk factor for stroke and myocardial infarction. N Engl J Med 1984;311:501–505.
161. Kannel WB, Wolf PA, Castelli WP, D'Agostino RB. Fibrongen and risk of cardiovascular disease: the Framingham study. J Am Med Assoc 1987;258:1183–1186.
162. Alderson MR. Season and mortality. Health Trends 1985;17:87–96.
163. Miller GJ. Ethnicity, lipoproteins and haemostatic factors. In Cruickshank JK, Beevers DG (Eds): Ethnic Factors in Health and Disease. London, Wright, 1989;280–288.
164. de Simone G, Devreux RB, Chien S, Alderman MH, Atlas SA, Laragh JH. Relation of blood viscosity to demographic and physiologic variables and to cardiovascular risk factors in apparently normal adults Circulation 1990;81:107–117.
165. Sane DC, Stump DC, Topol EJ et al. Racial differences in responses to thrombolytic therapy with recombinant tissue-type plasminogen activator: increased fibrin(ogen)olysis in blacks. Circulation 1991;83:170–175.
166. Visudhiphan S, Poolsuppasit S, Piboonnukarintr O, Tumliang S. The relationship between high fibrinolytic activity and daily capsicum ingestion in Thais. Am J Clin Nutr 1982;35:1452–1458.
167. Kantha SS. Dietary effects of fish oils on human health: a review of recent studies. Yale J Biol Med 1987;60:37–44.
168. Iso H, Folsom AR, Wu KK et al. Haemostatic variables in Japanese and caucasian men. Plasma fibrinogen, factor VIIc, factor VIIIc and von Willebrand factor and their relations to cardiovascular disease risk factors. Am J Epidemiol 1989;130:925–934.
169. Kannell WB, D'Agostino RB, Belanger AJ. Fibrinogen, cigarette smoking and the risk of cardiovascular disease: insights from the Framingham study. Am Heart J 1987;13:1006–1010.
170. Rival J, Riddle JM, Stein PD. Effects of chronic smoking on platelet function. Thromb Res 1987;45:75–85.
171. Davis JW, Shelton L, Watanabe IS, Arnold J. Passive smoking affects endothelium and platelets. Arch Intern Med 1989;149:386–389.
172. Jakubowski JA, Vaillancourt R, Deykin D. Interaction of ethanol, prostacyclin and aspirin in determining human platelet activity in vitro. Arteriosclerosis 1988;8:436–441.
173. Gorelick PB. The status of alcohol as a risk factor for stroke. Stroke 1989;20:1607–1610.
174. Ferguson EW, Bernier LL, Banta GR, Yu-Yahiro J, Schoomaker EB. Effects of exercise and conditioning on clotting and fibrinolytic activity in men. J Appl Physiol 1987;62:1416–1421.
175. Gris JC, Schved JF, Feugeas O et al. Impact of smoking, physical training and weight reduction on factor VII, PAI–1 and haemostatic markers in sedentary men. Thromb Haemost 1990;64:516–520.
176. Shi F, Hart RG, Sherman DG, Tegeler CH. Stroke in the People's Republic of China. Stroke 1989;20:1581–1585.
177. Balarajan R. Ethnic differences in mortality from ischaemic heart disease and cerebrovascular disease in England and Wales. Br Med J 1991;302:560–564.
178. John S, Prasad KMS, Krishnaswami S. Early and long term results following valve replacements in the young with advanced rheumatic heart disease. In Bodnar E (Ed): Surgery for Heart Valve Disease. London, ICR Publishers, 1990;44–53.
179. Davenport WD, Ball CR. Diet-induced atrial endothalial damage. Atherosclerosis 1981;40:145–152.
180. Batist G, Bothe A, Bern M, Bistrian BR, Blackburn GL. Low antithrombin III in morbid obesity: return to normal with weight reduction. J Parenteral Enteral Nutr 1983;7:447–449.
181. Zbinden G. Evaluation of thrombogenic effect of drugs. Annu Rev Pharmacol Toxicol 1976;16:177–188.
182. Collaborative Group for the Study of Stroke in Young Women: Oral contraception and increased risk of cerebral ischaemia or thrombosis. N Engl J Med 1973;288:871–878.
183. Collaborative Group for the Study of Stroke in Young Women: oral contraceptives and stroke in young women; associated risk factors. J Am Med Assoc 1975;231:718–722.

184. Yeh TJ, Anabtawi IN, Cornett VE, Ellison RG. Influence of rhythm and anticoagulation upon the incidence of embolisation associated with Starr-Edwards prostheses. Circulation 1967;35/36(Suppl I):I–77-I–81.
185. Friedli B, Aerichide N, Grondin P, Campeau L. Thromboembolic complications of heart valve prostheses. Am Heart J 1971;81:702–708.
186. Cleland J,. Molloy PJ. Thromboembolic complications of the cloth-covered Starr-Edwards prostheses, no 2300 aortic and no 6300 mitral. Thorax 1973;28:41–47.
187. Fuster V, Pumphrey CW, McGoon MD, Chesebro JH, Pluth JR, McGoon DC. Systemic thromboembolism in mitral and aortic Starr-Edwards prostheses: a 10–19 year follow-up. Circulation 1982;66(Suppl I):I–157-I–161.
188. Miller DC, Stinson EB, Jamieson SW, Baumgartner WA, Shumway NE. Ten to fifteen year reassessment of the performance characteristics of the Starr-Edwards model 6120 mitral valve prosthesis. J Thorac Cardiovasc Surg 1983;85:1–20.
189. Miller DC, Oyer PE, Mitchell RS et al. Peformance characteristics of the Starr-Edwards model 1260 aortic valve prosthesis beyond ten years. J Thorac Cardiovasc Surg 1984;88:193–207.
190. Bjørk VO, Henze A. Ten years' experience with the Bjørk-Shiley tilting disc valve. J Thorac Cardiovasc Surg 1979;78:331–342.
191. Bloomfield P, Kitchin AH, Wheatley DJ, Walbaum PR, Lutz W, Miller HC. A prospective evaluation of the Bjørk-Shiley, Hancock and Carpentier-Edwards heart valve prostheses. Circulation 1986;73:1213–1222.
192. Butchart EG, Lewis PA, Bethel JA, Breckenridge IM. Adjusting anticoagulation to prosthesis thrombogenicity and patient risk factors: recommendations for the Medtronic Hall valve. Circulation 1991;84(Suppl IV):61–69.
193. Nair CK, Mohiuddin SM, Hilleman DE et al. Ten-year results with the St Jude Medical prosthesis. Am J Cardiol 1990;65:217–225.
194. Czer LSC, Chaux A, Matloff JM et al. Ten year experience with the St Jude Medical valve for primary valve replacement. J Thorac Cardiovasc Surg 1990;100:44–55.
195. Edmiston WA, Harrison EC, Duick GF, Parnassus W, Lau FYK. Thromboembolism in mitral porcine valve recipients. Am J Cardiol 1978;41:508–511.
196. Jamieson WRE, Janusz MT, Miyagishima RT et al. Embolic complications of porcine heterograft cardiac valves. J Thorac Cardiovasc Surg 1981;81:626–631.
197. Oyer PE, Stinson EB, Miller DC, Jamieson SW, Mitchell RS, Shumway NE. Thromboembolic risk and durability of the Hancock bioprosthetic cardiac valve. Eur Heart J 1984; 5(Suppl D):81–85.
198. Cohn LH, Allred EN, DiSesa VJ, Sawtelle K, Shemin RJ, Collins JJ. Early and late risk of aortic valve replacement. J Thorac Cardiovasc Surg 1984;88:695–705.
199. Thulin LI, Bain WH, Huysmans HH et al. Heart valve replacement with the Bjørk-Shiley Monostrut valve: early results of a multicentre clinical investigation. Ann Thorac Surg 1988;45:164–170.
200. Horstkotte D. Personal communication.
201. Sanfilippo AJ, Abascal VM, Sheehan M et al. Atrial enlargement as a consequence of atrial fibrillation. A prospective echocardiographic study. Circulation 1990;82:792–797.
202. Sherrid MV, Clark RD, Cohn K. Echocardiographic analysis of left atrial size before and after operation in mitral valve disease. Am J Cardiol 1979;43:171–178.
203. Ruocco NA, Most AS. Clinical and echocardiographic risk factors for systemic embolisation in patients with atrial fibrillation in the absence of mitral stenosis. J Am Coll Cardiol 1986;7:165A.
204. Adams PC, Cohen M. Chesebro JH, Fuster V. Thrombosis and embolism from cardiac chambers and infected valves. J Am Coll Cardiol 1986;8:76B–87B.
205. Virchow R. Gesammelte abhandlungen zur Wissenschaftlichen medizin. IV Thrombose und embolie. Gefassentzundung und Septische Infektion, Frankfurt, Meidinger,1856.
206. Hylen JC. Mechanical malfunction and thrombosis of prosthetic heart valves. Am J Cardiol 1972;30:396–404.
207. Food and Drug Administration: Replacement Heart Valves; guidance for data to be submitted to the Food and Drug Administration in support of applications for premarket approval. US FDA, May 1990.
208. Swier P, Bos WJ, Mohammed SF, Olsen DB, Kolff WJ. An in vitro test model to study the performance and thrombogenicity of cardiovascular devices. ASAIO Trans 1989;35:683–687.
209. Lewis JMO, Macleod N. A blood analogue for the experimental study of flow-related thrombosis at prosthetic heart valves. Cardiovasc Res 1983;17:466–475.
210. Nelson RM, Noyes HE. Blood culture studies in normal dogs and dogs in haemorrhagic shock. Surgery 1954;35:782–785.
211. Das SK, Rush BF. Normal bacterial flora in dog blood. Surg Forum 1965;16:74–75.
212. Jones RD, Akao M, Cross FS. Bacteremia and thrombus accumulation on prosthetic heart valves in the dog. J Surg Res 1969;9:293–300.

213. Aasen AO, Resch F, Semb BJ et al. Development of a canine model for long-term studies after mitral valve replacement with the Hall-Kaster prosthesis. Eur Surg Res 1980;12:199–207.
214. Blackstone EH, Kirklin JW. Death and other time-related events after valve replacement. Circulation 1985;72:753–767.
215. Lindblom D. Long-term clinical results after aortic valve replacement with the Bjørk-Shiley prosthesis. J Thorac Cardiovasc Surg 1988;95:658–667.
216. Abernathy WS, Willis PW. Thromboembolic complications of rheumatic heart diseases. Cardiovasc Clin 1973;5:131–175.
217. Cerebral Embolism Task Force. Cardiogenic brain embolism. The second report of the Cerebral Embolism Task Force. Arch Neurol 1989;46:727–743.
218. Ryder SJ, Bradley H, Brannan JJ, Turner MA, Bain WH. Thrombotic obstruction of the Bjørk-Shiley valve: the Glasgow experience. Thorax 1984;39:487–492.
219. Grunkemeier GL, Rahimtoola SH. Artificial heart valves. Annu Rev Med 1990;41:251–263.
220. DeWall R, Pelletier LC, Panebianco A et al. Factors influencing thromboembolic complications in Omniscience cardiac valve patients. Eur Heart J 1984;5(Suppl D):53–57.
221. Callaghan JC, Coles J, Damle A. Six year clinical study of use of the Omniscience valve prosthesis in 219 patients. J Am Coll Cardiol 1987;9:240–246.
222. Fananapazir L, Clarke DB, Dark JF, Lawson RAM, Moussalli H. Results of valve replacement with the Omniscience prosthesis. J Thorac Cardiovasc Surg 1983;86:621–625.
223. Lawson RAM. Personal communication.
224. Landefeld CS, Goldman L. Major bleeding in outpatients treated with wafarin: incidence and prediction by factors known at the start of outpatient therapy. Am J Med 1989;87:144–152.
225. Mattle H, Kohler S, Huber P, Rohner M, Steinsiepe KF. Anticoagulation-related intracranial extracerebral haemorrhage. J Neurol Neurosurg Psych 1989;52:829–837.
226. Loeliger EA, van Duk-Weirda CA, van den Besselaar AMHP, Broekmans AW, Roos J. Anticoagulant control and the risk of bleeding. In Meade TW (Ed): Anticoagulants and Myocardial Infarction: A Reappraisal. London, Wiley, 1984;135–177.
227. Bonchek LI. Discussion of Moreno-Cabral RJ, McNamara JJ, Mamiya RT, Brainard SC, Chung GKT. Acute thrombotic obstruction with Bjørk-Shiley valves. J Thorac Cardiovasc Surg 1978;75:321–330.
228. Bjørk VO, Henze A. Encapsulation of the Bjørk-Shiley aortic disc valve prosthesis caused by the lack of anticoagulation treatment. Scand J Thorac Cardiovasc Surg 1973;7:17–20.
229. Gray LA, Fulton RL, Srivastava TN, Flowers NC. Surgical treatment of thrombosed Bjørk-Shiley aortic valve prosthesis. J Thorac Cardiovasc Surg 1976;71:429–432.
230. Wright JO, Hiratzka LF, Brandt B, Doty DB. Thrombosis of the Bjørk-Shiley prosthesis: illustrative cases and review of the literature. J Thorac Cardiovasc Surg 1982;84:138–144.
231. Kontos GJ, Schaff HV, Orszulak TA, Puga FJ, Pluth JR, Danielson GK. Thrombotic obstruction of disc valves: clinical recognition and surgical management. Ann Thorac Surg 1989;48:60–65.

Chapter 2.5

Scintigraphic and Haematological Detection of Thrombosis and Increased Embolic Risk

Jesse E. Adams III and Allan S. Jaffe

Highly accurate, reliable and rapid detection of thrombi and emboli is essential to the proper management of many groups of patients with cardiovascular disease, including those with prosthetic heart valves. Although thromboembolic complications associated with prosthetic valves have decreased in incidence over the past 30 years, life threatening events of this kind still occur with all types of replacement valves[1,2]. Attempts to estimate when thrombus formation begins are problematical, since the time from the onset of thrombus formation to clinical symptoms is highly variable. Depending on the size, location and underlying aetiology of the thrombotic process, patients may present with acute haemodynamic symptoms or a subacute course that persists for weeks or months prior to detection[3,4].

This diversity of presentations has implications for the haematological and scintigraphic detection of thromboembolic complications because the rate of incorporation and/or dissolution of platelets, fibrin and other components decrease with time, modulating the sensitivity of these techniques substantially. Nonetheless, results with these techniques in experimental models and some clinical situations suggest that extending their use to patients with prosthetic valves is possible. These haematological and scintigraphic methods will be reviewed in the light of the sparse data available in patients with prosthetic valves. It must be appreciated that most experimental models in which these techniques have been evaluated use protocols that induce fresh and thus more active thrombi, which are not generally representative of thrombi on a prosthesis or in the left atrium. In addition the animal models employed may have physiology at variance with that of humans. For example, thrombolysis in the dog is accelerated in comparison to man. Accordingly, such approaches will require additional refinement before they become applicable to the detection of thrombi on prosthetic valve surfaces in humans.

Thrombus formation within the heart, if large enough, can be detected by various visualisation techniques, including angiography, computerised tomography scanning and echocardiography (see Chapter 2.6). In addition, various components of the thrombus can be radiolabelled, directly or with the use of antibody probes, and peptides unique to thrombus formation or degradation can be detected in plasma.

THROMBUS FORMATION

Endothelium is normally resistant to thrombosis. This is due to the presence of antiaggregatory and vasodilator prostaglandins, local inhibition of thrombin by thrombomodulin, acting with its endothelial cofactor protein C, and the elaboration of both heparin and plasminogen activators in response to fibrin deposition[5]. Thus, on vascular surfaces the initiation of thrombosis, by platelet adhesion and aggregation, and its subsequent sustainment can only occur at sites of intimal damage or endothelial dysregulation. Intimal damage not only eliminates processes that inhibit thrombosis but also unmasks aggregatory and vasoconstrictor prostaglandins, serotonin, collagen and tissue factor, leading to further platelet aggregation and increased coagulation[6].

Once a platelet plug is formed, the phospholipid portion of the platelet membrane activates coagulation further by serving as a template for the activation of prothrombin with factors V and X[7]. The thrombin generated by prothrombin activation not only stimulates further platelet aggregation but also converts fibrinogen into fibrin. Fibrinogen circulates as two stranded symmetrical half-molecules composed of three polypeptide chains designated alpha, beta and gamma. The half-molecules are joined at the amino terminal ends by disulphide bridges with the chains oriented in an antiparallel manner[8]. The initial action of thrombin on fibrinogen is to cleave fibrinopeptide A (FPA), a 16 amino acid peptide, from each alpha chain and then fibrinopeptide B (FPB), a 14 amino acid peptide, from the beta chain (Fig. 2.5–1). This results in what is known as fibrin monomer, which is then capable of polymerising spontaneously end to end[9]. The morphological alteration produced after the release of FPA and FPB allows the D (peripheral) and E (central) regions of adjacent fibrin monomers to align in an overlapping fashion. The initial interaction of D and E regions on adjacent molecules occurs by noncovalent binding but, in the presence of factor XIII and calcium, lateral covalent crosslinking of fibrin monomers occurs leading to a stable fibrin polymer. The growth of the fibrin matrix occurs in both a linear and a branching

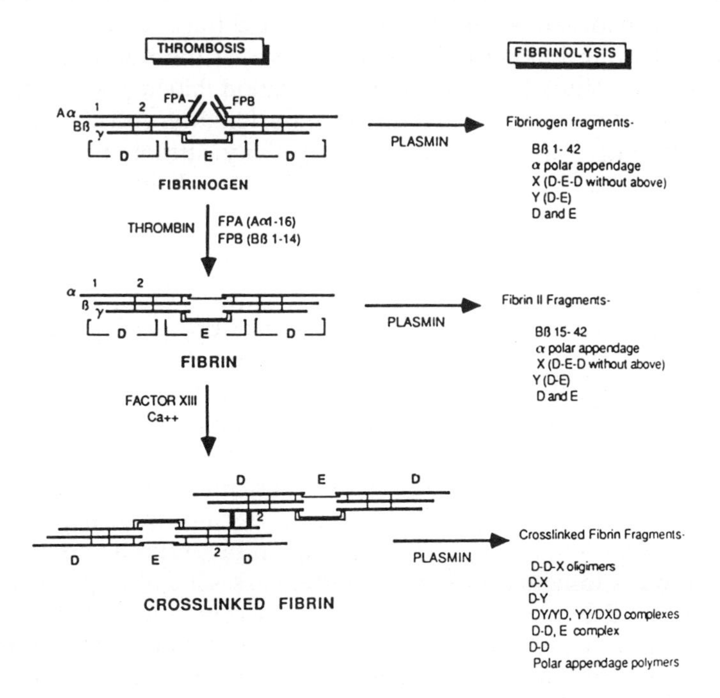

Figure 2.5–1. The origin of thrombin mediated and fibrinolytic fragments. From Jaffe et al[9] with permission.

fashion, forming a three dimensional structure that provides much of the stability of the clot. Subsequently, cross-linking occurs between the alpha chains as well, stabilising the clot still further.

The local plasmin generation results in the hydrolysis of fibrinogen, fibrin monomer and fibrin polymer. Because one of the early sites of plasmin degradation is between amino acid 42 and 43 on the beta chain, plasmin forms a product known as B β 1–42 prior to removal of FPB (the first 14 amino acids on the β chain and β 15–42 thereafter. When plasmin acts on cross-linked fibrin, degradation products are formed that contain cross-linked D-sites (so called D-dimer). An immunoassay using antibodies specific for these D-D sites has been developed[10].

SCINTIGRAPHIC DETECTION OF THROMBOSIS

Many of the components involved in thrombus formation and/or dissolution can be radiolabelled for scintigraphic visualisation. The utility of such approaches depends on the half-life of the component of interest, its ability to retain an appropriate radiolabel and its affinity for thrombus. The efficacy and safety of each technique depend on factors such as the amount of blood required for labelling, radiation dosimetry and the tissue distribution and half-life of the radiopharmaceutical employed. For successful visualisation a radioactivity ratio of at least 2 to 1 between the thrombus and the background blood must be achieved. For this reason tracers that remain in the circulation tend to inhibit imaging whilst those with short plasma half-lives are often more suitable; these include FAB′ monovalent fragments to components of the beta chain of fibrin, antibodies to fragment E1 and radiolabelled tissue plasminogen activator. The blood pool can be labelled with a second tracer and then subtracted to correct for the background blood pool radioactivity[11]. If the tracer of interest binds avidly to thrombus but tends to persist in the circulation, blood pool subtraction may improve sensitivity but the technique is cumbersome, lengthy, and at times technically challenging. Furthermore if an increase in sensitivity attributable to background subtraction is offset in part by a decrease in specificity, overall diagnostic accuracy may be unchanged[12].

Indium-labelled platelets

Indium-labelled platelets are very useful for imaging purposes because platelets are essential to both the initial formation of thrombus and its continued propagation. However the platelet content of thrombi varies considerably, arterial thrombi tending to be much more platelet-rich than venous thrombi. ^{111}Indium is an attractive label[13]. It has a half-life of 2.8 days and its electron capture decay results in the cascade emission of two abundant gamma rays at 173 and 247 KEV. These photons account for 87% of the released energy and are in the range easily detectable by conventional gamma cameras. The long half-life of indium allows multiple scans to be performed over a period of several days without additional dosing, permitting assessment of platelet accumulation and life span and delineation of slower platelet incorporation into thrombi.

Many labelling techniques have been reviewed recently[14,15], but most modern techniques permit nearly normal platelet structure and function to be maintained. In general, indium remains complexed to the platelet with only five to 10 per cent being released into the blood pool after labelling.

The disadvantages of indium-labelled platelet scintigraphy are twofold. Firstly, the sequestration of radioactive platelets in the spleen imposes limits on sequential studies (to avoid excessive splenic radiation) and may hinder visualisation of the inferior aspect of the heart unless special views are obtained. Secondly, labelled platelets remain in the blood pool for a prolonged period, reducing the thrombus-to-background activity ratios essential to proper visualisation of thrombus. This has lead some to advocate background subtraction to optimise sensitivity[11]. Despite these limitations, indium-labelled platelets have been used successfully to identify thrombus formation in many situations, including the left ventricle, the left atrium, the pulmonary and coronary circulations and the surface of prosthetic valves.

Size is not the most important determinant of thrombus visualisation with radiolabelling. Although a larger thrombus is often easier to visualise[16,17], if platelet incorporation is not brisk, there may be insufficient uptake of tracer irrespective of size. Recently formed clots, whether small or large, incorporate new material more rapidly and are thus easier to identify scintigraphically. This is an important issue in patients with prosthetic valves, where thrombus formation is often subacute or chronic and thus more difficult to identify scintigraphically. With ^{111}indium platelet scintigraphy, this difficulty can sometimes be addressed by imaging over a longer period, to compensate for the slower incorporation of platelets. Another difficulty in the detection of prosthetic valve thrombosis is that imposed by the motion of cardiac structures and the larger blood pool which together create greater and more variable background activity.

Since indium-labelled platelets allow thrombus visualisation by incorporating themselves in an active thrombus, there has been concern that anticoagulants might decrease the sensitivity of this approach. Experimentally induced venous thrombi and pulmonary emboli cannot be visualised after heparin administration because of reduced platelet incorporation into the thrombus and thus reduced thrombus/blood ratios of the tracer. This effect can be reversed by protamine[18]. Sulfinpyrazone, aspirin plus dipyridamole and warfarin seem to have similar effects, judging from studies of ^{111}indium-labelled platelet uptake in patients with left ventricular thrombi. In the absence of antithrombotic therapy, left ventricular thrombi were unchanged in size and activity, as assessed by the incorporation of ^{111}indium-labelled platelets. In contrast, patients treated with anticoagulants developed either negative or equivocal scans, even though the size of the thrombus remained constant as assessed by echocardiography. In a study by Stratton and Ritchie, sulfinpyrazone had the most marked effect (in five of seven patients), but aspirin and dipyridamole or warfarin also diminished or extinguished indium uptake in over 50 per cent of patients[19]. Other investigators have reported similar findings[20,21].

Ezekowitz and others compared the diagnostic efficacy of ^{111}indium-labelled platelet scintigraphy with venography for the diagnosis of lower extremity venous thrombosis[20]. Prior to treatment, the sensitivity and specificity of platelet scintigraphy was excellent, 93% and 97% respectively. After treatment with heparin, sensitivity fell to 43% and specificity to 67% due to decreased platelet incorporation. Similarly, Yamada and co-workers found that 10 of 11 patients with left ventricular mural thrombi, treated with warfarin, reverted from positive to negative indium scans within two to six weeks, whereas the thrombi of 8 of 9 patients not treated with warfarin remained scintigraphically detectable. When one patient, whose indium-labelled platelet scan had reverted to negative on treatment, discontinued his medication the scan once again became positive.

Studies directly relevant to patients with prosthetic valves

There have been both experimental and clinical studies evaluating the potential applicability of ^{111}indium platelet scintigraphy for detection of intracardiac thrombi. In a study by Kessler and associates[22], indium-labelled platelets were employed in an attempt to identify a possible cardiac source of emboli in patients with acute cerebrovascular accidents. Ten patients, who had carotid artery disease but no cardiac disease by history or two-dimensional echocardiography, had normal platelet scans. In contrast, 13 of the 27 (48.1%) patients with cardiovascular disease diagnosed clinically or by echocardiography had abnormal scintigrams. Platelet accumulation was detected in the left atrium in three, in the left ventricle in nine and on the aortic valve in one patient. The authors concluded that the use of indium-labelled platelets was a useful diagnostic tool in patients with a presumed cardiac source of emboli, potentially including those with prosthetic valves. These findings are consistent with the reports of others who have been able to demonstrate ventricular as well as atrial thrombi in patients with known cardiovascular disease[19,21–26]. However before attributing an embolus to an identified thrombus within the heart, other possible sources of emboli should be excluded.

The only publication focusing solely on patients with prosthetic valves is that of Acar and associates[27]. They studied 45 prosthetic valves in 41 patients, who had suffered one or more embolic events (mean 2.3) suspected to be secondary to prosthetic valve thrombosis. Only two had evidence of prosthetic valve dysfunction on transthoracic echocardiography. Indium-labelled platelets were injected at a mean of 32 ± 25 days after the last embolic event and images were obtained serially for 5 days. Twenty-four of 41 patients (58.5%) had abnormal accumulation of the tracer at the site of the prosthetic valve. Most developed positive scintigrams by 72 hours, but optimum sensitivity was achieved only at 96 hours, consistent with a relatively indolent process and full anticoagulation. Prosthetic valve thrombosis was documented in ten patients either at surgery or at autopsy. Eight of these thrombi were also demonstrated by the positive ^{111}indium platelet scans. The authors concluded that the indium-labelled platelet scans were useful, especially if transoesophageal echocardiography produced negative or uncertain results.

An understanding of Acar's findings depends in part on experimental studies in animals. Although it would be attractive to think that only thrombosed prosthesis are associated with positive ^{111}indium scintigrams, it appears from experimental work that many prostheses accumulate radiolabelled platelets, at least in the early postoperative period (see also Chapters 2.4, 3.1 and 3.4). DeWangee and co-workers investigated the accumulation of ^{111}indium-labelled platelets in a dog model both immediately and several weeks after prosthetic valve implantation[28–30]. In tissue blocks from five dogs with Bjørk-Shiley valves explanted from the mitral position, indium-labelled platelet deposition was observed on the sewing ring of the prosthesis and on the perivalvular tissue within 24 hours of implantation. In addition, tissue sample analysis showed a significant, two- to threefold increase in platelet deposition in skeletal muscle, kidney and lung, probably due to microemboli despite heparinisation during surgery[28].

In a subsequent study, it was also documented that platelet deposition could be detected in 11 dogs with bovine pericardial bioprostheses in the mitral position, at one, 14 and 20 days after implantation[29]. Again, the sewing ring and perivalvular tissues were the sites of maximum platelet deposition. In decreasing magnitude the muscles, lungs and kidneys of these animals also manifested significant tracer deposition secondary to microemboli. The extent of extracardiac deposition diminished within 30 days, despite the absence of anticoagulation. The administration of dipyridamole did not decrease the sensitivity of scintigraphy, despite the reduction in platelet deposition observed on tissue analysis[30]. Whether treatment with dipyridamole would diminish indium uptake further in anticoagulated patients with prosthetic valves is unclear. Although Dewangee and his coauthors concluded that this technique was a sensitive marker for the detection of platelet deposition on prosthetic valves and might permit evaluation of the effects of antiplatelet drugs, their data also suggest that positive images may occur as part of the 'normal' incorporation process or 'healing' of the sewing ring and adjacent perivalvular tissues (see Chapters 2.4 and 3.4).

Studies potentially relevant to patients with prosthetic valves

In view of the paucity of studies focusing on the detection of thrombus formation on prosthetic heart valves, it may be possible to gain some insights from investigations of the small, platelet-rich thrombi that form in coronary arteries. In this situation also detection is complicated by the substantial background activity within the cardiac chambers. However coronary artery thrombi differ in two important respects. Firstly, they are more acute and turnover is more rapid initially than in many prosthetic valve thrombi. Incorporation of fibrin into coronary thrombus continues for many hours[31,32] and it is likely but unproven that platelet incorporation occurs at a similar rate. Secondly, spontaneous lysis probably occurs with greater frequency in coronary arteries than on prosthetic valves. Nonetheless, some of the principles established in this area are likely to lead to insights into the issues related to detection of prosthetic valve thrombi as well.

Studies employing ^{111}indium-labelled platelets to detect coronary artery thrombi have been performed in both animal models and in humans. In dogs with extensive coronary thrombi induced by electrical trauma, ^{111}indium-labelled platelets administered 30–60 minutes after thrombus formation localised in the occluded artery and were easily detected externally. In four dogs in which labelled platelets were injected 22 hours after thrombus formation, detectable platelet accumulation did not occur despite the presence of thrombus confirmed at autopsy. There were no false-positive results in dogs after 'sham' surgery. Thus the rapid early turnover of coronary artery thrombi allowed clear visualisation with labelled platelets, but as thrombus turnover diminished, accumulation in the thrombus could no longer be distinguished from that in the blood pool over short imaging intervals[33].

These considerations led Fox[11] and Bergmann[34] and their co-workers to employ ^{99m}technetium labelled red cells to permit subtraction of blood pool activity, in the hope of increasing the sensitivity of identification of coronary thrombi. With this technique, blood pool radioactivity was estimated by measurement of ^{99m}technetium red cell activity in the carotid artery. The relation between ^{99m}Tc and ^{111}indium activity was determined to subtract blood pool activity within the heart. Any excess ^{111}indium activity remaining was attributed to uptake in the thrombus rather than in the blood pool itself. In an initial animal study, it was possible with this modified technique to identify rapidly and accurately acute coronary thrombi and their dissolution with intracoronary streptokinase[33]. In a subsequent, clinical study of 24 patients, nine of whom had suffered acute myocardial infarction, distinct foci of indium-labelled platelet accumulation in the acute ischaemic zones were documented with the aid of blood pool subtraction, despite the fact that all patients received low dose subcutaneous heparin. ^{111}Indium was injected as soon as possible after admission. Images were positive in seven of eight patients at the time of the early scan (mean = 5.6 ± 3.3 hours) and in eight of nine patients during subsequent imaging (mean = 23.6 ± 1.9 hours). Only one of fifteen control patients without coronary thrombi demonstrated a cardiac focus of tracer accumulation which represented either a false-positive or an occult thrombus. Whether, as reported by others, more false-positive results will occur with this method of blood pool subtraction is unclear.

In six patients undergoing coronary angioplasty, ^{111}indium platelet scintigraphy failed to detect platelet deposition at the site of the angioplasty, perhaps because of anticoagulation[35]. It would be of interest to know whether blood pool subtraction could improve these results.

Conclusions regarding the use of ^{111}indium labelled platelets for the diagnosis of prosthetic valve thrombosis must be viewed as preliminary. With blood pool subtraction, there is hope that sensitivity may improve sufficiently that detection may be possible even in anticoagulated patients. However this technique is likely to remain inferior to transoesophageal echocardiography (Chapter 2.6) for three reasons: (a) detection of 'chronic' thrombus requires 2 – 4 days, (b) splenic radiation dose is substantial and (c) scintigraphy is more expensive than echocardiography. Nevertheless the technique may have value in some research applications to quantitate platelet deposition on prosthetic surfaces and in other viscera.

Monoclonal antibodies

Many receptors are expressed on the surface of platelets. Recently, monoclonal antibodies directed against these receptors have been developed. Those employed thus far for imaging have been directed against the IIb/IIIa glycoprotein receptor (the platelet fibrinogen receptor) or against proteins expressed on the platelet surface after degranulation. The former have been designated 50H.19, 7E3 and P256 and the latter S–12, W–40, and anti-PADGEM. Som and associates used 50H.19 labelled with ^{99m}technetium to label peripheral, pulmonary and right ventricular thrombi in dogs. Fibrin rich, recently formed thrombi were visualised successfully by two to three hours after injection of the radioligand[36]. Similar results have been reported with 7E3[37], an antibody which has been used to block the platelet fibrinogen receptor in vivo.

In studies with the ^{111}indium-labelled FAB′ fragment of P256, thrombi induced in the veins of mice were detected at one and 48 hours in all animals. In a clinical study, the same labelled fragment was used successfully to diagnose postoperative deep vein thrombosis and pulmonary embolism after hip replacement[28]. Sensitivity was modest in those patients who were not receiving anticoagulants. So far, this technique has not been evaluated for the detection of intracardiac thrombosis.

The glycoproteins expressed on the cell surface of platelets following degranulation have also served as an epitope for scintigraphy with labelled monoclonal antibodies. In unstimulated platelets, GMP 140 is located in the alpha-granule membrane. With activation, it is expressed on the plasma cell membrane[39]. Monoclonal antibodies (S–12 and W–40) are directed against unique epitopes on GMP 140[40] and it appears that the anti-PADGEM antibodies (antibodies against Platelet Activation-Dependent Granule-External-Membrane protein) are also directed at GMP 140. Because they are directed towards this activation-specific protein, antibodies have a high specificity for binding to activated platelets and thus can be used to image vascular thrombi and sites of vascular injury. FAB′ S12 labelled with ^{99m}technetium manifests significant injured-to-normal tissue activity ratios in rabbits after aortic injury, suggesting that it may be valuable for the imaging of platelet rich thrombi[41]. Anti-PADGEM labelled with ^{123}iodine has been used to image deep vein thrombi in baboons and to follow the decrease in thrombus size in response to streptokinase[42]. The detection of intracardiac thrombus with these agents has not been reported as yet.

Fibrin directed thrombus detection

The fibrin component of thrombus can be used for labelling also. There are multiple sites involved in the formation, stabilisation and/or dissolution of clots which can provide for the binding of an appropriately labelled radioligand. Although these techniques have not been investigated for detection of thrombosis on prosthetic valves, they appear potentially useful in this application.

Fibrinogen labelled with iodine or gallium and ^{99m}technetium has been employed in the past for thrombus imaging and to determine the rate of thrombus formation and/or dissolution. Radiolabelled fibrinogen is taken up briskly immediately after thrombus formation and continues to be incorporated into coronary artery thrombi for up to 72 hours in experimental studies, indicating the dynamic balance between formation and dissolution in such thrombi[31,32]. Although the rate of incorporation may vary depending upon the type of thrombus formed (platelet rich or fibrin rich) and its site, remodelling and the prolonged time course of thrombus turnover are common to most thrombi. Therefore, labelled fibrinogen and/or its products may be capable of detecting thrombi for prolonged periods of time. Fibrinogen labelled with ^{131}iodine permits detection of intracardiac thrombi in both dogs and humans, although in general this technique appears less promising for this application than imaging with ^{111}indium platelets[43,44]. Kaufman and associates reported that ^{131}I fibrinogen is not as sensitive as labelled platelets for the detection of fresh thrombi in a model of thrombosis induced by carotid arterial injury[44]. This lack of sensitivity combined with technical issues related to fibrinogen labelling have reduced the enthusiasm for iodine labelled fibrinogen imaging. Although perhaps a better label, ^{123}I is quite expensive. Its usefulness has been demonstrated in the detection of deep venous thrombosis, where diagnostic accuracy was 90%, although most patients required imaging at 24 hours for proper identification of thrombus. False-negative results were sometimes obtained in patients treated with heparin[45].

Recently there has been a resurgence of interest in imaging with fibrinogen. ^{67}Gallium can be complexed with deferoxamine (DFO), a bi-directional metal chelating agent[14,46]. Incorporation of the water soluble polymer dialdehyde starch (DAS) between the gallium and DFO improves stability and clotability. This combination has been used to visualise deep venous thrombi[39]. The technique properly identified 10 of

15 patients (10 of 17 studies) with suspected deep venous thrombosis and 2 of 9 pulmonary emboli documented by ventilation/perfusion scans.

Antibodies, in many instances monoclonal, to components of fibrin are now being utilised increasingly for visualisation of thrombi and are much more promising than the older techniques with fibrinogen. Most studies have used radiolabelling with ^{111}indium or ^{99m}technetium. Both tracers are efficient radiolabels for venous thrombi, although thrombus/blood and thrombus/muscle ratios tend to be higher with ^{99m}technetium[48]. Two types of monoclonal antibodies have been used for imaging: (a) those specific for epitopes on the beta chain of fibrin but not fibrinogen (that is, after the first 14 amino acids of the beta chain (FPB), have been removed by the action of thrombin) and (b) antibodies to neoepitopes in the D region after cross-linked fibrin is proteolysed by plasmin.

These antibodies do not cross-react with fibrinogen or other components of the thrombus and have been configured either as whole antibodies, as FAB or as FAB′ monovalent fragments. Monovalent FAB′ fragments may prove preferable since they avoid the platelet activation that can occur with large immunoglobulins. They are also cleared more rapidly from the blood stream, resulting in decreased background radioactivity, earlier visualisation and possibly improved sensitivity. In binding studies in vitro, antibodies specific for the amino terminus of the beta chain of fibrin labelled with ^{125}I, have been shown to accumulate and permit visualisation of human thrombi in rabbit jugular veins[49]. The sensitivity of this approach with the beta chain antibody has been confirmed by imaging residual left anterior coronary artery thrombi after reperfusion in dogs given intracoronary injections of labelled monoclonal antibody[50]

However, heparin reduces not only thrombus size but also the binding of most fibrin monoclonal antibodies. In dogs, this effect is greater on platelet antibodies directed at the platelet fibrinogen receptor than on the beta chain antifibrin antibody[51], but effects may vary with different antifibrin antibodies. The fibrin-specific monoclonal antibody that binds to an epitope somewhere on the 15 to 21 region of the amino terminus of the beta chain (GC4) has been employed for the detection of venous thrombi in dogs, as has a monoclonal antibody to a neoepitope in the D region of fibrin exposed by the action of plasmin (T2GIs)[52]. Binding of the D specific antibody to three hour thrombi was less than with the beta chain antibody, but it was greater in three day old thrombi. Thus, it appears that the sensitivity of scintigraphic detection with these antibodies may depend on the age of the thrombus.

Surprisingly, relative binding of the beta chain antibody is enhanced by heparin, in contrast to the binding of almost all other antifibrin monoclonal antibodies, antiplatelet monoclonal antibodies and indium labelled antibodies[52]. Fragment E (see below) appears to be the only other peptide whose binding is accentuated by heparin. The mechanism for this augmentation is currently unknown but could be the result of protection of the epitope from being covered with more thrombus, so called 'blanketing'. The D region antibody FAB′ fragment also has been employed to image fresh thrombi in dogs two to four hours after injection of indium labelled material[53]. These results are comparable to those using other beta chain FAB′ fragments in both rabbits and dogs. Some acute thrombi can be visualised at four hours, but some require up to 24 hours after injection[54].

There are sparse clinical data in patients. Alavi and others studied 31 patients with

^{111}indium labelled beta chain FAB′ fragments and compared the results with those of contrast venography. Antibody thrombus imaging was highly sensitive for the detection of venous thrombi in the lower extremities. However, as in animal studies, there was a lower detection rate in 16 patients concomitantly receiving heparin[55]. Other fibrin-specific imaging modalities are currently under investigation. Radiolabelled tissue plasminogen activator (t-PA) has a high specificity for fibrin (in distinction to urokinase and streptokinase) and has been used successfully to visualise deep vein thrombi in rabbits[56]. Radiolabelled t-PA was found to be equal to radiolabelled fibrinogen for thrombus detection, but required significantly less time (1/50) because of its very short half-life in blood (67 seconds). Fragment E, which is produced by plasmin digestion of cross linked fibrin, binds to fibrin dimers and polymers but not to fibrin or fibrin monomers[14]. Its rapid clearance from blood may allow improved detection of thrombi. Furthermore, heparin does not decrease binding of fragment E to thrombus but may enhance blood clearance, theoretically further improving thrombus detection. Unfortunately, fragment E requires laborious preparation and appears to bind only transiently to thrombus.

Thus, both antifibrin and antiplatelet monoclonal antibodies can be used for thrombus imaging. At present, neither have been investigated for visualisation of prosthetic valve thrombosis, but both methods have the potential to identify thrombus in this situation accurately in an acceptably short period of time. Whether they will require subtraction of blood pool activity for optimum sensitivity remains unclear.

HAEMATOLOGICAL DETECTION OF THROMBOSIS

Routine measurements of coagulation factors and fibrinogen are of no value in the detection of thrombus whilst measurements of platelet activity such as platelet factor 4 (PF4) and beta thromboglobulin (BTG) are excessively sensitive and indiscriminative, being influenced by intramuscular injections, catheter insertions, therapeutic interventions and thrombus formation in parts of the body other than the area of interest[57]. To some extent this problem is common to all haematological markers of thrombosis. However, some newer techniques may provide improved sensitivity and specificity.

The method for measurement of human FPA was developed by Nossel and associates[58]. This small, 16 amino acid peptide is a sensitive and specific marker of thrombin activity. The assay for FPA requires acquisition of samples with atraumatic venipuncture and strict quality control to avoid confounding thrombin activation. Furthermore, unless an assay for the carboxy terminal portion of the molecule is used, fibrinogen and other fibrinogen fragments that contain FPA must be removed before assay[9]. In addition, some minor fragments such as elastase and plasmin-derived short alpha chain fragments can account for a small percentage of FPA immunoreactivity[59]. Nonetheless, the method is sensitive enough to detect thrombus in patients with acute myocardial infarction for example[60]. In patients admitted early after acute transmural myocardial infarction, presumably with fresh thrombi, FPA was elevated to 55.5 ± 14.7 ng/ml (normal less than 2.0 ng/ml). If, as suggested by Nossel, 4ng/ml FPA are elaborated in plasma from the breakdown of 1 mg fibrinogen, and given the three to five minute half-life of FPA, marked elevations must be indicative of very marked thrombin activity and continuing incorporation of fibrin into thrombi[58]. Ten hours after infarction, FPA falls to 4.9 ± 1.9 ng/ml indicating reduced thrombus turnover and reduced fibrin deposition.

These data are consistent with those of others in patients with acute infarction[61] and patients with venous and arterial thrombi[62,63]. It is of interest that these patients with marked elevations of FPA and acute infarction had little evidence of spontaneous fibrinolysis, as assessed by the infrequent and modest elevations of D-dimer. Only patients with severe complications of infarction, indicating either more extensive thrombosis or the involvement of other noncardiac vascular beds, manifested substantial elevations of D-dimer[64].

Assay of FPA has been used in the evaluation of patients with prosthetic valves. Pengo and associates assessed FPA levels in 38 patients with mechanical and 20 patients with bioprosthetic heart valves[65]. The level of FPA in their control population composed of healthy subjects was found to be 1.02 ng/ml, using an amino terminal assay. The mean level of FPA in anticoagulated patients with bioprosthetic valves was 1.41 ng/ml; higher than the control group but statistically not significantly different ($p=0.08$ – Fig. 2.5–2). The mean FPA level in patients with mechanical valves (mainly first generation tilting disc valves) was significantly higher than controls (1.82 ng/ml – $p<0.01$). As expected, those with lower intensity anticoagulation had the highest levels of FPA. Among the five patients with previous thromboembolic complications, FPA levels were significantly elevated at 2.65 ng/ml in those with 'adequate' anticoagulation as assessed by prothrombin time, and slightly higher at 2.74 ng/ml in those who were

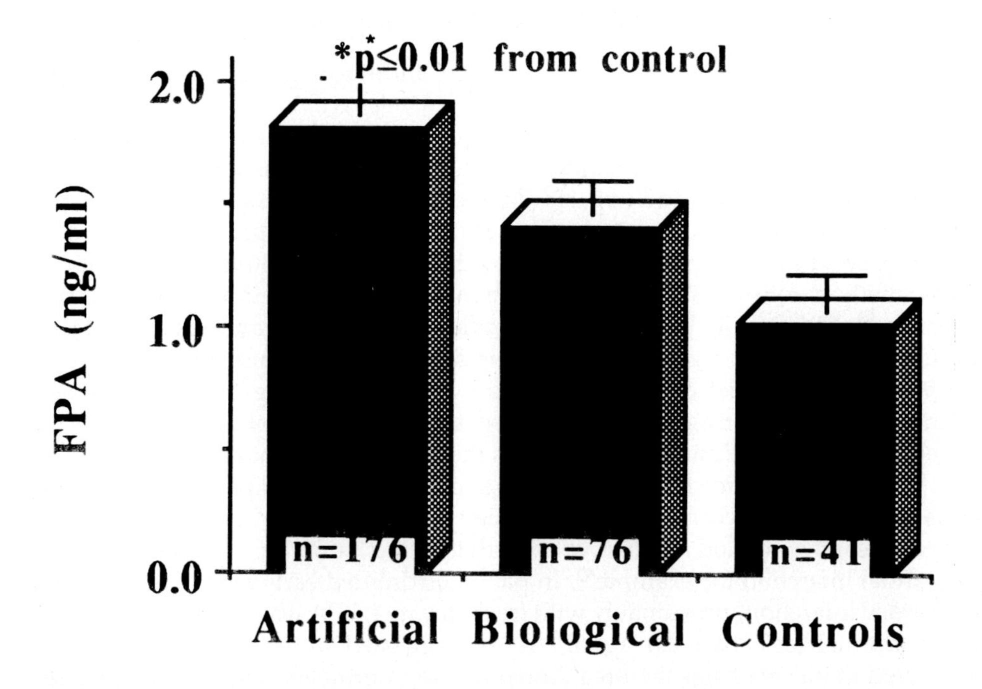

Figure 2.5–2. FPA levels in patients with mechanical and biological prosthetic valves as compared with control. From Pengo et al[65] with permission.

'underanticoagulated'. However, the predictive value of FPA for thromboembolism was not investigated.

These data suggest that prosthetic surfaces induce thrombin activity, and that this activity is greater with some mechanical valves than it is with bioprostheses. The authors concluded that, if normalisation of FPA is taken as the therapeutic endpoint, mechanical heart valves may require a higher level of anticoagulation than is often prescribed. However, the implication that regulation of FPA in this manner would reduce thromboembolic complications remains unconfirmed (see also Chapter 3.4). It is possible that the increased values in patients with such complications are the result of thrombus formation, rather than an indication of baseline thrombogenicity.

Unfortunately, levels of FPA are elevated in many situations associated with blood clotting or tissue destruction, and this reduces its potential for investigating specific groups of patients. In a study by Feinberg and associates, FPA was found to be markedly elevated in acute stroke, requiring a month to return to normal[66]. Despite evidence of thrombosis, markers of fibrinolysis such as D-dimer were only mildly elevated in these patients, indicating a relative paucity of intrinsic fibrinolysis. The B beta-fibrinopeptides were also normal in all patients throughout the study[66]. FPA levels have also been found to be elevated in pulmonary embolism[67] and atrial fibrillation[68].

Heparin potentiates the action of antithrombin III at least one hundredfold in antagonising the action of thrombin. When the genesis of thrombin activity takes place intravascularly and antithrombin III is present in adequate amounts, the administration of heparin should result in a prompt decline of FPA due to its short half-life in plasma. This is the response to heparin administration in acute myocardial infarction[61]. However, some patients require very high doses, suggesting that heparin, in some circumstances, may not be an ideal thrombin inhibitor. This has led to the investigation of other thrombin inhibitors such as hirudin[69].

Until recently, FPA was the only available in vivo marker with which to assess thrombin activity. In the late 1970s an assay for the F1.2 fragment of prothrombin was developed and published by Lau and co-workers[70]. It measures a fragment removed by activation of prothrombin by the prothrombinase complex and is thus an indirect measure of factor X activation and activity. Since prothrombin activity results in thrombin activation, it is also an indirect measure of thrombin activity. Additional validation is required to establish the extent to which changes in this marker parallel those of FPA. For example, do spurious elevations due to in vitro artefacts occur as easily as with FPA, and do processes other than Factor X activation (e.g., the action of plasmin) induce elevations directly? Once these questions are answered, F1.2 measurement may in future augment our ability to identify thrombosis in vivo.

Another approach is the development of antibodies to thrombin-antithrombin III complexes. Preliminary data appear similar to those with FPA, but these complexes are unlikely to be as sensitive as FPA to in vitro artefacts and they have a long half-life in plasma[71]. Unfortunately, at present the assay for these complexes is based on separate antibodies to thrombin and antithrombin III, rather than specific antibodies to the complex itself.

Crosslinked fibrin degradation products (XL-FDP), also known as D-dimer are markers of fibrinolysis. Since the presence of fibrinolysis implies intravascular thrombosis, the presence of fibrinolytic activity has been used as marker of thrombosis.

All markers of fibrinolysis are apt to be less sensitive than more direct measures of thrombosis since some thrombotic processes are associated with impaired fibrinolysis (e.g., acute infarction and stroke). In addition, many assay configurations use a specific antibody as a capture for D-dimer but a less specific antibody as a tag. It has been shown that in the presence of marked fibrinogenolysis, material that cross-reacts with the non-specific tag can be captured with cross-linked material, resulting in spurious increases[72]. Several monoclonal antibodies, specific for the gamma-gamma cross-link site on fibrin have been employed in clinical studies. In one study ninety-six percent of patients with ventilation/perfusion scans highly suggestive of pulmonary embolism also had high concentrations of XL-FDPs and there was a direct correlation between the probability of pulmonary embolism as assessed by ventilation/perfusion scans and the extent of elevation of XL-FDPs. However, 43% of patients with normal or low probability scans also had elevations of XL-FDPs, probably due to blood clotting and fibrinolysis associated with their underlying illness[73]. Similar results in pulmonary embolism have been reported by others[74]. In experimental animals, thrombi have been successfully demonstrated using D dimer radiolabelled with ^{131}I[75].

β 15–42 is another marker of the dissolution of fibrin after FPB has been removed. Since the 42/43 bond is a common early site for the action of plasmin on fibrin, β 15–42 should be a sensitive marker for fibrinolysis and thus indirectly of thrombosis. It is elevated physiologically after exercise and during pregnancy and pathologically in patients with malignancy, pancreatitis, and liver disease. In thrombotic disorders levels are raised in pulmonary embolism, deep venous thrombosis, arterial embolism and disseminated intravascular coagulation. A further rise is seen after administration of heparin and thrombolytic therapy. As a marker, at present it appears less sensitive than D-dimer[9]. It is, however, of use in evaluating the relative extent of fibrin dissolution compared to fibrinogen dissolution in vivo. In 28 patients treated with streptokinase for acute myocardial infarction, the effect of streptokinase on fibrinogen predominated early, but over time fibrinolysis became more extensive and fibrinogen degradation less apparent, perhaps due to fibrinogen depletion[76].

Although further studies are required, these assays are exciting new techniques for the diagnosis of thrombosis. Their applicability to the detection of increased thrombotic and embolic risk in patients with prosthetic valves remains to be determined.

DETECTION OF EMBOLISM

Although some thrombi and emboli may have catastrophic consequences, others may be difficult to detect. If only sudden neurological events and symptomatic occlusions of visceral and peripheral arteries are considered, the overall incidence of systemic embolism is likely to be grossly under-estimated, since many small emboli are clinically silent (Chapters 1.2 and 1 .3). Visceral and skeletal muscle microemboli have been identified in the early postoperative period in animals with prosthetic mitral valves using radioactive labelling of platelets[28–30]. Although sensitive and very useful for quantitation of microemboli in animals, this technique has not yet been used clinically.

Microangiography has been used for the diagnosis of retinal embolism. Unfortunately, there are no published data specific to prosthetic valves. In most studies fluorescein has been used as the contrast agent although some have used indocyanine green. Since indocyanine green is more tightly bound to protein, it does not leak into the choroid and retina to the same extent as fluorescein[77]. In retinal microangiography, visualisation depends on the fluorescent nature of the dye when it comes into contact with specific wavelengths of light. Extravasation of dye presumably reflects disruption of microvascular integrity and is more likely to occur with small molecules not tightly bound to larger proteins. Arruga and associates investigated 70 patients with retinal embolism, and found that cholesterol and fibrin-platelet emboli were commoner than calcific emboli. They hypothesised that the former probably originated from carotid atheroma, while the latter probably had a cardiac source[78]. Younge noted that calcific retinal emboli usually came from diseased native heart valves, whereas emboli composed of synthetic materials were infrequent and originated from disintegrating prosthetic valves[79].

Retinal emboli that affect vision are associated with a significantly decreased life expectancy because of the likelihood of severe underlying heart disease[80]. No controlled studies of retinal microangiography have been undertaken in asymptomatic patients with prosthetic valves in an attempt to quantify microembolism. Indeed such studies may be difficult to accomplish because of the short lifespan of retinal emboli.

Recently, microemboli have been detected in some patients with prosthetic aortic valves using transcranial Doppler to 'observe' the middle cerebral artery for periods up to one hour. The significance of these microemboli remains uncertain but preliminary data suggest that the presence of very frequent microemboli may be associated with an increased risk of larger symptomatic emboli[81] (see also Chapter 2.4 for further discussion of this phenomenon).

REFERENCES

1. Forbes CD, Prentice CRM. Thrombus formation and artificial surfaces. Br Med Bull 1978;34:201–207.
2. Grunkemeier GL, Rahimtoola S. Artificial heart valves. Annu Rev Med 1990;41:251–263.
3. Kontos GJ, Schaff HV, Orszulak TA, Puga FJ, Pluth JR, Danielson GK. Thrombotic obstruction of disc valves: Clinical recognition and surgical management. Ann Thor Surg 1989;48:60–65.
4. Wright JO, Hiratzka LF, Brandt B, Doty DB. Thrombosis of the Bjørk-Shiley prosthesis. J Thorac Cardiovas Surg 1982;84:138–144.
5. Adams PC, Badimon JJ, Badimon L, Chesebro JH, Fuster V. Role of platelets in atherogenesis: Relevance to coronary arterial restenosis after angioplasty. In Mehta JL (Ed.): Thrombosis and Platelets in Myocardial Ischemia. Philadelphia, F.A. Davis Company, 1987;49–71.
6. Tracy PB. The role of endothelium in the expression of procoagulant activity. Coron Art Dis 1991;2:146–151.
7. Walsh PN, Schmaier AH. Platelet-coagulant protein interactions. In Colman RW, Hirsh J, Marder VJ, Salzman EW (Eds.): Hemostasis and Thrombosis. Philadelphia, JB Lippincott Company, 1987;689–709.
8. Mosesson MW. Fibrin polymerization and its regulatory role in haemostasis. J Lab Clin Med 1990;116:8–17.
9. Jaffe AS, Eisenberg PR, Wilner GD. In vivo assessment of thrombosis and fibrinolysis during acute myocardial infarction. In Brown EB (Ed.): Progress in Hematology. Orlando, Grune and Stratton, 1987:71–89.
10. Rylatt DB, Blake AS, Cottis LE, et al. An immunoassay for human D dimer using monoclonal antibodies. Thromb Res 1983;31:767–778.
11. Fox KAA, Bergmann SR, Mathias CJ, et al. Scintigraphic detection of coronary artery thrombi in patients with acute myocardial infarction. J Am Coll Cardiol 1984;4(5):975–986.
12. Machac J, Vallabhajosula S, Goldman ME, et al. Value of blood-pool subtraction in cardiac indium–111-labelled platelet imaging. J Nuc Med 1989;30:1445–1455.
13. Thakur ML, Welch MJ, Joist JH, Coleman RE. Indium–111 labelled platelets: Studies on preparation and evaluation of in vitro and in vivo functions. Throm Res 1976;9:345–357.

14. Knight LC. Radiopharmaceuticals for thrombus detection. Semin Nucl Med 1990;20:52–67.
15. DeWangee MK. Methods of assessment of thrombosis in vivo. Ann N Y Acad Sci 1987;516:541–571.
16. Ezekowitz MD, Wilson DA, Smith EO, et al. Comparison of indium–111 platelet scintigraphy and two-dimensional echocardiography in the diagnosis of left ventricular thrombi. N Eng J Med 1982;306:1509–1513.
17. Seabold J, Bruch P, Ponto J, et al. Sensitivity and specificity of In–111 platelet scintigraphy and two-dimensional echocardiography for detection of left ventricular thrombi: clot size threshold. J Am Coll Cardiol 1985;5:389(abstract).
18. Moser KM, Spragg RG, Bender F, Konopka R, Hartman MT, Fedullo P. Study of factors that may condition scintigraphic detection of venous thrombi and pulmonary emboli with indium–111-labelled platelets. J Nucl Med 1980;21:1051–1058.
19. Stratton JR, Ritchie JL. The effects of antithrombotic drugs in patients with left ventricular thrombi: Assessment with indium–111 platelet imaging and two-dimensional echocardiography. Circulation 1984;69:561–568.
20. Ezekowitz MD, Pope CF, Sostman HD, et al. Indium–111 platelet scintigraphy for the diagnosis of acute venous thrombosis. Circulation 1986;73:668–674.
21. Yamada M, Onishi K, Fukunami M, et al. Assessment of warfarin therapy under full dose using indium–111 platelet scintigraphy in patients with intracardiac thrombi. Jpn Circ J 1988;52:1357–1364.
22. Kessler C, Henningsen H, Reuther R, Kimming B, Rösch M. Identification of intracardiac thrombi in stroke patients with indium–111 platelet scintigraphy. Stroke 1987;18:63–67.
23. Vandenberg BF, Seabold JE, Conrad GR, et al. 111 In-Labelled platelet scintigraphy and two-dimensional echocardiography for detection of left atrial appendage thrombi. Circulation 1988;78:1040–1046.
24. Stratton JR, Ritchie JL. 111 In platelet imaging of left ventricular thrombi. Circulation 1990;81:1182–1189.
25. Bellotti P, Claudiani PBF, Chiarella F, et al. Activity of left ventricular thrombi of different ages. Assessment with indium-oxine platelet imaging and cross-sectional echocardiography. Eur Heart J 1987;8:855–860.
26. Yamada M, Hoki N, Ishikawa K, et al. Detection of left atrial thrombi in man using indium–111 labelled autologous platelets. Br Heart J 1984;51:298–305.
27. Acar J, Vahanian A, Dorent R, et al. Detection of prosthetic valve thrombosis using indium–111 platelet imaging. Eur Heart J 1990;11:389–398.
28. DeWangee MK, Kaye MP, Fuster V, Rao SA. Noninvasive radioisotope technique for detection of platelet deposition in mitral valve prosthesis and renal microembolism in dogs. Trans Am Soc Artif Intern Organs 1980;26:475–480.
29. DeWangee MK, Trastsek VF, Tago M, Kaye M. Radioisotope techniques for noninvasive detection in bovine-tissue mitral-valve prostheses and in vitro quantification of visceral microembolism in dogs. Invest Radiol 1984;19:535–542.
30. DeWangee MK, Fuster V, Rao SA, Forshaw PL, Kaye MP. Noninvasive radioisotope technique for detection of platelet deposition in mitral valve prostheses and quantification of visceral microembolism in dogs. Mayo Clin Proc 1984;58:307–314.
31. Moschos C, Oldewurtel HA, Haider B, Regan TJ. Effect of coronary thrombus age on fibrinogen uptake. Circulation 1976;54:653–656.
32. Salami A, Oliver C, Lee J, Sherman L. Continued incorporation of circulating radiolabelled fibrinogen into preformed coronary thrombi. Circulation 1977;56:213–217.
33. Riba AL, Thakur ML, Gottshalk A, Zaret BL. Imaging experimental coronary artery thrombosis with Indium–111 platelets. Circulation 1979;60:767–775.
34. Bergmann SR, Lerch RA, Mathias CJ, Sobel BE, Welch MJ. Noninvasive detection of coronary thrombi in In–111 platelets: Concise communication. J Nucl Med 1983;24:130–135.
35. Callahan RJ, Bunting RW, Block PC, Boucher CA, McKusick KA, Strauss HW. Evaluation of platelet deposition at the site of coronary angioplasty using indium–111 labelled platelets. J Nucl Med 1983;24:60(abstract).
36. Som P, Oster ZH, Zamora PO, et al. Radioimmunoimaging of experimental thrombi in dogs using technetium-^{99m}-labelled monoclonal antibody fragments reactive to human platelets. J Nucl Med 1986;27:1315–1320.
37. Oster ZH, Som P. Editorial: Of monoclonal antibodies and thrombus-specific imaging. J Nucl Med 1990;31:1055–1058.
38. Stuttle AWJ, Klosok J, Peters AM, Lavender JP. Sequential imaging of post-operative thrombus using the In–111-labelled platelet-specific monoclonal antibody P256. Br J Radiol 1989;62:963–969.
39. Stenberg PE, McEver RP, Shuman MA, Jacques YV, Bainton DF. A platelet alpha-granule membrane protein (GMP–140) is expressed on the plasma membrane after activation. J Cell Biol 1985;101:880–886.

40. McEver RP, Martin MN. A monoclonal antibody to a membrane glycoprotein binds only to activated platelets. J Biol Chem 1984;259:9799–9804.
41. Miller DD, Boulet A, Garcia O, et al. Technetium-^{99m} monoclonal S–12 antibody imaging of in vivo platelet activation after balloon arterial injury in an experimental atherosclerotic model. J Nucl Med 1989;30:787(abstract).
42. Palabrica T, Konstam MA, Furie BC, et al. Localization of venous thrombi with anti-PADGEM antibodies specific for activated platelets. Circulation 1987;76(Suppl IV):202(abstract).
43. Frisbie JH, Tow DE, Sasahara AA, Barsamian EM, Parisi AF. Noninvasive detection of intracardiac thrombosis. Circulation 1976;53:988–991.
44. Kaufmann HH, Woo J, Anderson JH, Cannon DC, Handel SF, Hevezi JM. Radioiodinated fibrinogen for clot detection in a canine model of cervical carotid thrombosis. J Nucl Med 1978;19;370–376.
45. DeNardo GL, DeNardo SJ, Carretta RF, et al. Correlation of bioscintigraphy, contrast venography, and iodine–125 fibrinogen uptake test. Clin Nucl Med. 1985;10:880–883.
46. Ohmomo Y, Yokoyama A, Suzuki J, et al. Ga–67-labelled human fibrinogen: A promising new imaging agent. Eur J Nucl Med 1982;7:458–461.
47. Yamamoto K, Senda M, Fujita T, et al. Positive imaging of venous thrombi and thromboemboli with Ga–67 DFO-DAS-fibrinogen. Eur J Nucl Med 1988;14:60–64.
48. Knight LC, Maurer AH, Ammar IA, Epps LA, Dean RT, Berger HJ. Comparison of Tc-^{99m} and In-^{111} labelled antifibrin antibodies in a thrombus model. J Nucl Med 1988;29:746(abstract).
49. Liau C, Haber E, Matsueda GR. Evaluation of monoclonal antifibrin antibodies by their binding to human blood clots. Thromb Haemostas 1987;57:49–54.
50. Kanke M, Yasuda T, Matsueda G, et al. Detection of residual coronary thrombi ater reperfusion of experimental myocardial infarction using In–111 labelled monoclonal antifibrin antibody. J Nucl Med 1988;27:910(abstract).
51. Saito T, Powers J, Nossiff ND, et al. Radioimmunoimaging of experimental thrombi in dogs using monoclonal antifibrin (AF) and antiplatelet (AP) antibodies: Effect of heparin on uptake by pulmonary emboli (PE) and venous thrombi (VT). J Nucl Med 1988;29:825(abstract).
52. Rosebrough SF, McAfee JG, Grossman ZD, et al. Thrombus imaging: A comparison of radiolabelled GC4 and T2G1s fibrin-specific monoclonal antibodies. J Nucl Med 1990;31:1048–1054.
53. Knight LC, Maurer AH, Ammar IA, et al. Tc–99m antifibrin Fab' fragments for imaging venous thrombi: evaluation in a canine model. Radiology 1989;173:163–169.
54. Knight LC, Maurer AH, Ammar IA, Shealy DJ, Mattis JA. Evaluation of Indium–111-labelled anti-fibrin antibody for imaging vascular thrombi. J Nucl Med 1988;29:494–502.
55. Alavi A, Gupta N, Berger H, Palevsky H, Jatlow A, Kelley M. Detection of venous thrombosis with In–111 labelled antifibrin (59D8) antibody imaging. J Nucl Med 1988;29:825(abstract).
56. Orlandi C, Austin ML, Blaser CB, Morser J, Thoolen MJ, Liberatore FA. Rapid clot uptake of radiolabelled tissue plasminogen activator (tPA) in an animal model of deep vein thrombosis. J Nucl Med 1989;30:787(abstract).
57. Jaffe AS, Lee RG, Perez JE, Geltman EM, Wilner GD, Sobel BE. Lack of elevation of platelet factor IV in plasma from patients with myocardial infarction. J Am Coll Cardiol 1984;4:653–659.
58. Nossel HL, Yudelman I, Canfield RE, et al. Measurement of fibrinopeptide A in human blood. J Clin Invest 1974;54:43–53.
59. Eisenberg PR, Sherman L, Rich M, et al. Importance of continued activation of thrombin reflected by fibrinopeptide A to the efficacy of thrombolysis. J Am Coll Cardiol 1986;7:1255–1262.
60. Eisenberg PR, Sherman LA, Schectman K, Perez J, Sobel BE, Jaffe AS. Fibrinopeptide A: a marker of acute coronary thrombosis. Circulation 1985;71:912–918.
61. Mombelli G, Im Hof V, Haeberli A, Straub PW. Effect of heparin on plasma fibrinopeptide A in patients with acute myocardial infarction. Circulation 1984;69:684–689.
62. Yudelman IM, Nossel HL, Kaplan KL, Hirsh J. Plasma fibrinopeptide A levels in symptomatic venous thromboembolism. Blood 1978;51:1189–1195.
63. Nossel HL, Butler VP, Canfield RE, Yudelman I, Kalliope-Spanondis MT, Soand T. Potential use of fibrinopeptide A measurement in the diagnosis and management of thrombosis. Thromb Diathes Haemorrh. 1975;33:426–434.
64. Eisenberg PR, Sherman LA, Perez J, Jaffe AS. Relationship between elevated plasma levels of crosslinked fibrin degradation products (XL-FDP) and the clinical presentation of patients with myocardial infarction. Thromb Res 1987;46:109–120.
65. Pengo V, Peruzzi P, Baca M, et al. The optimal therapeutic range for oral anticoagulant treatment as suggested by fibrinopeptide A (FPA) levels in patients with heart valve prostheses. Eur J Clin Invest 1989;19:181–184.
66. Feinberg WM, Bruck DC, Ring ME, Corrigan JJ. Haemostatic markers in acute stroke. Stroke 1989;20:592–597.

67. Yudelman I. Indices of fibrinogen proteolysis and platelet activation during the resolution of pulmonary embolism. Thromb Haemost 1987;57:11–16.
68. Uno M, Tsuji H, Sawada S, Toyoda T, Nakagawa M. Fibrinopeptide A (FPA) levels in atrial fibrillation and the effects of heparin administration. Jpn Circ J 1988;52:9–12.
69. Markwardt F, Nowak G, Sturzebecher J, Vogel G. Clinico-pharmacological studies with recombinant hirudin. Thromb Res 1988;52:393–400.
70. Lau HK, Rosenberg JS, Beeler DL, Rosenberg RD. The isolation and characterization of a specific antibody population directed against the prothrombin activation fragments F2 and F1+2. J Biol Chem 1979;254:8751–8761.
71. Gulba DC, Barthels M, Reil G, Moller W, Jost S, Lichten PR. Thrombin antithrombin III complex: a sensitive and specific predictor for early reocclusion after thrombolysis for myocardial infarction. Circulation 1988;78(suppl II):130(abstract).
72. Eisenberg PR, Jaffe AS, Stumpt DC, Collen D, Bovill EG. Validity of enyzme-linked immunosorbent assays of cross-linked fibrin degradation products as a measure of clot lysis. Circulation 1990;82:1159–1168.
73. Rowbotham BJ, Egerton-Vernon J, Whitaker AN, Elms MJ, Bunce IH. Plasma cross linked fibrin degradation products in pulmonary embolism. Thorax 1990;45:684–687.
74. Goldhaber SZ, Vaughan DE, Tumeh SS, Loscalzo J. Utility of cross-linked fibrin degradation products in the diagnosis of pulmonary embolism. Am Heart J 1988;116:505–508.
75. Walker KZ, Khafgi F, Bautovich GJ, Boniface GR, Bundesen PG, Rylatt DB. Anti-fibrin monoclonal antibodies for radioimmunodetection: Preliminary assessment in a rat model. Thromb Res 1988;52:269–278.
76. Eisenberg PR, Sherman LA, Jaffe AS. Differentiation of fibrinolysis from fibrinogenolysis with Bβ 1–42 and Bβ 15–42. Circulation 1986;74 (Suppl II):245.
77. McDonnell PJ, Flower R, Green R. Platelet-fibrin embolism in a rhesus macaque: Angiographic and pathologic studies comparing fluorescein and indocyanine green. Am J Vet Res 1983;44:1385–1391.
78. Arruga J, Sanders M. Ophthalmologic findings in 70 patients with evidence of retinal embolism. Ophthalmology 1982;89:1336–1347.
79. Younge BR. The significance of retinal emboli. J Clin Neurol Ophthalmol 1989;9:190–194.
80. Howard RS, Russell RWR. Prognosis of patients with retinal embolism. J Neurol Neuorosurg Psych 1987;50:1142–1147.
81. Berger M, Davis D, Lolley D, Rams J, Spencer M. Detection of subclinical microemboli in patients with prosthetic aortic valves. J Cardiovasc Technol 1991;9:282–283.

Chapter 2.6

Ultrasonic Detection of Increased Embolic Risk

Alan G. Fraser

Echocardiography is now a very powerful tool for detecting intracardiac sources of emboli. The incorporation of more ultrasonic elements into standard commercially-available transducers has produced better lateral resolution. New echocardiographic approaches and in particular transoesophageal echocardiography which images the heart with a reduced depth of field, have allowed higher ultrasonic frequencies to be used, resulting in better axial resolution. Thus, most cardiac ultrasound systems can be used to identify masses $\geqslant$ 2 mm in diameter, and with transoesophageal imaging masses $\geqslant$ 1 mm may be detected. The ultrasonic diagnosis of the type of tissue constituting a mass is more problematical, and to a large extent still depends on the clinical context and associated abnormalities. In future, however, it is possible that the use of tissue characterisation to study the pattern of backscattered ultrasonic signals returning from solid structures may facilitate the differentiation of fresh or old thrombus from vegetation or pannus.

In patients with valve disease and suspected emboli, the present range of echocardiographic approaches and techniques allows very full investigation of possible sources within the heart. In the past, a major problem for studying patients with prosthetic valves or annular rings was that these foreign bodies masked all onward transmission of ultrasound. Precordial echocardiography allows only one aspect of a prosthetic aortic or mitral valve to be imaged, but any prosthetic valve should be studied by at least two ultrasonic approaches. The development of transoesophageal echocardiography has overcome this problem, so it is now an invaluable and essential investigation in all patients with suspected dysfunction of a prosthetic valve.

Many of the echocardiographic indicators of increased embolic risk apply equally to patients with disease of native valves, and those with prosthetic valves. They will, therefore, be considered together. Ultrasonic techniques can also be used in the operating theatre to reduce the risk of perioperative embolism, and these applications will be reviewed first.

INTRAOPERATIVE STUDIES

Intracardiac thrombus

If there is loosely attached thrombus within one of the cardiac chambers, it may be dislodged by handling the heart. If this occurs prior to aortic cross-clamping while the heart is still ejecting, embolism may result. In patients with mitral valve disease, thrombus within the left atrium may be identified by intraoperative transoesophageal or epicardial echocardiography during pre-bypass imaging of the mitral valve to assess its suitability for a reconstruction procedure. Transoesophageal echocardiography is also useful for excluding atrial thrombus in patients being considered for balloon mitral valvotomy as an alternative to surgery; thrombus in the left atrium or the left atrial appendage is a contraindication to balloon valvotomy, because of the risk of embolism[1].

In patients undergoing left ventricular aneurysmectomy, or operative removal of mural thrombus from the site of an extensive infarct in the left ventricle, thrombus can be identified by epicardial echocardiography with the ultrasonic transducer in a sterile bag placed directly on the surface of the beating heart. This information may assist the surgeon in selecting a safe site for ventriculotomy, in order to reduce the risk of dislodging or breaking up the thrombus before it is removed (see fig. 2.6–4).

Aortic atheroma

In patients with extensive atherosclerosis of the ascending aorta, atheromatous material or overlying thrombus may be dislodged from the wall of the aorta during cardiac surgery, at the time of cannulation or aortic cross-clamping. Obviously, this may result in perioperative cerebral embolism. In order to reduce this risk by selecting a site which is free from significant atheroma, some surgeons now perform epivascular ultrasound studies[2,3]. The ascending aorta can be imaged either before or after pericardiotomy, with a probe placed directly over the right ventricular outflow tract and then on the ascending aorta to scan in successive short-axis planes. In addition, when the transducer is placed on the right side of the ascending aorta and directed towards the left shoulder, the ascending aorta and arch can be displayed in their long axis.

In one study of 50 patients, the echocardiographic prevalence of severe atheroma in the ascending aorta was 58%[2]; in comparison, visual inspection and palpation identified atherosclerosis in only 24%. As a result these authors modified their surgical approach in 24% of patients[2,3]. However, definite proof that this technique can reduce perioperative neurological complications of cardiopulmonary bypass is awaited.

Air embolism

Ultrasonic imaging is a very sensitive technique for detecting air retained in the cardiac chambers or trapped between trabeculae within the heart after cardiopulmonary bypass[4]. Epicardial echocardiography can therefore be used to ensure that adequate de-airing has been performed. The echoes produced by microbubbles of air are relatively large and often sparsely distributed, and they appear dissimilar from the pattern produced by spontaneous echocardiographic contrast (see below). As well as arising within the left atrium or ventricle, they may be seen entering the left atrium from the pulmonary veins immediately after bypass in many patients who have had an uncomplicated procedure. In one series of 79 patients undergoing cardiopulmonary bypass for a variety of indications, microbubbles were observed within the left ventricle in 49%[5]. The clinical significance of these echoes is not known. It has been suggested that they may be a cause of multiple small emboli, but in a study of 34 patients with a 41% incidence of microbubbles, there was no correlation between echocardiographic abnormalities and the development of encephalopathy after bypass surgery[6].

Fat embolism

Intraoperative transoesophageal echocardiography has been used during orthopaedic surgery, to monitor the occurrence or absence of fat embolism. During procedures which increase intramedullary pressure within long bones, such as drilling of a femur before inserting a nail, intramedullary fat or marrow may be released into the circulation. The resulting systemic venous emboli can be detected as they pass to the pulmonary circulation, if flow within the right atrium and right ventricle is monitored using a transoesophageal probe[7]. The phenomenon may account for peri-operative 'fat' embolism to the lungs, or paradoxical embolism if the pressures in the right atrium and ventricle are (or become) elevated in a patient who has a patent oval foramen. Observations from intraoperative monitoring may lead orthopaedic surgeons to modify their operative techniques in order to reduce post-operative morbidity, for example by drilling 'escape' holes into the shaft of the femur to prevent excessive rises in intramedullary pressure.

SOURCES OF EMBOLISM OR INCREASED EMBOLIC RISK

Using echocardiography it is possible with considerable confidence to identify a wide variety of sources of thromboembolism, and other abnormalities which have been associated in clinical studies with increased risk of embolism. Intracardiac sources of non-thrombotic emboli such as tumours or vegetations can also be demonstrated. The most common conditions and risk factors are listed in Table 2.6–1; less frequent causes have been reviewed elsewhere[8,9].

Table 2.6–1
Causes of systemic embolism or increased embolic risk which are identifiable with echocardiography

thrombus in left atrium
thrombus in left atrial appendage
thrombus in left ventricle or left ventricular aneurysm
atrial septal aneurysm
patent oval foramen (paradoxical embolism)
spontaneous echocardiographic contrast in left atrium
abnormal mechanical function of left atrial appendage
enlarged left atrium
calcified mitral annulus
rheumatic mitral stenosis
mitral valve prolapse
calcific aortic stenosis
prosthetic mitral or aortic valve
pannus or thrombus on prosthetic valve or sewing ring
intracardiac tumour (especially myxoma)
papillary tumour (fibroelastoma)
infective endocarditis (vegetations on native or prosthetic valve)
atheromatous plaques and/or thrombus in the thoracic aorta

Patent foramen ovale

From a study of 965 autopsies, the prevalence of patent foramen ovale within a normal population was estimated to be 30%[10]. Such 'probe patent' oval fossa defects may overestimate the clinical incidence of patency *in vivo*, however, since contrast echocardiographic studies in 176 adults in two series suggested a patent foramen ovale in only 8.5%[11,12]. Nonetheless, a significant proportion of adults will shunt from right to left across a patent foramen ovale when the filling pressure of the right heart is elevated. The commonest physiological cause of this event is during the Valsalva manoeuvre, for example when straining. Transient reversed flow may also occur in normal subjects as a phasic phenomenon during each cardiac cycle[13]. In pathological conditions, right-to-left shunting has been shown to occur after acute right ventricular infarction[14]. It may also occur soon after cardiac surgery in patients who have significant heart failure or right ventricular dysfunction, or chronic respiratory disease, and it may be exacerbated by ventilation with positive end-expiratory pressure. Acutely, these factors may be associated with paradoxical embolism in patients who develop venous thrombosis due to immobility. Chronically, the conditions for paradoxical embolism may persist in patients who have persistently elevated filling pressures of the right heart, for example if pulmonary hypertension fails to improve while filling pressures of the left heart fall after mitral valve replacement. Such a risk could be avoided by routine suturing of the atrial septum in any patient with a patent foramen ovale. If the problem is suspected before cardiac surgery in a patient who is unlikely to have an atriotomy with inspection of the atrial septum, then the integrity of the septum can be checked beforehand by non-invasive investigations. Obviously, such tests should also be performed routinely in any patient who is being investigated for a potential source of systemic embolism.

The diagnosis of a patent foramen ovale is made best by echocardiography. It is difficult to study the atrial septum in detail from the precordium, but the thin septum primum in the oval fossa may be shown from a subxiphoid approach[15]. In adults, the flap of the oval fossa is seen well only on transoesophageal echocardiography. Since the potential communication runs from an inferior position on the right side of the atrial septum, to a superior one on the left side, this is seen best using a biplane or multiplane transoesophageal probe imaging in the longitudinal axis. In horizontal planes superior to the limbus of the septum secundum, a fluid-filled space may be seen within the atrial septum between its primum and secundum components. Colour flow mapping may show flow within this space, but usually the diagnosis of a patent foramen ovale can be confirmed only by using colour flow mapping[16] or contrast echocardiography[11] during a manoeuvre designed to increase the right atrial pressure temporarily. Opacification of the superior vena cava and right atrium is achieved by injecting a bolus of echocardiographic contrast material rapidly into a peripheral vein in the upper limbs. Agents which can be used include sonicated radiological contrast media, echocardiographic contrast media[17], and hand-agitated saline containing microbubbles of air. The patient is instructed to perform a Valsalva manoeuvre when the contrast is injected, and to release the intrathoracic pressure while the right atrium is opacified. The appearance of more than 3–5 bubbles within the left heart within 2–3 beats confirms the presence of a patent foramen. The diagnosis can be made using either transthoracic[18] or transoesophageal imaging (Fig. 2.6–1).

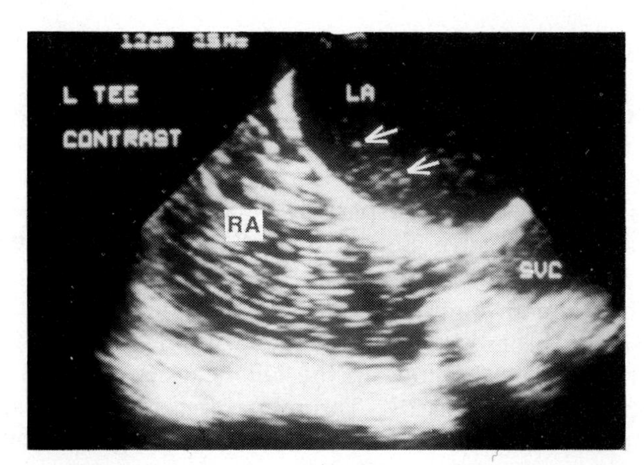

Fig. 2.6–1: Cross-sectional image in the longitudinal axis obtained during transoesophageal echocardiography in a patient with a suspected patent oval foramen. The superior vena cava (SVC) and the right atrium (RA) are opacified by echocardiographic contrast, and during the Valsalva manoeuvre a few bubbles (arrow) are observed within the left atrium (LA), confirming the diagnosis and raising the possibility of paradoxical embolism.

These diagnostic techniques are used by anaesthetists in patients undergoing neurosurgery, in whom there is a risk of air embolism into the venous circulation during craniotomy; in the presence of a patent foramen ovale, this venous air may reach the cerebral arterial circulation. A patient at particular risk can be identified by (intraoperative) transoesophageal studies[19], and the operative approach can then be modified. Similar techniques are used to identify divers who may be at risk of paradoxical gas embolism if they develop decompression sickness[20]. In a study of young patients with stroke, Lechat and co-authors found a patent foramen ovale but no other cardiac abnormality or potential explanation for systemic embolism in 40%, compared with an incidence of patent foramen ovale of 10% in controls[12]. Cases of paradoxical coronary arterial embolism have also been described[21].

In patients with heart valve disease but no history suggestive of embolism, the clinical significance of a patent foramen ovale is uncertain. For example, it is not known if routine surgical closure of a patent foramen would be advisable in a patient having an isolated aortic valve replacement, when the atrium would not normally be opened. Since patency of the foramen ovale is so common in a healthy population, it has been estimated that it might be a purely coincidental finding in one third of all young adults with an unexplained stroke[9].

Intracardiac thrombus

Echocardiography can usually differentiate between normal blood which is sonolucent, and intracavitary thrombus which reflects ultrasound back to the transducer. Possible exceptions are fibrin clot which may be almost sonolucent[22], and very recent thrombus, but in one experimental study thrombus was detected by echocardiography within 45–180 minutes of ligating a coronary artery and injecting a sclerosing agent subendocardially[23]. Chronic laminar thrombus may be distinguished since it is relatively echo-dense and may contain regions of calcification. Nonetheless, when using echocardiography it may be difficult and sometimes impossible to determine whether a small mobile mass is composed of thrombus or other tissue such as a vegetation.

The appearances of *large* thrombi within the left atrium are very specific and may be shown from the precordium using cross-sectional imaging in up to 99% of cases[24]), but transthoracic imaging is relatively insensitive for detecting *small* or flat atrial thrombi, which are easily missed[25], especially in patients with marked atrial enlargement or a prosthetic mitral valve. Sensitivities of between 38% and 61% have been reported[24,26–28].

In patients with rheumatic mitral valve disease, and in others with atrial fibrillation, the commonest site of thrombus within the left atrium is the appendage. In autopsy studies of mitral stenosis, thrombus in the left heart is confined to the left atrial appendage in about 50% of cases[29]. Thrombus at this site is usually missed on transthoracic echocardiography[24,30], but with transoesophageal echocardiography the appendage can be imaged in almost all patients and thrombus can be detected with very high sensitivity and specificity[25,31]. Thus a transoesophageal study should be performed in all patients in whom there is strong clinical suspicion of embolism but

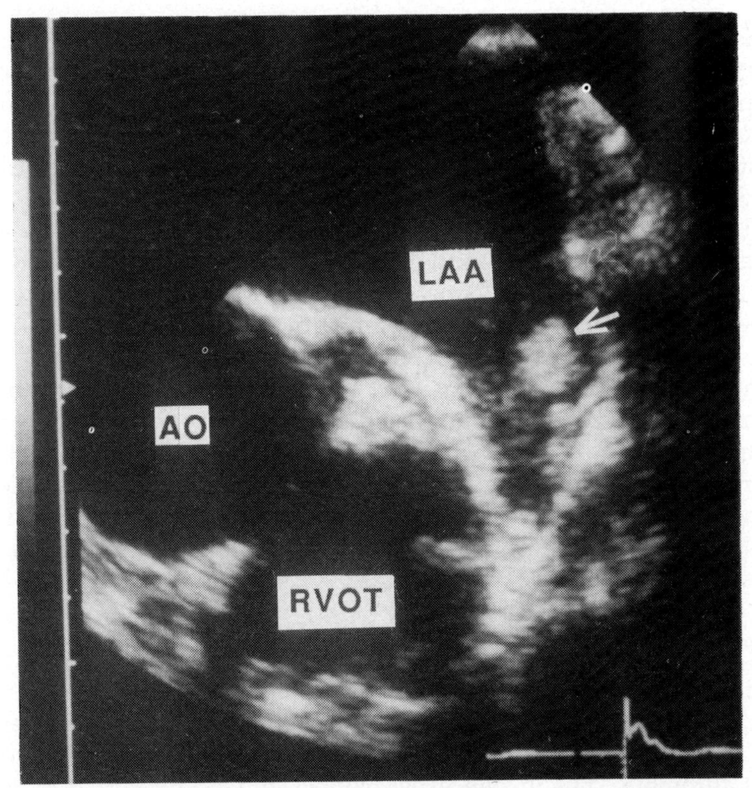

Fig. 2.6–2: Transverse transoesophageal image demonstrating a thrombus (arrow) in the left atrial appendage (LAA). There is associated spontaneous echocardiographic contrast at the tip of the appendage, indicating stagnant flow. AO = proximal ascending aorta (at level of the origin of the left main coronary artery, which can be seen between the aorta and the left atrial appendage); RVOT = right ventricular outflow tract, just proximal to the pulmonary valve.

transthoracic echocardiography is normal, especially if there are risk factors for a cardiogenic source of embolism such as atrial fibrillation. It is impossible to 'exclude' (as much as this can ever be done) a cardiac source of embolism without undertaking such a study. The outline of a normal left atrial appendage is indented by the pectinate muscles, but thrombus is usually distinguished without difficulty as a large filling defect within the cavity of the appendage (Fig. 2.6–2). If the left atrium is very large, the appendage may be shown better in the longitudinal axis, using a biplane probe. A single plane (transverse) transducer may also miss laminar thrombus applied to the roof or the floor of the left atrium (Fig. 2.6–3).

A rare but dramatic cause of thromboembolism from the left atrium is ball thrombus. The echocardiographic features are instantly recognisable and almost always apparent on precordial imaging[32]. Early surgery is mandatory in affected patients because the risk of embolism is particularly high; up to 54% in the cases reviewed by Schechter[33]. Another unusual cause of thromboembolism can occur in patients after cardiac transplantation, in whom transoesophageal echocardiography may demonstrate thrombus at the site of the atrial suture line[34]. Recently, it has been suggested that highly mobile filamentous strands on the mitral valve may be a source of embolism[35].

Precordial echocardiography is particularly useful for detecting left ventricular thrombus, which occurs most frequently at the site of an anterior infarction, in a left ventricular aneurysm[36], or at the apex. The sensitivity of transthoracic imaging for

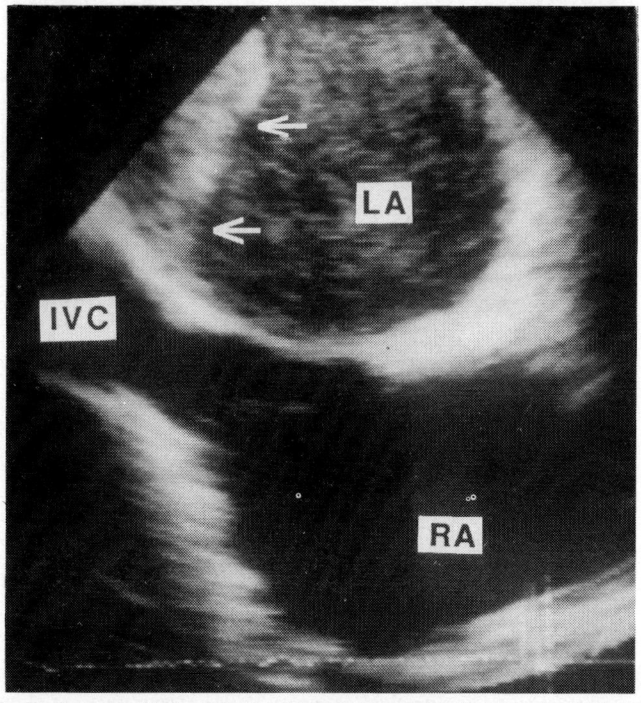

Fig. 2.6–3: Longitudinal image obtained during biplane transoesophageal echocardiography in a patient with rheumatic mitral stenosis. There is dense echo contrast within the left atrium (LA) and a laminar thrombus (arrows) adherent to the floor of the atrium. This was not apparent on imaging in transverse planes, which failed to reveal that percutaneous valvotomy was contraindicated because of the risk of embolism. RA = right atrium; IVC = inferior vena cava.

detecting thrombus at these sites is about 90%[37–39], while these regions are demonstrated rather poorly or not at all on transoesophageal echocardiography[25]. When diagnostic images cannot be obtained from the precordium, a transoesophageal probe can be used to study the ventricles in transgastric imaging planes, but the study may be incomplete even when a biplane probe is used.

Ventricular thrombus usually arises on an akinetic scar related to previous myocardial infarction, but it can also occur at the left ventricular apex in patients with a dilated left ventricle and low cardiac output, or at the site of an apical vent after cardiac surgery. The characteristics of a left ventricular thrombus should be studied carefully, since its appearance correlates with the risk of embolism. For example, Visser and associates reported an embolic rate of 88% in patients whose thrombus protruded into the cavity of the left ventricle (compared with 18% in patients with 'flat' thrombi), and

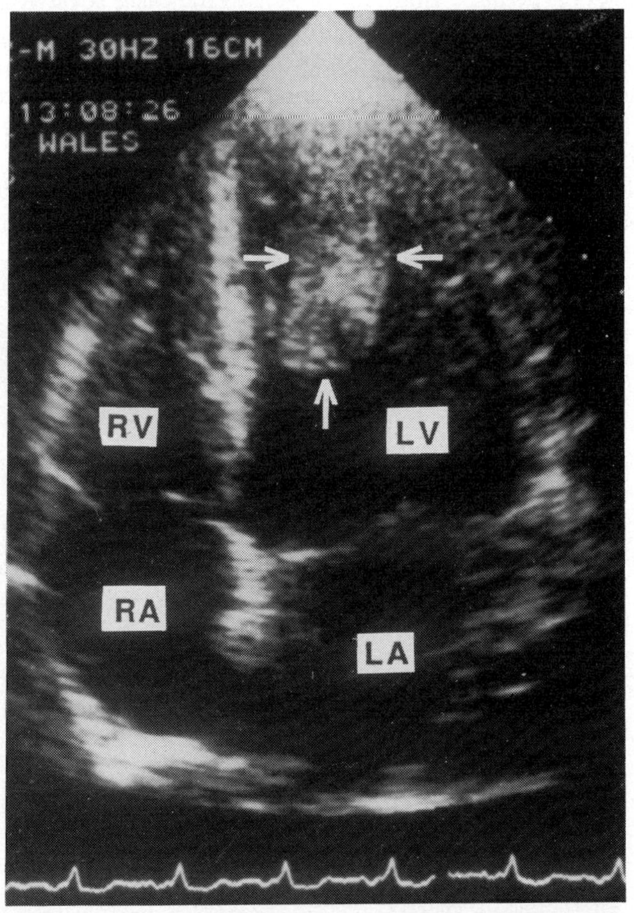

Fig. 2.6–4: Transthoracic apical four-chamber image in a patient who suffered two separate embolic events (to the mesenteric and cerebral circulations) following an acute anterior myocardial infarction. There is a large pedunculated thrombus (arrows) within the left ventricle, adherent to the site of the infarct at the apex. It was subsequently removed at open heart surgery, using epicardial echocardiography to select the site of the left ventriculotomy. RV = right ventricle; LV = left ventricle; RA = right atrium; LA = left atrium.

a rate of 58% when the thrombus was mobile (compared with 3% when it was immobile)[40]. An example of a protruding and mobile thrombus is shown in Fig. 2.6–4. Rare causes of left ventricular thrombus causing embolism, which can be identified by echocardiography, include thrombosis on a ruptured false tendon[41].

In patients with suspected pulmonary embolism, transthoracic echocardiography may show thrombus within the right atrium or ventricle. Thrombus in the main pulmonary artery or within a major pulmonary artery can be identified on transoesophageal echocardiography[42], or by intravascular ultrasonic imaging[43]. Recently, there have been several reports of paradoxical embolism confirmed by echocardiography, for example by demonstrating thrombus straddling the atrial septum.

Thrombosis of prosthetic valves

In most patients with thrombosis of a prosthetic valve, symptoms of impaired haemodynamic performance will predominate. Thus, suspicion of valve thrombosis as a possible source of systemic emboli will be reinforced strongly by coincidental symptoms suggesting obstruction, especially if the history of heart failure is acute (see also Chapters 2.4 and 5.1). Conventional transthoracic Doppler studies can demonstrate significant obstruction of a prosthetic valve if the velocity of flow across the valve is substantially increased compared with previous reference values for the same valve in that patient. Using the modified Bernoulli equation, the estimated pressure drop across the valve can be estimated from the peak velocity, or alternatively the effective orifice area of the valve can be calculated using either the Holen-Hatle or

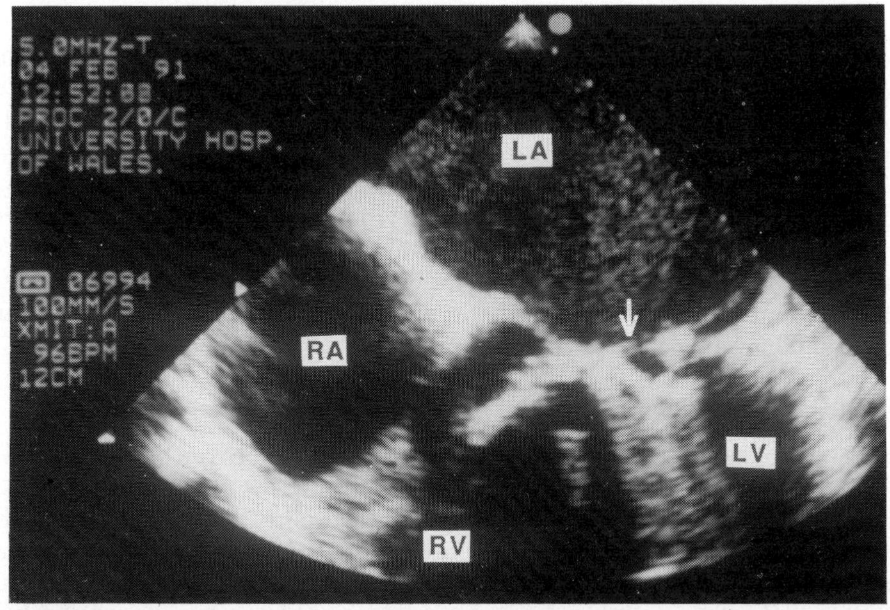

Fig. 2.6–5: Transoesophageal four-chamber image in a patient with a prosthetic mitral valve who presented with cerebral embolism. Although the valve was not obstructed, thrombus was observed on the posterior surfaces of the sewing ring and disc, and within the orifices of the valve (arrow). This is difficult to demonstrate on a still-frame, since the masses were very mobile. There is also spontaneous echo contrast within the left atrium. Abbreviations as in Fig. 2.6–4.

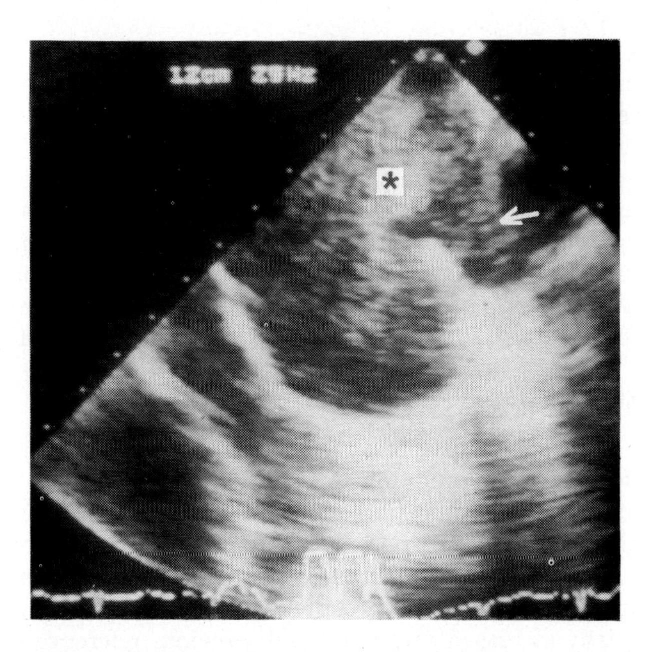

Fig. 2.6–6: Spontaneous echocardiographic contrast within the left atrium, seen during a transoesophageal study. Blood entering the atrium from the left upper pulmonary vein (arrow) is relatively sonolucent and causes a swirling pattern of the contrast (asterisk) within the atrium, so that it appears to radiate from the infolded wall of the atrium between the orifices of the vein and the left atrial appendage. Doppler studies in this patient showed low velocities of flow at the junction of the appendage with the left atrium.

the continuity equation. In patients presenting with heart failure, a thrombus may be extremely large and yet still not apparent from the precordium. As discussed more fully in Chapter 5.1, transoesophageal echocardiography should therefore be performed in any patient with suspected embolism and a prosthetic valve. Embolism may also occur from valve thrombosis which is not causing obstruction (Fig. 2.6–5), and from thrombus on an annular ring in a patient who has undergone mitral valve repair even when this is the only prosthetic material which has been inserted. Transoesophageal imaging is so detailed that individual sutures can be seen, but these are readily differentiated from thrombus because of their multiple number, their regularly spaced locations around the sewing ring, and their lack of mobility.

Spontaneous echocardiographic contrast

Sometimes blood itself may be echogenic. Particulate echoes can be identified within a cardiac chamber or large blood vessel, moving like wisps of smoke in a constantly changing pattern of swirls and eddies which is determined by the currents of blood flow (Fig. 2.6–6). This phenomenon has been called spontaneous echocardiographic contrast, and it is most likely to be observed when high ultrasonic frequencies are used. Thus, it is rarely seen in adults when imaging the heart from the precordium, but not infrequently identified during transoesophageal echocardiography[44,45] which uses higher frequencies (usually $\geq$ 5MHz). The 'spontaneous' echoes are not caused by high gain settings of the ultrasound machine, although they may be missed if the gain settings are low.

Table 2.6–2
Anatomical sites and conditions associated with spontaneous echocardiographic contrast

LEFT ATRIUM (including left atrial appendage) in
- atrial fibrillation
- mitral stenosis
- mitral valve replacement
- during balloon mitral valvotomy

LEFT ATRIAL APPENDAGE (as the only site) in
- atrial fibrillation
- isolated electromechanical dissociation ('standstill' of LAA)

LEFT VENTRICLE in
- anterior infarction (at apex)
- left ventricular aneurysm
- grossly enlarged and hypokinetic heart
- during balloon aortic valvotomy

AORTA in
- aortic aneurysm
- enlarged aorta with extensive atheroma or reduced cardiac output
- aortic dissection (usually in false lumen)
- systemic cooling on cardiopulmonary bypass

CORONARY ARTERIES in
- Kawasaki's disease

SYSTEMIC VEINS in
- venous disease (e.g. varicose veins)
- circumstances of reduced velocity of flow (e.g. SVC during a Valsalva manoeuvre, IVC in constrictive pericarditis)

RIGHT ATRIUM in
- rheumatic tricuspid stenosis
- obstructed prosthetic tricuspid valve
- Fontan circulation (especially if RA-PA conduit is obstructed)

LAA left atrial appendage, RA right atrium, PA pulmonary artery, SVC superior vena cava, IVC inferior vena cava

Since the original description in 1975[46], spontaneous echocardiographic contrast has been observed in most parts of the circulation including those sites listed in Table 2.6–2. It is found most frequently within the left atrium or the left atrial appendage, especially in patients with mitral valve disease or a mitral prosthesis[47–50]. It is particularly common in patients who have atrial fibrillation and an enlarged atrium, but it can also occur in those who are in sinus rhythm[44,45]. It may be seen within the right atrium, for example in tricuspid stenosis or when there is abnormal flow after a Fontan procedure[51] (see also Chapter 4.2). It can occur within the left ventricle in dilated cardiomyopathy or myocardial infarction[52], or it may be localised in a left ventricular aneurysm; it is most likely to be observed at the apex where the pattern may reveal stagnating flow[53]. Spontaneous echocardiographic contrast may also be seen within a dilated, aneurysmal or atherosclerotic aorta[54] and in the false lumen of an aortic dissection[55]. It is identified as a normal phenomenon within systemic veins[56], particularly when flow is slow or almost stationary[57]. It has been observed entering the inferior vena cava from the hepatic vein[58], and even in aneurysmal coronary arteries in a patient with Kawasaki's disease[59]. The circumstances common to all these situations are reduced or low velocities of flow, usually within enlarged cavities.

The mechanism(s) and precise pathophysiological significance of spontaneous echocardiographic contrast have not yet been determined. There may be several different causes. As already mentioned, the echoes seen in the hearts of patients after cardiopulmonary bypass are probably caused by air. It was suggested originally that spontaneous contrast might also be caused by bubbles, produced by microcavitation in the vicinity of a high velocity jet, by the release of oxygen from haemolysed red cells, or by the absorption of gas from the bowel[58], but these hypotheses have not been substantiated. In patients with typical spontaneous echocardiographic contrast, the echo 'particles' are smaller and more numerous than those occurring after bypass surgery, and it is likely that they are caused by aggregates of red blood cells and/or platelets. Echo contrast is found *in vitro* in citrated blood in proportion to its haematocrit when it is left to stand, and it is abolished by agitating the blood[22]. This pattern is exaggerated in blood taken from patients with myeloma, who have increased numbers of rouleaux of red blood cells, and it is reduced after lysis of the red cells[60]. *In vivo*, spontaneous contrast in the ventricle clears on ectopic or mechanical stimulation and during the infusion of dopamine[52], and it is related inversely to the velocity of flow[61]. In one patient, echo contrast in the inferior vena cava disappeared after pericardiectomy[62]. All these observations point to aggregates of red cells as the predominant cause of spontaneous echo contrast. However, echo contrast is also demonstrable *in vitro* in platelet rich plasma in proportion to the size of the platelet aggregates[56], and spontaneous contrast has been induced experimentally *in vivo* by injecting adenosine diphosphate as a platelet aggregating agent[63]. Wolverson and associates reported that washed red cells were less echogenic than whole blood[57], so it may be that both red cells and platelets contribute to the presence of echo contrast.

Whatever the explanation for spontaneous contrast, it must account for very localised and also very rapid and transient appearances of the phenomenon. For example, it may be restricted to the immediate environs of an atrial septal aneurysm. It arises within the left atrium almost immediately after the mitral orifice is occluded during balloon valvotomy, again suggesting a relationship to slow or stagnating flow. It may also be seen within the aorta as a patient is cooled during cardiopulmonary bypass. It is possible to speculate that regions of low shear stress between the circulating blood and adjacent vascular endothelium lead to reduced EDRF (endothelial derived relaxant factor, the endogenous source of nitric oxide) activity, thereby allowing increased aggregation (see also Chapter 1.3). It is now appreciated that nitric oxide is also released from endocardium, so a similar phenomenon might account for the appearance of spontaneous echocardiographic contrast within the cardiac chambers. The inverse relationship between shear rate and red cell aggregation is well recognised[64,65], and in patients with mitral stenosis Beppu and associates found that the occurrence and density of spontaneous contrast in the left atrium correlated inversely with estimated shear rates[47]. Cellular properties also influence red cell aggregation. All these observations lead to the conclusion that spontaneous echocardiographic contrast may even in healthy subjects be a 'normal' phenomenon under particular circumstances.

Spontaneous contrast may not be a risk factor *per se*, but prospective[66] and retrospective[44] clinical studies have established that it is a marker of increased embolic risk. Daniel and co-workers found that 48% of 61 patients with spontaneous contrast within the left atrium had either atrial thrombus or a history of embolism, compared with 7% of patients with no echo contrast[44]. Perhaps the significance of spontaneous contrast is that it implies that the conditions are present in which thrombus may occur; indeed, contrast and thrombus are very often seen together. It is not yet known if spontaneous contrast is a cause of chronic microembolisation, nor is it clear if the diagnosis of spontaneous contrast without thrombus should influence management, for example by increasing levels of anticoagulation or adding additional antiplatelet treatment. When Castello and associates treated a patient with thrombus and spontaneous contrast with warfarin, they found that the thrombus resolved but the contrast remained[45]. However, antiplatelet treatment added to anticoagulation does reduce the incidence of systemic embolism in patients with some types of prosthetic valve[67] (see Chapters 3.1 and 3.4), and in a single case report platelet disaggregatory treatment (with trifluoperazine) led to clearing of spontaneous contrast within the left ventricle[68].

Function of the left atrial appendage

Using colour flow mapping and pulsed Doppler echocardiography, it is possible to assess the haemodynamic function of the left atrial appendage. In healthy subjects, the appendage fills passively during atrial diastole and contracts during atrial systole, and normal velocities of flow at the orifice of the appendage are about 0.4 m/s[69,70]. In patients with atrial fibrillation the velocities may be greatly diminished[69,71]. Initial evidence suggests that there is a correlation between low velocities of flow within the appendage, or poor contraction of the appendage, and the presence of thrombus or spontaneous contrast[70,71]. Abnormal function of the appendage has also been described in patients in sinus rhythm but with a history of embolism, suggesting that localised electromechanical dissociation of the appendage is possible and that it may be a risk factor for developing thrombus within the appendage[72]. Thus, a full echocardiographic study of the heart for potential risk factors for embolism should include an assessment of the function of the appendage. No prospective studies of anticoagulation based on these findings have been reported.

Atrial septal aneurysm

Improvements in the resolution of ultrasonic images of the atrial septum have led to increasing recognition *in vivo* of abnormal mobility of the atrial septum. This may range from a localised area of ballooning or bulging of the septum, due to redundancy of the valve of the foramen ovale, to prolapse of the whole of the atrial septum. The aetiology of atrial septal aneurysm is unknown, but an association with mitral valve prolapse[73] raises the possibility of an underlying abnormality of connective tissue in some patients. An abnormal pattern has been defined as the displacement with each beat of

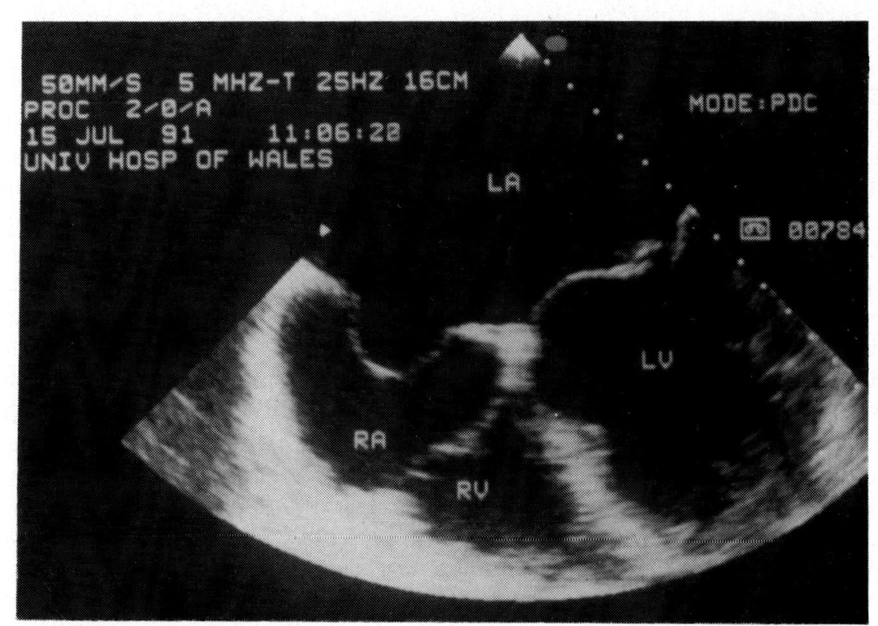

Fig. 2.6–7: Transoesophageal four-chamber view in a patient with an atrial septal aneurysm which in this plane involves the whole of the septum primum within the oval fossa. The width of the aneurysm is 2.8 cm and it is displaced towards the right atrium by 1.8 cm. Abbreviations as in Fig. 2.6–4.

a segment of the atrial septum, of more than 1.5 cm in width, towards the cavity of either atrium by more than 1.5 cm[74]. An example is shown in Fig. 2.6–7.

Atrial septal aneurysm was previously an incidental finding at autopsy in 1% of patients[75], but it is now also found in 0.25–1.2% of patients referred for echocardiography[76–78]. The significance of this finding is that it may be a risk factor for embolism[79]. There is a strong association between atrial septal aneurysm and atrial septal defect or patency of the oval foramen[77]. The condition is often entirely asymptomatic, but thrombus may be found on the atrial septum at the site of an aneurysm[75]. In a retrospective review, Schneider and associates found that 52% of patients with an aneurysm had previously suffered a stroke, and the incidence of stroke correlated with the thickness of the aneurysmal membrane (atrial septum) being 75% if the membrane was $\geqslant$ 5mm compared with 27% if it was $<$ 5mm[74]. In infants, atrial septal defects associated with an aneurysm often close spontaneously[80], but Brand and co-authors reported that more than two thirds of all children with a septal aneurysm still had an associated atrial septal defect[77]. In adults with atrial septal aneurysm, evidence of an atrial septal defect or a patent foramen ovale is found in about 80% of patients studied by transoesophageal echocardiography[74,81]. It has therefore been suggested that paradoxical embolism is the most likely mechanism for systemic embolism in these patients[81], and also that anticoagulation should be considered in all patients with septal aneurysm and probable systemic embolism[82].

Mitral valve prolapse

It has been stated that patients with mitral valve prolapse have a significant risk of systemic embolism[83], but the best studies of the clinical problems associated with incidentally discovered prolapse[84] have not confirmed this. It is possible that unselected series of patients favour those who present with systemic embolism and are found coincidentally to have prolapse. Nonetheless, abnormalities of the clotting mechanism (increased platelet aggregation rate, von Willebrand factor and fibrinopeptide A) have been reported in patients with mitral valve prolapse and systemic embolism[85] although not confirmed prospectively. Autopsy studies of patients with mitral valve prolapse who died suddenly have shown thrombus or fibrin deposits on the atrial surface of the hinge point of the posterior leaflet[86].

The challenge in assessing embolic risk in a patient with mitral valve prolapse arises firstly because of the difficulty of making an echocardiographic diagnosis, and secondly because the use of different echocardiographic approaches and criteria in different studies make it difficult to compare results. Transoesophageal studies using only a transverse transducer, such as that performed by Zenker and co-workers[87], probably overestimate the incidence of prolapse, because of the non-planar shape of the mitral annulus. Echocardiographic prolapse covers a wide spectrum, from mild billowing of the body of a leaflet which is almost certainly normal and probably confers no significant risk to the patient, to extreme prolapse of the edges and bodies of grossly myxomatous leaflets in a patient with associated severe regurgitation. Studies have defined echocardiographic characteristics which are risk factors for adverse outcome in mitral valve prolapse, but these characteristics do not predict cerebral embolic events[88,89]. Nevertheless, Barnett and associates suggested that in patients older than 45 years, mitral valve prolapse is a risk factor for cerebral ischaemia[90]. If there is indeed an association between prolapse and embolism, however, it seems likely that the absolute risk in young adults is very small – it has been estimated at 1 in 11,000 per year[9].

Calcification of the mitral annulus

An association between stroke and calcification of the mitral annulus has been reported[91], and perhaps thrombus may develop because a calcified annulus fails to contract and is thus relatively immobile. Alternatively, calcification of the annulus may be a marker of other conditions such as mitral stenosis or regurgitation[8]. In one series of 95 patients with stroke, calcification of the mitral annulus was found in 23% of those with clinical heart disease and in 4% of those who had otherwise normal hearts[92].

Endocarditis

Endocarditis may present with embolism, and once suspected, the source is revealed when echocardiography shows infective vegetations on a native or a prosthetic valve. The diagnosis may be made by precordial imaging but the transoesophageal approach is much more sensitive (Fig. 2.6–8)[93–96]. It can be difficult to distinguish between thrombus, vegetation, and a 'mass' caused by a small flail segment of a cusp, and so echocardiography should be used to search for related abnormalities including paraprosthetic regurgitation, mycotic abscesses and aneurysms, which would favour a diagnosis of endocarditis. The risk of embolism is probably greater in patients with large vegetations (for example, 47% when the vegetation was > 10mm in size, compared with 19% when it was ≤ 10mm, in the series of Mügge and associates[95]).

Non-bacterial thrombotic endocarditis is diagnosed rarely, but it has been estimated

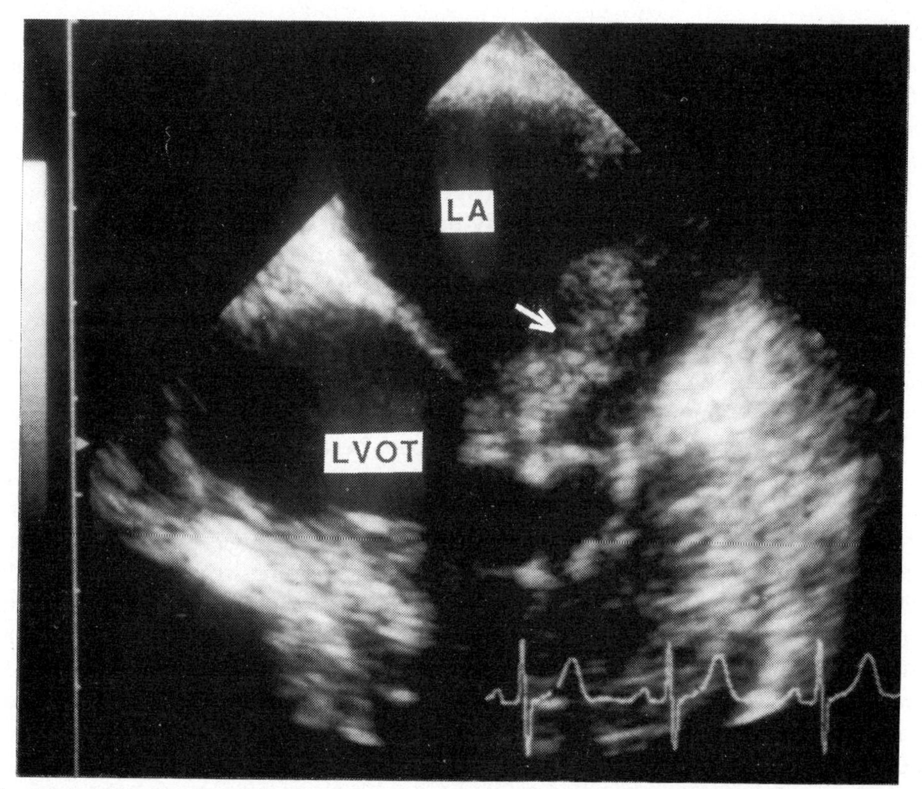

Fig. 2.6–8: Transoesophageal image obtained in a patient who was comatose and febrile, following an embolic stroke. Precordial echocardiography was unhelpful because the patient was obese, but transoesophageal echocardiography demonstrated a large vegetation (arrow) attached to the atrial surface of the anterior mitral leaflet. LA = left atrium; LVOT = left ventricular outflow tract.

to cause 27% of all ischaemic strokes occurring in patients with cancer[9]. It produces vegetations which can be diagnosed by echocardiography, as in infective endocarditis[97].

Cardiac tumours

About 30% of patients with a cardiac tumour present with embolism, and the vast majority will have a myxoma[98]. When this diagnosis is suspected, echocardiography is the investigation of choice[99]. Emboli can consist of myxomatous material or of thrombus from the surface of the tumour. Masses in the left heart are demonstrated as frequently by precordial as by transoesophageal echocardiography[25] but the attachments of an atrial myxoma may be shown more precisely by biplane transoesophageal imaging. The transoesophageal approach is also preferred for masses in the caval veins, and for right paracardiac masses[25].

Papillary tumours (also called fibroelastomas) are thought to be benign, and to arise from organised deposits of fibrin at the sites of minor endothelial damage[100]. They are found most frequently on the cardiac valves but they can occur at any site, and it has been suggested that they may be more common after previous cardiac surgery. They are diagnosed on precordial or transoesophageal echocardiography as small mobile

Table 2.6–3

Diagnostic Yield of Echocardiography in Suspected Embolism

First author	*Year*	*Reference*	*Number of patients*	*Prevalence of cardiac abnormalities* *Transthoracic echo (%)*	*Transoesophageal echo (%)*
Daniel	1989	108	186	26	54
Pop	1990	109	72	10	24
Cujec	1991	110	63	14	41
Pearson	1991	111	79	15	57
Lee*	1991	35	50	0	52

* patients in this study were selected on the basis of a negative transthoracic echocardiogram.

masses, usually attached to the edge of a leaflet[101,102]. Since they can cause systemic embolism[103] or coronary arterial embolism or obstruction, excision may be advisable even in the absence of symptoms.

Atrial enlargement

An enlarged left atrium (dimension > 4 cm) has been shown to be a risk factor for systemic embolism, for example in patients with atrial fibrillation and no mitral stenosis[104] and in patients with a prosthetic mitral valve[105]. Although some large studies have not found a statistically significant association with clinical events[106], asymptomatic cerebral infarcts have been detected by computed tomography in 26% of patients with atrial fibrillation and no valvular heart disease[107]. The prevalence of infarcts attributed to probable embolism was greatest (52%) in patients aged > 65 years who had a left atrial dimension > 5 cm[107]. Thus when echocardiography reveals an enlarged left atrium, even if it is the only abnormality, anticoagulation should be considered. This subject is discussed further in Chapter 1.3.

CLINICAL STUDIES OF PATIENTS WITH SUSPECTED EMBOLISM

Cardiogenic embolism has been estimated to account for about one sixth of all ischaemic strokes[8,9]. Four common conditions (atrial fibrillation, myocardial infarction, rheumatic heart disease, and prosthetic heart valves) together account for 90% of embolic strokes[8]. When a cardiac source is suspected, it may be detected by precordial echocardiography, but transoesophageal echocardiography is much more sensitive. This has been confirmed by several recent studies[35,108–111] which are summarised in Table 2.6–3. In another, smaller study of 13 patients, Tramarin and co-workers reported a diagnostic yield from the transoesophageal approach of 92%, compared with 15% from the precordium[112], but the consensus from the larger series is that a potential cause can be found in up to 50% of patients. In addition, transoesophageal echocardiography can demonstrate atherosclerotic plaques in the aorta, which are another potential embolic source[109].

Transoesophageal studies compare very favourably with the earlier experience of precordial echocardiography. The latter was especially disappointing in patients with no clinical evidence of cardiac disease. In precordial studies of patients with stroke, a possible cause of cardiogenic embolism (such as left atrial or left ventricular enlargement) may be found in 38–48%, but a definite source in as few as 3 or 4%[113,114]. Obviously, the diagnostic yield depends on the selection of patients and the interval between suspected embolism and subsequent echocardiography. With the precordial approach, the yield is particularly low if there is no clinical evidence of heart disease, but in such cases the transoesophageal approach has revealed a cardiac cause in 39% of patients (compared with 19% from the precordium)[111]. Earlier rather lukewarm recommendations for echocardiography in patients with suspected cardiogenic embolism, which were based on transthoracic imaging[115], need to be reconsidered in the era of transoesophageal studies. Particularly in patients with embolism and clinical evidence of heart disease, the evidence now supports a much greater use of transoesophageal echocardiography.

Some of the abnormalities reviewed in this chapter are difficult to diagnose. It is therefore important that a careful study is performed by an experienced investigator. Nonetheless, even with the techniques presently available, many echocardiographic examinations will not reveal an obvious underlying cause of previous embolism, perhaps because the conditions that created it were transient, or because the technique was insufficiently sensitive to detect very small thrombi in locations difficult to visualise. Further technical progress may improve the diagnostic accuracy. In the meantime, further prospective studies are required to investigate the clinical significance and possible therapeutic implications of echocardiographic features that appear to presage increased embolic risk in patients who have as yet not suffered any embolic events.

REFERENCES

1. Casale PM, Whitlow P, Currie PJ, Stewart WJ. Transesophageal echocardiography in percutaneous balloon valvuloplasty for mitral stenosis. Cleve Clin J Med 1989;56:597–600.
2. Barzilai B, Marshall WG, Saffitz JE, Kouchoukos N. Avoidance of embolic complications by ultrasonic characterization of the ascending aorta. Circulation 1989;80 (Suppl I):I–275–9.
3. Marshall WG, Barzilai B, Kouchoukos NT, Saffitz JE. Intraoperative ultrasonic imaging of the ascending aorta. Ann Thor Surg 1989;48:339–44.
4. Duff HJ, Buda AJ, Kramer R, Strauss HD, David TE, Berman ND. Detection of entrapped intracardiac air with intraoperative echocardiography. Am J Cardiol 1980;46:255–260.
5. Rodigas PC, Meyer FJ, Haasler GB, Dubroff JM, Spotnitz HM. Intraoperative 2-dimensional echocardiography: ejection of microbubbles from the left ventricle after cardiac surgery. Am J Cardiol 1982;50:1130–1132.
6. Topol EJ, Humphrey LS, Borkon AM, et al. Value of intraoperative left ventricular microbubbles detected by transesophageal two-dimensional echocardiography in predicting neurologic outcome after cardiac operations. Am J Cardiol 1985;56:773–5.
7. Wenda K, Henrichs KJ, Biegler M, Erbel R. (Detection of bone marrow embolism in femoral intramedullary nailing using transesophageal echocardiography.) Unfallchirurgie 1989;15:73–6.
8. Cerebral Embolism Task Force. Cardiogenic brain embolism. Arch Neurol 1986;43:71–84.
9. Cerebral Embolism Task Force. Cardiogenic brain embolism. The second report of the Cerebral Embolism Task Force. Arch Neurol 1989;46:727–43.
10. Hagen PT, Scholz DG, Edwards WD. Incidence and size of patent foramen ovale during the first 10 decades of life: an autopsy study of 965 normal hearts. Mayo Clin Proc 1984;59:17–20.
11. Lynch JJ, Schuchard GH, Gross CM, Wann LS. Prevalence of right-to-left atrial shunting in a healthy population: detection by Valsalva maneuver contrast echocardiography. Am J Cardiol 1984;53:1478–80.

12. Lechat P, Mas JL, Lascault G, et al. Prevalence of patent foramen ovale in patients with stroke. N Eng J Med 1988;318:1148–52.
13. Langholz D, Louie EK, Konstadt SN, Rao TLK, Scanlon PJ. Transesophageal echocardiographic demonstration of distinct mechanisms for right to left shunting across a patent foramen ovale in the absence of pulmonary hypertension. J Am Coll Cardiol 1991;18:1112–7.
14. Manno BV, Bemis CE, Carver J, Mintz GS. Right ventricular infarction complicated by right to left shunt. J Am Coll Cardiol 1983;1:554–7.
15. Bierman FZ, Williams RG. Subxiphoid two-dimensional imaging of the interatrial septum in infants and neonates with congenital heart disease. Circulation 1979;60:80–90.
16. Mügge A, Daniel WG, Klopper JW, Lichtlen PR. Visualization of patent foramen ovale by transesophageal color-coded Doppler echocardiography. Am J Cardiol 1988;62:837–8.
17. Feinstein SB, Cheirif J, Ten Cate FJ et al. Safety and efficacy of a new transpulmonary ultrasound contrast agent: initial multicenter clinical results. J Am Coll Cardiol 1990;16:316–24.
18. Kronik G, Mösslacher H. Positive contrast echocardiography in patients with patent foramen ovale and normal right heart haemodynamics. Am J Cardiol 1982;49:1806–9.
19. Cucchiara RF, Seward JB, Nishimura RA, Nugent M, Faust RJ. Identification of patent foramen ovale during sitting position craniotomy by transesophageal echocardiography with positive airway pressure. Anesthesiology 1985;63:107–9.
20. Moon RE, Camporesi EM, Kisslo JA. Patent foramen ovale and decompression sickness in divers. Lancet 1989;1:513–4.
21. Jungbluth A, Erbel R, Darius H, Rumpelt H-J, Meyer J. Paradoxical coronary embolism: case report and review of the literature. Am Heart J 1988; 116:879–85.
22. Sigel B, Coelho JCU, Spigos DG et al. Ultrasonography of blood during stasis and coagulation. Invest Radiol 1981;17:71–6.
23. Mikell FL, Asinger RW, Elsperger J, Anderson WR, Hodges M. Tissue acoustic properties of fresh left ventricular thrombi and visualization by two dimensional echocardiography: experimental observations. Am J Cardiol 1982;49:1157–65.
24. Shrestha NK, Moreno FL, Narciso FV, Torres L, Calleja HB. Two-dimensional echocardiographic diagnosis of left atrial thrombus in rheumatic heart disease. A clinicopathologic study. Circulation 1983;67:341–7.
25. Mügge A, Daniel WG, Haverich A, Lightlen PR. Diagnosis of noninfective cardiac mass lesions by two-dimensional echocardiography. Comparison of the transthoracic and transesophageal approaches. Circulation 1991;83:70–8.
26. Schweizer P, Bardos P, Erbel et al. Detection of left atrial thrombi by echocardiography. Br Heart J 1981;45:148–56.
27. Chiang CW, Pang SC, Lin FC et al. Diagnostic accuracy of two-dimensional echocardiography for detection of left atrial thrombus in patients with mitral stenosis. J Ultrasound Med 1987;6:525–9.
28. Roudant R, Gosse P, Aouizerate E, Dallocchio M. The diagnosis of intra-atrial masses with two-dimensional echocardiography: experience with 64 patients. Echocardiography 1987;4:431–6.
29. Jordan RA, Scheifley CH, Edwards JE. Mural thrombosis and arterial embolism in mitral stenosis. A clinicopathologic study of fifty-one cases. Circulation 1951;3:363–7.
30. Vandenberg BF, Seabold JE, Conrad GR et al. ^{111}In-Labelled platelet scintigraphy and two-dimensional echocardiography for detection of left atrial appendage thrombi. Studies in a new canine model. Circulation 1988;78:1040–6.
31. Aschenberg W, Schlüter M, Kremer P, Schröder E, Siglow V, Bleifeld W. Transesophageal two-dimensional echocardiography for the detection of left atrial appendage thrombus. J Am Coll Cardiol 1986;7:163–6.
32. Fraser AG, Angelini GD, Ikram S, Butchart EG. Left atrial ball thrombus: echocardiographic features and clinical implications. Eur Heart J 1988;9:672–7.
33. Schechter DC. Left atrial ball-valve thrombus. NY State J Med 1982;82:1831–8.
34. Angermann CE, Spes CH, Tammen AR, et al. Transthoracic and transesophageal echocardiographic findings after orthotopic heart transplantation. In: Erbel R, Khandheria BK, Brennecke R, Meyer J, Seward JB, Tajik AJ, eds. Transesophageal Echocardiography: a New Window to the Heart. Berlin: Springer-Verlag, 1989:330–8.
35. Lee RJ, Bartzokis T, Yeoh T-K, Grogin HR, Choi D, Schnittger I. Enhanced detection of intracardiac sources of cerebral emboli by transesophageal echocardiography. Stroke 1991;22:734–9.
36. Cabin HS, Roberts WC. Left ventricular aneurysm, intra-aneurysmal thrombus and systemic embolus in coronary heart disease. Chest 1980;77:463–9.
37. Stratton JR, Lighty GW, Pearlman AS, Ritchie JL. Detection of left ventricular thrombus by two-dimensional echocardiography: sensitivity, specificity, and causes of uncertainty. Circulation 1982;66:156–66.

38. Visser CA, Kan G, Meltzer RS, Lie KI, Durrer D. Long-term follow-up of left ventricular thrombus after acute myocardial infarction. Chest 1984;86:532–6.
39. Takamoto T, Kim D, Urie PM et al. Comparative recognition of left ventricular thrombi by echocardiography and cineangiography. Br Heart J 1985;53:36–42.
40. Visser CA, Kan G, Meltzer RS et al. Embolic potential of left ventricular thrombus after myocardial infarction: a two-dimensional echocardiographic study of 119 patients. J Am Coll Cardiol 1985;5:1276–80.
41. Mukai S, Fuseno H, Nakamura M, Yoxhikawa J, Shomura T. Dilated cardiomyopathy complicated by a pedunculated and mobile left ventricular thrombus on ruptured false tendons. Chest 1991;99:1042–3.
42. Nixdorff U, Erbel R, Drexler M, Meyer J. Detection of thromboembolus of the right pulmonary artery by transesophageal two-dimensional echocardiography. Am J Cardiol 1988;61:488–9.
43. Görge G, Erbel R, Schuster S, Ge J, Meyer J. Intravascular ultrasound in diagnosis of pulmonary embolism. Lancet 1991;337:623–4.
44. Daniel WG, Nellessen U, Schröder E et al. Left atrial spontaneous echo contrast in mitral valve disease: an indicator for an increased thromboembolic risk. J Am Coll Cardiol 1988;11:1204–11.
45. Castello R, Pearson AC, Labovitz AJ, Lenzen P. Prevalence and clinical implications of atrial spontaneous contrast in patients undergoing transesophageal echocardiography. Am J Cardiol 1990;65:1149–53.
46. Schuchman H, Feigenbaum H, Dillon JC, Chang S. Intracavitary echoes in patients with mitral prosthetic valves. J Clin Ultrasound 1975;3:107–10.
47. Beppu S, Nimura Y, Sakakibara H, et al. Smoke-like echo in left atrial cavity in mitral valve disease: its features and significance. J Am Coll Cardiol 1985;6:744–9.
48. Iliceto S, Antonelli G, Sorino M, Biasco G, Rizzon P. Dynamic intracavitary echoes in mitral stenosis. Am J Cardiol 1985;55:603–6.
49. Garcia-Fernandez MA, Moreno M, Banuelos F. Two-dimensional echocardiographic identification of blood stasis in the left atrium. Am Heart J 1985;109:600–1.
50. Chen YT, Kan MN, Chen JS, et al. Contributing factors to formation of left atrial spontaneous echo contrast in mitral valvular disease. J Ultrasound Med 1990;9:151–5.
51. Stümper O, Sutherland GR, Geuskens R, Roelandt JRTC, Bos E, Hess J. Transesophageal echocardiography in evaluation and management after a Fontan procedure. J Am Coll Cardiol 1991;17:1152–60.
52. Mikell FL, Asinger RW, Elsperger J, Anderson WR, Hodges M. Regional stasis of blood in the dysfunctional left ventricle: echocardiographic detection and differentiation from early thrombosis. Circulation 1982;66:755–63.
53. Delemarre BJ, Bot H, Visser CA, Dunning AJ. Pulsed Doppler echocardiographic description of a circular flow pattern in spontaneous left ventricular contrast. J Am Soc Echo 1988;1:114–118.
54. Castello R, Pearson AC, Fagan L, Labovitz AJ. Spontaneous echocardiographic contrast in the descending aorta. Am Heart J 1990;120:915–9.
55. Panidis IP, Kotler MN, Mintz GS, Ross J. Intracavitary echoes in the aortic arch in type III aortic dissection. Am J Cardiol 1984;54:1159–60.
56. Mahony C, Elion JL, Fischer PLC. A computerized analysis of platelet aggregation detected by ultrasound. Thrombosis Research 1989;55:351–60.
57. Wolverson MK, Nouri S, Joist JH, Sundaram M, Heiberg E. The direct visualization of blood flow by real-time ultrasound: clinical observations and underlying mechanisms. Radiology 1981;140:443–8.
58. Meltzer RS, Lancée CT, Swart GR, Roelandt J. Spontaneous echocardiographic contrast on the right side of the heart. J Clin Ultrasound 1982;10:240–2.
59. Gow RM, Smallhorn JF, Rowe RD. Dynamic intracoronary echoes in Kawasaki's disease. Am J Cardiol 1987;59:170.
60. Sigel B, Coelho JCU, Schade SG, Justin J, Spigos DG. Effect of plasma proteins and temperature on echogenicity of blood. Invest Radiol 1982;17:29–33.
61. Machi J, Sigel B, Beitler JC, Coelho JCU, Justin JR. Relation of in vivo blood flow to ultrasound echogenicity. J Clin Ultrasound 1983;11:3–10.
62. Hjemdahl-Monsen CE, Daniels J, Kaufman D, Stern EH, Teichholz LE, Meltzer RS. Spontaneous contrast in the inferior vena cava in a patient with constrictive pericarditis. J Am Coll Cardiol 1984;4:165–7.
63. Mahony C, Evans JM, Spain C. Spontaneous contrast and circulating platelet aggregates. [Abstract] Circulation 1989;80:II–1.
64. Wells RE. Rheology of blood in the microvasculature. N Eng J Med 1964;270:832–9.
65. Schmid-Schönbein H, Gaehtgens P, Hirsch H. On the shear rate dependence of red cell aggregation in vitro. J Clin Invest 1968;47:1447–54.
66. Black IW, Hopkins AP, Lee LCL, Walsh WF, Jacobson BM. Left atrial spontaneous echo contrast: a clinical and echocardiographic analysis. J Am Coll Cardiol 1991;18:398–404.

67. Stein B, Fuster V, Israel DH et al. Platelet inhibitor agents in cardiovascular disease: an update. J Am Coll Cardiol 1989;14:813–36.
68. Mahony C, Sublett KL, Harrison MR. Resolution of spontaneous contrast with platelet disaggregatory therapy (Trifluoperazine). Am J Cardiol 1989;63:1009–10.
69. Pozzoli M, Smyllie JH, Roelandt JRTC. Atrial lesions. In: Sutherland G, Roelandt JRTC, Fraser AG, Anderson RH, eds. Transesophageal Echocardiography in Clinical Practice. London, Gower Medical Publishing 1991:4.1–4.14.
70. Pollick C, Taylor D. Assessment of left atrial appendage function by transesophageal echocardiography. Implications for the development of thrombus. Circulation 1991;84:223–31.
71. Suetsugu M, Matsuzaki M, Toma Y, et al. (Detection of mural thrombi and analysis of blood flow velocities in the left atrial appendage using transesophageal two-dimensional echocardiography and pulsed Doppler flowmetry.) J Cardiol 1988;18:385–94.
72. Pozzoli M, Tramarin R, Torbicki A, et al. Standstill of left atrial appendage: a new Doppler sign of thromboembolic risk? [Abstract] Eur Heart J 1989;10 (suppl):206.
73. Rahko PS, Xu QB. Increased prevalence of atrial septal aneurysm in mitral valve prolapse. Am J Cardiol 1990;66:235–7.
74. Schneider B, Hanrath P, Vogel P, Meinertz T. Improved morphologic characterization of atrial septal aneurysm by transesophageal echocardiography: relation to cerebrovascular events. J Am Coll Cardiol 1990;16:1000–9.
75. Silver MD, Dorsey JS. Aneurysms of the septum primum in adults. Arch Pathol Lab Med 1978;102:62–5.
76. Hanley PC, Tajik AJ, Hynes JK, et al. Diagnosis and classification of atrial septal aneurysm by two-dimensional echocardiography: report of 80 consecutive cases. J Am Coll Cardiol 1985;6:1370–82.
77. Brand A, Keren A, Branski D, Abrahamov A, Stern S. Natural course of atrial septal aneurysm in children and the potential for spontaneous closure of associated septal defect. Am J Cardiol 1989;64:996–1001.
78. Katayama H, Mitamura H, Mitani K, Nakagawa S, Kimura M. (Incidence of atrial septal aneurysm: echocardiographic and pathologic analysis.) J Cardiol 1990;20:411–21.
79. Gallet B, Malergue MC, Adams C et al. Atrial septal aneurysms - a potential cause of systemic embolism. An echocardiographic study. Br Heart J 1985;53:292–7.
80. Shiraishi I, Hamaoka K, Hayashi S, Koh E, Onouchi Z, Sawada T. Atrial septal aneurysm in infancy. Pediatr Cardiol 1990;11:82–5.
81. Zabalgoitia-Reyes M, Herrera C, Gandhi DK, Mehlman DJ, McPherson DD, Talano JV. A possible mechanism for neurologic ischemic events in patients with atrial septal aneurysm. Am J Cardiol 1990;66:761–4.
82. Belkin RN, Kisslo J. Atrial septal aneurysm: recognition and clinical relevance. Am Heart J 1990;120:948–57.
83. Wolf PA, Sila CA. Cerebral ischemia with mitral valve prolapse. Am Heart J 1987;113:1308–15.
84. Devereux RB, Kramer-Fox R, Brown WT et al. Relation between clinical features of the mitral prolapse syndrome and echocardiographically documented mitral valve prolapse. J Am Coll Cardiol 1986;8:763–72.
85. Zuppiroli A, Cecchi F, Ciaccheri M et al. Platelet function and coagulation studies in patients with mitral valve prolapse. Clin Cardiol 1986;9:487–92.
86. Chesler E, King RA, Edwards JE. The myxomatous mitral valve and sudden death. Circulation 1983;67:632–9.
87. Zenker G, Erbel R, Kramer G, et al. Transesophageal two-dimensional echocardiography in young patients with cerebral ischemic events. Stroke 1988;19:345–8.
88. Nishimura RA, McGoon MD, Shub C, Miller FA, Ilstrup DM, Tajik AJ. Echocardiographically documented mitral valve prolapse. Long-term follow-up of 237 patients. N Eng J Med 1985;313:1305–9.
89. Marks AR, Choong CY, Sanfilippo AJ, Ferré M, Weyman AE. Identfication of high-risk and low-risk subgroups of patients with mitral-valve prolapse. N. Eng J Med 1989;320:1031–6.
90. Barbett HJM, Boughner DR, Taylor DW, Cooper PE, Kostuk WJ, Nichol PM. Further evidence relating mitral-valve prolapse to cerebral ischemic events. N Eng J Med 1980;302:139–44.
91. De Bono DP, Warlow CP. Mitral-annulus calcification and cerebral or retinal ischaemia. Lancet 1979;2:383–5.
92. Greenland P, Knopman DS, Mikell FL et al. Echocardiography in diagnostic assessment of stroke. Ann Intern Med 1981;95:51–3.
93. Erbel R, Rohmann S, Drexler M, et al. Improved diagnostic value of echocardiography in patients with infective endocarditis by transoesophageal approach. A prospective study. Eur Heart J 1988;9:45–53.
94. Daniel WG, Schröder E, Mügge A, Lichtlen PR. Transesophageal echocardiography in infective endocarditis. Am J Cardiac Imaging 1988;2:78–85.
95. Mügge A, Daniel WG, Frank G, Lichtlen PR. Echocardiography in infective endocarditis: reassessment

of prognostic implications of vegetation size determined by the transthoracic and the transesophageal approach. J Am Coll Cardiol 1989;14:631–8.
96. Taams MA, Gussenhoven EJ, Bos E, et al. Enhanced morphological diagnosis in infective endocarditis by transoesophageal echocardiography. Br Heart J 1990;63:109–13.
97. Lopez JA, Fishbein MC, Siegel RJ. Echocardiographic features of nonbacterial thrombotic endocarditis. Am J Cardiol 1987;59:478–80.
98. Blondeau P. Primary cardiac tumors – French studies of 533 cases. Thorac Cardiovasc Surg 1990;38(Suppl 2):192–195.
99. Salcedo EE, Adams KV, Lever HM, Gill CC, Lombardo H. Echocardiographic findings in 25 patients with left atrial myxoma. J Am Coll Cardiol 1983;1:1162–6.
100. Pomerance A. Papillary "tumours" of the heart valves. J Pathol Bacteriol 1981;81:135–40.
101. McFadden PM, Lacy JR. Intracardiac papillary fibroelastoma: an occult cause of embolic neurological deficit. Ann Thorac Surg 1987;43:667–9.
102. Lewis NP, Williams GT, Fraser AG. Unusual and intraoperative epicardial echocardiographic features of a papillary tumour of the aortic valve. Br Heart J 1989;62:470–4.
103. Fowles RE, Miller DC, Egbert BM, Fitzgerald JW, Popp RL. Systemic embolization from a mitral valve papillary endocardial fibroma detected by two-dimensional echocardiography. Am Heart J 1981;102:128–30.
104. Cabin HS, Clubb KS, Hall C, Perlmutter RA, Feinstein AR. Risk for systemic embolization of atrial fibrillation without mitral stenosis. Am J Cardiol 1990;65:1112–6.
105. Burchfiel CM, Hammermeister KE, Krause-Steinrauf H et al. Study on valvular heart disease: left atrial dimension and risk of systemic embolism in patients with a prosthetic heart valve. J Am Coll Cardiol 1990;15:32–41.
106. Peterson P, Kastsrup J, Helweg-Larsen S, Boysen G, Gotfredsen J. Risk factors for thromboembolic complications in chronic atrial fibrillation: the Copenhagen AFASAK Study. Arch Int Med 1990;150:819–21.
107. Feinberg WM, Seeger JF, Carmody RF, Anderson DC, Hart RG, Pearce LA. Epidemiologic features of asymptomatic cerebral infarction in patients with non-valvular atrial firbillation. Arch Intern Med 1990;150:2340–4.
108. Daniel WG, Engberding R, Erbel R et al. Transesophageal echocardiography in arterial embolism and cerebral ischemic events – a European multicenter study in patients without pre-known cardiac disease. [Abstract] Eur Heart J 1989;10 (Abstract Supp):204.
109. PopG, Sutherland GR, Koudstaal PJ, Sit TW, de Jong G, Roelandt JRTC. Transesophageal echocardiography in the detection of intracardiac embolic sources in patients with transient ischemic attacks. Stroke 1990;21:560–5.
110. Cujec B, Polasek P, Voll C, Shuaib A. Transesophageal echocardiography in the detection of potential cardiac source of embolism in stroke patients. Stroke 1991;22:727–33.
111. Pearson AC, Labovitz AJ, Tatineni S, Gomez CR. Superiority of transesophageal echocardiography in detecting cardiac source of embolism in patients with cerebral ischemia of uncertain aetiology. J Am Coll Cardiol 1991;17:66–72.
112. Tramarin R, Torbicki A, Franchini M et al. Transesophageal echocardiography in the definition of intracardiac sources of emboli in patients with recent ischemic stroke. G Ital Cardiol 1990;20:713–9.
113. Come PC, Riley MF, Bivas NK. Roles of echocardiography and arrhythmia monitoring in the evaluation of patients with suspected systemic embolism. Ann Neurol 1983;13:527–31.
114. Good DC, Frank S, Verhulst S, Sharma B. Cardiac abnormalities in stroke patients with negative arteriograms. Stroke 1986;17:6–11.
115. Knopman DS, Anderson DC, Asinger RW, Greenland P, Mikell F, Good DC. Indications of echocardiography in patients with ischemic stroke. Neurology 1982;32:1005–11.

Part 3

Postoperative management

Chapter 3.1

Platelet Inhibitor Drugs after Prosthetic Heart Valve Replacement

Valentin Fuster and Douglas H. Israel

The pathogenesis of prosthetic valve thrombosis and thromboembolism is related both to the activation of the coagulation system and to platelet function. The role of the coagulation cascade and the prophylactic use of anticoagulants is discussed in detail in other chapters. This chapter focuses on:

- The role of platelet activation in the pathogenesis of thromboembolism in patients with prosthetic heart valves.
- The physiology of platelet adhesion and aggregation.
- The pharmacology of platelet inhibitors.
- The use of platelet inhibitor therapy for the prevention of thromboembolic complications in prosthetic heart valve replacement.
- Recommendations for antithrombotic therapy.

PATHOGENESIS OF VALVE THROMBOSIS AND THROMBOEMBOLISM

The pathogenesis of valve thrombosis and thromboembolism begins with intra-operative and early postoperative activation of platelets and the coagulation system. Platelets are activated by exposed prosthetic surfaces, including the sewing ring, sutures and the prosthesis itself, as well as by perivalvular surfaces denuded of endothelium[1,2]. An additional factor may be the activation of platelets by the surfaces of the cardiopulmonary bypass circuit[3]. Such early platelet deposition may be imaged on the sewing ring by indium^{111} labelled platelet scintigraphy within 24 hours of surgery in dogs, whether a mechanical or bioprosthetic heart valve is used[1,2]. The intrinsic clotting system is activated in the early post-operative period by contact exposure to prosthetic or damaged native tissue surfaces. In addition, platelet membrane phospholipids serve as a catalytic surface for the generation of thrombin, which then functions to further activate platelets.

Other factors contribute to a thrombogenic milieu in the early post-operative period. These include lack of anticoagulation immediately following surgery, low cardiac output, arrhythmias and the relatively hypercoagulable state seen following major surgery (see also Chapter 3.4). The clinical relevance of these factors is corroborated by the greater incidence of thromboembolic events observed in many studies within the first three months of mechanical or bioprosthetic valve replacement[4–7].

A decrease in thromboembolic risk after this early period may occur due to endothelialisation of exposed perivalvular and prosthetic surfaces. However, there is a substantial chronic risk that is related to the characteristics of the prosthesis, the adequacy of antithrombotic therapy and abnormalities of cardiac rhythm and blood flow[8]. Haemodynamic abnormalities promoting thrombosis and embolism include both stasis, which is more related to fibrin generation, and turbulence, which may preferentially promote platelet activation[9].

Adequate and consistent anticoagulation appears to be the most important modifying factor in preventing thromboembolic complications. Nevertheless, even when this is achieved, there is a substantial residual risk of systemic embolism[8]. This seems to apply particularly to patients with older mechanical heart valves with more thrombogenic prosthetic materials or very turbulent blood flow patterns. With these prostheses, platelet activation may have major pathogenic significance. Because shortened platelet survival is directly related to prosthetic surface area[10–13], and because there are data to show that platelet inhibitor therapy can normalise platelet survival[10,13,14], there is a rationale for the use of platelet inhibitors in combination with oral anticoagulants to decrease the risk of embolism in patients with the more thrombogenic valves. The physiology of platelet activation and pharmacology of platelet inhibitors are discussed in detail below.

PHYSIOLOGY OF PLATELET ADHESION AND AGGREGATION

Platelets are small fragments of cytoplasm without a nucleus, enclosed with a phospholipid membrane. They contain vasoactive, proaggregant and mitogenic factors in their dense granules and alpha granules. The well characterised interaction of platelets with vascular subendothelium is of primary importance in haemostasis and, under pathological conditions, contributes to thrombogenesis and atherogenesis[15]. Activation of platelets and thrombosis involves platelet adhesion, platelet aggregation, activation of the coagulation system and the activation of endogenous inhibitors of thrombosis[15]. A detailed knowledge of the processes of platelet adhesion and aggregation is fundamental to the understanding of the pharmacology of platelet inhibitors.

Platelet adhesion occurs when there is exposure of subendothelial constituents, especially collagen and fibronectin. This adhesion is mediated by the binding of these elements to platelet surface glycoprotein receptors and is dependent in part on circulating von Willebrand factor (vWF) which also has a role in platelet aggregation. Glycoprotein Ia promotes binding to collagen, particularly at lower shear rates[16]. Glycoprotein Ib binds to vWF and may be more important in platelet adhesion under high shear conditions[17], as found with haemodynamic turbulence due to a mechanical prosthesis. Glycoprotein IIb/IIIa binds vWF and fibrinogen and is essential for both platelet adhesion and aggregation.

The adhesion of platelets to artificial surfaces is less well understood, but appears to depend on an interaction between platelet glycoprotein receptors and plasma proteins, such as fibrinogen adsorbed onto the prosthetic surface[18]. Platelet adherence to artificial surfaces is enhanced in turbulent flow conditions[19]. This effect may be due partly to physical trauma to platelets and red blood cells, resulting in the release of adenosine diphosphate (ADP)[20,21], and partly to other physical and chemical interactions between platelets, red blood cells and leucocytes[22]. Following activation, platelets extend pseudopodia due to the association of actin filaments, and spread out into a thin film that completely carpets the injured or prosthetic surface[23].

Platelet aggregation occurs soon after platelet adhesion in the presence of various thrombogenic stimuli. This process depends upon the binding of an agonist such as

ADP, serotonin, thromboxane A_2 (TXA_2), collagen or thrombin with a receptor complex on the platelet membrane[15]. Signal transduction by the agonist-receptor complex appears to act via a final common pathway, the hydrolysis of membrane phosphatidylinositol by phospholipase C, leading to the mobilisation of calcium from dense tubules[15]. The increase in cytoplasmic calcium activates three metabolic processes that amplify the process of platelet activation and result in aggregation:

1. *Secretion of ADP.* Soon after platelets contract or change their shape, they release the contents of their granules including ADP. Once ADP is secreted, it binds to membrane receptors on other platelets and induces a conformational change, again by the action of phospholipase C on phosphatidylinositol. This change in shape leads to exposure of an active site on glycoprotein IIb/IIIa that binds to fibrinogen and vWF in the presence of calcium ions, and bridges neighbouring platelets to one another[23–26]. The fibrinogen receptor mechanism plays a central role in platelet aggregation regardless of the agonist[25,26]. In patients with a prosthetic heart valve, the role of ADP may be very important because it is released not only from platelets, but also from red blood cells when there is haemolysis due to excessively turbulent blood flow.

2. *Activation of arachidonic acid metabolism.* The increase in cytoplasmic calcium that occurs with platelet activation also results in liberation of arachidonic acid from platelet membrane phospholipid by phospholipase A[27]. Arachidonic acid is converted by platelet cyclo-oxygenase to the labile prostaglandin intermediates PGG_2 and PGH_2. PGH_2 is converted by platelet thromboxane synthase to TXA_2, a potent vasoconstrictor and agonist of aggregation that acts by the common mechanism of activating the platelet fibrinogen receptor. Arachidonic acid released from the platelet membrane may also be metabolised by endothelial cells. The final product of such metabolism is prostacyclin (PGI_2), a potent inhibitor of platelet adherence and aggregation[28]. Prostacyclin appears to increase platelet levels of cyclic adenosine monophospate (cAMP) by increasing the activity of its synthetic enzyme, adenyl cyclase[29]. Cyclic AMP is a major inhibitor of platelet activation by all agonists[30] and its level is modulated by the availability of adenosine[31], the activity of adenyl cyclase, and the activity of phosphodiesterase, the enzyme that degrades cAMP[15].

3. *Collagen and thrombin.* These extrinsic platelet activators result in platelet activation and aggregation via the same metabolic pathways described above[15]. Collagen may be particularly important in triggering calcium release in platelets in pathological situations, where it is exposed in high local concentrations, such as rupture of an atherosclerotic plaque. Thrombin plays a fundamental part in thrombogenesis because it has a pivotal role in both platelet aggregation and the synthesis of fibrin, which is important to stabilise platelet aggregates.

PHARMACOLOGY OF PLATELET INHIBITORS

Given the complexities of platelet activation, there exists the possibility to inhibit platelet function by interfering at many different levels. Currently available platelet inhibitor agents may be broadly considered in four categories: (a) drugs that inhibit the arachidonic acid pathway, (b) drugs that modulate platelet cAMP levels, (c) drugs that inhibit the synthesis or action of thrombin, and (d) drugs with less clearly defined mechanisms. This section of the chapter considers currently available drugs with clinical applications, but also briefly describes newer drugs and experimental approaches, particularly those which may have clinical relevance to the patient with a prosthetic heart valve.

A) Inhibitors of arachidonic acid metabolism.

Cyclo-oxygenase inhibitors. Aspirin, the most widely used platelet inhibitor, acts by irreversibly acetylating platelet cyclo-oxygenase, resulting in inhibition of TXA_2 induced platelet aggregation for the life of the platelet[32]. Acetylation of vascular cyclo-oxygenase also occurs, but is not irreversible because endothelial cells may synthesise more of the enzyme. However, this effect requires many hours, and the former notion that very low dose aspirin may inhibit platelet function while sparing the synthesis of prostacyclin is probably incorrect[33]. Long term administration of aspirin at doses of 1 mg/kg daily, roughly the equivalent of one baby aspirin per day, effectively inhibits both platelet and vascular cyclo-oxygenase function in humans[34].

The daily administration of very low dose aspirin, such as 20–50 mg daily, may result in 90–98% inhibition of platelet TXA_2 production within 3–7 days of beginning therapy[35]. This emphasises an important point when very low doses are used; acetylation of cyclo-oxygenase is cumulative and requires several doses. Therefore such therapy should be preceded by a loading dose. In addition, when very low doses are used, gastric absorption may not be completely reliable. The minimum dose of aspirin with the most consistently beneficial effects in numerous clinical trials has been 160–325 mg/day[36,37]. This dose has not been associated with a greater incidence of gastric bleeding or other side effects than placebo in major clinical trials. Gastric side effects, including gastrointestinal bleeding due to the inhibition of synthesis of protective prostaglandins by the stomach, are however significant at higher doses of aspirin such as 900–1300 mg/day[38,39].

Other non-steroidal anti-inflammatory drugs also function as cyclo-oxygenase inhibitors. However, most are competitive inhibitors, and so differ in their potency and duration of action[40]. Experimental evidence supports a possible role for ibuprofen as an alternative agent in patients intolerant of aspirin[41]. As yet, no clinical trials have been completed with non-steroidal anti-inflammatory agents. In addition, the various agents cannot be assumed to be equivalent; for example indomethacin may inhibit platelet function, but appears to increase coronary vascular resistance and exacerbate myocardial ischaemia by other mechanisms[42].

Agents that modify platelet membrane phospholipid. The omega–3 fatty acids, eicosapentaenoic acid (EPA) and docosahexaenoic acid (DHA) are present in high concentrations in salt water fish. When large amounts of fish are consumed, EPA and DHA are incorporated into the membranes of platelets and other cells, where they compete with arachidonic acid as substrates for cyclo-oxygenase and other enzymes. When EPA is acted upon by cyclo-oxygenase, it is converted ultimately to thromboxane A_3 (TXA_3), which unlike its counterpart TXA_2, has no platelet agonist activity[43,44]. The final result of the metabolism of EPA by endothelial cells is prostaglandin I3, which, like PGI_2, is a potent vasodilator and platelet inhibitor[43,44]. The net result of the biochemical modifications is thus a shift in the haemostatic balance away from thrombosis and vasoconstriction. DHA has independent and less well understood platelet inhibitor properties, and may serve as a storage form for EPA via retroconversion[44].

Whereas the consumption of fish in large quantities has potent effects on platelet function, inflammatory and immune function and possibly atherogenesis[43,44], it remains to be seen whether moderate fish consumption has clinically relevant antithrombotic effects. High dose EPA and DHA, as consumed in concentrated fish oil capsules, should be considered a pharmacological agent rather than a dietary supplement, and cannot be recommended at present on the basis of the available data.

Inhibitors of thromboxane synthase. Imidazole containing structures with thromboxane synthase blocking activity have been developed with the hope of suppressing TXA_2 synthesis while shunting the endoperoxide intermediates PGG_2 and PGH_2 to the endothelial cells to be utilised in the synthesis of prostacyclin[45]. Clinical results have been somewhat disappointing, possibly because the endoperoxide intermediates PGG_2 and PGH_2 themselves have platelet agonist effects[46,47].

Thromboxane and prostaglandin endoperoxide receptor blockers. An alternative to the inhibition of thromboxane synthase would be to block the receptors for TXA_2 or its endoperoxide precursors[48]. The combination of a thromboxane synthase inhibitor with TXA_2 and endoperoxide receptor blockers could theoretically inhibit platelet function while sparing or enhancing PGI_2, but this requires further testing[49].

Drugs that modulate platelet cAMP levels

Dipyridamole. Dipyridamole increases platelet cAMP levels, probably via two mechanisms. First, dipyridamole is a platelet phosphodiesterase inhibitor and so decreases the enzymatic destruction of cAMP[50]. In addition, dipyridamole is a powerful inhibitor of vascular and erythrocyte uptake of adenosine, resulting in increased plasma adenosine levels[50,51]. This mechanism may be responsible for the vasodilatory effects of dipyridamole. Increased plasma adenosine levels may stimulate platelet adenyl cyclase, and so dipyridamole both increases synthesis and decreases breakdown of platelet cAMP. At very high doses experimentally, dipyridamole inhibits platelet adhesion to collagen and subendothelium[52,53].

However, the most important effect of dipyridamole is to inhibit platelet activation by prosthetic surfaces, and this effect occurs readily at doses used clinically[50,54]. In experimental animals dipyridamole at a dose of 10 mg/kg daily prevents thromboembolism from prosthetic surfaces[54], and doses of 5–7 mg/kg daily normalise platelet survival in patients with artificial heart valves and arteriovenous shunts[10,11,55]. As discussed below, there is evidence to show that this normalisation of platelet survival (or decrease in platelet consumption) is associated with a statistically significant reduction in the thromboembolism associated with some prosthetic heart valves.

Major side effects of dipyridamole include epigastric pain or nausea which may occur in up to 10% of patients when high doses are used. These effects may be prevented or lessened by initiating therapy with a lower dose and administering the drug with meals. Headache is another common side effect, due to the vasodilator action of dipyridamole, and rarely a coronary steal syndrome may occur with worsening of angina pectoris.

Triflusal. Triflusal is a new platelet inhibitor that is a weaker cyclo-oxygenase inhibitor than aspirin[56], but a strong inhibitor in vitro of phosphodiesterase[57]. Clinical experience with this agent is limited, but in a recent trial the combination of triflusal and dipyridamole compared favourably to low dose aspirin and dipyridamole in the prevention of occlusion in aorto-coronary vein grafts[58].

Prostacyclin and oral analogues. Prostacyclin is perhaps the most potent available platelet inhibitor. Infusion of prostacyclin inhibits the interaction of platelets with synthetic surfaces and preserves platelet number and function during cardiopulmonary bypass[59,60]. However, its utility is limited by its rapid chemical degradation, instability at neutral pH and its tendency to cause hypotension at platelet inhibitory doses. Iloprost, a stable analogue of prostacyclin, may be even more potent in increasing platelet levels of cAMP and inhibiting platelet aggregation in response to agonists, but clinical experience with this agent is limited[61]. Ciprostene is another stable prostacyclin analogue for which preliminary data appear to show a reduction in ischaemic events following angioplasty[62]. More work is needed to confirm this effect and to define its clinical role as a platelet inhibitor.

Thrombin inhibitors

Heparin. Heparin is a well known intravenous anticoagulant that works by increasing antithrombin III activity and so decreases the production of thrombin. Thus heparin indirectly reduces platelet deposition by decreasing synthesis of one of the major platelet agonists. The platelet inhibitory effect of heparin is dose dependent, requiring doses up to 250 units/kg in an experimental angioplasty model[63]. Furthermore, the effects of heparin are complex and may be inconsistent due to the molecular heterogeneity of the commercially available preparations[64] (see Chapter 3.2).

Other antithrombin agents. Hirudin is a natural anticoagulant isolated from the salivary secretions of the leech, and currently produced by recombinant DNA technology. Hirudin prevents the activation of clotting factors V, VIII and XIII thus inhibiting the synthesis of thrombin. It is also a potent noncovalent and irreversible inhibitor of thrombin, including its platelet agonist activity[65]. Hirudin inhibits platelet aggregation much more strongly than high dose heparin in the pig carotid angioplasty model[66], probably by displacing thrombin from its binding sites on platelets[67]. However, the inhibition of platelet thrombi with hirudin requires a five-fold greater level of thrombin inhibition than is required to inhibit the formation of fibrin thrombi[65]. Substantial experimental data now support a major role for hirudin, administered at doses sufficient to prolong the activated partial thromboplastin time to 2–3 times control[66], and preliminary human studies have begun.

Synthetic peptide inhibitors of thrombin have also been shown experimentally to produce potent thrombin and platelet inhibition exceeding the effects of heparin in a variety of experimental models[68]. Further experimental work and clinical testing will be required to further define the safety and efficacy of these compounds and their therapeutic role in patients with cardiovascular disease.

Drugs with other mechanisms

Sulfinpyrazone. Sulfinpyrazone appears to be a competitive inhibitor of cyclo-oxygenase, but the exact mechanism of its antiplatelet activity remains uncertain[69]. Sulfinpyrazone inhibits platelet secretion and aggregation both in vitro and in vivo, but only at very high doses[70,71]. Its inhibitory effect on collagen-induced platelet aggregation in rabbits persists for many hours after the drug is cleared from the blood, and has been postulated to be due to active drug metabolites[72]. Sulfinpyrazone has been shown to inhibit thrombus formation on subendothelium, and to protect endothelium from chemical injury in vitro[73,74]. However, as is the case for dipyridamole, the effect of sulfinpyrazone appears more consistently beneficial on artificial intravascular surfaces.

Sulfinpyrazone has been shown to normalise platelet survival in patients with some mechanical heart valve prostheses[13], and to decrease the incidence of thrombotic events associated with arteriovenous shunts, both in experimental animals and patients[69,74]. In contrast, results with sulfinpyrazone have been inconsistent when the surface is biological[39,75–78]. Unlike aspirin, sulfinpyrazone has a minor inhibitory effect on gastric prostaglandin production, but it may exacerbate the symptoms of peptic ulcer disease[79]. Sulfinpyrazone also increases sensitivity to warfarin, frequently necessitating a reduction in dosage of oral anticoagulants. Thus careful attention should be paid to the prothrombin time when initiating therapy with sulfinpyrazone[79]. It may also potentiate the effectiveness of oral hypoglycaemic agents and as a uricosuric agent can potentially precipitate uric acid stones[79].

Ticlopidine. Ticlopidine is a potent platelet inhibitor whose peak effects are manifest 24–48 hours after beginning therapy and persist several days after discontinuing the drug[80]. Ticlopidine strongly inhibits ADP-induced platelet aggregation, and inhibits aggregation and release mediated by collagen, thrombin, arachidonic acid and adrenaline, while prolonging platelet survival[81]. The mechanism of action of ticlopidine is uncertain, but it may involve inhibition of membrane receptors for fibrinogen or vWF in the final stages of platelet aggregation. As indicated above, this represents a final common pathway for platelet aggregation, and this may explain the broad spectrum of antagonism by ticlopidine for all the platelet agonists.

A number of large scale clinical trials are now available to demonstrate the efficacy of ticlopidine as a platelet inhibitor in patients with unstable angina[82], in saphenous vein bypass grafting[83], and in reducing acute occlusion after coronary angioplasty[84]. Although there are some data to suggest that ticlopidine is more effective than aspirin in patients with transient cerebral ischaemia[85], further studies will be required to evaluate the relative efficacy of ticlopidine compared with aspirin, which only inhibits the TXA_2 mediated pathway of platelet aggregation.

Other agents. With the possible exception of ticlopidine, none of the currently available drugs interfere with all the metabolic pathways responsible for platelet aggregation, and none will prevent adherence of platelets to an injured biological or artificial surface. Because the final common step in platelet aggregation involves the binding of fibrinogen and vWF to glycoprotein IIb/IIIa receptors on neighbouring platelets, one approach has been to develop monoclonal antibodies directed against glycoprotein IIb/IIIa or vWF[86,87]. Experimental studies show that this approach leads to powerful platelet inhibition in the setting of reocclusion prevention following thrombolysis[88], and preliminary investigation has begun in humans. The very high potency of these agents may preclude their chronic use. Nonetheless, they may be useful for short term therapy in patients at very high risk for thrombotic events.

PLATELET INHIBITOR THERAPY IN HEART VALVE REPLACEMENT

While platelets have an important role in the pathogenesis of thromboembolism related to heart valve prostheses, oral anticoagulant therapy comprises the cornerstone of antithrombotic therapy. Although data are limited, antiplatelet agents appear ineffective as monotherapy, particularly in patients with older mechanical prostheses. However, in selected cases, the use of platelet inhibitors in combination with oral anticoagulants has resulted in a significantly lower incidence of thromboemboli.

Platelet inhibitors alone

Mechanical Prostheses (Table 3.1–1). There is no randomised placebo controlled trial testing the use of platelet inhibitors alone as an antithrombotic regimen in mechanical heart valve replacement. However, in one prospective randomised trial involving over 250 patients with aortic or mitral Starr-Edwards valves, oral anticoagulation with warfarin was compared to a platelet inhibitor regimen including dipyridamole and aspirin, or pentoxifylline and aspirin[89]. The incidence of thromboembolism over a 2 year follow-up period in the groups receiving either combination of platelet inhibitors was significantly greater than that observed in the warfarin treated patients (dipyridamole/aspirin, 13.6%; pentoxifylline/aspirin 10.5% versus warfarin 4.1%). In a non-randomised series, the use of dipyridamole alone (100 mg/day) in a small group of patients with Starr-Edwards valves was associated with a high rate of thromboembolism (10 episodes per 100 patient years)[90], and this regimen has not undergone further evaluation.

The use of aspirin at a dose of 1.3 gm/day[89] was associated with an acceptable incidence of embolic events (2.6 episodes per 100 patient years). However in this series, patients receiving no antithrombotic drug had a relatively low incidence of 4 embolic events per 100 patient years. Thus, the favourable outcome in the group receiving aspirin may have been attributable to lower risk characteristics of this cohort. In another non-randomised series of patients with Starr-Edwards aortic valves, aspirin alone at a dose of 1gm/day was associated with fewer emboli than historical controls receiving anticoagulants as long as sinus rhythm was present[91]. However, patients with atrial fibrillation had a high risk of embolism on aspirin alone. The combination of aspirin 1gm/day plus dipyridamole 100mg/day in patients with Bjørk-Shiley aortic valves resulted in no reduction in systemic embolism, the incidence being identical to that in patients receiving no antithrombotic therapy[92,93].

Table 3.1–1
Platelet inhibitors alone for mechanical prosthetic heart valves

Study	*Drug*	*TE(%/yr)*
Dale et al (1977)[108]	ASA (100 mg/d)	15
Salazar et al (1984)[94]	ASA (1000 mg/d)	29 (pregnancy)
Chaux et al (1984)[96]	ASA (975 mg/d) +D (275 mgs/d)	7
Mok et al (1985)[89]	ASA (1000 mg/d) +D (275 mg/d)	7

Abbreviations: ASA = aspirin D = dipyridamole

Treatment with platelet inhibitors alone resulted in a devastating incidence of thromboembolic complications in a non-randomised series of pregnant women with predominantly caged ball or first generation tilting disc prostheses in either mitral or aortic position[94]. There was a 29% incidence of systemic embolism, and a 4.4% incidence of fatal valve thrombosis in 68 women treated with aspirin (1 gram/day), dipyridamole (400 mg/day), or both, compared with a 2.3% incidence of embolism in women treated with warfarin, and an 8.3% incidence (one patient) in women treated with subcutaneous heparin in the first trimester and final two weeks of pregnancy with oral anticoagulation in the interim period (see also Chapter 4.1).

Very limited information is available concerning the use of platelet inhibitors in patients with St. Jude valves. While low rates of embolism have been reported in two tiny series of patients with these valves in the aortic position[95], there was an embolic incidence of 6.5% per year reported in another non-randomised series of patients with St. Jude aortic valve replacement[96]. In a series of 52 young Saudi Arabian patients in sinus rhythm with a St. Jude aortic prosthesis treated with aspirin, there were no systemic emboli reported, but valve thrombosis occurred at a rate of 2.1% per year[97].

Data from non-randomised series suggest that platelet inhibitors alone may afford adequate protection for some children with mechanical prosthetic valves, particularly in the aortic position and with sinus rhythm[98–100]. Even with the implantation of Starr-Edwards or Bjørk-Shiley prostheses, no occurrence of valve thrombosis or systemic embolism was reported in these 3 series of 93 children[98–100]. In one of these reports, children with mitral replacements had an identical rate of thromboembolism (2.3% per year) whether warfarin or aspirin/dipyridamole was administered[99]. However, no data are available to assess the incidence of atrial fibrillation amongst the two groups, or the adequacy and consistency of anticoagulation in the group given warfarin. In another very small series, 25% of children with Bjørk-Shiley or St. Jude mitral valve replacements treated with aspirin experienced valve thrombosis requiring emergency reoperation[100]. Thus, the use of platelet inhibitors in children with aortic valve replacement appears promising, but these data must be considered preliminary, pending further randomised trials with larger numbers of patients (see also Chapter 4.2).

Bioprostheses. Very few studies have examined the use of platelet inhibitors in heart valve replacement with bioprostheses, and none have been randomised or placebo controlled. In series of patients with porcine mitral or aortic valve replacement and atrial fibrillation, the incidence of thromboembolic events varied from 0.3 to 1.3 events per 100 patient years when aspirin was given in doses ranging from 500 mg every other day to 1 gm daily[101,102]. For patients in sinus rhythm with porcine mitral, aortic or double valve replacement, no emboli were reported in 23–32 months of follow up when aspirin was administered in doses of 500 mg every other day to 1 gm daily[101,102]. Though inconclusive, these data suggest a possible role for aspirin in prophylaxis of systemic embolism in bioprostheses.

Combined anticoagulant and platelet inhibitor therapy (Table 3.1–2)

The relatively high risk of systemic embolism, observed in recipients of certain types of mechanical prostheses despite the use of anticoagulants, led to the evaluation of combined therapy with warfarin and platelet inhibitors. The pathophysiological

Table 3.1–2
Antithrombotic therapy in patients with mechanical prosthestic heart valves*

Study	*Methods*	*Follow-up (yr)*	*Treatment group*	*Dose (mg/day)*	*Patient (no.)*	*Thrombo-embolic events (%/yr)*
Sullivan[103]	Prospective,	1	A/C + placebo		84	14
	randomised		A/C + D	400	79	1
Kasahara[104]	Prospective,	1 to 3	A/C		39	21
	randomised	(mean 30 mo)	A/C + D	400	40	5
Groupe PACTE[107]	Prospective,	1	A/C		154	5
	randomised		A/C + D	375	136	3
Rajah[105]	Prospective,	1 to 2	A/C		87	13
	randomised		A/C + D	300	78	4
Dale[108]	Prospective,	1	A/C + placebo		38	9
	randomised		A/C + ASA	1,000	39	2
	blind		ASA	1,000	77	15
Altman[109]	Prospective,	2	A/C		65	20
	randomised		A/C + ASA	500	57	5

*A/C = anticoagulant; ASA = aspirin, D = dipyridamole. (Reproduced from Fuster V, Chesebro JH. Antithrombotic therapy: role of platelet inhibitor drugs; management of arterial thromboembolic and atherosclerotic disease. Mayo Clin Proc 1981; 56: 265-273, by permission of the Mayo Foundation.)

rationale for such a combination rests on the documentation of increased platelet consumption, as reflected by a measured decrease in platelet survival, in older mechanical valves[10–13]. Platelet survival in these studies was particularly shortened in patients with double valve replacement, probably due to their greater prosthetic surface area, and in patients with a prior history of embolism[10–13]. The administration of dipyridamole at a dose of 400 mg/day was found to be effective in normalising platelet survival[10].

As a result, five randomised controlled trials have been conducted comparing the antithrombotic efficacy of warfarin plus dipyridamole (5–6 mg/kg/day) versus warfarin alone in recipients of caged ball or first generation tilting disc valves. In three trials[103–105], combination therapy was significantly better than warfarin alone, resulting in a 70–92% reduction in embolic events. In two other trials, the addition of dipyridamole to warfarin resulted in a 40–50% decrease in embolic episodes when compared to warfarin therapy alone. However, with the relatively low event rates characteristic of more recently operated patients (perhaps due to higher anticoagulation intensity – see Chapter 3.4), the differences in these two trials did not achieve statistical significance[106,107]. The results of one trial testing the combination of sulfinpyrazone with warfarin appears to suggest a protective effect for patients in whom the platelet survival time was shown to be normalised[14].

However, the importance of normalised platelet survival with the administration of a platelet inhibitor as a marker for efficacy in preventing embolism is unclear. For example, 500–1,000 mg. aspirin daily did not normalise platelet survival in patients with mechanical prostheses[10], but did lead to a decrease in systemic embolism in three trials[106,108,109] when combined with warfarin. However, this combination can cause a significant increase in serious haemorrhage, particularly with the higher levels of anticoagulation used in the USA for some years (see Chapters 3.3 and 3.4), and is not recommended. These studies have all been conducted in recipients of caged ball or early first generation tilting disc valves which have been associated with the highest risk of thromboembolism. No data are currently available to assess whether the combination of platelet inhibitors with anticoagulants is beneficial in reducing the risk of thromboembolism in patients with more recently developed mechanical valves.

RECOMMENDATIONS FOR ANTIPLATELET THERAPY

Mechanical prostheses

All patients with mechanical prostheses should be treated with anticoagulants as described in Chapter 3.4. Low risk patients may be treated with anticoagulants alone. High risk patients include those with mechanical valves implanted before the mid–1970s, or those with prior embolic complications. Such patients should receive oral anticoagulants with the addition of dipyridamole 100 mg four times daily. Patients with intolerable side effects from dipyridamole may be treated with sulfinpyrazone, 200 mg four times daily in addition to warfarin. The addition of sulfinpyrazone to warfarin may prolong the prothrombin time, requiring careful monitoring and frequently a reduction in the warfarin dose.

Patients with haemorrhagic complications who have been receiving higher intensity anticoagulation with warfarin should have their intensity reduced (INR 2.0–3.0), in combination with dipyridamole, when anticoagulation is resumed. Investigation of the source of bleeding should be undertaken (see Chapter 5.4).

While antiplatelet agents alone are not advisable as sole antithrombotic therapy in the patient with a mechanical prosthesis, in the event that an absolute contraindication to oral anticoagulant therapy develops after implantation, the combination of dipyridamole 100 mg four times daily with sulfinpyrazone 200 mg four times daily, or aspirin 325 mg daily may be tried empirically.

Patients with recurrent systemic emboli despite maximal safe antithrombotic therapy with oral anticoagulants and platelet inhibitors should be investigated for possible hypercoagulability (see Chapter 1.5) and any remediable cause treated. Otherwise reoperation may be required, particularly if there is evidence of thrombus on the prosthesis or tissue overgrowth from the sewing ring (see Chapters 2.4, 2.6 and 5.2).

Platelet inhibitors are not approved for use during pregnancy; the effects of dipyridamole and sulfinpyrazone are unknown, and aspirin may cause premature closure of the ductus arteriosus because of its prostaglandin inhibitor effects. Anticoagulation management in pregnancy is discussed in Chapter 4.1.

Bioprostheses

Patients with bioprosthetic heart valves in normal sinus rhythm should ideally receive low intensity anticoagulant therapy to an INR of 2.0–3.0, beginning as soon as possible after surgery and continuing 3 months post-operatively. Following this period, aspirin may be considered in order to further decrease the low risk of systemic embolism in patients without other indications for chronic oral anticoagulation. Patients with bioprosthetic valves in atrial fibrillation, with left atrial thrombus discovered during surgery, or with a previous history of thromboembolism should receive long term anticoagulation. High dose warfarin for 3 months (INR 3.0–4.5) and low dose warfarin thereafter (INR 2.0–3.0) may be the safest approach but so far there are no data to support this recommendation.

REFERENCES

1. Dewanjee MK, Fuster V, Rao SA, Forshaw PL, Kaye MP. Non-invasive radioisotopic technique for detection of platelet deposition in mitral valve prosthesis and quantification of visceral microembolism in dogs. Mayo Clin Proc 1983;58:307–314.
2. Dewanjee MK, Trastek VF, Tago M. Radioisotopic techniques for non-invasive detection of platelet deposition in bovine mitral valve prostheses and quantitation of visceral microembolism in dogs. Invest Radiol 1984;6:535–542.
3. Becker RM, Smith MR, Dobell ARC. Effects of platelet inhibition on platelet phenomenon in cardiopulmonary bypass in pigs. Ann Surg 1974;179:52–57.
4. Edmunds LH. Thrombotic and bleeding complications of prosthetic heart valves. Ann Thorac Surg 44:430–445,1987.
5. Hertzer R, Topalidis T, Borst HG. Thromboembolism and anticoagulation after isolated mitral valve replacement with porcine heterografts. In: Cohn LH, Gallucci V (eds). Cardiac Bioprostheses. Proceedings, Second International Symposium on Cardiac Bioprostheses. New York: Yorke Medical Books, 1982;170–172.
6. Ionescu MI, Smith DR, Hasan SS, Chidambaram M. Tandon AP. Clinical durability of the pericardial xenograft valve: ten years experience with mitral replacement. Ann Thorac Surg 1982;34:265–277.
7. Oyer PE, Stinson EB, Griep RB, Shumway NE. Valve replacement with the Starr-Edwards and Hancock prostheses: comparative analysis of late morbidity and mortality. Ann Surg 1977;186:301–309.
8. Fuster V, Pumphrey CW, McGoon MD, Chesebro JH, Pluth JR, McGoon DC. Systemic thromboembolism in mitral and aortic Starr-Edwards prostheses. A 10–19 year follow-up. Circulation 1982;66(suppl I):157–161.
9. Virchow R, Gesammelte abhandlungen zur wissenshaftlichen medizin. IV. Thrombose und embolie. Gefassentzundung und septische infektion. Frankfurt, Meidinger, 1856.
10. Harker LA, Slichter SJ. Studies of platelet and fibrinogen kinetics in patients with prosthetic heart valves. N Engl J Med 1970;238:1302–1305.
11 Weily HS, Steele PP, Davies H, Pappas G, Genton E. Platelet survival in patients with substitute heart valves. N Engl J Med 1974;290:534–537.
12. Weily HS, Genton E. Altered platelet function in patients with prosthetic mitral valves: effects of sulfinpyrazone therapy. Circulation 1970;42:967–972.
13. Steele PM, Weily HS, Davies H, Pappas G, Genton E. Platelet survival time following aortic valve replacement. Circulation 1975;51:358–362.
14. Steele PP, Rainwater J, Vogel R. Platelet suppressant therapy in patients with prosthetic cardiac valves: Relationship of clinical effectiveness to alteration of platelet survival time. Circulation 1979;60:910–913.
15. Stein B, Fuster V, Israel DH, Cohen M, Badimon L, Badimon JJ, Chesebro JH. Platelet inhibitor agents in cardiovascular disease: An update. J Am Coll Cardiol 1989;14:813–836.
16. Nieuwenhuis HK, Sixma JJ. Platelet receptors. Proceedings European Conference on Antiplatelet Therapy: A twenty year experience. Florence, March 1987.
17. Hawiger J. Formation and regulation of platelet and fibrin haemostatic plug. Human Pathol 1987;18:111–122.
18. Lindon JN, Collins REC, Coe NP, Jasoda A, Brier-Russel D, Merril EW, Salzman EW. In-vivo assessment in sheep of thromboresistant materials by determination of platelet survival. Circ Res 1971;46:84- 90.
19. Stein PD, Sabbah HN. Measured turbulence and its effect on thrombus formation. Circ Res 1974;35:608–614.
20. Moritz MW, Reimers RC, Baker RK, Sutera SP, Joist JH. Role of cytoplasmic and releasable ADP in platelet aggregation induced by laminar shear stress. J Lab Clin Med 1983;101:537–544.

21. Reimers RC, Sutera SP, Joist JH. Potentiation by red blood cells of shear-induced platelet aggregation: relative importance of chemical and physical mechanisms. Blood 1984;64:1200–1206.
22. Joist JH, Pennington DG. Platelet reactions with artificial surfaces. Trans Am Soc Artif Intern Organs 1987;33:341–344.
23. Escolar G, Krumwiede M, White JG. Organisation of the actin cytoskeleton of resting and activated platelets in suspension. Am J Pathol 1986;123:86–94.
24. Peerschke EIB. The platelet fibrinogen receptor. Semin Hematol 1985;22:241–259.
25. Shattil SJ, Brass LP. Induction of the fibrinogen receptor on human platelets by intracellular mediators. J Biol Chem 1987;992–1000.
26. Coller BS. Activation affects access to the platelet receptor for adhesive glycoproteins. J Cell Biol 1986;103:451–456.
27. Lagarde M. Control mechanisms of platelet aggregation with special reference to eicosanoids and related components. Proceedings European Conference on Antiplatelet Therapy: A twenty year experience. Florence, March 1987.
28. Moncada S, Vane JR. Arachidonic acid metabolites and the interactions between platelets and blood vessel walls. N Engl J Med 1979;300:1142–1147.
29. Tateson JE, Moncada S, Vane JR. Effects of prostacyclin (PGX) on cyclic AMP concentrations in human platelets. Prostaglandins 1977;13:389–97.
30. Gerrard JM, White JF. Prostaglandins and thromboxanes: 'middlemen' modulating platelet function in haemostasis and thrombosis. Prog Hemost Thromb 1978;4:87–125.
31. Sattini A, Rall T. The effect of adenosine and adenine nucleotides on the cyclic adenosine 3′–5′ phosphate content of guinea pig cerebral cortex slices. Mol Pharmacol 1970;6:13–23.
32. Roth GL, Majerus PW. The mechanism of the effect of aspirin on human platelets. I. Acetylation of a particulate fraction protein. J Clin Invest 1975;56:624–632.
33. Kyrle PA, Eichler HG, Jager U, Lechner K. Inhibition of prostacyclin and thromboxane A_2 generation by low-dose aspirin at the site of plug formation in man in vivo. Circulation 1987;75:1025- 1029.
34. Weksler BB, Pett SB, Alonso D, et al. Differential inhibition by aspirin of vascular and platelet prostaglandin sythesis in atheroslerotic patients. N Engl J Med 1983;308:800–805.
35. Patrono C, Ciabattoni G, Patrignani P, et al. Clinical pharmacology of platelet cyclo-oxygenase inhibition. Circulation 1985;54:528–532.
36. Lewis HD, Davis JW, Archibald DG, et al. Protective effects of aspirin against acute myocardial infarction and death in men with unstable angina. Results of a Veterans Administration Cooperative Study. N Engl J Med 1983;309:396–403.
37. ISIS–2 (Second International Study of Infarct Survival) Collaborative Group. Randomised trial of intravenous streptokinase, oral aspirin, both, or neither among 17,187 cases of suspected acute myocardial infarction: ISIS–2. Lancet 1988;2:349–360.
38. Graham DY, Smith LJ. Aspirin and the stomach. Ann Intern Med 1986;104:390–398.
39. Cairns JA, Gent M, Singer J, et al. Aspirin, sulfinpyrazone, or both in unstable angina. N Engl J Med 1985;313:1369–1375.
40. Simon LS, Mills JA. Non-steroidal anti-inflammatory drugs. N Engl J Med 1980;312:1179–1185.
41. Lam JYT, Dewanjee MK, Badimon L, Fuster V. Ibuprofen: A potent antithrombotic agent for arterial injury after balloon angioplasty. J Am Coll Cardiol 1987;9(suppl A):64A.
42. Friedman PL, Brown EJ, Gunther S. Coronary vasoconstrictor effect of indomethacin in patients with coronary artery disease. N Engl J Med 1981;305:1171–1175.
43. Von Schacky C. Prophylaxis of atherosclerosis with marine omega–3 fatty acids. A comprehensive strategy. Ann Intern Med 1987;107:890–899.
44. Leaf A, Weber PC. Cardiovascular effects of n–3 fatty acids. N Engl J Med 1988;318:549–557.
45. FitzGerald GA, Reilly IA, Pedersen AK. The biochemical pharmacology of thromboxane synthase inhibition in man. Circulation 1985;72:1194–1201.
46. Reuben SR, Kuan P, Cairns T, Gysle OH. Effects of dazoxiben and exercise performance in chronic stable angina. Br J Clin Pharmacol 1983;15(suppl 1):83S–86S.
47. Thaulow E, Dale J, Myhre E. Effects of a selective thromboxane synthetase inhibitor, dazoxiben, and of acetylsalicyclic acid on myocardial ischemia in patients with coronary artery disease. Am J Cardiol 1984;53:1255–1258.
48. Saussy DL Jr, Mais DE, Knapp DR, Halushka PV. Thromboxane A_2 and prostaglandin endoperoxide receptors in platelets and vascular smooth muscle. Circulation 1985;72:1202–1207.
49. Gresele P, Van Houtte E, Arnout J, Deckmyn H, Vermylen J. Thromboxane synthase inhibition combined with thromboxane receptor blockade. A step forward in antithrombotic strategy. Thromb Haemost 1984;52:364.
50. FitzGerald GA. Dipyridamole. N Engl J Med 1987;316:1247–1257.
51. Crutchley DJ, Ryan US, Ryan JW. Effects of aspirin and dipyridamole on the degradation of adenosine diphosphate by cultured cells derived from bovine pulmonary artery. J Clin Invest 1980;66:29–35.

52. Cazenave J-P, Packham MA, Kinlough-Rathbone RL, Mustard RF. Platelet adherence to the vessel wall and to collagen-coated surfaces. Adv Exp Med Biol 1978;102:31–49.
53. Kinlough-Rathbone RL, Groves HM, Cazenave J-P, Richardson M, Mustard JF. Effect of dipyridamole and aspirin on platelet adherence to damaged rabbit aortas in-vitro and in-vivo (Abstract). Fed Proc 1978;37:260.
54. Harker LA, Hanson SR, Kirkman TR. Experimental arterial thromboembolism in baboons. Mechanism, quantitation, and pharmacologic prevention. J Clin Invest 1979;64:559–569.
55. Harker LA. Platelet survival time: Its measurement and use. Prog Hemost Thromb 1978;4:321–347.
56. Albors M, Castellarnau C, Vila L, Sola J, Rutllant M. Inhibition of thromboxane production and platelet function by triflusal in healthy volunteers. Rev Pharmacol Clin Exp 1987;4:11–19.
57. Garcia-Rafanell J, Ramis J, Gomez L, Forn J. Effect of triflusal and other salicylic acid derivatives on cyclic AMP levels in rat platelets. Arch Intern Pharmacodyn Ther 1986;284:155–159.
58. Guiteras P, Altimiras J, Aris A, et al. Prevention of aortocoronary vein-graft attrition with low-dose aspirin and dipyridamole versus triflusal and dipyridamole: a randomized, double-blind, placebo-controlled trial. Eur Heart J 1989;12:159–166.
59. Coppe D, Sobel M, Seavans L, Levine F, Salzman E. Preservation of platelet function and number by prostacyclin during cardiopulmonary bypass. J Thorac Cardiovasc Surg 1981;81:274–278.
60. Smith MC, Danviriyasup K, Crow, JW. Prostacyclin substitution for heparin in long-term hemodialysis. Am J Med 1982;73:669–678.
61. Fisher CA, Kappa JR, Sinha AK, Cottrell ED, Reiser HJ, Addonizio VP. Comparison of equimolar concentrations of iloprost, prostacyclin, and prostaglandin E_1 on human platelet function. J Lab Clin Med 1987;109:184–90.
62. Raizner A, Hollman J, Demke D, Wakefield L. Beneficial effects of ciprostene in PTCA: A multicenter, randomized, controlled trial (abstract). Circulation 1988;78(suppl II):290.
63. Heras M, Chesebro JH, Penny WJ, et al. Importance of adequate heparin dosage in arterial angioplasty in a porcine model. Circulation 1988;78:654–660.
64. Salzman EW, Rosenberg RD, Smith MH, Lindon JN, Favreau L. Effect of heparin fractions on platelet aggregation. J Clin Invest 1980;65:64–73.
65. Markwardt F, Nowick G, Sturzebecker J. Pharmacokinetics of anticoagulant effects of hirudin in man. Thromb Haemost 1984;52:160- 163.
66. Heras M, Chesebro JH, Penny WJ et al. Effects of thrombin inhibitors on the development of platelet-thrombus deposited during angioplasty in pigs. Heparin versus hirudin, a synthetic thrombin inhibitor. Circulation 1989;79:657–665.
67. Tam SW, Fenton JW, Detwiler TC. Dissociation of thrombin from platelets by hirudin. J Biol Chem 1979;254:8723–8725.
68. Hanson SR, Harker LA. Interruption of acute platelet-dependent thrombosis by the synthetic antithrombin D-phenylalanyl-L-prolyl-L-arginyl chloromethyl ketone. Proc Natl Acad Sci USA 1988;85:3184-3188.
69. Hanson SR, Harker LA, Bjornsson TD. Effect of platelet-modifying drugs on arterial thromboembolism in baboons. Aspirin potentiates the anti-thrombotic actions of dipyridamole and sulfinpyrazone by mechanism(s) independent of platelet cyclo-ozygenase inhibition. J Clin Invest 1985;75:1591–1599.
70. Packham MA, Mustard JF. Pharmacology of platelet-affecting drugs. Circulation 1980;62(suppl V):26–41.
71. Butler KD, Wallis RB, White AM. A study of the relationship between ex-vivo and in-vivo effects of sulphinpyrazone in the guinea pig. Haemostasis 1979;8:353–360.
72. Baumgartner HR. Effects of acetylsalicylic acid, sulfinpyrazone and dipyridamole on platelet adhesion and aggregation in flowing native and anticoagulated blood. Haemostasis 1979;8:340–352.
73. Harker LA, Harlan JM, Ross R. Effect of sulfinpyrazone on homocysteine-induced endothelial injury and arteriosclerosis in baboons. Circ Res 1983;53:731–739.
74. Kaegi A, Pineo GF, Shimizu A, Trivedi H, Hirsh J, Gent M. Arteriovenous-shunt thrombosis: Prevention by sulfinpyrazone. N Engl J Med 1974;290:304–306.
75. Report from the Anturane Reinfarction Italian Study: Sulfinpyrazone in post-myocardial infarction. Lancet 1982;1:237–242.
76. Baur HR, Van Tassel RA, Pierach CA, Gobel RL. Effects of sulfinpyrazone on early graft closure after myocardial revascularization. Am J Cardiol 1982;49:420–424.
77. Canadian Cooperative Study Group: A randomized trial of aspirin and sulfinpyrazone in threatened stroke. N Engl J Med 1978;299:53- 59.
78. Goldman S, Copeland J, Moritz T, et al. Improvement in early saphenous vein graft patency after coronary artery bypass surgery with antiplatelet therapy: results of a Veterans Administration Cooperative Study. Circulation 1988;77:1324–1332.
79. Fuster V, Adams PC, Badimon JJ, Chesebro JH. Current concepts of thrombogenesis: Platelet inhibitor drugs' role in coronary artery disease. Prog Cardiovasc Dis 1987;5:325–346.

80. O'Brien JR. Ticlopidine, a promise for the prevention and treatment of thrombosis and its complications. Haemostasis. 1983;13:1–54.
81. Lee H, Paton RC, Ruan C. The in-vitro effect of ticlopidine on fibrinogen and factor VIII binding to human platelets (abstract). Thromb Haemost 1981;46:67.
82. Violi F, Scrutinio D, Cimminiello C, et al. S.T.A.I. (Study of Ticlopidine in Unstable Angina) (abstract). J Am Coll Cardiol 1989;13(suppl A):238A.
83. Limet R, David JL, Magotteaux P, Larock MP, Rigo P. Prevention of aorta-coronary bypass graft occlusion. J Thorac Cardiovasc Surg 1987;94:773–783.
84. White CW, Chaitman B, Lassar TA. et al. Antiplatelet agents are effective in reducing the immediate complications of PTCA: Results from the ticlopidine multicenter trial (abstract). Circulation 1987;76(suppl IV):400.
85. Molony B. Ticlopidine in the prevention of stroke: A multicenter study (abstract). In: Proceedings of the Symposium, Newer Strategies in the Management of Thrombotic Disorders. Chicago, Loyola University 1987;35.
86. Hanson SR, Pareti FI, Ruggeri ZM, et al. Effects of monoclonal antibodies against the platelet glycoprotein IIb/IIIa complex on thrombosis and haemostasis in the baboon. J Clin Invest 1988; 81:149- 158.
87. Badimon L, Badimon JJ, Chesebro JH, Fuster V. Inhibition of thrombus formation: Blockage of adhesive glycoprotein mechanisms versus blockage of the cyclo-oxygenase pathway (abstract). J Am Coll Cardiol 1988;11(suppl A):30A.
88. Gold HK, Coller BS, Yasuda T, et al. Rapid and sustained coronary artery recanalization with combined bolus injection of recombinant tissue-type plasminogen activator and monoclonal antiplatelet GPIIb/IIIa antibody in a canine preparation. Circulation 1988;77:670–677.
89. Mok DK, Boey J, Wang R, et al. Warfarin versus dipyridamole-aspirin and pentoxifylline-aspirin for the prevention of prosthetic heart valve thromboembolism: a prospective randomized clinical trial. Circulation 1985;82:1059–1063.
90. Moggio RA, Hammond GL, Stansel HC Jr, Glen WWL. Incidence of emboli with cloth covered Starr-Edwards valve without anticoagulation and with varying forms of anticoagulation: Analysis of 183 patients followed for three and a half years. J Thorac Cardiovasc Surg 1978;75:296–299.
91. Dale J, Myhre E. Can acetylsalicylic acid alone prevent arterial thromboembolism? A pilot study in patients with aortic ball valve prostheses. Acta Med Scand Suppl 1981;645:73–78.
92. Bjørk VO, Henze A. Ten years experience with the Bjørk-Shiley tilting disk valve. J Thorac Cardiovasc Surg 1979;78:331–339.
93. Bjørk VO, Henze A. Management of thromboembolism after aortic valve replacement with the Bjørk-Shiley tilting disc valve. Scand J Thorac Cardiovasc Surg 1975;9:183–191.
94. Salazar E, Zajarias A, Gutierrez N, Iturbe I. The problem of cardiac valve prostheses, anticoagulants and pregnancy. Circulation 1984;70(Suppl I):169–177.
95. Gill CC. Clinical evaluation of the St. Jude medical valve: The small aortic root. In DeBakey ME (Ed.): Advances in Cardiac Valves, Clinical Perspectives. New York, Yorke Medical Books, 1983;173–177.
96. Chaux A, Czer LSC, Matloff JM, DeRobertis MA, Steward ME, Bateman TM. The St Jude Medical bileaflet valve prosthesis. A five year experience. J Thorac Cardiovasc Surg 1984;88:706–717.
97. Ribeiro PA, Al Zaibag MA, Idris M, et al. Antiplatlet drugs and the incidence of thromboembolic complications of the St. Jude Medical aortic prosthesis in patients with rheumatic heart disease. J Thorac Cardiovasc Surg 1986;91:92–98.
98. Verrier ED, Tranbaugh RF, Soifer SJ. Aspirin anticoagulation in children with mechanical aortic valves. J Thorac Cardiovasc Surg 1986;92:1013–1020.
99. Makhlouf E, Friedli B, Oberhansli I. Prosthetic heart valve replacement in children. J Thorac Cardiovasc Surg 1987;93:80–95.
100. Bradley LM, Midgley FM, Watson DC. Anticoagulation therapy in children with mechanical prosthetic cardiac valves. Am J Cardiol 1985;56:533–535.
101. Nunez L, Aguado GM, Celemin D, Iglesias A, Larrea JL. Aspirin or coumadin as the drug of choice for valve replacement with porcine bioprosthesis. Ann Thorac Surg 1982;33:354–358.
102. Nunez L, Aguado FM, Larrea JL, Celemin D, Oliver J. Prevention of thromboembolism using aspirin after mitral valve replacement with porcine bioprosthesis. Ann Thorac Surg 1984;37:84–87.
103. Sullivan JM, Harken DE, Gorlin R. Effect of dipyridamole on the incidence of arterial emboli after cardiac valve replacement. Circulation 1969;39/40(suppl I):149–153.
104. Kasahara T. Clinical effect of dipyridamole ingestion after prosthetic heart valve replacement – especially on the blood coagulation system. J Jpn Assoc Thorac Surg 1977;25:1007–1021.
105. Rajah SM, Sreeharan N, Joseph A, Watson DA. Prospective trial of dipyridamole and warfarin in heart valve patients (abstract). Acta Thera (Brussels) 1980;6:54.
106. Chesebro JH, Fuster V, McGoon DC, et al. Trial of combined warfarin plus dipyridamole or aspirin

therapy in prosthetic heart valve replacement: danger of aspirin compared with dipyridamole. Am J Cardiol 1983;51:1537–1541.

107. Groupe de recherche PACTE. Prevention des accidents thrombemboliques systemiques chez les porteurs de prostheses valvulaires artificielles: essai cooperatif controle du dipyridamole. Coeur 1978;9:915–969.
108. Dale J, Myhre E, Storstein O, Stormorken H, Efskind L. Prevention of arterial thromboembolism with acetylsalicylic acid. A controlled clinical study in patients with aortic ball valves. Am Heart J 1977;94:101–111.
109. Altman R, Boullon F, Rouvier J, Raca R, de la Fuente L. Aspirin and prophylaxis of thromboembolic complications in patients with substitute heart valves. J Thorac Cardiovasc Surg 1976;72:127–129.

Chapter 3.2

Pharmacology of Anticoagulants

Philip A. Routledge and Hamsaraj G. M. Shetty

Since the introduction of anticoagulants for clinical use 50 years ago, effective treatment and prevention of thromboembolic diseases has saved the lives of thousands of patients. The use of anticoagulants has steadily increased because of advances in surgical management of valvular and ischaemic heart disease and perhaps also because of a greater awareness of conditions and diseases predisposing to thromboembolism.

All anticoagulants have a narrow therapeutic index (margin of safety) and therefore a knowledge of the various factors which determine the response to these drugs is necessary for safe and rational therapy. This chapter will review the mechanisms of action, pharmacokinetics, adverse effects and drug interactions of heparin and warfarin.

HEPARIN

Heparin is a water soluble mucopolysaccharide with anticoagulant properties. McLean in 1916 discovered the anticoagulant activities of heparophosphatides from liver[1]. In 1918 Howell and Holt, who extended McLean's study, extracted an anticoagulant from liver and named it heparin because of its abundance in liver[2]. Jorpes elucidated its chemistry and purification[3] and Crafoord introduced it for clinical use as an anticoagulant to prevent postoperative thrombosis[4]. The requirement of the presence of a plasma co-factor for its anticoagulant effect was recognised by Brinkhous[5]. This co-factor is now recognised to be antithrombin III. Further understanding of the structure and mechanism of action of heparin led to the introduction of low molecular weight heparins with the hope of reducing adverse effects associated with unfractionated heparin[6,7].

Porcine gut and bovine lung tissues are the main sources of commercially produced heparin. It is a complex linear polysaccharide containing alternating glucosamine and glucuronic acid residues, with forms of variable molecular weights ranging from 2,000 to 40,000 daltons (mean 15,000 daltons). The low molecular weight heparins (mean molecular weight 3,200–6,500 daltons) are prepared from naturally occurring heparin by fractionation, enzymatic degradation or chemical modification[7].

Mechanism of action[7]

Antithrombin III, a glycosylated, single chain polypeptide synthesised in the liver, inhibits coagulation factors thrombin (II), Xa, IXa, XIa, XIIa and kallikrein. Heparin increases the rate of the thrombin – antithrombin reaction about 1000 fold. Inhibition of thrombin and factor Xa account for most of the anticoagulant effect of heparin. Heparin molecules containing less than 18 monosaccharide units (3000 to 4000 daltons) do not enhance the inhibition of thrombin by antithrombin and probably act by inhibiting Xa.

In low doses heparin produces its anticoagulant effect by inhibiting Xa via antithrombin and this is the rationale for low dose, prophylactic heparin therapy. In high doses, the anticoagulant effect of heparin is partly mediated by heparin co-factor II which is homologous to antithrombin III. Heparin co-factor II inhibits thrombin only (and not other coagulation factors), and has a lower affinity for heparin than antithrombin III.

Heparin produces prolongation of activated partial thromboplastin time, thrombin time and to a lesser extent prothrombin time, through enhancement of the inhibition of thrombin and Xa by anti-thrombin. In high doses it prolongs bleeding time by inhibiting platelet aggregation (see also Chapter 3.1). Heparin clears lipaemic plasma by releasing lipoprotein lipase into the circulation and the latter then hydrolyzes triglycerides to glycerol and free fatty acids. Discontinuation of heparin may result in rebound hyperlipaemia.

Pharmacokinetics[8]

Heparin is not absorbed from the gastro-intestinal tract. It can be administered by intravenous infusion, intermittent intravenous or deep subcutaneous injections. Intravenous heparin produces an anticoagulant effect immediately, whereas subcutaneous injections result in considerable variation in bioavailability and delay in onset of action ranging from 20 to 60 minutes. The peak activity occurs in three to four hours after subcutaneous injection with both standard and low molecular weight heparins. The bioavailability of low molecular weight heparin is greater when given subcutaneously, almost 100% as against 20–30%. Increasing skin fold thickness has been shown to be associated with decreasing absorption of standard heparin, but its effect on the absorption of low molecular weight heparin is not known[10].

Heparin is highly protein bound and its volume of distribution appears to be restricted to the intravascular space. Standard heparin does not cross the placenta and does not appear in breast milk. Although there is insufficient information about the low molecular weight heparins in this regard, one of them (CY 216), has been reported not to cross the placenta[11].

The half-life of heparin ranges between one and two hours, but shows considerable inter-individual variation. This variation is as great for some of the low molecular weight heparins as for standard heparin. It has been reported that the half-life increases with increasing dose. One study has shown that the half-life increases from 56 minutes to 152 minutes when the dose of heparin is increased from 100 to 400 units/Kg[12]. The half-life of low molecular weight heparin is not dose dependent and is approximately twice as long as that of standard heparin[13]. After subcutaneous injection of low molecular weight heparins, plasma heparin concentrations can be detected for up to 24 hours. In patients with pulmonary embolism, the half-life of heparin may be shorter whereas in patients with cirrhosis of the liver or renal insufficiency it may be prolonged.

Heparin is removed from the blood either by the reticuloendothelial system and endothelial cells (a saturable mechanism, but the major clearance mechanism when low doses of unfractionated heparin are administered) or by renal excretion. Unfractionated heparin in high doses and low molecular weight heparins are mainly removed by renal excretion, which is non-saturable.

Adverse effects

Haemorrhage

The incidence of bleeding varies between 9.5 and 24 per 1000 patient days (3.46%/pty and 8.76%/pty, respectively) and severe bleeding between 3 and 5.3 per 1000 patient days (1.1%/pty and 1.9%/pty, respectively)[15–17]. The risk of bleeding appears to be increased by the presence of severe cardiac or hepatic disease, acute renal disease, poor general condition, and in women aged over 60 years. The intensity of anticoagulation also is an important risk factor, with the patients who have kaolin cephalin clotting time (KCCT) of three or more times normal having an eight-fold increase in the risk of bleeding[17]. Intermittent as against continuous intravenous administration is associated with a higher frequency of bleeding[19,20].

It was hoped that low molecular weight heparins would reduce the risk of bleeding since they produce less anti-aggregating effect on platelets and on theoretical grounds should produce less haemorrhage. Although some studies have indicated that the low molecular weight heparins are associated with a risk of bleeding similar to that of standard heparin, one recent study has claimed that low molecular weight heparins produce significantly less haemorrhagic complications when used for prevention of postoperative deep vein thrombosis[21].

Thrombocytopenia[22]

Heparin-induced thrombocytopenia (HITP) has been reported in 10% (range 0–30%) of patients receiving heparin therapy, and of these nearly 10% have been shown to develop thromboembolic complications. The route of administration and the dose of heparin do not appear to be the predisposing factors for HITP but patients receiving bovine lung heparin have been shown to have a three- to four-fold increase in the risk of developing HITP when compared with those receiving porcine intestinal mucosal heparin.

Two types of HITP occur. The first type occurs three to five days after initiation of treatment and results in platelet counts usually above 50×10^9/L. Most of these patients are asymptomatic and the platelet count often returns to normal in spite of continuation of heparin therapy. It is rarely associated with thromboembolism and is thought to be due to heparin-induced platelet aggregation.

The second type of thrombocytopenia occurs after about six days of treatment and often results in a profound decrease in platelet count. Thromboembolic complications occur in 50% of patients and these are more likely to occur when the platelet counts are lower. IgG – mediated thromboxane A_2 production resulting in platelet aggregation and consumption is thought to be the mechanism underlying this adverse effect. In patients who develop this serious form of thrombocytopenia, heparin should be discontinued. Although experience is limited, some studies have reported improvement in thrombocytopenia and reduction in thromboembolic complications after administration of low molecular weight heparins. In one patient, however, low molecular weight heparin produced a recurrence of HITP[23]. Platelet transfusions are not recommended. A prostacyclin analogue, iloprost, has been shown to prevent recurrence of HITP in patients who require reexposure to heparin[24]. Plasmapheresis has been used to treat HITP successfully in one patient[25]. Thrombolytic therapy with intravenous streptokinase has been employed to treat thrombosis and embolism secondary to HITP[26]. The overall incidence of thrombocytopenia appears to be reduced with low molecular weight heparins compared with standard heparin[27]. Although rare, heparin therapy has been occasionally associated with thrombosis in the presence of normal absolute platelet counts[28].

Osteoporosis

The incidence of heparin-induced osteoporosis is unknown. It has been reported most often in pregnant women[29]. It is recognised that osteoporosis is unlikely to occur in patients receiving less than 15,000 units of heparin per day for up to 6 months[29], but one patient receiving 5000 units of heparin twice daily for nine months has been reported to develop this adverse effect[30]. The mechanism underlying osteoporosis is unknown. Increased osteoclastic and reduced osteoblastic activity, a heparin-induced collagenase effect and abnormalities of vitamin D metabolism are some of the explanations suggested[31]. There is limited evidence that this adverse effect is reversible[32].

Other adverse effects[33]

Hypersensitivity reactions such as urticaria, conjunctivitis, bronchospasm and anaphylaxis occur rarely. Other rare adverse effects include skin necrosis, priapism and lipodystrophy[33].

WARFARIN

In the 1920s a new cattle disease causing bleeding, often fatal, appeared on the prairies of North Dakota and in Alberta, Canada. This disease was called "sweet clover disease" as its origin was traced to improperly cured feed material made from the common varieties of sweet clover (Melilotus alba and Melilotus officianalis). Veterinarians Schofield and Roderick recognised that the disease was reversible and the latter, after a thorough study of the disease, concluded that the coagulation defect was due to a "prothrombin deficit". Link and his associates were successful in isolating the haemorrhagic agent, dicoumarol, from the improperly cured sweet clover hay[34]. A number of new coumarins were synthesised in Link's laboratory (Fig. 3.2–1). Of these, coumarin no. 42, was 5–10 times more effective than dicoumarol, and Link named it warfarin (for the Wisconsin Alumni Research Foundation). Warfarin sodium was investigated in man by Shapiro and it was introduced for clinical use as an anticoagulant in the late 1940s. The transformation of a 'cow poison' to a 'rat poison' and then to one of the most useful and widely used drugs in humans is one of the most fascinating stories in the annals of clinical pharmacology[34].

Warfarin is a racemic mixture of two optical isomers, R- and S-warfarin, as it has an asymmetrical carbon at the 3- position. Racemic warfarin is usually administered as the sodium salt which is highly water soluble.

Mechanism of action[35]

Warfarin acts by inducing a functional deficiency of reduced vitamin K, the active hydroxyquinone form of vitamin K. Factors II, VII, IX and X are dependent on reduced

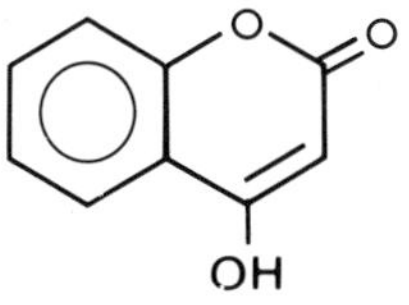

4 - HYDROXY COUMARIN

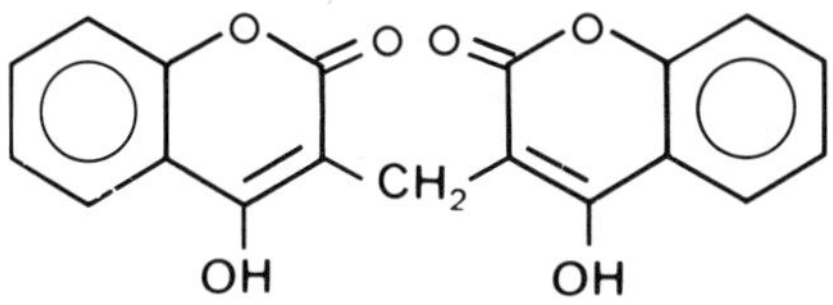

DI COUMAROL

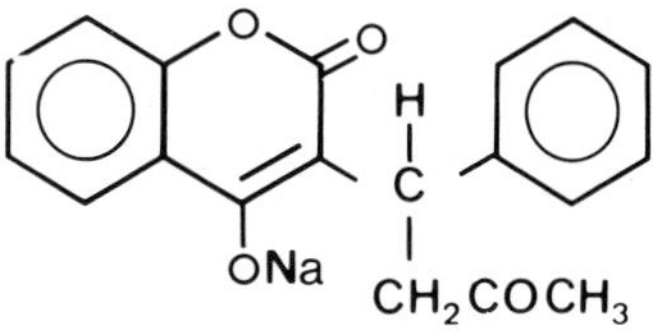

WARFARIN SODIUM

Figure 3.2–1 Chemical structure of coumarin anticoagulants

vitamin K for carboxylation of ten or more glutamic acid residues at their amino-terminal ends by a microsomal enzyme, carboxylase. This carboxylation is necessary for their normal synthesis. It also endows them with their biological activity by conferring upon them the ability to bind calcium, which in turn enables them to bind to phospholipid-containing membranes. The carboxylation reaction is coupled to an epoxidase of vitamin K which catalyses the oxidation of reduced vitamin K to inactive vitamin K epoxide. An epoxide reductase regenerates the active form of vitamin K (reduced vitamin K) with reduced nicotinamide adenine dinucleotide (NADH) as a co-factor. This step is blocked by warfarin and other anticoagulants of coumarin type, resulting in a functional deficiency of reduced vitamin K (Fig. 3.2–2). S-warfarin is at least five times more potent than R-warfarin in this regard.

In therapeutic doses, warfarin decreases the synthesis of factors II, VII, IX and X by 30 to 50% and reduces the biological activity of these factors to 10 to 40% of normal. It has no effect on fully carboxylated factors II, VII, IX and X and therefore does not produce an immediate anticoagulant effect. The delay in the onset of the anticoagulant effect is dependent on the rate of clearance of the fully carboxylated factors and the time required for the undercarboxylated factors to reach a new steady state. The half-life of factor VII is approximately six hours, factor IX, 24 hours, factor X, 36 hours and factor II, 50 hours.

Pharmacokinetics[36,37]

Absorption

Warfarin sodium, when given orally, is completely absorbed from the stomach and

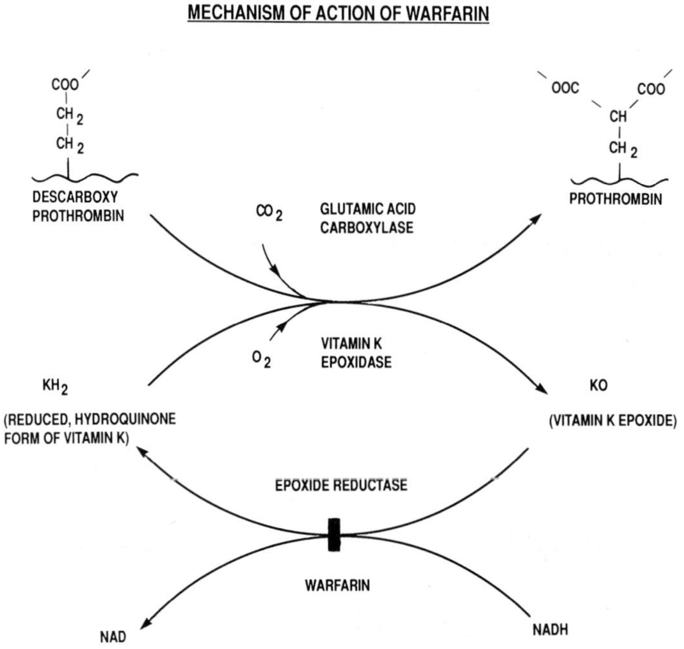

Figure 3.2–2 Mechanism of action of warfarin

proximal small intestine and is 100% bioavailable[38]. Peak plasma concentration occurs between 0.3 and four hours. Food decreases the rate but not the extent of absorption[39]. Because of complete absorption from the stomach and proximal small intestine, resistance to treatment due to decreased absorption is rare and has not been observed even in patients who have had extensive ileal resection[40]. Selective malabsorption of warfarin, in the absence of clinical and biochemical evidence of malabsorption, has been reported to be associated with the articular form of Danlos' syndrome[41]. Cholestyramine binds to warfarin in the gut and produces resistance to warfarin, in part by impairing absorption. This interaction can be reduced by administering the two drugs 3 to 6 hours apart[42]. Resistance to warfarin due to impaired absorption has also been reported in patients with malabsorption syndromes and with concurrent administration of liquid paraffin laxatives and excessive amounts of antacids such as magnesium trisilicate (See also Table 3.2-1).

Distribution

Warfarin is highly protein bound (99%), binding almost entirely to albumin[43]. The apparent volume of distribution ranges between 7.6 L and 13.9 L in an adult[44,45]. The volumes of distribution of R and S enantiomers are similar[46]. Warfarin crosses the placental barrier[47] but is secreted into breast milk in trace amounts insufficient to have a measurable anticoagulant effect in infants breast-fed by mothers receiving the drug[48].

As warfarin is highly albumin bound, it might be expected that the free fraction would increase in hypoalbuminaemic states. It has been shown that this does indeed occur, together with an increase in the rate of clearance and a shortening of the half-life in idiopathic hypoalbuminaemia[49]. Similarly in hypoalbuminaemia associated with the nephrotic syndrome, a twofold increase in free fraction and a threefold increase in clearance has been observed[50]. These changes, however, were not associated with major changes in anticoagulant response.

Protein binding is decreased in patients with chronic renal failure[51] and this may result in a transient increase in sensitivity to warfarin, but not at steady state. Drugs displacing warfarin from its binding sites could theoretically increase the sensitivity to the drug, but only temporarily and the significance of this effect has probably been overstated.

Metabolism

Warfarin is metabolised by the cytochrome P450 enzyme system in the liver[52], and only small traces of the unmetabolised drug appear in urine. The average rate of clearance from plasma is 0.2 litre/hour/70 Kg[53]. The half-life ranges from 20 to 60 hours (mean 40 hours). It therefore takes about a week for steady state to be reached and relatively little fluctuation occurs in plasma concentration during the daily dosing interval. The duration of action ranges between two and five days.

R and S warfarin exhibit substrate stereospecificity and are metabolised by different pathways. R warfarin is mainly metabolised by reduction of the acetyl side chain into secondary warfarin alcohols that are excreted via the kidneys. S warfarin, on the other hand, is metabolised by oxidation of the coumarin ring to 7-hydroxy-s-warfarin which is excreted mainly by the liver into the bile and stool[54]. The half-life of R-warfarin is longer than that of S-warfarin[36].

In patients with hepatic impairment, decreased metabolism of warfarin and decreased synthesis of coagulation factors may result in increased sensitivity to the drug. The increased sensitivity of the elderly to warfarin is probably due to pharmacodynamic factors[55], but one study has shown a slightly decreased clearance of racemic drug in this age group[56]. Short term administration of alcohol results in a decrease in factors II, VII and X, and it presumably increases warfarin sensitivity[57]. However, meal time wine (20oz. daily) has been found to have no effect on the sensitivity to warfarin[58]. Chronic cigarette smoking, which may induce oxidative enzymes, has no apparent effect on warfarin metabolism[59].

Inhibition of the P450 microsomal enzyme system by concomitantly administered drugs may reduce warfarin metabolism and thus enhance drug effect. This effect may be stereoselective in the case of some drugs[54,59]. The induction of microsomal enzymes by certain drugs may enhance the metabolism of warfarin and diminish drug effect. Drugs which induce or inhibit microsomal enzymes and thereby interact with warfarin are listed in Table 3.2-1.

Excretion

Warfarin is almost totally cleared by hepatic metabolism and the metabolites are excreted through the kidney. These metabolites have very low anticoagulant effect and

Table 3.2–1

Interactions of Drugs with Warfarin

1. Potentiation of anticoagulant effect:

i) BY INHIBITION OF MICROSOMAL ENZYMES: The enantiomer whose metabolism is inhibited is indicated in parentheses when known.

Allopurinol	Disulfiram	Metronidazole (S)
Amiodarone (S,R)	Enoxacin (R)	Omeprazole (R)
Azapropazone (S)	Erythromycin	Oxyphenbutazone (S)
Cimetidine (R)	Fluconazole	Phenylbutazone (S)
Ciprofloxacin	Fluvoxamine	Sulphinpyrazone
Co-trimoxazole (S)	Ketoconazole	Sulphonamides

ii) DECREASED AVAILABILITY OF VITAMIN K:

Aminoglycoside antibiotics	Tetracyclines
Cephalosporins	

iii) INCREASED CATABOLISM OF VITAMIN K DEPENDENT FACTORS:
Thyroid compounds

iv) MECHANISM UNKNOWN:

Acetyl salicyclic acid (>1.5 Gm/day)	Flurbiprofen	Nalidixic acid
Aminosalicyclic acid	Gemfibrozil	Norfloxacin
Anabolic steroids and androgens	Glucagon	Ofloxacin
Azapropazone	Ifosamide/Mesna	Phenytoin
Bezafibrate	Indomethacin	Quinidine
Chloramphenicol	Isoniazid	Sulindac
Clofibrate	Itraconazole	Tamoxifen
Danazol	Lovastatin	Topical Salicylates
Diflunisal	Mefenamic acid	Vitamin E
Disopyramide	Miconazole	

2. Diminution of Anticoagulant Effect

i) BY INDUCTION OF MICROSOMAL ENZYMES:

Aminoglutethimide	Carbamazepine
Barbiturates/Primidone	Gintethimide
	Rifampicin

ii) BY DECREASING ABSORPTION AND/OR INTERRUPTION OF ENTEROHEPATIC CIRCULATION:

Cholestyramine	Colestipol

iii) DUE TO INCREASED AVAILABILITY OF VITAMIN K:
Nutritional preparations eg: Parenteral feeds

iv) DUE TO DECREASED CATABOLISM OF VITAMIN K-DEPENDENT FACTORS:

Carbimazole	Thiouracils

v) DUE TO INCREASED SYNTHESIS OF CLOTTING FACTORS:
Oestrogens

vi) MECHANISM UNKNOWN:

Griseofulvin	6-Mercaptopurine
Haloperidol	Phenytoin (may also potentiate)

therefore impairment of renal function is unlikely to alter significantly their pharmacokinetics or effects[51]. Age-related decline in renal function has no effect on warfarin sensitivity.

Pharmacodynamic factors affecting response to warfarin[37]

Genetic factors

It has been observed that the variance of warfarin half-life is much greater in fraternal than in identical twins[60]. Warfarin resistance, inherited as an autosomal dominant trait, is associated with normal pharmacokinetics but a marked increase in the requirement of vitamin K has been described[61].

Vitamin K excess or deficiency

Dietary deficiency is a rare cause of increased sensitivity to warfarin, and may occur in the presence of small bowel disease. In patients who have dietary deficiency of vitamin K, broad spectrum oral antibiotics which deplete intestinal bacterial sources of vitamin K, may increase the sensitivity to warfarin. Alpha-tocopherol in large doses antagonises the action of vitamin K and may increase the sensitivity to warfarin[62]. Surreptitious intake of vitamin K in the form of health foods[63] or weight-reducing diets[64] has been reported to be associated with warfarin resistance. Similarly enteral feeds containing large amounts of phytomenadione (vitamin K_1) have also been shown to cause resistance to warfarin[65].

Variations in the levels of vitamin K dependent clotting factors

In the presence of liver disease, the synthesis of vitamin K-dependent clotting factors may be decreased, and this may result in increased sensitivity to warfarin. In hyperthyroid patients, the rate of decay of vitamin K-dependent factors is increased up to threefold. Warfarin therapy in such patients results in a greater fall in factors II and VIII, and an increase in sensitivity to the drug[66].

Investigation of patients with abnormal response to warfarin

Poor compliance, kinetic resistance, kinetic sensitivity, tissue resistance or tissue sensitivity may all cause an abnormal response to warfarin therapy. A recent study using algorithms to correlate plasma warfarin concentration and plasma warfarin clearance with the patient's International Normalised Ratio (INR), has described a method to identify the cause of abnormal warfarin responsiveness[67].

Adverse effects of warfarin[33]

Haemorrhage[33,68]

Warfarin therapy may be associated with bleeding due to a predisposing condition such as peptic ulcer, tumour, severe liver damage, an endogenous coagulation disturbance, thrombocytopenia or severe hypertension. Excessive anticoagulation due to poorly controlled treatment or a drug interaction enhancing the effect of warfarin may also result in haemorrhage. However bleeding may occur even when anticoagulation is not excessive.

Major bleeding has been reported in 4.4 to 8.2% of patients on warfarin. The risk of anticoagulant related death may be as high as 9% per year in elderly patients anticoagulated at the higher levels used in North America[71]. The incidence of bleeding increases with increasing duration of anticoagulant therapy: 1% at six months, 5% at one year, 7% at two and three years[72]. The risk is higher when the prothrombin time is prolonged beyond the therapeutic range[70] and in patients anticoagulated for cerebrovascular disease[71]. Age and sex do not appear to have any effect on the incidence of haemorrhage[69,73]. Although bleeding can occur in any part of the body, life-threatening haemorrhages are usually gastrointestinal or intracranial (see also Chapter 5.4).

Skin reactions[33]

Purpura and ecchymoses are common and pruritic, macular, papular, vesicular or urticarial lesions occur occasionally. A small proportion, 0.01 to 1% of patients develop potentially fatal skin infarction, mostly between the third and sixth days of treatment[74]. Obese, middle aged women are particularly prone to this adverse effect, and the infarction usually occurs in fatty tissues such as breasts, buttocks and thighs[74]. Histopathological examination of the involved areas shows thrombus in the dermal capillaries and vessels, coagulation necrosis and haemorrhage. The vessel walls, perivascular tissues and the arteries are generally not affected[74]. The aetiology of skin infarction is unknown. A number of pathophysiological mechanisms have been suggested, including hypersensitivity, thrombosis, haemorrhage, factor VII deficiency, protein C deficiency and a direct toxic effect of warfarin[74].

Protein C is an inhibitor of coagulation, as it inactivates activated factors V and VIII. It also facilitates fibrinolysis in vivo. Warfarin therapy results in a decreased production of protein C which is vitamin K-dependent. As protein C levels fall more rapidly than those of factors IX, X and prothrombin, a temporary hypercoagulable state results. This hypercoagulable state, which reaches a maximum by the second or third day of warfarin therapy, is thought to be the cause of skin necrosis[75]. One study has shown that protein C deficient patients are likely to be predisposed to warfarin skin necrosis. Eleven out of 13 patients in this study who had warfarin necrosis were found to have protein C levels ranging from 23 to 69% after they had recovered from the necrosis and when they were not on warfarin[76]. In patients who develop skin necrosis, warfarin should be discontinued, vitamin K given and heparin used instead[74]. It has been suggested that avoidance of large loading doses and overlapping of heparin and warfarin therapy for three to four days may reduce the risk of skin necrosis[74].

Adverse effect on foetus

If given in the first trimester of pregnancy, warfarin may cause chondrodysplasia punctata (characterised by 'punched out' lesions in ossification centres) and absence of the spleen. The incidence of embryopathy is less than 5%[77,78]. Irrespective of the stage of pregnancy, warfarin therapy has been reported to cause microcephaly, optic atrophy, cranial nerve palsies, and hydrocephalus[79]. A high rate of spontaneous abortion has also been described with warfarin therapy but the condition for which the patient is receiving anticoagulant therapy may also be contributory in some cases (see also Chapter 4.1).

Other adverse effects[33]

Hypersensitivity reactions (for example vasculitic skin lesions), fever, vomiting, nausea, diarrhoea, alopecia, priapism, eosinophilia, feeling of coldness, cholesterol embolism, hepatic cell necrosis and cholestatic jaundice are all rare adverse effects of warfarin.

Drug interactions[80–90]

A number of drugs interact with warfarin and result in either enhancement or diminution of its anticoagulant effect. Table 3.2-1 lists the drugs interacting with warfarin and the mechanisms involved. Some drugs may interact by more than one mechanism.

CONCLUSION

Anticoagulants are potentially life-saving drugs in many clinical situations. However, because of their narrow therapeutic index they can also cause potentially serious haemorrhagic complications. A thorough knowledge of pharmacokinetic and pharmacodynamic factors affecting the response to these drugs and careful monitoring of anticoagulant therapy (Chapter 3.3) are the cornerstones of optimal anticoagulant therapy.

REFERENCES

1. McLean. The thromboplastic action of cephalin. Am J Physiol 1916;41:250–257.
2. Howell WH. Heparin, an anticoagulant: preliminary communication. Am J Physiol. 1922;63:434–435.
3. Jorpes JE. The chemistry of heparin. Biochem J 1935;29:1817–1830.
4. Crafoord C. Preliminary report on post-operative treatment with heparin as a preventive of thrombosis. Acta Chir Scand 1937;79:407- 426.
5. Brinkhous KM, Smith HP, Warner ED, Seegers WH. The inhibition of blood clotting: an unidentified substance which acts in conjunction with heparin to prevent the conversion of prothrombin to thrombin. Am J Physiol 1939;125:683–687.
6. Kakkar VV, Djazqeri B, Fox J, Fletcher M, Scully MF, Westwick J. Low molecular weight heparin and prevention of post-operative deep vein thrombosis. Br Med J 1982;284:375–379.
7. Fareed J. Heparin, its fractions, fragments and derivatives. Some newer perspectives. Semin Thromb Hemost 1985;11:1–9.
8. Jackson CM. Mechanism of heparin action. Baill Clin Haematol 1990;3:483–504.
9. Boneu B, Caranobe C, Sie P. Pharmacokinetics of heparin and low molecular weight heparin. Baill Clin Haematol 1990;3:531–544.
10. Kroon C, De Boer A, Kroon JM, Schoenmaker HC, Vd Meer FJM, Cohen AF. Influence of skin fold thickness on heparin absorption. Lancet 1991;337:945–946.
11. Forestier F, Daffos F, Rainaut M, Toulemonde F. Low molecular weight heparin (C Y 216) does not cross the placenta during the third trimester of pregnancy. Thromb Haemost 1987;57:234(abstract).
12. Olsson P, Lagergren H, Ek S. The elimination from plasma of intravenous heparin. An experimental study on dogs and humans. Acta Med Scand 1963;173:619–630.
13. Bratt G, Törnbohm E, Lockner D, Bergström K. A human pharmacological study comparing conventional heparin and a low molecular weight heparin fragment. Thromb Haemost 1985;53:208–211.
14. De Swart CAM, Nijmeyer B, Roelofs JMM, Sixma JJ. Kinetics of intravenously administered heparin in normal humans. Blood. 1982;60:1251–1258.

15. Basu D, Gallus A, Hirsh J, Cade J. A prospective study of the value of monitoring heparin treatment with the activated partial thromboplstic time. N Engl J Med 1972;287:324–327.
16. Walker AMJ, Jick H. Predictors of bleeding during heparin therapy. JAMA. 1980;244:1209–1212.
17. Landefeld CS, Cook EF, Flatley M, Weisberg M, Goldman L. Identification and preliminary validation of predictors of major bleeding in hospitalized patients starting anticoagulant therapy. Am J Med 1987;82:703–713.
18. Jick H, Slone D, Borda IT, Shapiro S. Efficacy and toxicity of heparin in relation to age and sex. N Engl J Med 1968;279:284–286.
19. Mant MJ, O'Brien BD, Thong KL, Hammond GW, Birthwistle RV, Grace MG. Haemorrhagic complications of heparin therapy. Lancet 1977;1:1133–1135.
20. Glazier RL, Crowell EB. Randomized prospective trial of continuous vs intermittent heparin therapy. JAMA 1976;236:1365–1367.
21. Levine M, Hirsh J, Gent M, et al. Prevention of deep vein thrombosis after elective hip surgery. A randomized trial comparing low molecular weight heparin with standard unfractionated heparin. Ann Intern Med 1991;114:545–551.
22. Becker SP, Miller VT. Heparin-induced thrombocytopaenia. Stroke 1989;20:1449–1459.
23. Copplestone A, Oscier DG. Heparin-induced thrombocytopaenia in pregnancy. Br J Haematol 1987;65:248(abstract).
24. Addonizio VP Jr, Fisher CA, Kappa JR, Ellison N. Prevention of heparin-induced thrombocytopaenia during open heart surgery with iloprost (ZK 36374). Surgery 1987;102:796–807.
25. Vender JS, Mathew EB, Silverman IM, Konowitz H, Dau PC. Heparin- associated thrombocytopaenia: Alternative managements. Anaesth Analg 1986;65:520–522.
26. Mehta DP, Yder EL, Appel J, Bergsman KL. Heparin-induced thrombocytopaenia and thrombosis: reversal with streptokinase. A case report and review of literature. Am J Haematol 1991;36:275–279.
27. Mammen E. Why low molecular weight heparin? Semin Thromb Haemostas 1990;16(Suppl):1–4.
28. Phelan BK. Heparin-associated thrombosis without thrombocytopaenia. Ann Intern Med 1983;99:637–638.
29. Ginsberg JS, Hirsh J. Use of anticoagulants during pregnancy. Chest 1989;95:1565–1605.
30. Griffiths HT, Liv DTY. Severe heparin osteoporosis in pregnancy. Postgrad Med J 1984;60:424–425.
31. Avioli LV. Heparin-induced osteoporosis: an appraisal. Adv Exp Med Biol 1975;52:375–387.
32. Zimran A, Shilo S, Fisher D, Bob I. Histomorphometric evaluation of reversible heparin-induced osteoporosis in pregnancy. Arch Intern Med 1986;164:386–388.
33. Shetty HGM, Fennerty AG, Routledge PA. Adverse effects of anticoagulants. Adverse Drug Reactions Bulletin 1989;137:512–515.
34. Link KP. The discovery of dicoumarol and its sequels. Circulation 1959;19:97–107.
35. Suttie JW. The biochemical basis of warfarin therapy. Adv Exp Med Biol 1987;214:3–16.
36. Holford NHG. Clinical pharmacokinetics and pharmacodynamics of warfarin: understanding the dose-effect relationship. Clin Pharmacokinet 1986;11:483–504.
37. Shetty HGM, Fennerty AG, Routledge PA. Clinical pharmacokinetic considerations in the control of oral anticoagulant therapy. Clin Pharmacokinet 1989;16:238–253.
38. Deykin D. Warfarin therapy. N Engl J Med 1970;283:691–694, 801- 803.
39. Majerus PW, Broze GJ, Miletich JP, Tollefsen DM. Anticoagulant, thrombolytic and antiplatelet drugs. In Goodman Gilman A, Rall TW, Nies AS, Taylor P (Eds). The Pharmacological Basis of Therapeutics. 8th ed. New York: Pergamon Press 1990;1311–1331.
40. Kearns Jr PR, O'Reilly RA. Bioavailability of warfarin in a patient with severe short bowel syndrome. J Parenteral Enteral Nutr 1986;10:100–101.
41. Lefrere J, Guynon F, Horellou M, Conard J, Samama M. Selective malabsorption of anticoagulants. JAMA 1986;256:595.
42. Robinson DS, Benjamin DM, McCormack JJ. Interaction of warfarin and non-systemic gastrointestinal drugs. Clin Pharmacol Ther 1971;12:492–495.
43. O'Reilly RA. The binding of sodium warfarin to plasma albumin and its displacement by phenylbutazone. Ann NY Acad Sci 1973;226:293–308.
44. Slattery JT, Levy G, Jain A, McMahon FG. Effect of naproxen on the kinetics of elimination of and anticoagulant activity of a single dose of warfarin. Clin Pharmacol Ther 1979;25:51–60.
45. Toon S, Hopkins KJ, Garstang FM, Digret B, Rowland M. The warfarin-cimetidine interaction: stereo chemical considerations. Br J Clin Pharmacol 1986;21:245–246.
46. Hignite C, Uetrecht J, Tschariz C, Azarnoff D. Kinetics of R and S warfarin enantiomers. Clin Pharmacol Ther 1980;28:99–105.
47. Hall JG. Warfarin and foetal abnormality. Lancet 1976;1:1127.
48. L'e Orme M, Lewis PJ, de Swiet M, Serlin MJ, Sibeon R, Baty JD. May mothers given warfarin breast-feed their infants? Br Med J 1977;1:1564–1565.

49. Piroli RJ, Passananti GT, Shively CA, Vessel ES. Antipyrine and warfarin disposition in a patient with idiopathic hypoalbuminaemia. Clin Pharmacol Ther 1981;30:810–816.
50. Ganeval D, Fischer AM, Barre J, Pertuiset N, Dautzenberg MD. Pharmacokinetics of warfarin in nephrotic syndrome and effect on vitamin K-dependent clotting factors. Clin Nephrol 1986;25:75–80.
51. Aggeler PM, O'Reilly RA. Pharmacological basis of oral anticoagulant therapy. Thromb Diath Haemorrhag 1966;21(Suppl):227–256.
52. Brodie BB. Of mice, microsomes and man. Pharmacologist 1964;6:12- 26.
53. Andreasen P, Vessel E. Comparison of plasma levels of antipyrine, tolbutamide and warfarin after oral and intravenous administration. Clin Pharmacol Ther 1974;16:1059–1065.
54. Lewis RJ, Trager WF, Chan KK, et al. Warfarin: stereochemical aspects of its metabolism and the interaction with phenylbutazone. J Clin Invest 1974;53:1607–1617.
55. Routledge PA, Chapman PH, Davies DM, Rawlins MD. Factors affecting warfarin requirements – a prospective population study. Eur J Clin Pharmacol 1979;15:319–322.
56. Shepherd AMM, Hewick DS, Moreland TA, Stevenson IH. Age as a determinant of sensitivity to warfarin. Br J Clin Pharmacol 1977;4:315–320.
57. Reidler G. Einfluss des Alkohoh auf die antikoagulantien Therapie. Thromb Diath Haemorrh 1966;16:613(abstract).
58. O'Reilly RA. Lack of effect of fortified wine ingested during fasting and anticoagulant therapy. Arch Intern Med 1981;141:458–459.
59. Choonara I, Cholerton S, Hayes B, Breckenridge A, Park BK. Stereoselective interaction between R enantiomer of warfarin and cimetidine. Br J Clin Pharmacol 1986;21:271–277.
60. Vessel ES, Page JG. Genetic control of dicoumarol levels in man. J Clin Invest 1968;47:2657–2663.
61. O'Reilly RA. Vitamin K in hereditary resistance to oral anticoagulant drugs. Am J Physiol 1971;221:1327–1330.
62. Corrigan Jr JJ. The effect of vitamin E on warfarin induced vitamin K deficiency. Ann NY Acad Sci 1982;393:361–368.
63. O'Reilly RA, Rytand DA. 'Resistance' to warfarin due to unrecognised vitamin K supplementation. N Engl J Med 1980;303:361–368.
64. Qureshi GD, Reinders TP, Swint JJ, Slate MB. Acquired warfarin resistance and weight-reducing diet. Arch Intern Med 1981;141:507- 509.
65. Watson AJM, Pegg M, Green JRB. Enteral feeds may antagonise warfarin. Br Med J 1984;288:557.
66. Kellett HA, Sawers JSA, Boulton FE, Cholerton S, Park BK, Toft AD. Problems of anticoagulation with warfarin in hyperthyroidism. Quart J Med 1986;58:43–51.
67. Bentley DP, Backhouse G, Hutchings A, Haddon RL, Spragg B, Routledge PA. Investigation of patients with abnormal response to warfarin. Br J Clin Pharmacol 1986;22:37–41.
68. Levine MN, Raskob G, Hirsh J. Risk of haemorrhage associated with long term anticoagulant therapy. Drugs 1985;30:444–460.
69. Gurwitz JH, Goldberg RJ, Holden A, Knapic A, Ansell J. Age-related risks of long-term oral anticoagulant therapy. Arch Intern Med 1988;48:1733–1736.
70. Forfar JC. A 7 year analysis of haemorrhage in patients on long- term anticoagulant treatment. Br Heart J 1979;42:128–132.
71. Levine MN, Raskob G, Hirsh J. Risk of haemorrhage associated with long-term anticoagulant therapy in elderly patients after myocardial infarction. Chest 1989;95(Suppl):26S–36S.
72. Petty GW, Lennihan L, Mohr JP, Hauser WA, Weitz J, Owen J, Towey C. Complications of long-term anticoagulation. Ann Neurol 1988;23:570–574.
73. Sixty-plus Reinfarction Study Research Group: Risks of long-term oral anticoagulant therapy in elderly patients after myocardial infarction. Lancet 1982;1:64–68.
74. Cole MS, Minifee PK, Wolma FJ. Coumarin necrosis – a review of literature. Surgery 1988;103:271–276.
75. McGehee WG, Klotz TA, Epstein DJ, Rapaport SI. Coumarin necrosis associated with hereditary protein C deficiency. Ann Intern Med 1984;100:59–60.
76. Rose VL, Kwaan HC, Williamson K, Hoppensteadt D, Walenga J, Fareed J. Protein C deficiency and warfarin necrosis. Ann J Clin Pathol 1986;86:653.
77. Stevenson R, Burton M, Farlanto GJ, Taylor HA. Hazards of oral anticoagulants during pregnancy. JAMA 1980;243:1549–1551.
78. Cox DR, Martin L, Hall BD. Asplenia syndrome after foetal exposure to warfarin. Lancet 1977;2:1134.
79. Holzgreve W, Carey JC, Hall BD. Warfarin-induced fetal abnormalities. Lancet 1976;ii:914–915.
80. Serlin MJ, Breckenridge AM. Drug interaction with warfarin. Drugs 1983;25:610–620.
81. Littleton Jr F. Warfarin and topical salicylates. JAMA 1990;263:2888.
82. Yip ASB, Chow WH, Tai YT, Cheng KL. Adverse effect of topical methylsalicylate ointment on warfarin anticoagulation: an unrecognised potential hazard. Postgrad Med J 1990;66:367–369.
83. Hall G, Lind MJ, Huang M, et al. Intravenous infusions of ifosfamide/mensa and perturbation of warfarin anticoagulant control. Postgrad Med J 1990;66:860–861.

84. Linville T, Matanin D. Norfloxacin and warfarin. Ann Intern Med 1989;110:751–752.
85. Mott FE, Murphy S, Hunt V. Ciprofloxacin and warfarin. Ann Intern Med 1989;111:542–543.
86. Baciewicz AM, Morgan PJ. Ranitidine-warfarin interaction. Ann Intern Med 1990;112:76–77.
87. Leor J, Matetzki S. Ofloxacin and warfarin. Ann Intern Med 1988;109:761.
88. Ahmad S. Lovastatin-warfarin interaction. Arch Intern Med 1990;150:2407.
89. Yeh J, Soo S, Summerton C, Richardson C. Potentiation of warfarin by itraconazole. Br Med J 1990;301:669.
90. Toon S, Hopkins KJ, Garstang FM, Aarons L, Sedman A, Rowland M. Enoxacin-warfarin interaction: pharmacokinetic and stereochemical aspects. Clin Pharmacol Ther 1987; 42: 33–41

Chapter 3.3

Standardisation of Oral Anticoagulation Measurement and Management

Antonias M. H. P. van den Besselaar and Felix J. M. van der Meer.

Antithrombotic treatment with coumarin drugs must be monitored carefully. On the one hand, there is a minimal level below which anticoagulants fail to achieve satisfactory results[1], and on the other, the risk of bleeding increases with the intensity of anticoagulation[2]. The required minimal therapeutic level depends on the origin of the thromboembolic process and different target ranges have been recommended for various clinical states. At present, full international consensus on the therapeutic target ranges has not yet been achieved, though considerable progress has been made in recent years for most clinical conditions with the notable exception of prosthetic heart valves[3,4,5](see Chapter 3.4).

The prothrombin time (PT) is the primary measurement of monitoring of oral anticoagulant treatment. The prothrombin time, originally described by Quick and co-workers[6], is based on the tissue factor pathway of blood coagulation. The result of the PT test is strongly dependent on the nature of the tissue extract (thromboplastin) and the method used. Many modifications of the original Quick test have been applied for monitoring of oral anticoagulant treatment. In an attempt to standardise the PT test, results were initially expressed as percentage prothrombin activity. However, the percentage prothrombin activity read from a curve based on dilutions of normal plasma in saline was still dependent on the tissue extract used for the PT test[7]. Similarly, the expression of the PT as a ratio (patient's PT divided by the mean normal PT) depended strongly on the modification used.

The multiplicity of modifications of the PT test has contributed to the confusion about the optimum therapeutic target levels of oral anticoagulation[8]. The confusion could only be resolved with the introduction of an international standardisation system established by the World Health Organisation (WHO) and recommended by the International Committee for Standardisation in Haematology (ICSH) and the Scientific and Standardisation Committee of the International Society on Thrombosis and Haemostasis[9,10]. This system led to the definition of the International Normalised Ratio (INR), which should now be regarded as the recommended universal scale for intensity of oral anticoagulation (vide infra).

The quality of oral anticoagulant treatment is determined not only by the quality of laboratory measurements, but also by the physician's skill in dosage regulation, patient education, and last but not least, the organisational framework of patient management. Therapeutic quality assessment is an essential part of the control of oral anticoagulation treatment.

INTERNATIONAL STANDARDISATION

International standardisation of the PT could be achieved by relating any given test system to an established primary standard reference method. In 1977, a research standard prepared by the International Committee on Thrombosis and Haemostasis in collaboration with the National Institute of Biological Standards and Control (NIBSC) in London, was established by the WHO as the primary international reference preparation (IRP) for thromboplastin[11]. This material, coded 67/40, was prepared from human brain supplemented with adsorbed bovine plasma (combined reagent) and was to be used according to meticulously defined instructions[12].

A further advance in standardisation was the development of a model for the calibration of any PT test system in terms of the primary IRP, as proposed by Kirkwood[13]. In this model, a linear relationship was hypothesised between the logarithms of PTs obtained with the primary IRP method and the logarithms of PTs obtained with the test system (Fig. 3.3–1). Furthermore, the model required that a

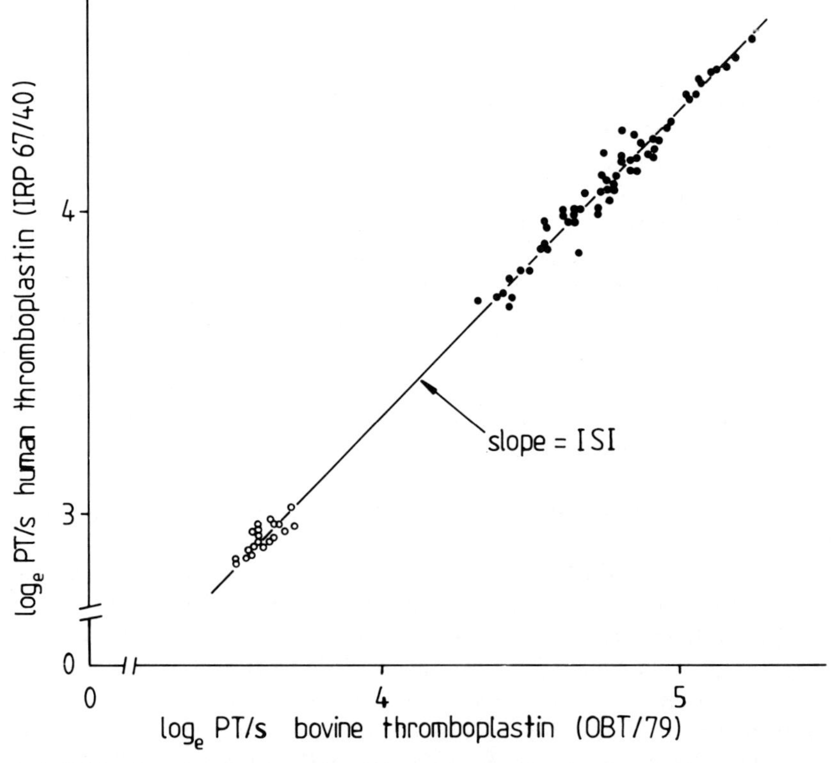

Figure 3.3–1: Calibration plot of the secondary reference preparation for thromboplastin, bovine, combined (coded OBT/79) against the primary International Reference Preparation (coded 67/40). The natural logarithms of the prothrombin times (PT) with the secondary preparation (OBT/79) are plotted along the horizontal axis and the natural logarithms of the PTs with the primary IRP are plotted along the vertical axis. Healthy individuals are represented by white circles and patients on stabilised oral anticoagulant treatment by black circles. The calibration line is calculated by orthogonal regression analysis. The ISI of the secondary preparation is the slope of the regression line. The data were obtained from the collaborative study for the calibration of secondary reference preparations[14].

single relationship be valid for fresh plasma specimens of normal individuals and fresh specimens of patients on stabilised oral anticoagulant treatment:

$$\log PT_{67/40} = a + c. \log PT_{test} \quad \text{(Equation 1)}$$

in which a and c are the intercept and slope of the calibration line, respectively. The model leads to a simple equation to transform a PT ratio (R = patient PT: mean normal PT) obtained with the working PT system into the PT ratio which would have been obtained had the primary IRP 67/40 been used:

$$R_{67/40} = R^{ISI} \quad \text{(Equation 2)}$$

in which ISI is the *international sensitivity index* of the working system. The ISI is equal to the slope c. $R_{67/40}$ is usually called the *international normalised ratio* (INR). The INR is the universal scale to express the PT for oral anticoagulant control. This calibration model was tested successfully in an international collaborative exercise organised by the European Community Bureau of Reference (BCR) and ICSH[14]. Consequently, this model was adopted by WHO[9].

Calibrations of other thromboplastins have been carried out in accordance with the WHO model[15–21]. However, the WHO model is empirical and for a particular

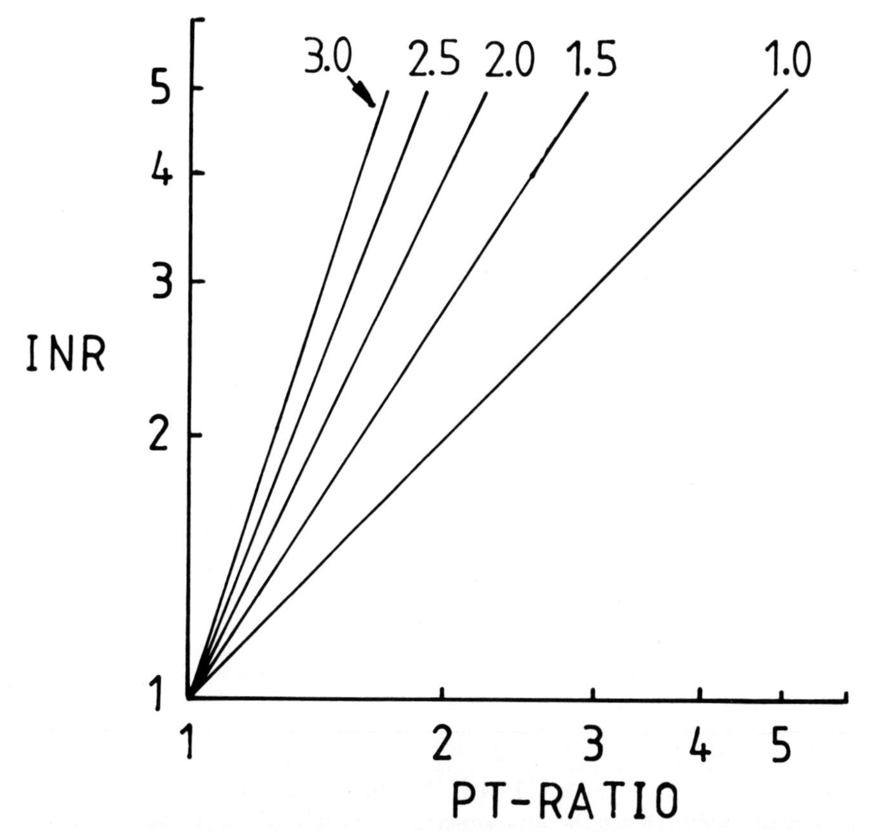

Figure 3.3–2: Relationships between PT ratio and INR for thromboplastins with different ISI. ISI values are shown with each line of relationship. Note that the scales are logarithmic.

combination of thromboplastins, a significant deviation from the model has been observed although a modified model could account for the experimental calibration data[22,23].

It is the thromboplastin manufacturers' responsibility to provide the calibration data for each batch of their material[10]. This can be done either by reporting an ISI value or providing a table in which the relationship between clotting time (ratio), percentage activity and INR is given.

If an anticoagulant clinic wants to report INR values for their patients but does not have a calculator with a power function (Equation 2), the measured PT ratio can be transformed to INR by means of a graph specific for the ISI of the reagent used (Fig. 3.3–2). ISI values of rabbit tissue thromboplastins on the North American market range between about 1.7 and 2.8. Clearly, reporting of a PT ratio obtained with a North American rabbit thromboplastin is not adequate unless the ISI of the reagent is reported as well.

The relationship between INR and the percentage prothrombin activity measured with Quick's rabbit brain thromboplastin is shown in Figure 3.3–3. For comparison, the relationship between INR and percentage Thrombotest activity is also given. At a given intensity of anticoagulation (INR), the percentage Thrombotest activity is always lower

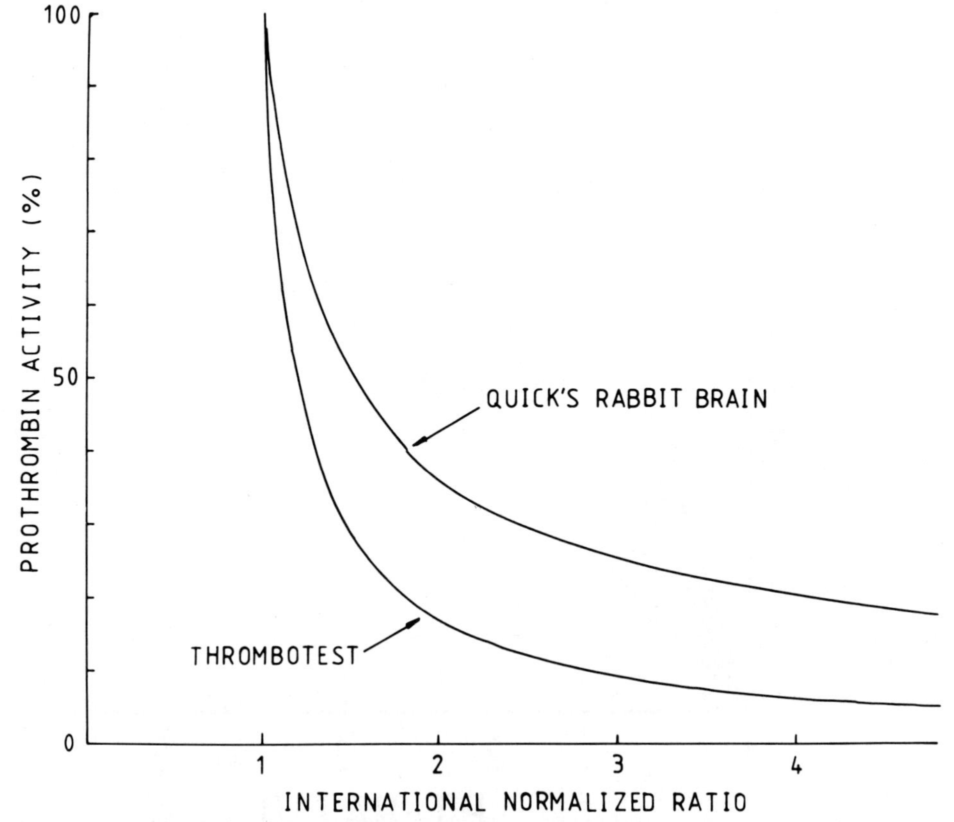

Figure 3.3–3: Relationships between INR and percentage prothrombin activity for two thromboplastin reagents. Rabbit brain thromboplastin was prepared and used as described by Quick[51]. Thrombotest (bovine brain thromboplastin) was obtained from Nycomed, Oslo, Norway[22].

Table 3.3–1
International Reference Preparations for Thromboplastins

Designation	*Species/composition*	*ISI*	*Available from*	*Ref.*
67/40	Human/combined	1.00	(Discontinued)	11, 12, 24
BCT/253	Human/plain	1.08	WHO	15, 24
BCT/099	Human/plain	1.05	BCR	14
BCT/441	Human/plain	1.04	ICSH	16
RBT/79	Rabbit/plain	1.41	WHO	14
CRM/149R	Rabbit/plain	1.34	BCR	21
OBT/79	Bovine/combined	1.01	WHO, BCR	14

ISI = International Sensitivity Index
WHO = World Health Organization
BCR = Community Bureau of Reference (Brussels)
ICSH = International Committee for Standardisation in Haematology

than the activity measured with Quick's reagent. It should be emphasised that the INR/ISI system can only be used in oral anticoagulant control. It has no significance in other applications of the PT test.

SELECTION OF THROMBOPLASTIN STANDARDS

The WHO model for thromboplastin calibration requires a hierarchy of standardisation. Secondary standards have been calibrated against the primary IRP in international collaborative exercises. The calibration of a thromboplastin is, in general, more precise when comparisons are made between similar preparations from the same species[9]. The secondary standards represent different species and types of reagents. It is suggested that laboratories and manufacturers use the secondary standard of the same species for the calibration of their materials[9]. The composition of the thromboplastin reagent has been shown to have considerable effect on the precision of calibration. Plain reagents (i.e. without addition of adsorbed plasma) should be calibrated against a plain secondary standard. Combined reagents should be calibrated against a combined standard. At present, only one combined standard (OBT/79) is available, as the primary IRP 67/40 has been discontinued[24]. The WHO standards are intended only for the calibration of national reference preparations. A supply is available to a limited number of national control laboratories[9]. The WHO standards are listed in Table 3.3–1. Secondary standards are also available from the BCR (Table 3.3–1).

These reference materials are intended to be more widely available to manufacturers of commercial or non-commercial thromboplastins. The BCR reference materials have been certified in terms of the primary WHO IRP 67/40. Manufacturers of thromboplastin are being urged to introduce a house standard or working reference preparation, which is a batch of thromboplastin set aside for the calibration of individual production batches. The calibration of the house standard should be performed by comparison with a (BCR) secondary standard. The calibrated house standard may then be used for the calibration of subsequent batches of the same production line. Batch-to-batch calibration may be carried out with pooled (either deep-frozen or lyophilised) instead of fresh plasmas.

THROMBOPLASTIN CALIBRATION IN THE NETHERLANDS

In the Netherlands, most anticoagulant clinics (Thrombosis Services) and hospitals presently use one brand of reagent: Thrombotest. A relatively small number of Centres are using different brands of thromboplastin. A few Centres are using chromogenic prothrombin time tests[25].

All thromboplastins used in The Netherlands for oral anticoagulant control are checked by a National Reference Laboratory founded by the Federation of Dutch Thrombosis Centres. The check involves assessment of the ISI, and for Thrombotest, the clotting times at given INR values. The Dutch Reference Laboratory receives all Thrombotest batches before introduction onto the Dutch market. Each batch is calibrated against a national reference batch that, in turn, is calibrated against the corresponding International Reference Preparation for thromboplastin, bovine, combined (OBT/79).

The calibration of each batch against the national reference batch is co-ordinated with the manufacturer's calibration, that is the same reference batch and the same set of three control plasmas are used. In addition, fresh patients' samples are used for the calibration. The clotting time determinations are performed by 10–12 collaborating Dutch laboratories (decentralised calibration). The clotting time data are returned to

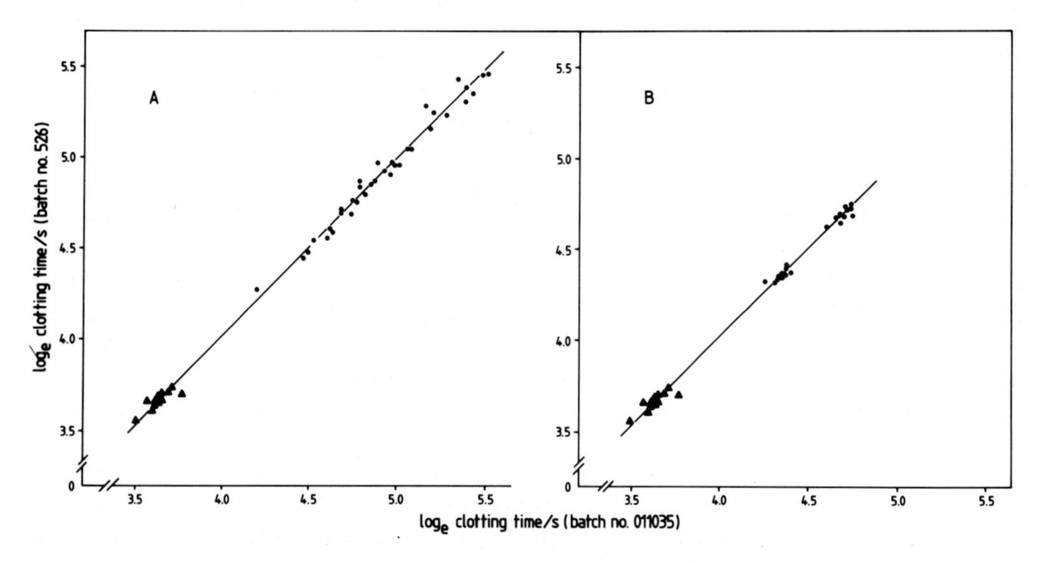

Figure 3.3–4: Batch-to-batch calibration of Thrombotest by the Dutch reference laboratory of anticoagulant control. The natural logarithms of the clotting times are plotted. Panel A: measurements of fresh patients' blood samples (black circles) and pooled normal control plasma (triangles). Panel B: measurements of three lyophilised control plasmas. Two lyophilised control plasmas were obtained from anticoagulated patients (black circles) and one was a pooled normal plasma (triangles). The measurements shown in panels A and B were determined by the same 12 laboratories collaborating in the calibration scheme.

Table 3.3–2
Mean and inter-batch variation of ISI values of 117 Thrombotest batches used in The Netherlands.

	Collaborating Dutch laboratories		*Manufacturer*
	Fresh samples	*Lyophilized samples*	*Lyophilized samples*
Mean ISI	0.97	0.98	0.99
Inter-batch CV(%)	3.5	2.8	2.5

CV = coefficient of variation
ISI values were determined with fresh patients' blood samples or with lyophilized pooled patients' plasmas, by a group of 10-12 collaborating Dutch laboratories. For comparison, the manufacturer's ISIs determined with the same lyophilized plasmas are given.

the central reference laboratory for calculation of the ISI and the relation between clotting times and INR values. An example is shown in Figure 3.3–4.

The precision of calibration is excellent (CV of the regression slope for each batch is about 1%) because of the high similarity of the Thrombotest batches. Mean ISI values and the inter-batch variation are given in Table 3.3–2. The inter-batch variation of the ISI depends on the samples used. With fresh patients' samples the interbatch CV is 3.5%, but with lyophilised plasmas it is 2.8%. In general, there is a good correlation between the ISIs calculated with the fresh patients' data and the ISIs calculated with the lyophilised control plasmas. A small but significant ISI difference between the fresh and lyophilised controls was observed. Similar differences have been observed previously[26], and may be explained by changes of clot formation induced by the lyophilisation process or the handling prior to this process. Nevertheless, the inclusion of lyophilised controls is recommended for quality assessment of the calibration procedure.

EFFECTS OF INSTRUMENTS

The thromboplastin standards issued by WHO and BCR have been calibrated by means of manual techniques, and the ISI values of the standards relate to the manual technique. However, more than 98% of larger hospital laboratories in the USA rely on instruments rather than manual methods for coagulation testing. In Europe, the proportion of laboratories using instruments is increasing. It is important to know the effect of different instruments on the PT, and more specifically, on the ISI used for oral anticoagulant control.

Several studies have shown that instruments may have a significant effect on the PT. Some studies indicate that the use of PT ratios (patient PT divided by mean normal PT) would eliminate some of the bias due to differences in the method (instrument) of clot detection[27]. More recent studies indicate that instruments may have a significant effect on the PT ratio and hence on the ISI[19,28,29,30]. The difference in ISI, observed between two photo-optical instruments could amount to approximately 10%[19]. It cannot be excluded that even greater differences in ISI between instruments will be detected[31]. These observations imply that the thromboplastin manufacturer should indicate the instrument(s) for which the stated ISI is valid. Preliminary results suggest that instrument-specific ISI values can allow determination of INR-equivalents with acceptable precision on lyophilised samples[28]. Conversely, INR equivalents assigned to lyophilised plasmas might be used for local calibration of thromboplastin-instrument systems. These questions are presently under investigation.

EXTERNAL QUALITY ASSESSMENT OF PT MEASUREMENTS

In many countries, national external quality assessment (EQA) programmes for the prothrombin time are being executed. In general, the results of EQA are presented according to the reagents used by the participants. A score is usually assigned to each participant on the basis of the consensus mean PT and the inter-laboratory variation[32]. It is not always possible to evaluate the results statistically when the number of participants using a particular brand of reagent is small. Several investigators have demonstrated that the PT differences between laboratories are mainly systematic[33].

Several countries have added the INR to their EQA programmes, including the United Kingdom, France, The Netherlands, and Switzerland. In general, the inclusion of INR in EQA programmes had an educational effect, because the participants were requested to use the INR/ISI system. The inter-laboratory variation of the INR gradually decreased when the participants became more familiar with the system. In the Netherlands, the INR was introduced in the EQA programme in 1985. In 1986, the mean interlaboratory variation of INR values was about 8% CV. The mean CV decreased to 5.8% in 1990 (Table 3.3–3).

An important source of variation is the mean normal PT (MNPT) used for calculation of the INR. Some laboratories use the MNPT given in the thromboplastin manufacturer's chart. The MNPT determined by the laboratory using fresh samples from healthy volunteers may be different from the manufacturer's value[30]. It is recommended that the MNPT is the geometric mean of 20 fresh plasmas obtained from healthy ambulant adults, by the same technique as used for the patients' samples[34]. It is not practical to determine MNPT for every new batch of reagent according to the recommended procedure. The procedure may be simplified by replacing the fresh

Table 3.3–3
Inter-laboratory variation of INR values in the Netherlands External Quality Assessment programme.

Year	*1986*	*1987*	*1988*	*1989*	*1990*
Mean CV (%)	8.0	7.0	6.9	6.4	5.8
n	126	134	136	138	141

CV = coefficient of variation
For each control sample, INR values were determined with Thrombotest. After exclusion of outliers, the CV was calculated. Each year, at least 40 control samples prepared from patients' plasma specimens were shipped to the participants of the programme.
The average number of participants reporting INR is given (n).

plasmas by a deep-frozen pooled normal plasma[3]. The use of lyophilised calibrated pooled normal plasmas for calculation of INR is under investigation[21].

The use of INR in EQA programmes has the potential advantage that results obtained with different reagent/instrument combinations could be pooled and a consensus mean INR could be calculated. This would also allow the assignment of scores to participants using a minority reagent, providing that the INR of the survey sample was the same for each reagent/instrument.

However, experience in the Netherlands and the United Kingdom with INR EQA programmes has shown that there are differences between results obtained with various thromboplastins. One possible explanation for a discrepancy is that of incorrect ISI assignation[35]. Another possibility is that of a bias introduced by the survey sample itself. The INR was intended for *fresh* samples of patients stabilised on oral anticoagulant therapy. The survey samples are not fresh and as they are lyophilised, the properties may have changed. A recent multi-centre study showed a small but significant difference in INR equivalent between a human and a rabbit thromboplastin used for assessment of the INR[21]. Furthermore, if the survey sample is derived from one single patient, differences in INR between thromboplastins may be due to biological variation. The effect of biological variation is readily appreciated when one observes the scatter of individual patients' points about the orthogonal regression line in a calibration plot (Fig. 3.3–1). If pooled patients' plasmas are used, the effect of biological variation is largely averaged out.

It is difficult to predict the inter-laboratory variation of INR among a group of laboratories using the same thromboplastin reagent. Some authors suggested a direct relationship between the CV of the INR and the ISI: CV(INR) = CV(PR) × ISI, in which CV(PR) is the inter-laboratory variation of the measured PT ratio[36]. Furthermore, they suggested that a low CV(INR) is associated with a low ISI. However, it may well be that CV(PR) and ISI are not independent. It has been suggested that when the ISI is decreased, the CV(PR) goes up[37]. The use of EQA data to determine which thromboplastin yields the highest precision, that is the lowest CV(INR), may not be appropriate, because different groups of laboratories are compared. When laboratories use different instruments and techniques, the comparison of thromboplastin may be biased[33]. In the authors' opinion, a fair comparison of thromboplastin reagents can be performed only if the reagents are tested by the same laboratories using the same techniques.

PRECISION OF THE INR

From the previous paragraphs it can be seen that the precision of the INR depends on the analytical precision of ISI and PT ratio. But even if the ISI and PT ratio were known without analytical error, there would still be variation of the INR, because the INR would still depend to some extent on the thromboplastin/instrument used. The residual variation of the INR is the result of biological variation of the individual patient's coagulation factors and inhibitors. This can be readily appreciated from the scatter of individual patient points in a calibration plot (Fig. 3.3–1).

The biological variation of the INR is a function of the difference between the working thromboplastin and the primary IRP 67/40. Thus, the true INR is best approximated with a thromboplastin similar to IRP 67/40[23,38]. According to Loeliger, calibration inaccuracy (ISI imprecision) plays only a minor role in the inter-thromboplastin variation of the INR within a single centre[38,39]. Under well controlled conditions the overall (including ISI imprecision, inter-laboratory variation of the PT ratio and biological variation) coefficient of variation of the INR is 11–13.5%, if thromboplastins of ISI ~ 1 are used[38,40].

THE FEDERATION OF DUTCH THROMBOSIS SERVICES

Building upon the model created in Utrecht by the late Professor F. L. J. Jordan in 1949, a nationwide system of regionally centralised anticoagulant control clinics for out-patients and home patients was developed in the Netherlands[2]. Each of the individual Dutch centres is called a Thrombosis Service. The critical element for success is the nurse who visits the patients, who is in close contact with each patient's referring physician and who relies for the regulation of the anticoagulant dosage on the centre's physician. Thirty thrombosis services formed the Federation of Dutch Thrombosis Services in 1971, and the number of members has grown to 72 in 1991. This organisation attempts to satisfy all demands for successful anticoagulant therapy in home and out-patients without loss of the patient-referring doctor relationship. At present the Dutch Thrombosis Services cover more than 90% of the country. About 250,000 patients are being treated by the 72 centres (total population of the Netherlands: 15 million). The great majority of the centres use the same modification of

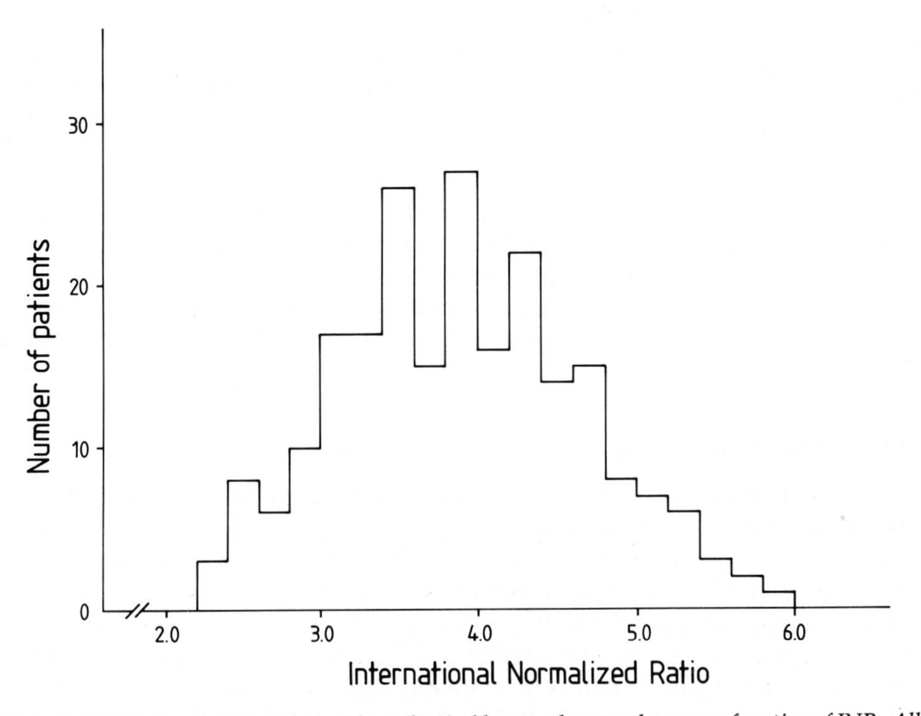

Figure 3.3–5: Histogram of patients with mechanical heart valve prostheses as a function of INR. All patients being treated by the Leiden Thrombosis Center on 1 January 1988 are included in the histogram. The therapeutic target intensity is 4.0 INR (range:3.2–5.3 INR).

the prothrombin time determination, namely the Thrombotest method according to Owren[41]. About 3.5 million PT determinations are performed annually.

THERAPEUTIC QUALITY ASSESSMENT

An important part of internal quality control in the anticoagulation clinic is the assessment of therapeutic control achieved in the patients under treatment. This type of self-audit has demonstrated that the quality of oral anticoagulant therapy may require considerable improvement, particularly in short term patients[42]. In some hospitals, under-anticoagulation is the main deficiency, most probably due to excessively cautious prescribing by junior staff concerned to avoid the risk of bleeding problems[43]. Unstable anticoagulation among out-patients, in contrast, is probably mainly due to poor compliance[44].

Therapeutic control of anticoagulation consists of continuous assessment of the proportion of time spent by each patient in the target INR range[45]. For an individual patient, PT determinations are performed at distinct time points or clinic visits, and no information is available about the anticoagulation intensity between the time points. Therefore, the proportion of time spent by the patient in the target INR range can only be approximated. If one is interested in the average therapeutic control of all patients, several methods are available to assess the proportion of time spent by these patients in the target range.

First, an assessment of the proportion of all satisfactory PT tests of a clinic's total patient population can be made. However, this results in underestimation of the clinic's performance because unstable patients are checked more frequently than stable patients[46]. Second, it is possible to make a correction for the frequency with which each patient's INR is checked, resulting in a higher estimate of adequate control[46]. Third, an assessment can be made of all patients at a certain point in time instead of a certain period of time[47]. This cross-section of all patients' files is considered to reflect the proportion of time spent by these patients in the target range[46]. To obtain this proportion, it is recommended to review all patients' last INR values at a certain point in time, i.e. one INR value per patient. The Federation of Dutch Thrombosis Services requests its members to perform such assessment of their patient populations twice a year.

The distribution of all patients' last INR values measured in patients with mechanical heart valve prostheses attending the Leiden Thrombosis Centre is shown in Figure 3.3–5. This Centre applied a therapeutic range of 3.2–5.3 INR for patients with artificial heart valves[46]. About 76% of these patients were in the 3.2–5.3 INR range. The maximum of the distribution was at about 3.8 INR, which is in good agreement with the target value (4.0 INR) for patients with mechanical heart valves recommended by the Federation of Dutch Thrombosis Services.

The proportion of time spent by each patient in the target range is correlated with the frequency of testing. This is to be expected because unstable patients are checked more frequently in an attempt to improve their therapeutic control. The mean percentage of INRs in the target range is plotted as a function of the number or clinic visits per year (Fig. 3.3–6). Patients checked 12–15 times per year have the highest percentage (80–85%) of their INRs in the target range. Most patients are checked less than 25 times per year. Very few patients have a percentage less than 60%.

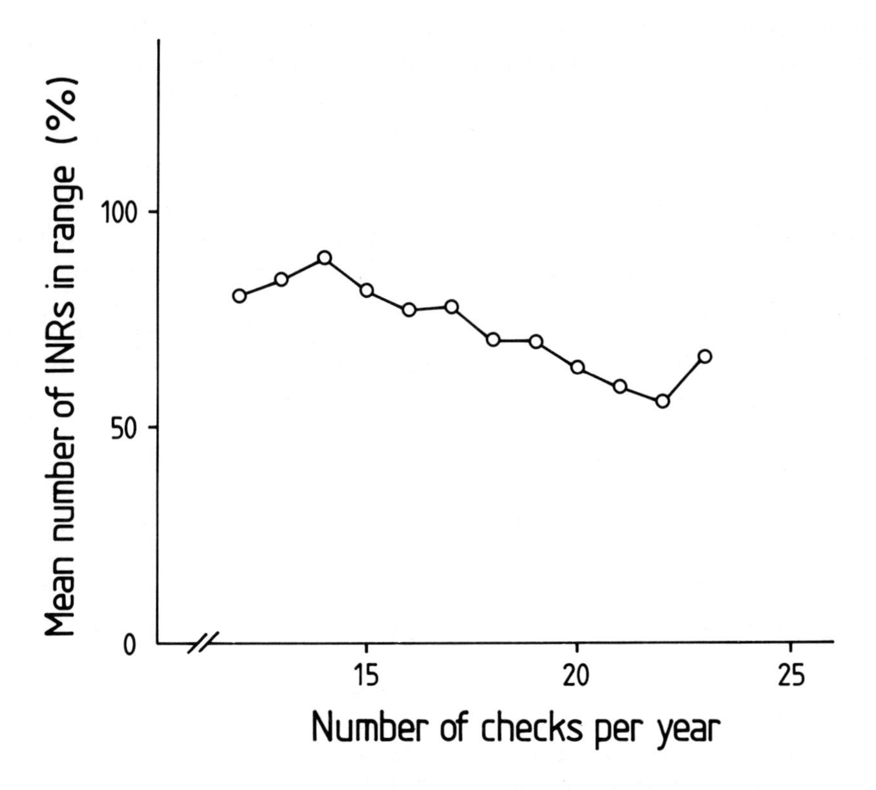

Figure 3.3–6: Proportion of INR values in the therapeutic range as a function of the number of checks per year. For each patient with a mechanical heart valve prosthesis treated by the Leiden Thrombosis Centre during 1987, the proportion of INR values in the 3.2–5.3 range was calculated. The mean proportion (in %) is plotted along the vertical axis.

The above mentioned recommended method of assessment of therapeutic control yields an overall view of a clinic's performance. The level obtained with this method depends on the type of patients, however. Conceptually, this assessment is targeted at patients who are on long-term anticoagulant therapy; this approach is less applicable to patients in the induction phase of therapy.

It should be emphasised that therapeutic control depends on many factors, the most important of which are laboratory control, patient compliance, physicians' dosage prescription, interaction with other drugs, intercurrent diseases and dietary changes. It is also clear that the proportion of patients' INR values in the target range depends on the target range per se. The wider the target range, the easier it is to keep the patient in the range. It is recommended that the target INR range is reported with each patient's INR values.

With increasing consensus on therapeutic target ranges, comparison of therapeutic control in different clinics will be more rewarding. Therapeutic control may reveal poor results in certain treatment groups and could demonstrate the effect of remedial strategies. It is recommended that quality assessment is performed at least once or twice a year. The proposed method is easy to perform and does not require expensive computer facilities.

Clinicians and investigators are also urged to assess their patients' therapeutic control according to the above method. Editors and reviewers of scientific papers on clinical trials of anticoagulated patients should insist on therapeutic control data being provided[45](see also Chapters 3.4 and 6.4).

CLINICAL TRIALS

Many clinical trials of oral anticoagulant treatment have been performed during the last 50 years. Unfortunately, the intensity of anticoagulation achieved in many of these trials cannot be assessed because no adequate information is available about the thromboplastins used. For example, in the report of a recent trial of anticoagulant therapy in pregnant women with artificial heart valves[48], referred to in Chapter 4.1, the authors stated that the prothrombin time was maintained between 2 and 2.5 times the control value. No information was given on the thromboplastin used and we can only guess about the intensity of anticoagulation.

In the Stroke Prevention in Atrial Fibrillation Study[49], described in detail in Chapter 1.2, conventional American rabbit brain thromboplastins are used to maintain the PT ratio between 1.3 and 1.8 times control. The majority of conventional North American thromboplastins have ISI values that range between 1.7 and 2.8[50]. Thus, the INR range equivalent to a PT ratio of 1.3 varies between 1.6–2.1 and that equivalent to a ratio of 1.8 between 2.7–5.2. As a consequence, two centres participating in the study could have dramatically different anticoagulant intensities, though their mean PT ratios may be the same. Such differences could make the interpretation of the trial results very difficult if not impossible.

SUMMARY

The prothrombin time (PT) test is the primary measurement in the laboratory control of oral anticoagulant treatment. The traditional expression of PT test results, either as percentage prothrombin activity or PT ratio, is inadequate for international communication and comparison because the values depend on the nature of the thromboplastin test system used. The WHO recommended universal scale of reporting PT results is based on calibration of local thromboplastin systems against an international reference preparation. This scale is the International Normalised Ratio (INR). Application of the INR scale in clinical practice should be encouraged by External Quality Assessment (EQA) schemes, which improve its precision. Therapeutic quality can be assessed by estimating the proportion of time that patients are within the target INR range. The overall performance of each anticoagulant clinic should be regularly measured in this way.

Many physicians are insufficiently aware of the different sensitivities of rabbit thromboplastins, which result in different anticoagulation intensities being employed in different clinics[50]. Improvement in the situation can only be achieved by continuous education. The more widespread use of the INR scale should facilitate international comparison of anticoagulation results and eventually consensus on optimal target values. The introduction of the INR to countries not already using it, particularly the USA, should be strongly encouraged by all physicians with an interest in anticoagulation and especially those undertaking the long-term management of patients with prosthetic heart valves. Not only will this facilitate comparison of results, but it should also offer greater safety for patients who travel frequently and may need to have their prothrombin time checked in different centres or even different countries.

REFERENCES

1. Wright IS. The use of the anticoagulants in the treatment of diseases of the heart and blood vessels. Ann Intern Med 1949;30:80–91.
2. Loeliger EA, van Dijk-Wierda CA, van den Besselaar AMHP, Broekmans AW, Roos J. Anticoagulant Control and the Risk of Bleeding. In Meade TW, ed. Anticoagulants and Myocardial Infarction, A Reappraisal. Chichester:John Wiley and Sons, 1984;135–177.
3. Loeliger EA, Poller L, Samama M, Thomson JM, van den Besselaar AMHP, Vermylen J, Verstraete M. Questions and answers on prothrombin time standardisation in oral anticoagulant control. Thromb Haemostas 1985;54:515–517.
4. Hirsh J, Poller L, Deykin D, Levine M, Dalen JE. Optimal therapeutic range for oral anticoagulants. Chest 1989;95 (Supplement):5S–11S.
5. British Society for Haematology, British Committee for Standards in Haematology, Haemostasis and Thrombosis Task force. Guidelines on oral anticoagulation:second edition. J Clin Pathol 1990;43:177–183.
6. Quick AJ, Stanley-Brown M. Bancroft FW. A study of the coagulation defect in hemophilia and in jaundice. Am J Med Sci 1935;190:501–511.
7. Conley CL, Morse WI. Thromboplastic factors in the estimation of prothrombin concentration. Am J Med Sci 1948;215:158–169.
8. Hirsh J, Levine M. Confusion over the therapeutic range for monitoring oral anticoagulant therapy in North America. Thromb Haemostas 1988;59:129–132.
9. WHO Expert Committee on Biological Standardisation. Requirements for thromboplastins and plasma used to control oral anticoagulant therapy. 33rd Report. Tech Rep Ser 687, Geneva, World Health Organisation, 1983:81–105.
10. Loeliger EA. ICSH/ICTH recommendations for reporting prothrombin time in oral anticoagulant control. Thromb Haemostas 1985;54:155–156.
11. WHO Expert Committee on Biological Standardisation. Standardisation in the control of anticoagulation (oral). 28th Report. Techn Rep Ser 610, Geneva, World Health Organisation, 1977:45–51.
12. Bangham DR, Biggs R, Brozovic M, Denson KWE. Calibration of five different thromboplastins using fresh and freeze-dried plasma. Thromb Diathes Haemorrh 1973;29:228–239.
13. Kirkwood TBL. Calibration of reference thromboplastins and standardisation of the prothrombin time ratio. Thromb Haemostas 1983;49:238–244.
14. Hermans J, van den Besselaar AMHP, Loeliger EA, van der Velde EA. A collaborative calibration study of reference materials for thromboplastins. Thromb Haemostas 1983;50:712–717.
15. Thomson JM, Tomenson JA, Poller L. The calibration of the second primary international reference preparation for thromboplastin (Thromboplastin, human, plain, coded BCT/253). Thromb Haemostas 1984;52:336–342.
16. Thomson JM, Darby KV, Poller L. Calibration of BCT/441, the ICSH reference preparation for thromboplastin. Thromb Haemostas 1986;55:379–382.
17. van den Besselaar AMHP, Hermans J, van der Velde EA, Bussemaker-Verduyn den Boer E, van Halem-Visser LP, Jansen-Grüter R, Loeliger EA. The calibration of rabbit tissue thromboplastins: experience of the Dutch reference laboratory for anticoagulant control. J Biol Stand 1986;14:305–317.
18. Palareti G, Coccheri S, Poggi M, Bonetti M, Cervi V, Mazzuca A, Savoia M, Veri L, Fiori F, Gaspari G, Palareti A. Oral anticoagulant therapy control: evidence that INR expression improves the inter-laboratory comparability of results. The Bologna oral anticoagulant control exercise. Thromb Haemostas 1987;905–910.
19. Poggio M. van der Besselaar AMHP, van der Velde EA, Bertina RM. The effect of some instruments for prothrombin time testing on the International Sensitivity Index (ISI) of two rabbit tissue thromboplastin reagents. Thromb Haemostas 1989;62:868–874.
20. Gugliemone HA, Vides MA. Prothrombin time in the monitoring of oral anticoagulant: a comparison of results using different thromboplastins. Ann Biol Clin 1990;48:547–550.
21. van den Besselaar AMHP, Bertina RM. Multi-Centre Calibration of the Second Reference Material for Thromboplastin, Rabbit, Plain, Coded CRM 149R. Thromb Haemostas 1991;65:263–267.
22. Gogstad GO, Wadt J, Smith P, Brynildsrud T. Utility of a modified calibration model for reliable conversion of thromboplastin times to International Normalised Ratios. Thromb Haemostas 1986;56:178–182.
23. Tomenson JA. A statistician's independent evaluation. In van den Besselaar AMHP, Gralnick HR,

Lewis SM, eds. Thromboplastin Calibration and Oral Anticoagulant Control. Boston:M Nijhoff Publishers 1984:87–108.
24. WHO Expert Committee on Biological Standardisation. 34th Report. Tech Rep Ser 700, Geneva, World Health Organisation, 1984:19.
25. Jonker JJC, Azar AJ, van Bergen PFMM, Klarenberg RA, Przespolewski EF. Laboratory and therapeutic control in the Thrombosis Centre Rotterdam using chromogenic prothrombin time tests. Res Clin Lab 1990;20:45–57.
26. Loeliger EA, van der Hoeff-van Halem R, van Halem LP. Thromboplastin calibration. Experience of the Dutch reference laboratory for anti-coagulant control. Thromb Haemostas 1978;40:272–287.
27. International Committee on Thrombosis and Haemostasis, International Committee for Standardization in Haematology. Prothrombin Time Standardization:Report of the Expert Panel on Oral Anticoagulant Control. Thromb Haemostas 1979;41:1073–1114.
28. van den Besselaar AMHP, Bertina RM. Standardization and quality control in blood coagulation assays. In Lewis SM, Verwilghen RL, eds. Quality Assurance in Haematology. London; Baillière Tindall, 1988:119–150.
29. Ray MJ, Smith IR. The dependence of the International Sensitivity Index on the Coagulometer used to perform the Prothrombin Time. Thromb Haemostas 1990;63:424–429.
30. Peters RHM, van den Besselaar AMHP, Olthuis FMFG. A multicentre study to evaluate method dependency of the International Sensitivity Index of bovine thromboplastin. Thromb Haemostas 1989;61:166–169.
31. Hawkins PL, Barrow DA, Maynard JR. A sensitive thromboplastin reagent prepared from rabbit brain tissue factor for monitoring oral anticoagulant therapy. Thromb Haemostas 1989;62:530.
32. Lewis SM. External Quality Assessment. In Lewis SM, Verwilghen RL, eds. Quality Assurance in Haematology. London; Baillière Tindall, 1988:151–175.
33. van den Besselaar AMHP. ISI value of thromboplastin. J Clin Pathol 1989;42:1118–1119.
34. Poller L, Hirsh J. A simple system for the derivation of International Normalized Ratios for the reporting of prothrombin time results with North American Thromboplastin Reagents. Am J Clin Pathol 1989;92:124–126.
35. Morrison M, Caldwell A, McQuaker G, Fitzsimons EJ. Discrepant INR values:a comparison between Manchester and Thrombotest reagents using capillary and venous samples. Clin Lab Haematol 1989;11:393–398.
36. Taberner DA, Poller L, Thomson JM, Darby KV. Effect of international sensitivity index (ISI) of thromboplastins on precision of international normalised ratios (INR). J Clin Pathol 1989;42:92–96.
37. Denson KWE. Thromboplastin – sensitivity, precision and other characteristics. Clin Lab Haematol 1988;10:315–328.
38. van den Besselaar AMHP. The International Normalized Ratio for Prothrombin Time testing. In Triplett DA, ed. Advances in Coagulation Testing: Interpretation and Application. Skokie: College of American Pathologists, 1986:357–364.
39. Loeliger EA. Critical remarks from a clinician's point of view. In van den Besselaar AMHP, Gralnick HR, Lewis SM, eds. Thromboplastin Calibration and Oral Anticoagulant Control. Boston; Martinus Nijhoff Publishers 1984:109–116.
40. Loeliger EA, van den Besselaar AMHP, Lewis SW. Reliability and clinical impact of the normalization of the prothrombin times in oral anticoagulant control. Thromb Haemostas 1985;53:148–154.
41. Owren PA. Thrombotest. A new method for controlling anticoagulant therapy. Lancet 1959:2:754–758.
42. Majumdar G, Payne RW. Quality of oral anticoagulant therapy. Clin Lab Haematol 1985;7:125–131.
43. Harries AD, Birtwell AJ, Jones DB. Anticoagulant control. Lancet 1981;1:1320.
44. Kumar S, Haigh JRM, Rhodes LE, Peaker S, Davies JA, Roberts BE, Feely MP. Poor compliance is a major factor in unstable outpatient control of anticoagulant therapy. Thromb Haemostas 1989;62:729–732.
45. van den Besselaar AMHP. Recommended method for reporting therapeutic control of oral anticoagulant therapy. Thromb Haemostas 1990;63:316–317.
46. van den Besselaar AMHP, van der Meer FJM, Gerrits-Drabbe CW. Therapeutic control of oral anticoagulant treatment in the Netherlands. Am J Clin Pathol 1988;90:685–690.
47. Loeliger EA. Laboratory control, optimal therapeutic ranges and therapeutic quality control in oral anticoagulation. Acta Haematol 1985;74:125–131.
48. Iturbe-Alessio I, Del Carmen Fonseca M, Mutchinik O, Santos MA, Zajarias A, Salazar E. Risks of anticoagulant therapy in pregnant women with artificial heart valves. N Engl J Med 1986;315:1390–1393.
49. Stroke Prevention in Atrial Fibrillation study group investigators. Preliminary report. N Engl J Med 1990;322:863–868.

50. van den Besselaar AMHP. Adoption and validation of the International Normalized Ratio for monitoring oral anticoagulant therapy: the situation in 1989. Res Clin Lab 1990;20:75–81.
51. Quick AJ. Hemorrhagic diseases and thrombosis. Philadelphia, Lea and Febiger, 1966: 391–395.

Chapter 3.4

Prosthesis-Specific and Patient-Specific Anticoagulation

Eric G. Butchart

From the very earliest experiences with artificial heart valves in the late 1950's, it was immediately apparent that one of the major problems that would have to be overcome was that of thrombus accumulation on the prosthesis[1]. The pathophysiological reaction to all inert foreign bodies is to attempt to encapsulate them and exclude them from contact with normal tissues[2]. With foreign bodies in the circulation, the process begins with progressive thrombus deposition, followed by organisation of the thrombus, fibrosis and eventually a covering of endothelium[3]. This process of progressive exclusion is modified by local blood flow conditions (Chapters 2.1 and 2.4), by the materials from which the foreign body is constructed (Chapter 2.3) and by anticoagulation[4]. In the case of early prosthetic heart valves, the body's attempts at encapsulation by initially covering the prosthesis with thrombus led to the catastrophic failure of many of these devices[1].

Eventually, improved designs and the use of oral anticoagulants which had been introduced in the early 1940's[5] substantially reduced the risk of thrombus formation on the prosthesis. The work of Nina Braunwald and her associates at the US National Heart and Lung Institute established the necessity for early anticoagulation to reduce the thickness of tissue overgrowth on the sewing ring[4] and other studies confirmed the necessity to prevent thrombus deposition on the smooth working surfaces (Chapter 2.3), but the search continued for a mechanical prosthesis which would not require long term anticoagulation. The introduction of cloth covering on the orifice and struts to stimulate endothelialisation[6–9] and later the employment of less thrombogenic materials[10], particularly pyrolitic carbon[11], both briefly increased hopes that long term anticoagulation could be avoided. Local anticoagulation of the prosthesis was evaluated experimentally[12] and clinically[12A] but never gained widespread acceptance.

Although there are no randomised prospective studies in the literature, many reports detail the advantages of anticoagulation versus no anticoagulation in reducing the incidence of embolism and valve thrombosis[13–24]. Lack of anticoagulation produced a high incidence of embolism with early ball valve prostheses[15], especially in the mitral position[14,25]. Modifications of these valves with cloth covering on the orifice and struts were promoted as not requiring long term anticoagulation but embolism persisted[17–19], they proved prone to thrombosis[26,27] and a new problem of cloth wear leading to cloth embolism and excessive haemolysis was introduced[28]. Attempts to manage early tilting disc valves without anticoagulation proved unsatisfactory[16,21,29] although some authors initially recommended no anticoagulation for aortic valve replacement in patients in sinus rhythm with good left ventricular function and no residual gradient[20]. The introduction of the first bileaflet valve (St. Jude Medical), with the perceived advantages of all-pyrolytic carbon construction and central laminar flow[30,31], again raised hopes that anticoagulation could be avoided, at least in aortic patients[22–24]. However, some studies showed the incidence of valve thrombosis to be unacceptably high when only antiplatelet drugs were used[22,23]. Embolic rates were low in one of these series[22] containing mainly young patients in sinus rhythm, underlining the distinction between thrombosis and embolism in some prostheses and the importance of patient-related factors in determining embolic rates (see Chapter 2.4).

A high proportion of patient-related risk factors may magnify differences in embolic rate with different management regimes. In a large series of St. Jude valves, in which almost half the patients had additional procedures (including coronary surgery and proximal aortic aneurysm surgery) embolic rates per patient-year with anticoagulation, antiplatelet drugs only or no anticoagulation were 2.6%, 9.2% and 15.6% respectively[24].

Some authors have theorised that anticoagulation could be withdrawn in some prostheses after endothelialisation of the sewing ring has taken place[20,32], but one study has documented a higher incidence of emboli in patients who had their anticoagulants discontinued than in those who had never been on anticoagulants[13]. However, this study was not randomised and selection bias cannot be excluded. It is nevertheless interesting that some of these patients suffered emboli soon after discontinuation of anticoagulants, raising the possibility of rebound hypercoagulability. Rebound hypercoagulability following cessation of anticoagulants is an entity the existence of which has been disputed for many years[33], but most of the evidence against rebound has come from series of patients anticoagulated for deep venous thrombosis[34] and the argument remains unresolved as far as prosthetic valve patients are concerned. Currently most surgeons and cardiologists recommend life-long anticoagulation for all mechanical prostheses although many issues remain to be resolved. The remainder of this chapter will be devoted to addressing these issues which can be summarised as follows:

- The interpretation of anticoagulation data in the literature and the need for standardisation.
- The objectives of anticoagulation.
- The value of early anticoagulation.
- The determination of the ideal level of anticoagulation for each prosthesis, patient and time frame.
- The necessity for supplementary antiplatelet agents for each prosthesis, patient and time frame.
- The place for fixed 'mini-dose' warfarin.
- The need for risk factor modification as an adjunct to anticoagulation.
- The need to promote patient compliance.

THE INTERPRETATION OF ANTICOAGULATION DATA

In the early days of anticoagulation for heart disease and subsequently for prosthetic heart valves, the level prescribed was largely arbitrary as there were no scientific data on which to base dose recommendation[35,36](see The Ideal Level of Anticoagulation, page 299). The inevitable result was that many patients received too much anticoagulation and the incidence of anticoagulant-related bleeding was high[25]. This led some surgeons to abandon anticoagulation altogether[25] and many physicians believed that a high complication rate from anticoagulation therapy was inevitable[37] with the probability of bleeding increasing with duration of therapy[38]. The spectre of anticoagulant-related bleeding has continued to have an adverse effect on the popularity of mechanical prostheses ever since[39,40]. With hindsight and the availability of more scientific data, this must be regarded as an over-reaction, for three reasons:

a) The incidence of anticoagulant-related bleeding is directly related to the level of anticoagulation[15,41–44] and the risk of serious bleeding is acceptably low with anticoagulation of low intensity[45–48].

b) Recently introduced methods of standardisation of anticoagulation measurement (see Chapter 3.3) using the International Normalised Ratio (INR)[49–52] have revealed a wide discrepancy between levels of anticoagulation prescribed[47,53,54]. Wide variation not only exists between countries[47,53], but also between institutions in the same country according to local prescribing practice[54] and the thromboplastin reagent used for measuring the prothrombin time[47,55].

c) In general, levels of anticoagulation traditionally employed in the USA for the last 20 years (INR 5.0 to 10.0) have clearly been far too high when assessed in terms of the risk of bleeding[47]. Furthermore, the increased risk of anticoagulant bleeding in the elderly demonstrated in the USA[41] is not seen when lower levels of anticoagulation are employed[45,46] (see also Chapter 4.3), nor does the risk of bleeding necessarily increase with duration of therapy at low intensity anticoagulation[46].

The implications are twofold. Firstly, older series of prosthetic valves from the two sides of the Atlantic Ocean are not comparable in terms of their incidence of embolism and valve thrombosis because they have been maintained at very different anticoagulation levels[54]. Future prosthetic valve series should specify anticoagulation levels actually achieved in internationally standardised terminology (see Chapters 3.3 and 6.4); the terms "adequate" and "inadequate" anticoagulation lack precision[56]. Secondly, the introduction of newer prostheses, whose design characteristics have led to lower thrombogenicity, should allow a reduction in anticoagulation levels, providing that these are scientifically determined (vide infra), with a consequent reduction in the risk of bleeding[57]. Ultimately it may be possible to lay the spectre of anticoagulant bleeding to rest and to show that the risk of thrombosis, embolism and bleeding in low thrombogenicity mechanical prostheses maintained on low levels of anticoagulation is no higher than that of bioprostheses without anticoagulation. No trials involving this type of comparison are yet available.

THE OBJECTIVES OF ANTICOAGULATION

Before discussing the most suitable level of anticoagulation for particular situations, it is important to clarify the aims of anticoagulation in general terms. Clearly, in order to minimise the risk of bleeding, the level of anticoagulation should be no higher than that required to achieve the primary aims.

The most important objective of anticoagulation is to prevent valve thrombosis. Although other factors play a part, the two major factors involved in the risk of valve thrombosis are the thrombogenicity of the prosthesis and the level of anticoagulation (Chapter 2.4). The lower the thrombogenicity of the prosthesis, the lower the level of anticoagulation likely to be required to prevent valve thrombosis[57]. The level of anticoagulation chosen must therefore be determined primarily by the thrombogenicity of the prosthesis. If a very high level of anticoagulation is required to prevent valve thrombosis, the risk of bleeding may be too high to contemplate its further use. In some prostheses complete prevention of thrombosis by anticoagulation may be impossible in all patients (Fig. 3.4–1).

The second objective of anticoagulation is the minimisation of embolism. It is essential to realise that embolism can only be *minimised* and not *prevented* by anticoagulation, since many, and possibly the majority of, emboli probably do not originate from the prosthesis itself (Chapter 2.4). Indeed, even in atrial fibrillation unrelated to valve disease, anticoagulation does not totally eliminate embolism originating from the left atrium[58–62].

Thus, the intensity of anticoagulation should be adjusted primarily to a level which will prevent valve thrombosis, then subsequently 'fine-tuned' to achieve a balance between the risk of embolism and the risk of bleeding[63], recognising that in some patients it will be impossible to *prevent* either of these complications[40]. Clearly when using a mechanical prosthesis of low thrombogenicity in a patient with no risk factors

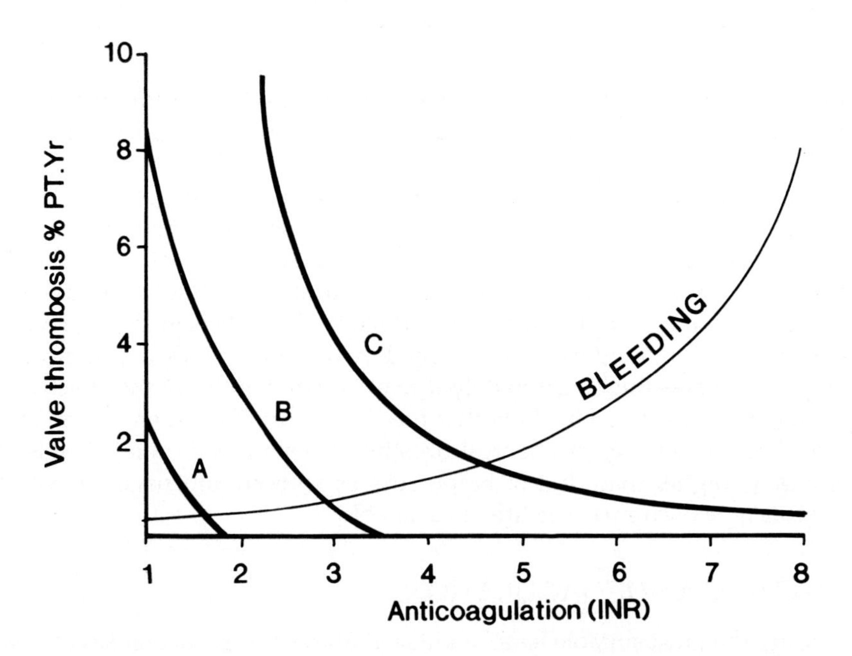

Figure 3.4–1 Effect of anticoagulation level on the incidence of valve thrombosis in three hypothetical prosthetic valves (A, B and C). In valve A (of low thrombogenicity), valve thrombosis can be effectively prevented by low intensity anticoagulation. In valve B (of moderate thrombogenicity) the same effect can only be achieved by higher levels of anticoagulation. In valve C (of high thrombogenicity) it is impossible to prevent valve thrombisis even with dangerously high levles of anticoagulation.

for embolism there will be the opportunity to employ lower levels of anticoagulation and minimise the risk of bleeding (vide infra).

The value of early anticoagulation

The problem of balancing the risks of embolism and bleeding is most acute in the early postoperative period (Chapter 1.7). In the first 24 hours after operation, there is a natural concern to minimise the risk of postoperative bleeding and tamponade. Consequently, the most common practice is to commence oral anticoagulation only after postoperative blood loss has stopped and the drainage tubes have been removed. Unfortunately this practice results in complete lack of anticoagulation for the first 24–36 hours and subtherapeutic levels for several days thereafter (Chapter 3.2), at a time when the risk of embolism is higher (Fig. 3.4–2) for several reasons[64]. The factors responsible for higher risk can be categorised according to Virchow's triad[65]:

a) *Surfaces in contact with the blood.* The operative site provides many rough surfaces on which thrombus may form; aortotomy or atriotomy suture lines, tissue adjacent to the annulus denuded of endothelium[66,67], transected papillary muscles and the sewing ring of the prosthesis[3,4,66] with its attendant suture

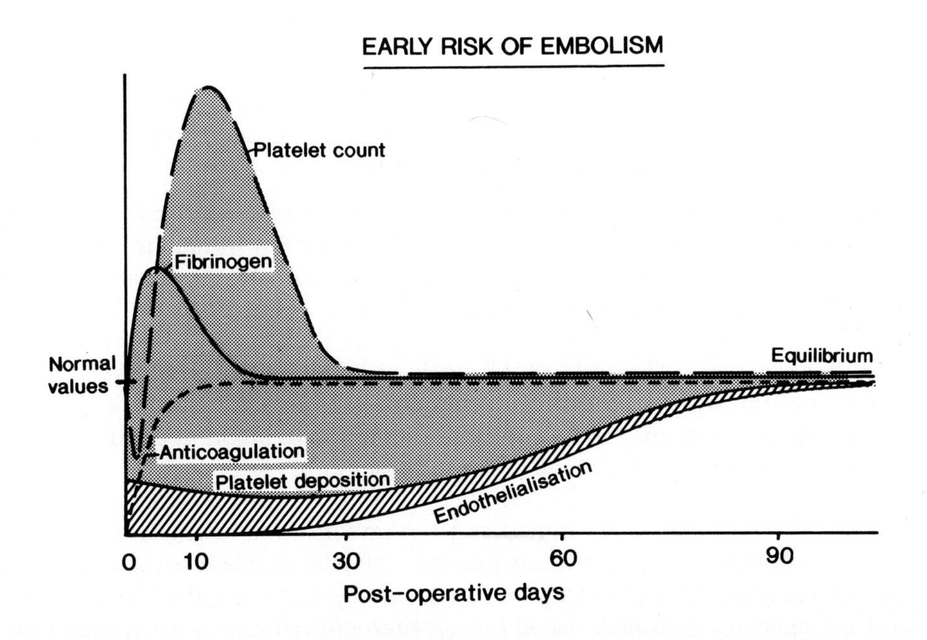

Figure 3.4–2(a) Diagrammatic representation of the factors involved in the early risk of embolism after heart valve replacement. 'Platelet deposition' (hatching) refers to the numbers of platelets found on the sewing ring of the prosthesis, gradually diminishing as endothelialisation proceeds. The shaded area is proportional to the risk of embolism. A state of 'equilibrium' is probably reached at about 90 days postoperatively.

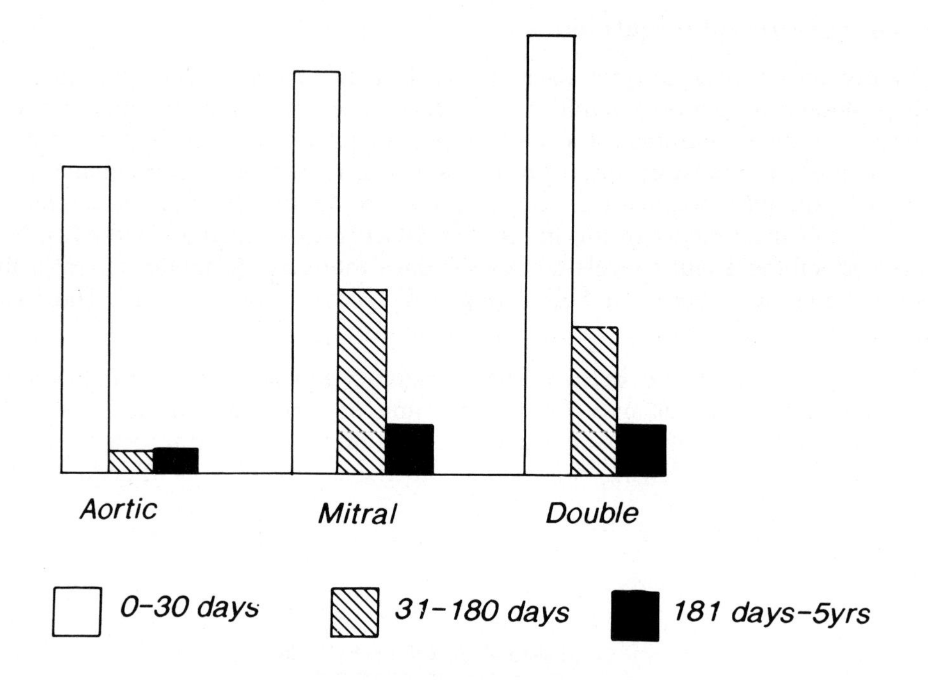

Figure 3.4–2(b) Relative risk of embolism in different time periods after operation. Based on data on the Medtronic Hall valve from Ref 54.

knots[68] and pledgets[69,70]. In addition to the effects of foreign material (Chapter 2.3), exposed collagen is a particularly powerful stimulator of platelet adhesion[71,72] and damaged endothelium may loose its natural local anticoagulant activity[73,74] and normal regulatory function[75,76].

b) *Blood flow conditions.* The early postoperative period may be complicated by low cardiac output which, especially if combined with atrial fibrillation and an enlarged left atrium, may induce relative stagnation of blood in proximity to the thrombogenic surfaces described above (Chapter 2.3).

c) *Enhanced coagulability.* Although platelet numbers and function are reduced immediately after cardiopulmonary bypass[77], platelet numbers are usually within the normal range by the third post operative day and thereafter both numbers and aggregability gradually rise to greater than normal levels, a response which lasts for up to three weeks[78]. Many patients commencing oral anticoagulants on the first postoperative day will not have achieved adequate anticoagulation levels before this rebound increase in platelet activity occurs, lending support to the use of antiplatelet drugs in the first few postoperative days[78] (vide infra).

Levels of the natural anticoagulant, antithrombin III, are depressed in the first three postoperative days[79,80] and for much longer and to a greater extent in the presence of bacterial infection[79]. Another natural anticoagulant, protein C, is depressed immediately after cardiopulmonary bypass and also at the onset of warfarin administration before the anticoagulant effect of warfarin is achieved[82,83]. Fibrinogen levels are elevated in the first few postoperative days[84], raising blood viscosity which my be further increased by overtransfusion of red cells[85] or excessive use of diuretics[86]. An inflammatory state postoperatively, in addition to raising fibrinogen levels[87], may have a generalised effect on endothelial cell function, depressing thrombomodulin activity and further increasing coagulability[74].

With factors from all three components of Virchow's triad in operation, it is not surprising to find that the incidence of embolism in the first 30 days after valve replacement is higher than the long term rate[64]. Disappointingly, this phenomenon has received scant attention in the literature and there are no controlled trials of early intravenous anticoagulation versus conventional oral anticoagulation, although some observational studies of various protocols exist[78,88–92].

Following the early work of Nina Braunwald and her associates on the prevention of excessive accumulation of thrombus on the sewing ring of valves implanted in animals, using low molecular weight dextran[4], some surgeons have used dextran clinically and found a reduction in the early embolic incidence[93]. More commonly used however is heparin, commenced on the day of operation[89,91], and in Japan particularly there appears to be enthusiasm for the use of antiplatelet drugs, either alone[78,92] or in combination with heparin and urokinase[88], until therapeutic levels of oral anticoagulation have been achieved. An observational study has shown the early use of heparin to be beneficial in eliminating embolism in the early postoperative period but no comparative data arising from conventional management were provided[89]. The recommendations for the use of antiplatelet agents in the immediate postoperative period have been mainly based on observations of platelet function rather than assessment of embolic incidence[78,88,92].

In one study intravenous warfarin, commenced within 18 hours of valve replacement and supplemented with heparin if a therapeutic level had not been achieved by the second postoperative day, was very effective in minimising early postoperative embolism with a low risk of bleeding, but again no comparative data were provided[90]. The rapid establishment of effective anticoagulation as soon as possible after operation is clearly a logical goal. However, further studies on this important aspect are required in order to determine the optimum combination of therapy.

THE IDEAL LEVEL OF ANTICOAGULATION

For many years recommendations concerning anticoagulation levels for patients with prosthetic heart valves have been largely arbitrary, based mainly on surveys of current practice and observational studies rather than scientific evaluation of different levels[91,94–101]. They have been graded as grade C recommendations (i.e. not supported by randomised trials)[102]. The current consensus view is to recommend an INR of 3.0 – 4.5 for all mechanical prosthetic valves[99,101]. In many instances, advice has come from haematologists who have based their recommendations on data relating to older prostheses[95,96,99] and assumed either that all prosthetic valves were equally thrombogenic, or that a uniform level should be recommended which would be high enough to reduce the risk of thrombotic and embolic complications even in patients with the most thrombogenic prostheses. This latter approach may simplify the management of anticoagulant clinics, which monitor patients receiving anticoagulation for many different prostheses and, of course, other medical conditions, but will not benefit the individual patient without risk factors for embolism who has a prosthesis of low thrombogenicity[57]. With a policy of uniform high level anticoagulation for all prosthetic valves in all clinical situations, such a patient may be exposed to an unnecessarily high risk of anticoagulant bleeding[57]. Clearly, what is required is a sliding scale of anticoagulation level according to prosthesis thrombogenicity and patient risk factors, taking into account temporal factors also. How should this be achieved?

In the past, much of the confusion surrounding anticoagulation intensity has stemmed from lack of standardisation of measurement (see Chapter 3.3). The acceptance of an international standard in anticoagulation measurement is an essential first step in formulating meaningful recommendations[49–52,99]. Henceforth in this chapter (and indeed throughout this book) anticoagulation level is expressed as the International Normalised Ratio (INR).

The determination of the optimum INR for each type of prosthesis and each group of patients according to their risk factors can only be achieved by trials of different levels of anticoagulation. Despite over 30 years of prosthetic valve implantation, this aspect of postoperative management has received little attention, mainly for reasons of history, early inaccuracy of tests and lack of standardisation. In addition many studies of older prostheses concluded that poor control of anticoagulation in individual patients was more important in determining the risk of embolism than the *target* range that was prescribed[32,103–105]. However this is not a valid argument against striving to set safer levels for the majority of patients, especially those with modern prostheses of low thrombogenicity.

Historically, following the isolation of dicumarol by Link and co-workers in 1940 and its subsequent introduction to clinical practice in the early 1940's[5], it was soon apparent that the drug and its later analogue, warfarin, could not be administered safely without regular prothrombin time estimations[35]. In treating embolism of cardiac origin, it was thought that a prothrombin time of more than twice normal would be required[36]. Initially this ratio appears to have been decided arbitrarily, but in the early 1950s it was confirmed that this intensity of anticoagulation resulted in the lowest incidence of thromboembolic complications after myocardial infarction; lower intensities were less effective and higher intensities produced a high incidence of bleeding without increasing the therapeutic effect[106]. Ten years later, when anticoagulation was required for prosthetic heart valves, it must therefore have seemed logical to use similar levels of anticoagulation, producing prothrombin times of approximately 'twice normal'. With the thromboplastin reagents used in the 1960s, prothrombin times two to two and a half times normal (a common recommendation) were equivalent to INRs in the range 2.8 – 3.6. In the early 1970s several commercial reagents were introduced in the USA, each relatively insensitive in comparison to those used in the 1960s[48]. As a result, prothrombin times two to two and a half times normal became equivalent to INRs in the range 5 – 10. This enormous increase in anticoagulation level appears to have gone largely unnoticed[48]. The high level of anticoagulation, perhaps arguably necessary for some early generation, highly thrombogenic prostheses, was perpetuated in the USA during the 1970s and 1980s despite the availability of less thrombogenic valves. Recently, the finding that lower INRs could be employed in many conditions without jeopardising antithrombotic effectiveness led to the questioning of these high levels[47,48]. In much of Europe meanwhile, a commercial test (Thrombotest) was being used to express the anticoagulant effect in a different way: as the percentage of normal coagulation activity remaining[107], but recommended percentages varied and different results were obtained depending on whether capillary or venous blood was used[107]. Furthermore, the logarithmic nature of the scale decreased the sensitivity of the measurement as anticoagulation increased. For example a Thrombotest of 5% is approximately equivalent to an INR of 4.8, whereas 4% is 5.8 and 3% is 7.4 (see Chapter 3.3).

Although its use continues in many European countries, the Thrombotest method was gradually superceded in the UK by the British Ratio (BR) and later the British Corrected Ratio (BCR) which gave numerical values in the therapeutic range similar to the recently adopted INR[95]. It seems likely that, before international standardisation was introduced, many clinicians believed that a BCR or INR of 2.0 meant the same as a prothrombin time of 'twice normal' as recommended in the USA. Hence, for many years British heart valve patients were maintained at an INR of 2.0 to 3.0 whilst American patients experienced INRs between 5.0 and 10.0 (vide infra).

This state of confusion partly explains the paucity of scientific data available on which to base reliable guidelines for specific prostheses or patient groups. For example, a prothrombin time of 'twice normal' in the USA may be equivalent to an INR of either 5.0 or 7.0 or to an intermediate value, depending on which commercial reagent has been used for the test[51]. If the laboratory changes its reagent without informing the clinician, an important increase or decrease in *real* anticoagulation may result whilst the prothrombin time remains 'twice normal'[47,48]. In 1980, a report was published comparing the long-term postoperative embolic incidence in two consecutive 7-year time periods, using the same prosthesis in the same institution and maintaining the prothrombin time at 'twice normal'[108]. The lower incidence of embolism in the second 7-year period was ascribed to a difference in patient risk factors, which may indeed have been part of the explanation. However, the incidence of anticoagulant-related bleeding in the second time period was more than double that in the first time period, implying a higher level of anticoagulation[108]. It is possible than an increase in mean INR, brought about by a change in reagent[47,48], was responsible at least in part for the observed reduction in embolic incidence, because the transition from first to second 7-year time period coincided approximately with the introduction of new commercial reagents in the USA[48].

Trials involving different levels of anticoagulation for prosthetic heart valves are few in number. A randomised comparison of low (INR 2.0 – 2.25) and moderate (INR 2.5 – 4.0) anticoagulation in the first three months after bioprosthetic valve replacement in a small number of patients failed to demonstrate any reduction in embolic incidence with the higher level of anticoagulation but revealed a significantly greater incidence of bleeding events[109]. Another small randomised study comparing INR 2.0 – 3.0 with INR 3.0 – 4.5 over a slightly longer period in Bicer tilting disc valves showed similar results[110], although the anticoagulant bleeding incidence may have been magnified and the embolic incidence lowered by the concomitant use of aspirin and dipyridamole in both groups of patients, rather blunting the impact of the investigation. Both of these randomised comparisons contained too few patients and too few events to reach any conclusion about the effect of anticoagulation level on embolic incidence.

A larger randomised trial from Saudi Arabia with longer follow-up, comparing a target INR of 2.65 with a target INR of 9.0 also showed an increased incidence of bleeding with the higher level of anticoagulation but no difference in embolic incidence[111]. However, the effect of anticoagulation on embolic incidence in this study is difficult to interpret. Although 'target' INRs were set, there appears to have been considerable variability in INR (as in most series[54]) and many patients had a low INR at the time of their embolic event. Interpretation is also confounded by the inclusion of five different prostheses of mixed vintage which yielded different embolic rates. Overall, the embolic rates were quite high for a young patient population (90% under the age of 40, 70% under 30), only 20% of whom were in atrial fibrillation, perhaps reflecting the effect of the older, more thrombogenic prostheses. In caged ball and caged disc valves, heavily represented in this series, thrombus formation on the cage occurs as a consequence of turbulence and flow separation and embolism is probably mainly due to thrombus dislodgement from the cage by occluder impact (see Chapter 2.4). It is possible that this type of thrombosis and embolism either cannot be greatly reduced even by high intensity anticoagulation, or is more sensitive to inadequately controlled anticoagulation[32,103–105]. It is interesting that the same group of Saudi Arabian surgeons report a much lower embolic incidence in a later group of patients who received only modern tilting disc and bileaflet valves, despite using only moderate levels of anticoagulation[112].

The experience from Saudi Arabia described above illustrates the problem imposed by other variables in a study designed primarily to investigate the effect of anticoagulation level. The different embolic rates of the various prostheses used reduced the ability to discern an effect of anticoagulation in the study as a whole. This underlines the importance of studying prostheses individually when attempting to define optimum anticoagulation levels, since it is likely that the 'optimum' will vary from one prosthesis to another, especially when comparing prostheses of different vintage and totally different design. Even so, patient risk factors need to be taken into consideration also.

With a large experience of one prosthesis (Medtronic Hall) implanted in one institution and subjected to two different mean anticoagulation levels, the Cardiff valve study was able to provide recommendations concerning the ideal level of anticoagulation for patients with isolated aortic or mitral valve replacement with this prosthesis[57]. Having already found a zero incidence of valve thrombosis despite low levels of anticoagulation[113] (mean INR 2.5), the level of anticoagulation was increased to a mean of 3.0 to determine the effect on embolism. In isolated mitral valve replacement, the risk of serious embolism (causing death or permanent disability) at 3 years was reduced ten-fold from 5% to 0.5% with a concomitant fall in minor embolism and only a small increase in the risk of bleeding (Fig. 3.4–3). It was felt that any further increase in INR would have been counterproductive and that a mean INR of 3.0 was therefore the ideal level for isolated mitral valve replacement.

In isolated aortic valve replacement the effect of increasing mean INR from 2.5 to 3.0 was quite different. Not only did the incidence of bleeding increase as expected, but the incidence of embolism rose also (Fig. 3.4–4). However, further analysis showed that

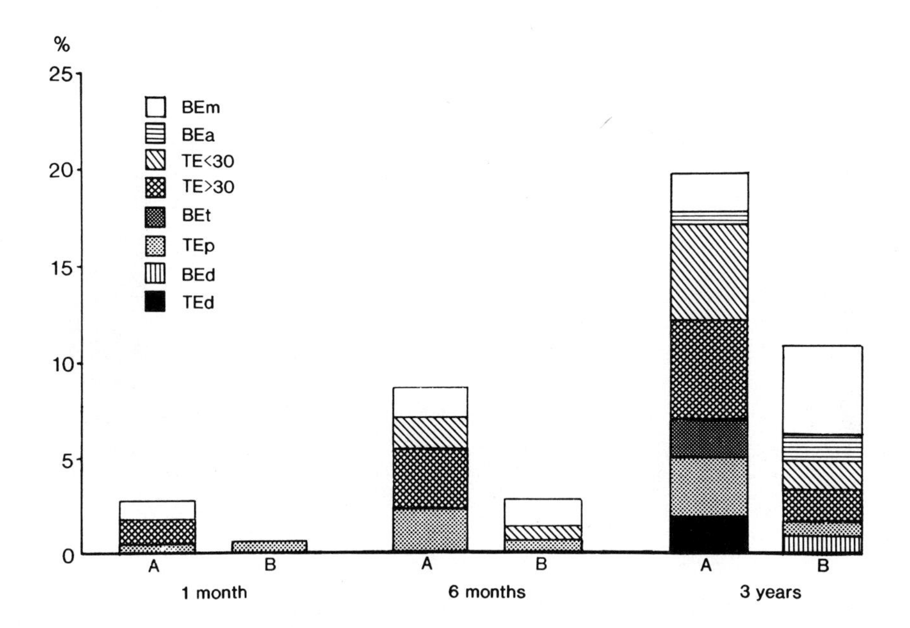

Figure 3.4–3 Effect of anticoagulaton level on cumulative embolic and bleeding risks 1 month, 6 months and 3 years after mitral valve replacement with the Medtronic Hall valve. A = low anticoagulation (mean INR 2.5). B = moderate anticoagulation (means INR 3.0).
TEd = Thromboembolic death. BEd = Bleeding death. TEp = Thromboembolic event with permanent deficit. BEt = Bleeding requiring hospital treatment. TE>30 = Transient thromboembolic event lasting more than 30 minutes. TE<30 = Transient thromboembolic event lasting less than 30 minutes. BEa = Bleeding causing anaemia. BEm = Minor bleeding.

the group of patients with higher anticoagulation also contained significantly more patients in atrial fibrillation and significantly more hypertensives. Extending the analysis to include other known stroke risk factors showed that all patients suffering emboli had one or more established stroke risk factors, and that patients who had none did not suffer any embolic episodes, irrespective of their level of anticoagulation. Thus patients who were aged less than 70, non-smokers, normotensive and in stable sinus rhythm gained nothing from higher anticoagulation and were exposed to a greater risk of bleeding. An INR of 2.5 was therefore thought to be high enough for isolated aortic valve replacement, on the basis that patients with risk factors did not appear to be protected from embolism by higher anticoagulation. The findings of this study also suggest that it may be possible to manage patients with no risk factors at even lower levels of anticoagulation (vide infra).

An analysis of the mitral embolic data according to known stroke risk factors yielded similar results. Twenty three of 183 patients in the low anticoagulation group (mean INR 2.5) and 4 of 162 patients in the moderate anticoagulation group (mean INR 3.0) suffered embolic events. Of these 27 patients, 24 (89%) were in atrial fibrillation at the

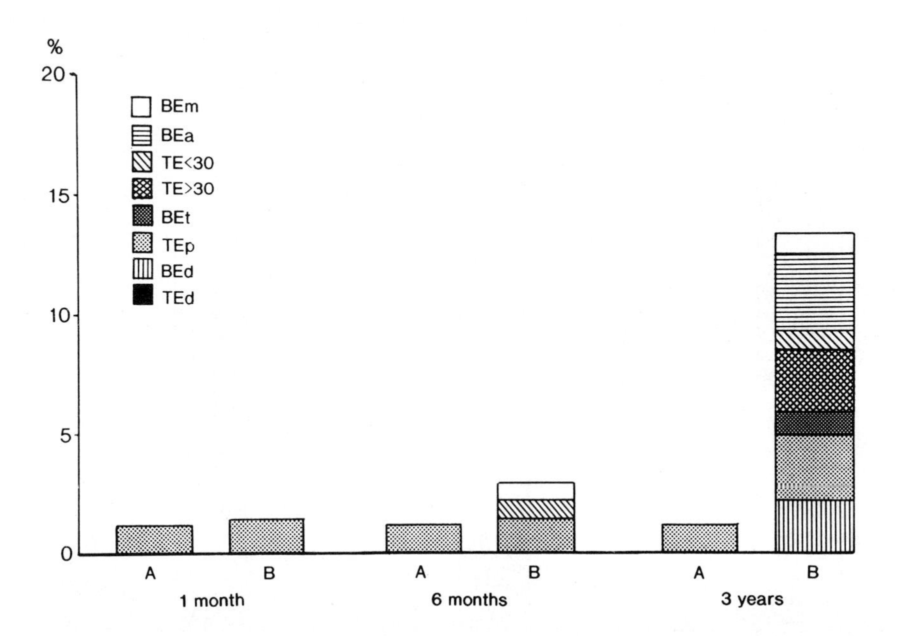

Figure 3.4–4. Effect of anticoagulation level on cumulative embolic and bleeding risks 1 month, 6 months and 3 years after aortic valve replacement with Medtronic Hall valve. A = low anticoagulation (mean INR 2.5). B = moderate anticoagulation (mean INR 3.0). Abbreviations. see Figure 3. Note: in both Figure 3 and Figure 4, anticoagulation level refers to the level actually achieved *rather than a target level.*

time of their event and 3 (11%) were in stable sinus rhythm. The 3 patients in sinus rhythm who suffered embolic events had certain features in common: they all experienced transient events with complete recovery, they all had one known stroke risk factor (either hypertension or cigarette smoking) and all were in the low anticoagulation group. Patients in sinus rhythm with no stroke risk factors suffered no embolic events irrespective of their anticoagulation level. All patients in sinus rhythm anticoagulated at a moderate level (mean INR 3.0) avoided embolism.

The dramatic fall in embolic risk in these mitral patients with increased anticoagulation was almost certainly due, at least in part, to the effect of anticoagulation on the embolic potential of atrial fibrillation, since it has been shown that anticoagulation will decrease the risk of embolism even in atrial fibrillation unassociated with valve disease[59–62](see also Chapter 1.2). This underlines the importance of considering patient-related factors in addition to the prosthesis when deciding on optimum anticoagulation levels.

It should be stressed that the optimum anticoagulation levels referred to above apply only to one prosthesis (Medtronic Hall). Unpublished data on anticoagulation levels for the St. Jude Medical aortic valve suggest that an INR in the range 2.0 – 3.0 should minimise the combined incidence of embolism and bleeding (Table 3.4–1)[114]. Using randomised trials of different anticoagulant levels, it should be possible to determine optimum levels for other prostheses. It is important to emphasise that the level of anticoagulation should be primarily set at a minimum level to prevent valve

Table 3.4–1
Thromboembolic (TE) and Severe Bleeding (B) Complications[1] Due to Anticoagulation Treatment in Patients with St. Jude Medical Aortic Valve Prostheses[2]
– Influence of target INR on the incidence of complications –

target INR	*period of follow-up*	*n*	*mean follow-up (months)*	*total FUM[3]*	*frequency* TE	B	TE+B	*linearised incidence* TE	B	*TEB Index[4]*
3.0–4.5	1980–1985	524	31.2	16,357	11	33	44	0.81	2.42	3.23
2.5–3.5	1986–1988	323	28.8	9,058	8	15	23	1.06	1.99	3.05
2.0–3.0	1988–1990	256	18.7	4,798	5	6	11	1.25	1.50	2.75

[1] Definition according to Ann Thorac Surg (1988) 46:275
[2] Patients who were not in sinus rhythm or who had significant left ventricular dysfunction on echocardiography were excluded from analysis
[3] FUM = follow-up months. Only the first thromboembolic episode was accounted. Patients with low intensity anticoagulation and a TE episode were put on so called "effective" anticoagulation (target INR 3.0–4.5)
[4] TEB index is the sum of TE and B incidence. For further details see Chapter – 6.4.

thrombosis and subsequently 'fine-tuned' to minimise both embolism and bleeding. It is probable therefore that higher levels of anticoagulation will be required for prostheses which, on currently available information, appear more prone to valve thrombosis[113,115]. Higher levels of anticoagulation may also be necessary in prostheses associated with turbulence-related and occluder impact embolism (for example caged ball and caged disc valves – see Chapter 2.4) although there is no definite evidence that higher levels are protective in these valves [111]. Indeed the addition of dipyridamole or ticlopidine to moderate levels of anticoagulation may be more beneficial in this situation (vide infra). Higher levels may be required in the first few postoperative months for all prosthetic valves until endothelialisation of the sewing ring has taken place, although in the absence of any information on this aspect in the literature, this must remain speculative.

Bioprostheses in general are considered to be less thrombogenic than mechanical prostheses[39]. However, they are not immune from thrombus deposition, both on the sewing ring and the leaflets[66], especially in the first three postoperative months, and even gross valve thrombosis may occur in porcine valves[116–119](see Chapter 2.4). In the mitral position the incidence of embolism differs very little from that seen with mechanical prostheses[40]. It is probably mainly associated with non-prosthetic risk factors, especially atrial fibrillation[40,119], as in mechanical prostheses (Chapter 2.4), and is not eliminated by anticoagulation[40].

Although the current consensus view is to anticoagulate all patients with bioprostheses in the first three months until the sewing has been endothelialised[100], there is no evidence to show that anticoagulation significantly reduces embolism during this period[40]. The trial of two different levels of anticoagulation in bioprostheses[109], referred to earlier, suggests that an INR in the range 2.0 – 2.25 is probably high enough for these valves. In this respect bioprostheses during the first three postoperative months might be considered equivalent to low thrombogenicity mechanical valves. In the presence of

Table 3.4–2
Tentative INR Recommendations

Prosthesis	AVR	MVR
Low thrombogenicity mechanical valves and bioprostheses	2.0–2.5	2.5–3.0
Mechanical valves with severe turbulence	3.0–3.5 + Antiplatelet therapy	
High thrombogenicity mechanical valves	3.5 – 4.0	

Patients with embolic risk factors – higher end of each range
– plus anti-platelet agents
(see text for explanation)

atrial fibrillation, left atrial thrombus or a history of embolism, long term anticoagulation should be recommended[100]. However the use of a bioprosthesis under such circumstances should be questioned. For patients in sinus rhythm with no stroke risk factors anticoagulation is unnecessary after the first three months, at least in the aortic position[100]. Long term anticoagulation for patients with mitral bioprostheses in sinus rhythm is probably also unnecessary[100,119], but the situation remains unclear since no satisfactory trials exist. The place of antiplatelet agents is discussed below.

A suggested protocol is detailed in Table 3.4–2, proposing anticoagulation levels that could be applied to groups of patients categorised according to their prosthesis and their risk factors. In addition it may also be possible eventually to 'personalise' anticoagulation levels for individual patients according to tests which measure various coagulability parameters (Chapters 1.5 and 2.5) or according to echocardiographic assessment of embolic risk (Chapter 2.6) or both. A prospective study is being undertaken in Cardiff to evaluate this approach.

Some attempts have already been made to place anticoagulant prescribing on a more scientific foundation using fibrinopeptide A measurements. Fibrinopeptide A is released when fibrinogen is converted to fibrin and has been used as a marker of in vivo thrombin activity. An Italian study found elevated levels in a small number of patients with a variety of different mechanical prostheses (mainly Sorin, Bjørk-Shiley and Lillehei-Kaster) anticoagulated in the INR range 3.0 – 4.5[120]. They found that fibrinopeptide A levels could only be lowered to values approaching those of normal controls by raising the INR to between 4.5 and 5.1. This is perhaps in keeping with the more thrombogenic nature of these prostheses of older design. However, they produced no evidence that decreased thrombin activity actually reduced the risk of embolism, nor did they provide information about patient risk factors. The latter is particularly relevant in this context as atrial fibrillation alone has been shown to be associated with relative hypercoagulability[121]. This study illustrates the danger of extrapolating laboratory data to clinical decision making without first correlating the laboratory findings with event incidence.

A small study from Romania correlating lowered anti-thrombin III levels with thromboembolic complications has suggested that low levels should be an indication for intensifying anticoagulant treatment[122]. This accords with the finding that antithrombin III levels are lowered in proportion to the severity of mitral stenosis[123]. Increased betathromboglobulin production from platelets (a measurement of ADP-induced platelet activation[124]) has also been advanced as an indication for increasing anticoagulation level, on the basis that normal values of betathromboglobulin can be restored by greater anticoagulation intensity in patients with prosthetic valves[125], presumably because decreased fibrin deposition on prosthetic and other surfaces diminishes platelet activation. However, others have shown that patients who suffered embolic events had elevated betathromboglobulin levels despite 'adequate' anticoagulation[126]. Further studies on both antithrombin III and betathromboglobulin are required.

High fibrinogen levels have been suggested as an indication for greater anticoagulation intensity and for supplementation with non-steroidal anti-inflammatory drugs[89]. This applies to the immediate postoperative period, when fibrinogen levels tend to be raised as part of a normal physiological response[84], and to the long term when raised levels may be associated with a variety of conditions[87]. For example, raised fibrinogen levels are found in diabetes, pregnancy and inflammatory conditions and in response to endotoxins, stress and high dietary fat intake[87]. Cigarette smoking also raises fibrinogen levels[127]. Because high fibrinogen levels increase blood viscosity[128] and coagulability[129], especially in conditions of sluggish flow, and are associated with greater risk of stroke[127,130,131], myocardial infarction[127,130,132] and thromboembolism after myocardial infarction[133], they should probably be taken into account in prosthetic heart valve patients. However, higher anticoagulation levels will not influence fibrinogen levels, nor the effect of fibrinogen on viscosity and platelets. There is evidence that the antiplatelet agent ticlopidine and some lipid-lowering drugs reduce fibrinogen levels (Chapter 1.5), but no studies have been conducted in patients with prosthetic valves.

THE PLACE OF SUPPLEMENTARY ANTIPLATELET DRUGS

Thrombus formation that takes place on the arterial side of the circulation, in high pressure/high flow conditions, involves mainly platelets and the surface in contact with the blood, with coagulation factors playing a lesser role[72,134]. Under these conditions, inhibition of platelet function may have a significant effect (Chapter 3.1). In contrast, under conditions of slow blood flow or relative stagnation on the venous side, coagulation factors play the most important part and platelets have a lesser role. Here, antiplatelet agents have little place and anticoagulation is the dominant effect required[134].

Following heart valve replacement a combination of 'arterial' and 'venous' conditions exist. Although blood flow through prosthetic valves may be rapid, especially in the aortic position, some types of prosthesis give rise to areas of relatively stagnant flow or turbulence (Chapter 2.1). Turbulence and flow separation, by increasing shear stresses cause red cell and platelet damage, liberating ADP, a potent stimulator of platelet aggregation (see Chapter 2.2). 'Venous' conditions also exist in the left atrium following mitral valve replacement, particularly when the left atrium is enlarged and/or fibrillating, or when the prostheses is relatively stenotic[135–137].

Platelet activity in relation to heart valve replacement is greatest in the first few weeks after operation[78]. Immediately after prosthetic valve replacement platelet survival is decreased and turnover greatly increased, in contrast to almost normal platelet kinetics after aortic homograft replacement[138]. During the first three weeks, platelet numbers[78], aggregability[78] and adhesiveness[139,140] are increased. For the first three months, the sewing ring is not fully endothelialised and susceptible to platelet deposition which gradually diminishes over this period[66,67]. Many of the emboli generated during these early postoperative weeks are probably predominantly platelet emboli[66,138].

Although some surgeons and cardiologists prescribe long term antiplatelet therapy in addition to anticoagulation for all patients with mechanical valves, antiplatelet drugs are not without side effects and up to 10% of patients are obliged to abandon them because of drug intolerance[91]. It is therefore rational to limit their use to situations where they are of proven effectiveness or where there is sufficient scientific basis to suggest a beneficial effect, as follows:

1. *The early postoperative period in all prostheses*, until the sewing ring is endothelialised, for the reasons outlined above. Dipyridamole inhibits platelet deposition on artificial surfaces when combined with anticoagulation[141] and has been shown to increase platelet survival[138] and reduce platelet aggregability[78] in the postoperative period. Its effects on platelet adhesiveness are less clear[141]. Some studies have shown an effect[140] whereas others have not[138]. Two Japanese studies have shown ticlopidine to be more effective than dipyridamole in suppressing platelet aggregability postoperatively[78,142]. Aspirin, although it has little effect on platelet survival or aggregability[138], effectively suppresses platelet adhesiveness[138,143] and this can be used to monitor dosage postoperatively[139]. Most surgeons prefer to avoid the combination of aspirin and warfarin, however, because of the increased risk of bleeding[144].

2. *In patients with stroke risk factors*, where antiplatelet agents have been shown to be beneficial or a scientific basis exists; for example diabetes[145], persistent cigarette smoking[146], atheroma involving the ascending aorta, carotid arteries and cerebral arteries [147–149] or surgery of the ascending aorta[150]. In these situations both aspirin and ticlopidine are probably more beneficial than dipyridamole[151], but both should probably be used only if the INR can be maintained at a low level (for example after aortic valve replacement) because of the increased risk of bleeding[144].

3. *In patients with concomitant coronary artery disease*. The case for antiplatelet agents in this situation is now well established, at least in the early postoperative months[91]. Long term therapy with aspirin may also be beneficial, especially if coronary risk factors persist postoperatively, because many of these factors are also stroke risk factors.

4. *In patients with older turbulent prostheses*. Much of the data demonstrating a reduction in embolic incidence and increased platelet survival when sulfinpyrazone or dipyridamole are added to anticoagulation are based on studies involving older prostheses associated with massive turbulence and flow separation, such as caged ball and caged disc valves[138,144,152–156]. Dipyridamole appears to work at least in part by inhibiting ADP-induced platelet aggregation[141]. This may explain its beneficial effect in turbulent prostheses, since turbulence and flow separation give rise to shear stresses which damage red cells and platelets liberating ADP[157]. Platelet survival time measurement in patients with these older prostheses should indicate which patients require antiplatelet therapy, since those with normal platelet survival seem less

susceptible to embolism[154]. There is no evidence in the literature to show that antiplatelet agents have any long term benefit in patients with modern prostheses. One randomised trial comparing dipyridamole, a related substance and placebo added to anticoagulation, failed to show any difference in platelet survival times in a study group in which tilting disc valves predominated[157A].

5. *In patients who have suffered emboli despite good anticoagulant control.* Although this is common practice, it is a recommendation[100] which is based on trials of warfarin versus warfarin plus dipyridamole in *primary* prevention rather than *secondary* prevention. Furthermore, all the trials involved older caged ball and caged disc valves[140,144,152,156]. There are no data in the literature on secondary prevention trials.

6. *For the long term management of bioprostheses.* For patients in sinus rhythm, even though the risk of embolism without anticoagulation is low, long term management with aspirin may provide additional protection[158], although it is possible that the risk of embolism is more dependent on non-prosthetic factors[150] (see paragraph 2 above). No randomised trials exist on which to base firm recommendations[100]. For further discussion of this subject see Chapters 2.4 and 3.1.

7. *In the management of children.* See Chapter 4.2.

FIXED 'MINI-DOSE' WARFARIN

Low dose warfarin (target INR 1.5–2.9) has been shown to be highly effective in preventing stroke in patients with non-rheumatic atrial fibrillation[62] and in recent years, the use of so-called 'mini-dose' warfarin in fixed dosage has been described in a number of clinical situations[159–162]. In these, it has been shown to be clinically effective with the additional advantages of ease of administration, avoidance of regular blood tests and, above all, reduced risk of bleeding[159,161,162]. A dose of 1 mg of warfarin in most patients does not prolong the prothrombin time beyond the normal range, but can significantly reduce factor VII levels when these are elevated[160] and may increase fibrinolysis[161]. This dose of warfarin has also been shown to exert a clinical effect even when the assays of vitamin K-dependent coagulation factors (II, VII, IX and X) do not differ from normal controls[162], so that a more subtle effect on prothrombin function seems likely at this reduced dose of warfarin[162].

Mini-dose (1 mg) warfarin has been shown to be effective in reducing the incidence of deep vein thrombosis[159,161] and thrombosis in central venous catheters[165]. A primary prevention of myocardial infarction trial is on-going in men with elevated factor VII levels, aiming at a mean INR of 1.5[163]. However, no trials have yet been undertaken in patients with prosthetic heart valves. Patients with prosthetic aortic valves of low thrombogenicity and no additional stroke risk factors would seem to be an ideal group for a prospective randomised trial between fixed mini-dose and conventionally administered warfarin. A pilot study of low dose warfarin (INR 1.5) before proceeding to fixed mini-dose warfarin would probably be prudent as a first step. If found to be safe and effective, fixed mini-dose warfarin would be particularly suitable for the management of elderly patients and patients in developing countries with limited facilities for anticoagulation control.

RISK FACTOR MODIFICATION

As discussed earlier, it is necessary to stratify patients into groups according to risk factors when making detailed recommendations about anticoagulation level. There is obvious benefit to be gained by being able to 'promote' patients to a lower risk group when they lose one or more risk factors, since less intense anticoagulation reduces the risk of bleeding[45–48]. Yet this is an aspect of postoperative management that has received little attention. An aggressive policy towards restoring sinus rhythm if possible[97] and treating hypertension[164,165] postoperatively may reduce the risk of stroke. Life-style advice should centre on the avoidance of cigarette smoking[166,167] which increases coagulability directly by raising fibrinogen levels[127], platelet aggregability[146,168–170] and red cell volume[86,171] and indirectly by raising plasma cholesterol and free fatty acids[172,173]. Advice should also include the avoidance of environmental tobacco smoke[174,175] and drugs that increase coagulability[176] (for example oral contraceptives[87,176–178]), the necessity for weight reduction in obesity[179] and the advisability of regular exercise[180,181].

Dietary advice is also important, since it has been shown that ADP-induced platelet aggregation (a dominant effect in turbulent prostheses) is increased in experimental animals fed on a diet rich in saturated fatty acids[182]. Electron microscopy studies have also shown that experimental animals fed on a high animal fat, high carbohydrate, low protein diet develop atrial endothelial damage, which predisposes to atrial thrombosis[183]. Vegetable and fish oils rich in polyunsaturated fatty acids in contrast have an antithrombotic effect[182]. Fish oils appear to exert their effect mainly by inhibiting platelet aggregation although some of the antithrombotic action may be due to increased levels of anti-thrombin III and reduced levels of fibrinolytic enzyme inhibitors[184]. Both fish oils and aspirin inhibit platelet thromboxane A_2 formation and their effects in this respect are additive[182].

As yet, no trials of dietary supplementation of anticoagulant control have been conducted after heart valve replacement, but this seems to be an area which merits further study. Indeed, the whole question of risk factor reduction after heart valve surgery is a subject that merits at least as much attention as coronary risk factor reduction.

PATIENT COMPLIANCE

The co-operation of the patient is absolutely essential for good anticoagulant control, especially if a narrow range of anticoagulant level is to be achieved. The advantages of home prothrombin time estimation and autoregulation of anticoagulation are explained in Chapters 3.5 and 3.6 , but are likely to be available only to a minority of patients. Before the patient leaves hospital, it is important that a full explanation of anticoagulant therapy is given, including the dietary factors and drugs (including alcohol) that can modify the effect of warfarin (see Chapter 3.2). Change of diet when the patient returns home often results in a change in dose requirement[15,90], and the first few weeks of anticoagulation after leaving hospital must be monitored very closely[90]. In elderly or forgetful patients, a close relative should be involved in explanations and in dispensing the medication. Avoidance of different doses on alternate days (a common practice in some anticoagulant clinics) helps to eliminate another source of error, when the patient cannot remember which dose was taken the previous day.

In Japan, the drug bucolome which competes with warfarin for albumin-binding sites, is used in many centres on the basis that it 'smooths out' the peaks and troughs of

INR values seen on many patients' anticoagulant charts, and allows more sophisticated control within a narrow range[185–186]. Further trials of this drug would seem to be worthwhile.

REFERENCES

1. Lefrak EA, Starr A. Historic aspects of cardiac valve replacement. In Lefrak EA, Starr A: Cardiac Valve Prostheses, New York, Appleton Century Crofts, 1979;3–37.
2. Walter JB, Israel MS. General Pathology. London, Churchill 1964.
3. Berger K, Sauvage LR, Wood SJ, Wesolowski SA. Sewing ring healing of cardiac valve prostheses. Surgery 1967;61:102–117.
4. Bonchek LI, Braunwald NS. Modification of thrombus formation on prosthetic heart valves by the administration of low molecular weight dextran. Ann Surg 1967;165:200–205.
5. Link KP. The discovery of dicumarol and its sequels. Circulation 1959;19:97–107.
6. Braunwald NS, Bonchek LI. Prevention of thrombus formation on rigid prosthetic heart valves by the ingrowth of autogenous tissue. J Thorac Cardiovasc Surg 1967;54:630–638.
7. Braunwald NS, Morrow AG. Tissue ingrowth and the rigid heart valve. J Thorac Cardiovasc Surg 1968;56:307–322.
8. Braunwald NS, Bull BS. Factors controlling the development of tissue layers on fabrics. In Brewer LA (Ed):Prosthetic Heart Valves. Springfield. Charles C Thomas, 1969;228–242.
9. Palmer TE, Lautsch EV, Sanmarco ME, Davila JC. A non-thrombogenic, non-anticoagulant dependant mitral valve prosthesis. Circulation 1967;35/36 Suppl I:42–47.
10. Gott VL. Synthetic materials for valve construction. Adv Cardiol 1972;7:12–24.
11. Bokros JC. Carbon in prosthetic devices. Biomed Mater Res Symp Trans 1978;2:32–36.
12. Schwartz ML, Sheldon DS, Dorman F, Blackshear PL, Varco RL, Buchwald H, Nicoloff DM. Local anticoagulation of prosthetic heart valves. Circulation 1973;47/48 Suppl III:85–89.

12A. Mobin-Uddin K, Utley JR, Bryant LR, Dillon M, Weiss DL: Experimental and clinical evaluation of heparin-impregnated cloth-covered cardiac valves used without systemic anticoagulation. Ann Thorac Surg 1974; 17: 351–359.

13. Duvoisin GE, Brandeburg RO, McGoon DC. Factors affecting thromboembolism associated with prosthetic heart valves. Circulation 1967;35/36 Suppl I:70–76.
14. Yeh TJ, Anabtawi IN, Cornett VE, Ellison RG. Influence of rhythm and anticoagulation upon the incidence of embolization associated with Starr-Edwards prostheses. Circulation 1967;35/36 SupplI:77–81.
15. Gadboys HL, Litwak RS, Niemetz J, Wisch N. Role of anticoagulants in preventing embolization from prosthetic heart valves. J Am Med Assoc 1967;202:134–138.
16. Bjørk VO, Henze A. Management of thromboembolism after aortic valve replacement with the Bjørk-Shiley tilting disc valve. Scand J Thorac Cardiovasc Surg 1975;9:183–191.
17. Larsen GL, Alexander JA, Stanford S:Thromboembolic phenomena in patients with prosthetic aortic valves who did not receive anticoagulants. Ann Thorac Surg 1977;23:323–326.
18. Limet R, Lepage G, Grondin CM. Thromboembolic complications with the cloth-covered Starr-Edwards aortic prosthesis in patients not receiving anticoagulants. Ann Thorac Surg 1977;23:529–533.
19. Moggio RA, Hammond GL, Stansel HC, Glenn WWL. Incidence of emboli with cloth covered Starr-Edwards valve without anticoagulation and with varying forms of anticoagulation. J Thorac Cardiovasc Surg 1978;75:296–299.
20. Thomsen PB, Alstrup P. Thromboembolism in patients without anticoagulants after aortic valve replacement with the Lillehei-Kaster disc valve. Thorac Cardiovasc Surgeon 1979;27:313–315.
21. Tanaka N, Yamaguchi T, Ohno T, Ohori K, Kitano I, Abe T, Komatsu S. The results of long term follow-up study for 445 cases of valve replacement with various kinds of cardiac prostheses, with or without postoperative anticoagulant therapy (English abstract). Nippon Kyobu Geka Gakkai Zasshi 1983;31:152–160.
22. Ribeiro PA, Al Zaibag M, Idris M, Al Kasab S, Davies G, Mashat E, Wareham E, Al Fagih M. Antiplatelet drugs and the incidence of thromboembolic complications of the St. Jude Medical aortic prosthesis in patients with rheumatic heart disease. J Thorac Cardiovasc Surg 1986;91:92–98.
23. Hartz RS, LoCicero J, Kucich V, DeBoer A, O'Mara S, Meyers SN, Michaelis LL. Comparative study of warfarin versus antiplatelet therapy in patients with a St. Jude Medical valve in the aortic position. J Thorac Cardiovasc Surg 1986;92:684–690.
24. Myers ML, Lawrie GM. Crawford ES, Howell JF, Morris GC, Glaeser DH, DeBakey ME. The St. Jude prosthesis: analysis of the clinical results in 815 implants and the need for systemic anticoagulation.
25. Effler DB, Favaloro R, Groves LK. Heart valve replacement: clinical experience. Ann Thorac Surg 1965;1:4–24.

26. Smithwick W, Kouchoukos NT, Karp RB, Pacifico AD, Kirklin JW. Late stenosis of Starr-Edwards cloth-covered prostheses. Ann Thorac Surg 1975;20:249–255.
27. Stein DW, Rahimtoola SH, Kloster FE, Selden R, Starr A. Thrombotic phenomena with non-anticoagulated composite-strut aortic prostheses. J Thorac Cardiovasc Surg 1976;71:680–684.
28. Warnes CA, McIntosh CL, Roberts WC. Wear of the metallic studs on the composite seat of 2320 Starr-Edwards aortic valve and its clinical consequences. Am J Cardiol 1983;52:1062–1065.
29. Foreman R, Beck W, Barnard CN. Results of valve replacement with the Lillehei-Kaster disc prosthesis. Am Heart J 1977;94:282–286.
30. Emery RW, Nicoloff DM. St. Jude Medical cardiac valve prosthesis: in vitro studies. J Thorac Cardiovasc Surg 1979;78:269–276.
31. Yoganathan AP, Chaux A, Gray RJ, De Robertis M, Matloff JM. Flow characteristics of the St. Jude Prosthetic valve: an in vitro and in vivo study. Artif Organs 1982;6:288–294.
32. Friedli B, Aerichide N, Grondin P, Campeau L. Thromboembolic complications of heart valve prostheses. Am Heart J 1971;81:702–708.
33. Editorial: Risks of suddenly stopping anticoagulants. Br Med J 1971;1:485–486.
34. Shetty HGM, Fennerty AG, Routledge PA. Clinical pharmacokinetic considerations in the control of oral anticoagulant therapy. Clin Pharmacokin 1989;16:238–253.
35. Barker NW, Hines EA, Kvale WF, Allen EV. Dicumarol: its action, clinical use and effectiveness as an anticoagulant drug. Am J Med 1947;3:634–642.
36. Wright IS, Foley WT. Use of anticoagulants in the treatment of heart disease. Am J Med 1947;3:718–739.
37. Nitter-Hauge S, Dale J. High complication and failure rates of anticoagulant therapy are unavoidable. Z Kardiol 1986, 75 (Suppl 2):293–297.
38. Petitti DB, Strom BL, Melmon KL. Duration of warfarin anticoagulant therapy and the probabilities of recurrent thromboembolism and haemorrhage. Am J Med 1986;81:255–259.
39. Jamieson WRE. Bioprostheses are superior to mechanical prostheses. Z Kardiol 1986;75 (Suppl 2):258–271.
40. Edmunds LH Jr. Thrombotic and bleeding complications of prosthetic heart valves. Ann Thorac Surg 1987;44:430–445.
41. Coon WW, Willis PW. Haemorrhagic complications of anticoagulant therapy. Arch Intern Med 1974;133:386–392.
42. Kase CS, Robinson RK, Stein RW, DeWitt LD, Hier DB, Harp DL, Williams JP, Caplan LR, Mohr JP. Anticoagulant-related intracerebral haemorrhage. Neurology 1985;35:943–948.
43. Levine MN, Raskob G, Hirsh J. Haemorrhagic complications of long term anticoagulant therapy. Chest 1989;95 (Suppl):26S–36S.
44. Landefeld CS, McGuire E, Rosenblatt MW. A bleeding risk index for estimating the probability of major bleeding in hospitalized patients starting anticoagulant therapy. Am J Med 1990;89:569–578.
45. Forfar JC. A 7-year analysis of haemorrhage in patients on long term anticoagulant treatment. Br Heart J 1979;42:128–132.
46. Second report of the Sixty Plus Reinfarction Study Research Group: Risks of long term oral anticoagulant therapy in elderly patients after myocardial infarction. Lancet 1982;1:64–68.
47. Hirsh J. Is the dose of warfarin prescribed by American physicians unnecessarily high? Arch Intern Med 1987;147:769–771.
48. Hirsh J, Levine M. Confusion over the therapeutic range for monitoring oral anticoagulant therapy in North America. Thromb Haemost 1988;59:129–132.
49. WHO Expert Committee on Biological Standardization: Requirements for thromboplastins and plasma used to control oral anticoagulant therapy. 33rd Report Tech Rep Ser 687, Geneva, World Health Organisation, 1983;81–105.
50. Loeliger EA. ICSH/ICTH recommendations for reporting prothrombin time in oral anticoagulant control. Thromb Haemost 1985;54:155–156.
51. Poller L. A simple nomogram for the derivation of International Normalised Ratios for the standardisation of prothrombin times. Thromb Haemost 1988;60:18–20.
52. Loeliger EA, Poller L, Samama M, Thomson JM, van den Besselaar AMHP, Vermylen J, Verstraete M. Questions and answers on prothrombin time standardisation in oral anticoagulant control. Thromb Haemost 1985;54:515–517.
53. Poller L, Taberner DA. Dosage and control of oral anticoagulants: an international survey. Br J Haematol 1982;51:479–485.
54. Butchart EG, Lewis PA, Kulatilake ENP, Breckenridge IM. Anticoagulation variabililty between centres: implications for comparative prosthetic valve assessment. Eur J Cardiothorac Surg 1988;2:72–81.
55. Bloom AL. The need for standardisation of anticoagulation management. In Rabago G, Cooley DA (Eds):Heart Valve Replacement. New York, Futura, 1987;319–333.

56. McGoon DC. The risk of embolism following valvular operations: how does one know? J Thorac Cardiovasc Surg 1984;88:782–786.
57. Butchart EG, Lewis PA, Bethel JA, Breckenridge IM. Adjusting anticoagulation to prosthesis thrombogenicity and patient risk factors: recommendations for the Medtronic Hall valve. Circulation 1991; 84(Suppl III): 61–69.
58. Lodder J, Dennis MS, van Raak L, Jones LN, Warlow CP. Co-operative study on the value of long term anticoagulation in patients with stroke and non-rheumatic atrial fibrillation. Br Med J 1988;296:1435–1438.
59. Lundstrom T, Ryden L. Haemorrhagic and thromboembolic complications in patients with atrial fibrillation on anticoagulant prophylaxis. J Intern Med 1989;255:137–142.
60. Petersen P, Boysen G, Godtfredsen J, Andersen ED, Andersen B. Placebo-controlled randomised trial of warfarin and aspirin for prevention of thromboembolic complications in chronic atrial fibrillation. Lancet 1989;1:175–179.
61. SPAF Study Group Investigators: Preliminary report of the Stroke Prevention in Atrial Fibrillation Study. N Engl J Med 1990;322:863–868.
62. BAATAF Investigators:The effect of low-dose warfarin on the risk of stroke in patients with non-rheumatic atrial fibrillation. N Engl J Med 1990;323:1505–1511.
63. Paulker SG, Eckman MH, Levine HJ. A decision analytic view of anticoagulant prophylaxis for thromboemolism in heart disease. Chest 1989;95 (Suppl):161S – 169S.
64. Butchart EG. Thrombosis, embolism and bleeding. In Bodnar E, Frater RWM (Eds):Replacement Heart Valves, Philadelphia, Pergamon Press, 1991; 77–97.
65. Virchow R. Gesammelte abhandlungen zur wissenschaftlichen medizin. IV Thrombosis und embolie. Gefassentzundung und septische infektion. Publ Meidinger, Frankfurt, 1856.
66. Dewanjee MK, Trastek VF, Tago M, Torianni M, Kaye MP. Noninvasive radio-isotopic technique for detection of platelet deposition on bovine pericardial mitral valve prostheses and in vitro quantification of visceral embolism in dogs. Trans Am Soc Artif Intern Organs 1983;29:188–193.
67. Dewanjee MK. Methods of assessment of thrombosis in vivo. Ann NY Acad Sci 1987;516:541–571.
68. Dahlke H, Dociu N, Thurau K. Thrombogenicity of different suture materials as revealed by scanning electron microscopy. J Biomed Mater Res 1980;14:251–268.
69. Starek PJK. Technical aspects of uncomplicated valve replacement. In Starek PJK (Ed):Heart Valve Replacement and Reconstruction. Chicago, Year Book Medical, 1987;61–79.
70. Butchart EG. The potential complications of heart valve replacement and their prevention: technical considerations. In Rabago G, Cooley DA (Eds):Heart Valve Replacement. New York, Futura, 1987;31–53.
71. Badimon L, Badimon JJ, Turitto VT, Fuster V. Thrombosis: studies under flow conditions. Ann NY Acad Sci 1987;516:527–540.
72. Vermylen J, Verstraete M, Fuster V. Role of platelet activation and fibrin formation in thrombogenesis. J Am Coll Cardiol 1986;8 (Suppl):2B – 9B.
73. Esmon CT. The regulation of natural anticoagulant pathways. Science 1987;235:1348–1352.
74. Esmon NL. Thrombomodulin. In Collier BS (Ed): Progress in Haemostasis and Thrombosis, Volume 9. Philadelphia, WB Saunders Co, 1989;29–55.
75. Vanhoute PM. Endothelium and control of vascular function. Hypertension 1989;13:658–667.
76. Henderson AH. Endothelium in control. Br Heart J 1991;65:116–125.
77. Kesteven PJL. Haemostatic changes during cardiopulmonary bypass. Perfusion 1990;5 (Suppl):9–19.
78. Takayama T. Antithrombogenic therapy based on the study of the change of the platelet aggregability and blood coagulability in the early period after prosthetic valve replacement (English abstract). Nippon Kyobu Geka Gakkai Zasshi 1985;33:14–24.
79. Schipper HG, Roos J, van den Meulen F, ten Cate JW. Antithrombin III deficiency in surgical intensive care patients. Thromb Res 1981;21:73–80.
80. Buller HR, ten Cate JW. Acquired antithrombin III deficiency: laboratory diagnosis, incidence, clinical implications and treatment with antithrombin III concentrate. Am J Med 1989;87 (Suppl 3B):44S–48S.
81. Knobl PN, Zilla P, Fasol R, Muller MM, Vukovich TC. The protein C system in patients undergoing cardiopulmonary bypass. J Thorac Cardiovasc Surg 1987;94:600–605.
82. Verstraete M. Prevention of thrombosis in arteries: novel approaches. J Cardiovasc Pharamcol 1985;7 (Suppl 3):S191-S205.
83. Weiss P, Soff GA, Halkin H, Seligsohn U. Decline of proteins C and S and Factors II, VII, IX and X during the initiation of warfarin therapy. Thromb Res 1987;45:783–790.
84. Chakrabarti R, Hocking ED, Fearnley GR. Reaction pattern to three stresses:electroplexy, surgery and myocardial infarction of fibrinolysis and plasma fibrinogen. J Clin Pathol 1976;22:659–662.
85. Toghi H, Yamanouchi H, Murakami M, Kameyama M. Importance of the haematrocrit as a risk factor in cerebral infarction. Stroke 1978;9:369–374.
86. Harrison MJG, Pollock S, Thomas D, Marshall J. Haematrocrit, hypertension and smoking in patients

with transient ischaemic attacks and in age and sex matched controls. J Neurol Neurosurg Psych 1982;45:550–551.
87. DiMinno G, Cerbone AM. Fibrinogen: a coagulation protein in the cardiovascular risk factor profile. In Crepaldi G, Grotto AM, Manzato E, Baggio G (Eds): Atherosclerosis VIII. Amsterdam, Elsevier, 1989;469–474.
88. Kudoh T. Antithromboembolic treatment after cardiac valve replacement. Jpn Circ J 1984;48:1169–1171.
89. Baudet E. Anticoagulation and prosthetic heart valves. In Horstkotte D, Loogan F (Eds): Update in Heart Valve Replacement. Darmstadt, Steinkopf Verlag, 1986;109–115.
90. Thulin LI, Olin CL. Initiation and long term anticoagulation after heart valve replacements. Arq Bras Cardiol 1987;49:265–268.
91. Penny WJ, Chesebro JH, Heras M, Fuster V. Antithrombotic therapy for patients with cardiac disease. Curr Prob Cardiol 1988;7:433–513.
92. Kudo T. Current topics of anticoagulant therapy and antiplatelet therapy after cardiac valve replacement (English abstract). Kyobu Geka 1988;41:644–648.
93. Akins CW. Anticoagulation after heart valve replacement at the Massachusetts General Hospital. Personal communication (letter, Feb 1991).
94. Bodnar AG, Hutter AM. Anticoagulation in valvular heart disease preoperatively and postoperatively. Cardiovasc Clin 1984;14:247–264.
95. Poller L. Therapeutic ranges in anticoagulant administration. Br Med J 1985;290:1683–1686.
96. Loeliger EA. Laboratory control, optimum therapeutic ranges and therapeutic quality control in oral anticoagulation. Acta Haematol 1985;74:125–131.
97. Kadish SL, Lazar EJ, Frishman WH. Anticoagulation in patients with valvular heart disease, atrial fibrillation or both. Cardiol Clin 1987;5:591–628.
98. Fuster V, Badimon L, Badimon JJ, Chesebro J. Prevention of thromboembolism induced by prosthetic valves. Semin Thromb Hemost 1988:14:50–58.
99. Hirsh J, Poller L, Deykin D, Levine M, Dalen JE. Optimal therapeutic range for oral anticoagulants. Chest 1989, 95 (Suppl):5S–11S.
100. Stein PD, Kantrowitz A. Antithrombotic therapy in mechanical and biological prosthetic heart valves and saphenous vein bypass grafts. Chest 1989, 95 (Suppl):107S–117S.
101. BCSH Haemostasis and Thrombosis Task Force. Guidelines on oral anticoagulation:second edition. J Clin Pathol 1990;43:177–183.
102. Sackett DL. Rules of evidence and clinical recommendations on the use of antithrombotic agents. Chest 1989, 95 (Suppl):2S–4S.
103. Barnhorst DA, Oxman HA, Connolly DC, Pluth JR, Danielson GK, Wallace RB, McGoon DC. Long term follow-up of isolated replacement of the aortic or mitral valve with the Starr-Edwards prosthesis. Am J Cardiol 1975, 35:228–233.
104. Pumphrey CW, Fuster V, Chesebro JH. Systemic thromboemolism in valvular heart disease and prosthetic heart valves. Mod Concepts Cardiovasc Dis 1982, 51:131–136.
105. Edmunds LH Jr. Thromboembolic complications of current cardiac valvular prostheses. Ann Thorac Surg 1982, 34:96–106.
106. Wright IS, Beck DF, Marple CD. Myocardial infarction and its treatment with anticoagulants. Lancet 1954;1:92–95.
107. Owren PA. Thrombotest: a new method for controlling anticoagulant therapy. Lancet 1959;2:754–758.
108. McManus Q, Grunkemeier GL, Lambert LE, Teply JF, Harlan BJ, Starr A. Year of operation as a risk factor in the late results of valve replacement. J Thorac Cardiovasc Surg 1980;80:834–841.
109. Turpie AGG, Gunstensen J, Hirsh J, Nelson H, Gent M. Randomised comparison of two intensities of oral anticoagulant therapy after tissue valve replacement. Lancet 1988;1:1242–1245.
110. Altman R, Rouvier J, Gurfinkel E, D'Ortencio O, Manzanel R, de la Fuente L, Favaloro RG. Comparison of two levels of anticoagulant therapy in patients with substitute heart valves. J Thorac Cardiovasc Surg 1991;101:427–431.
111. Saour JH, Sieck JO, Mamo LAR, Gallus AS. Trials of different intensities of anticoagulation in patients with prosthetic valves. N Engl J Med 1990;322:428–432.
112. Saour JN, Sieck JO, Mammo LAR, Gallus AS. Anticoagulation and prosthetic heart valves (letter). N Engl J Med 1990;323:756–757.
113. Butchart EG, Lewis PA, Grunkemeier GL, Kulatilake N, Breckenridge IM. Low risk of thrombosis and serious embolic events despite low intensity anticoagulation. Circulation 1988;78 (Suppl I): 66–77.
114. Horstkotte D. Recommended anticoagulation levels for the St Jude Medical prosthesis in the aortic position. Personal communication (letter, June,1991).
115. Grunkemeier GL, Rahimtoola SH. Artificial heart valves. Annu Rev Med 1990;41:251–263.
116. Hetzer R, Hill JD, Kerth WJ, Wilson AJ, Adappa MG, Gerbode F. Thrombosis and degeneration of Hancock valves: clinical and pathological findings. Ann Thorac Surg 1978;26:317–322.
117. Thiene G, Bortolotti U, Panizzon G, Milano A, Gallucci V: Pathological substrates of thrombus

formation after heart valve replacement with the Hancock bioprosthesis. J Thorac Cardiovasc Surg 1980; 80: 414–423.
118. Craver JM, Jones EL, McKeown P, Bone DK, Hatcher CR, Kandrach M: Porcine cardiac xenograft valves: analysis of survival, valve failure and explantation. Ann Thorac Surg 1982; 34: 16–21.
119. Croft CH, Buja LM, Floresca MZ, Nicod P, Estrera A: Late thrombotic obstruction of aortic bioprostheses. Am J Cardiol 1986; 57: 355–356.
120. Pengo V, Peruzzi P, Baca M, Marzari A, Zanon F, Schivapappa L, Dalla S. The optimal therapeutic range for oral anticoagulant treatment as suggested by fibrinopeptide A levels in patients with heart valve prostheses. Eur J Clin Invest 1989;19:181–184.
121. Kumagai K, Fukunami M, Ohmori M, Kitabatake A, Kamada T, Hoki N. Increased intracardiovascular clotting in patients with chronic atrial fibrillation. J Am Coll Cardiol 1990;16:377–380.
122. Bedeleanu D, Vlaicu R, Roman S, Cucuianu M. Antithrombin III in patients with prosthetic cardiac valves. Rev Roum Med 1983;21:169–173.
123. Fukuda Y, Kuroiwa Y, Okumiya K et al. Hypercoagulability in patients with mitral stenosis. Jpn Circ J 1980;44:867–874.
124. Pengo V, Boschello M, Prandoni P, Schivazappa L, Girolami A. Betathromboglobulin and platelet factor 4 release by ADP contact with native whole blood. Thromb Res 1985;39:645–650.
125. Russo R, Prandoni P, Pengo V, Boschello M, Compostella L, Schivazappa L. Effetto del livello di anticoagulazione sulla concentrazione plasmatica della betatromboglobulina nei pazienti con protesi valvolare cardiaca in trattamento con warfarina. Minerva Cardioangiologica 1984;32:387–391.
126. Pumphrey CW, Dawes J. The platelet release reaction in cardiovascular disease: evaluation of betathromboglobulin as a marker of a prothrombotic state. Eur Heart J 1984;5 (Suppl D):7–11.
127. Kannell WB, D'Agostino RB, Belanger AJ. Fibrinogen, cigarette smoking and the risk of cardiovascular disease: insights from the Framingham Study. Am Heart J 1987;113:1006–1010.
128. Wells RE, Gawronski TH, Cox PJ, Perera RD. Influence of fibrinogen on flow properties of erythrocyte suspensions. Am J Physiol 1964;207:1035–1040.
129. Meade TW, Vickers MV, Thompson SG, Seghatchian MJ. The effect of physiological levels of fibrinogen on platelet aggregation. Thromb Res 1985;38:527–534.
130. Wilhelmsen L, Svardsudd K, Korsan-Bengsten K, Larsson B, Welin L, Tibblin G. Fibrinogen as a risk factor for stroke and myocardial infarction. N Engl J Med 1984;311:501–505.
131. Coull BM, Beamer N. de Garmo P et al. Chronic blood viscosity in subjects with acute stroke, transient ischaemic attack and risk factors for stroke. Stroke 1991;22:162–168.
132. Meade TW, Mellow S, Brozovic M et al. Haemostatic function and ischaemic heart disease: principal results of the Northwick Park Heart Study. Lancet 1986;2:533–537.
133. Fulton RM, Duckett K. Plasma fibrinogen and thromboemboli after myocardial infarction. Lancet 1976;2:1161–1164.
134. Drouet L, Caen JP. Current perspectives in the treatment of thrombotic disorders. Semin Thromb Haemost 1989;15:111–122.
135. Tsuyuguchi N. Shigeta H, Hashimoto M et al. Two dimensional echocardiographic study on left atrial thrombi in patients with a mitral prosthetic valve. J Cardiogr 1983;13:923–933.
136. Daniel WG, Nellessen U, Schroder E, Nonnast-Daniel B, Bednarski P, Nikutta P, Lichtlen PR. Left atrial spontaneous echo contrast in mitral valve disease: an indicator for increased thromboembolic risk. J Am Coll Cardiol 1988;11:1204–1211.
137. Chen YT, Kan MN, Chen JS et al. Contributing factors to formation of left atrial spontaneous echo contrast in mitral valvular disease. J Ultrasound Med 1990; 9: 151–155.
138. Harker LA, Slichter SJ. Studies of platelet and fibrinoen kinetics in patients with prosthetic heart valves. N Engl J Med 1970;283:1302–1305.
139. Wyss M, Diez C, Balavoine JF, Martin D, Bouvier CA. Prevention of thromboembolic complications of valve prostheses by agents affecting platelet function. Eur J Cardiol 1978;8:337–347.
140. Kasahara T. Clinical effect of dipyridamole ingestion after prosthetic valve replacement (English abstract). J Jpn Assoc Thorac Surg 1977;25:1007–1021.
141. Fitzgerald GA. Dipyridamole. N Engl J Med 1987;316:1247–1257.
142. Saito H. Evaluation of antiplatelet drugs on platelet function: comparison between ticlopidine and dipyridamole after prosthetic valve replacement. Kokyu To Junkan 1989;37:87–92.
143. Weiss HJ, Aledort LM, Kochura S. The effect of salicylates on the haemostatic properties of platelets in man. J Clin Invest 1968;47:2169–2180.
144. Chesebro JH, Fuster V, Elveback LR et al. Trial of combined warfarin plus dipyridamole or aspirin therapy in prosthetic heart valve replacement: danger of aspirin compared with dipyridamole. Am J Cardiol 1983;51:1537–1541.
145. Mayne EE, Bridges JM, Weaver JA. Platelet adhesiveness, plasma fibrinogen and factor VIII levels in diabetes mellitus. Diabetologia 1970;6:436–440.

146. Davis JW, Davis RF. Prevention of cigarette smoking-induced platelet aggregate formation by aspirin. Arch Intern Med 1981;141:206–207.
147. Barnett HJM. Aspirin in stroke prevention: an overview. Stroke 1990;21 (Suppl IV): 40–43.
148. Gent M, Easton JD, Hachinksi VC et al. The Canadian American Ticlopidine Study in thromboembolic stroke. Lancet 1989;1:1215–1220.
149. Hass WK, Easton JC, Adams HP et al. A randomised trial comparing ticlopidine hydrochloride with aspirin for the prevention of stroke in high risk patients. N Engl J Med 1989;321:501–507.
150. David TE, Ho WIC, Christakis GT. Thromboembolism in patients with aortic porcine bioprostheses. Ann Thorac Surg 1985;40:229–233.
151. Acheson J, Danta G, Hutchinson EC. Controlled trial of dipyridamole in recent cerebral vascular disease. Br Med J 1969;1:614–615.
152. Sullivan JM, Harken DE, Gorlin R. Effect of dipyridamole on the incidence of arterial emboli after cardiac valve replacement. Circulation 1969;39/40 (Suppl I):149–153.
153. Weily HS, Genton E. Altered platelet function in patients with prosthetic mitral valves. Circulation 1970;42:967–972.
154. Steele P, Rainwater J, Vogel R. Platelet suppressant therapy in patients with prosthetic cardiac valves: relation of clinical effectiveness to alteration of platelet survival time. Circulation 1979;60:910–913.
155. Lee G, Joye JA, Rose A, DeNardo S, Kozina JA, Mason DT. Evaluation of platelet kinetics following porcine and mechanical valve replacement. Clin Cardiol 1981;4:11–14.
156. Chesebro JH, Adams PC, Fuster V. Antithrombotic therapy in patients with valvular heart disease and prosthetic valves. J Am Coll Cardiol 1986;8:41B–56B.
157. Stein PD, Sabbah HN. Haemorheology of turbulence. Biorheology 1980;17:301–319.
157A. Schbath J, Boissel JP, Mathy B, Ville D, Benveniste E, Sanchini B. Drugs effect on platelet survival time: comparison of two pyrimido-pyrimidine derivatives in patients with aortic or mitral replacement. Thromb Haemost 1984;51:45–49.
158. Nunez L, Aguado GM, Larrea JL, Celemin D, Oliver J. Prevention of thromboembolism using aspirin after mitral valve replacement with porcine bioprostheses. Ann Thorac Surg 1984;37:84–87.
159. Poller L, McKernan A, Thomson JM, Elstein M, Hirsch PJ, Jones JB. Fixed minidose warfarin: a new approach to prophylaxis against venous thrombosis after major surgery. Br Med J 1987;295:1309–1312.
160. Poller L, MacCallum PK, Thomson JM, Kerns W. Reduction of factor VII coagulant activity, a risk factor for ischaemic heart disease, by fixed dose warfarin: a double blind crossover study. Br Heart J 1990;63:231–233.
161. MacCallum PK, Thomson JM, Poller L. Effects of fixed minidose warfarin on coagulation and fibrinolysis following major gynaecological surgery. Thromb Haemost 1990;64:511–515.
162. Bern MM, Lokich Jj, Wallach SR et al. Very low doses of warfarin can prevent thrombosis in central venous catheters: a randomised prospective trial. Ann Intern Med 1990;112:423–428.
163. Meade TW. Low-dose warfarin and low-dose aspirin in the primary prevention of ischaemic heart disease. Am J Cardiol 1990;65:7C–11C.
164. Wolf PA, Kannel WB, Cupples LA, D'Agostino RB. Risk factor interaction in cardiovascular and cerebrovascular disease. In Furlan AJ (Ed):The Heart and Stroke. London, Springer-Verlag, 1987; 331–355.
165. McMahon S, Peto R, Cutler J. Blood pressure, stroke and coronary heart disease. Part 1: prolonged differences in blood pressure: prospective observational studies corrected for the regression dilution bias. Lancet 1990;335:765–774.
166. Wolf PA, D'Agostino RB, Kannel WB, Bonita R, Belaner AJ. Cigarette smoking as a risk factor for stroke. The Framingham Study. J Am Med Assoc 1988;259:1025–1029.
167. Shinton R, Beevers G. Meta-analysis of relation between cigarette smoking and stroke. Br Med J 1989;298:789–794.
168. Levine PH. An acute effect of cigarette smoking on platelet function: a possible link between smoking and arterial thrombosis. Circulation 1973;48:619–623.
169. Bierenbaum ML, Fleischman AI, Stier A, Somol H, Watson PB. Effect of cigarette smoking upon in vivo platelet function in man. Thromb Res 1978;12:1051–1057.
170. Modesti PA, Abbate R, Gensini GF, Colella A, Serneri GGN. Platelet thromboxane A_2 receptors in habitual smokers. Thromb Res 1989;55:195–201.
171. Smith JR, Landaw SA. Smokers' polycythaemia. N Engl J Med 1978;298:6–10.
172. Criqui MH, Wallace RB, Heiss G, Mischkel M, Schonfeld G, Jones GTL. Cigarette smoking and plasma high-density lipoprotein cholesterol. Circulation 1980;62 (Suppl IV):70–76.
173. Muscat JE, Harris RE, Haley NJ, Wynder EL. Cigarette smoking and plasma cholesterol. Am Heart J 1991;121:141–147.
174. Davis JW, Shelton L. Watanabe IS, Arnold J. Passive smoking affects endothelium and platelets. Arch Intern Med 1989;149:386–389.
175. Glantz SA, Parmley WW. Passive smoking and heart disease. Circulation 1991;83:1–12.

176. Zbinden G. Evaluation of thrombogenic effects of drugs. Annu Rev Pharmacol Toxicol 1976;16:177–188.
177. Collaborative Group for the Study of Stroke in Young Women: Oral contraception and increased risk of cerebral ischaemia or thrombosis. N Engl J Med 1973;288:871–878.
178. Collaborative Group for the Study of Stroke in Young Women: Oral contraceptives and stroke in young women; associated risk factors. J Am Med Assoc 1975;231:718–722.
179. Batist G, Bothe A, Bern M, Bistrian BR, Blackburn GL. Low antithrombin III in morbid obesity: return to normal with weight reduction. J Parent Ent Nutr 1983;7:447–449.
180. Ferguson EW, Bernier LL, Banta GRF, Yu-Yahiro J, Schoomaker EB. Effects of exercise and conditioning on clotting and fibrinolytic activity in man. J Appl Physiol 1987;62:1416–1421.
181. Gris JC, Schved JF, Feugeas O et al. Impact of smoking, physical training and weight reduction on FVII, PAI–1 and haemostatic markers in sedentary men. Thromb Haemost 1990;64:516–520.
182. Hornstra G. Effect of dietary lipids on arterial thrombus formation: rationale for the support of drug therapy by diet. Semin Thromb Hemost 1988;14:59–65.
183. Davenport WD, Ball CR. Diet-induced atrial endothelial damage: a scanning electron-microscopic study. Athererosclerosis 1981;40:145–152.
184. Goodnight S, Fisher M, Fitzgerald GVA, Levine PH. Assessment of the therapeutic use of dietary fish oil in atherosclerotic vascular disease and thrombosis. Chest 1989, 95 (Suppl);19S–25S.
185. Washio M, Sakashita S, Nakamura C et al. A new anticoagulant medication in cardiac valve replacement. J Cardiovasc Surg 1978;19:455–463.
186. Sakashita I, Ohtani S, Nakamura C, Washio M. Clinical evaluation of a new anticoagulant therapy in prosthetic valve replacement. Jpn Heart J 1978;19:324–331.

Chapter 3.5

Patient-regulated Anticoagulation

Ari Schachner, Ehud Deviri and Shai Shabat

Three decades after the first successful clinical implantation of a prosthetic heart valve, thromboembolism and anticoagulant related haemorrhage remain the major complications after valve replacement with a mechanical prosthesis[1]. As the optimum method of anticoagulation with coumarin is yet to be defined, there is little doubt that inappropriate management of life-long anticoagulant therapy is the most important, treatment-related risk factor in determining the rate of thromboembolic and bleeding complications in patients with mechanical prostheses[2–5].

The risks of valve thrombosis, thromboembolism and the bleeding complications of anticoagulant therapy deter many surgeons from implanting mechanical prostheses. The incidence of these complications, however, varies with the intensity of anticoagulation (Chapter 3.4) and with the quality of anticoagulation control, a factor that is influenced not only by scientific methods but by the relevant health care system and, in broader terms, by the prevailing socio-economical circumstances.

For these reasons a policy was developed and pursued in Tel Aviv to encourage the patient to take an active role in the maintenance of the therapeutic level of anticoagulation. In the last twenty years, a patient self-regulation method has been used to simplify the anticoagulant regimen and to increase its efficacy[6].

According to this routine, each patient who is discharged after heart valve replacement is provided with an anticoagulation booklet that contains guidance on recommended doses and monthly control tables (Fig. 3.5–1). As the concept of INR (Chapter 3.3) had not been introduced at the time when this policy was started, the level of anticoagulation was, and still is, defined in terms of prothrombin time. The change to INR is currently under consideration.

A daily prothrombin time (Quick test) is obtained during the immediate postoperative days. When the appropriate maintenance dose is established, this is recorded in the guidance table together with the corrective doses, according to the fluctuations of the prothrombin values. The target therapeutic range, prothrombin time 20–30% (equivalent to INR 2.5–4.0) is clearly marked in the guide table. During hospitalisation, the patient and close family members are thoroughly familiarised with the programme, and after several explanatory sessions, their comprehension is checked. One copy of the guidance table is kept in the patient's records for further evaluation.

For supervision of the effectiveness of treatment, monthly control tables are used. The patient records his daily dose, and at the bottom of the weekly column, the results of weekly prothrombin time tests are entered. If the results differ from the advised target therapeutic range, the patient immediately corrects the dose of anticoagulant drug according to the guidance table, and has another test taken within 48 hours. As a further precaution, the patient and his family physician are instructed regarding drugs

Beilinson Medical Center

Name ____________

Address ____________

I.C. ____________

Month ____________

Operation ____________

Prosthesis ____________

Date operation ____________

Drugs ____________

Prothrombin time	1	2	3	4	5	6	7
50–60%	15	12.5	10	7.5	5	5	5
40–50%	12.5	10	7.5	7.5	5	5	5
30–40%	12.5	7.5	5	5	5	5	5
20–30%	5	5	5	5	5	5	5
15–20%	2.5	5	5	5	5	5	5
15%		2.5	5	5	5	5	5

Prothr. time at discharge 28%
Daily dose 5mg

Beilinson Medical Center

July 1989

Antigoagulation therapy

Name

I. C.

☐ Digoxin ☐ Diuretics

☐ Antibiotics ☐ Blockers

☐ Salicylates ☐ Coumadin

Associated medicaments

☐ Slow k ☐

☐ ☐

Suggestions

Day	Date	Dosage	Date	Dosage	Date	Dosage	Date	Dosage	Date	Dosage	Date	Dosage
Sun.			2	5	9	5	16	12.5	23	5	30	5
Mon.			3	5	10	5	17	10	24	5	31	5
Tus.			4	5	11	5	18	7.5	25	5		
Wed.			5	5	12	5	19	7.5	26	5		
Thu.			6	5	13	5	20	5	27	5		
Fri.			7	5	14	5	21	5	28	5		
Sat.	1	5	8	5	15	5	22	5	29	5		
P. T.			25%		28%		45%		30%		25%	
Hb												

Figure 3.5–1: Above: A sample guidance table. Note the shaded target effective range. Below: A sample monthly control sheet.

and substances that act antagonistically or synergistically with the anticoagulant agent prescribed (Chapter 3.2).

Patients are asked to carry out prothrombin tests twice weekly during the first three months after surgery, and weekly for the following three month period. Once an acceptable level of anticoagulation is achieved without frequent fluctuations, and after the patient has adjusted to the system, monthly prothrombin time tests are recommended. The control tables are collected by the Cardiac Surgery Department each month, and after evaluation, those patients with unacceptable levels of anticoagulation are advised by telephone, or requested to attend the out-patient clinic.

It became obvious soon after introducing this method that a large proportion of the patient population were unable or unwilling to participate in the scheme. Nonetheless, because of the apparent theoretical advantages, the programme has been continued and every effort has been made over the years to enrol as many patients as possible. As a result, a mixed cohort of patients has emerged in which both self-regulation and hospital-based regulation of anticoagulation are represented. At the end of 1990, it was felt that the amount of follow up data would justify the assessment of long term clinical outcome depending on the mode of anticoagulant regulation. Therefore, a total of 120 patients comprising four groups of 30 patients each, were selected randomly by a computer. They had all undergone single heart valve replacement with mechanical prosthetic valves at the Beilinson Medical Center over the period 1975–1990. The four groups within which the random selection was completed were (a) aortic or (b) mitral valve replacement with a Medtronic Hall and (c) aortic or (d) mitral valve replacement with a Bjørk-Shiley prosthesis (Table 3.5–1).

Patients with Bjørk-Shiley prostheses where selected from 1975 onwards, while those with Medtronic Hall prostheses from 1980 onwards. The age of the patients ranged from 6 to 76 years. Seventy-three (61%) were males, 47 (39%) were females. There was no statistically significant difference in sex, age or incidence of atrial fibrillation among the various groups. The total follow up for the 120 patients was 875 patient/years, the mean follow up for the entire group was 7.29 years.

Each patient provided the following information: a) compliance with the anticoagulant treatment, b) usage of the patient-regulated anticoagulation system, c) thromboembolic complications, d) haemorrhagic complications and e) evidence of any grossly abnormal anticoagulation: Quick's prothrombin time below 20% (INR > 4.0) or above 50% (INR < 1.5). Thromboembolic and haemorrhagic complications were defined according to the recently introduced reporting guidelines[7]. The relationship between usage of the patient-regulated anticoagulation system and the rates of thromboembolism, haemorrhagic complications, and inadequate anticoagulation state, was examined.

Table 3.5–1
Composition of Study Groups

	Bjørk-Shiley			*Medtronic Hall*			*Total of Both Prostheses*		
	NU	*U*	*TOTAL*	*NU*	*U*	*TOTAL*	*NU*	*U*	*TOTAL*
Aortic	11	19	30	14	16	30	25	35	60
Mitral	17	13	30	19	11	30	36	24	60
Total	28	32	60	33	27	60	61	59	120

NU = Non-users of the self-regulation system
U= Users of the self-regulation system

Anticoagulation regime

Of the 120 randomly selected patients, only one neglected all regular control of prothrombin level. Fifty-nine (49.2%) used the patient-regulated anticoagulation method ('users'). The remaining 60 patients had their anticoagulation levels regulated by their cardiologists or family physicians ('non-users') (Table 3.5–1).

The percentage usage of patient-regulated anticoagulation was not statistically different among the four patient groups. There was also no difference in the percentage usage of the patient-regulated system in males or females. However, there was a highly significant difference in the mean follow up period; 5.7 years for 'users' and 8.4 years for'non-users' ($p<0.0005$). It is difficult to interpret this difference between the randomly selected two groups, especially since the Medtronic Hall group with a potentially shorter follow up had somewhat less 'users' than the Bjørk-Shiley cohort.

Embolism

Twenty-eight patients suffered a single thromboembolic episode (3.2% per patient/year); of these, 16 made a complete recovery following the event (1.8% per patient/year), and 12 had residual damage (1.4% per patient/year). Twenty-four (85%) of these 28 patients did not use the self-controlled anticoagulation system. The rate of thromboembolic complications in the 'non-users' group was 4.7% per patient/year, compared to 1.1% per patient/year in the group using the patient-regulated anticoagulation method ($p<0.0005$) (Fig. 3.5–2).

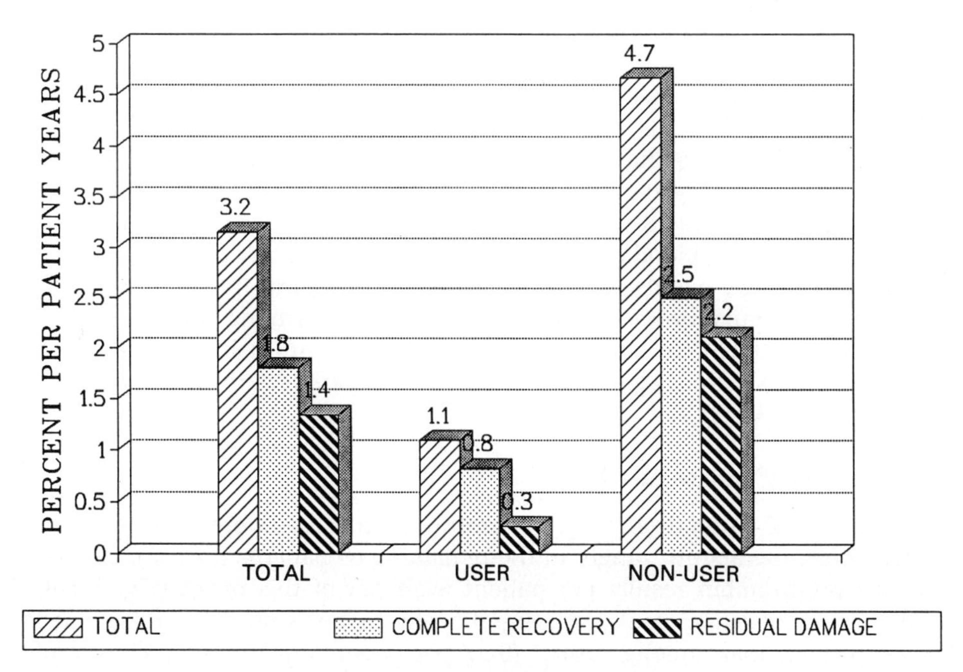

Figure 3.5–2: Diagram showing total thromboembolic events among 'users' and 'non-users' of patient-regulated anticoagulation regimen.

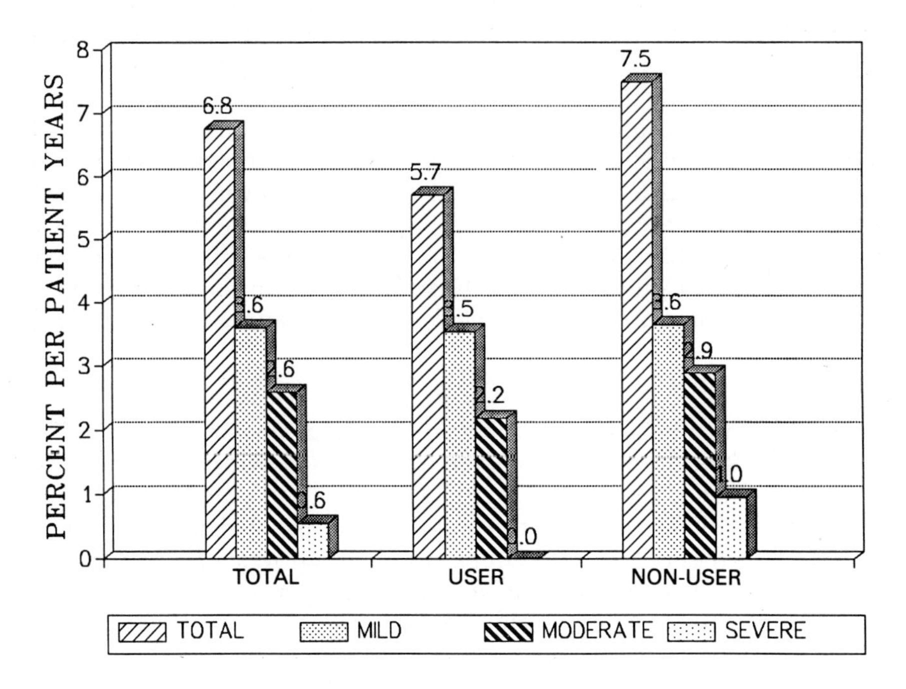

Figure 3.5–3: Diagram showing total haemorrhagic events among 'users' and 'non-users' of patient-regulated anticoagulation regimen.

Bleeding complications

There were a total of 60 haemorrhagic events (6.8% per patient/year). Of these, 32 were mild, not requiring treatment (3.6% per patient-year), 23 moderate, requiring hospitalisation or treatment with iron supplements (2.6% per patient-year), and five were severe, requiring blood transfusions or surgery (0.6% per patient-year). The rate for all haemorrhagic events was significantly lower among patients using patient-regulated anticoagulation (5.7% per patient-year) than among non-users (7.5% per patient-year) ($p<0.05$). In addition, none of the patients using the self-controlled method had a severe haemorrhagic event, compared with five events among 'non-users' (Fig. 3.5–3).

Achieved level of anticoagulation

In 51 of the 120 patients (42.5%), the prothrombin values were never grossly out of the prescribed therapeutic range. In the remaining 69 patients (57.5%), between one and nine prothrombin results per patient were out of this range (Fig. 3.5–4). The number of out-of-range results was significantly higher among 'non-users' (average 2.9 per patient) than among 'users' (0.53 per patient) ($p<0.0005$). The number of abnormal results was significantly higher in females than in males (2.4 vs. 1.3 per patient, $p<0.01$), and higher in patients with mitral than in those with aortic valve

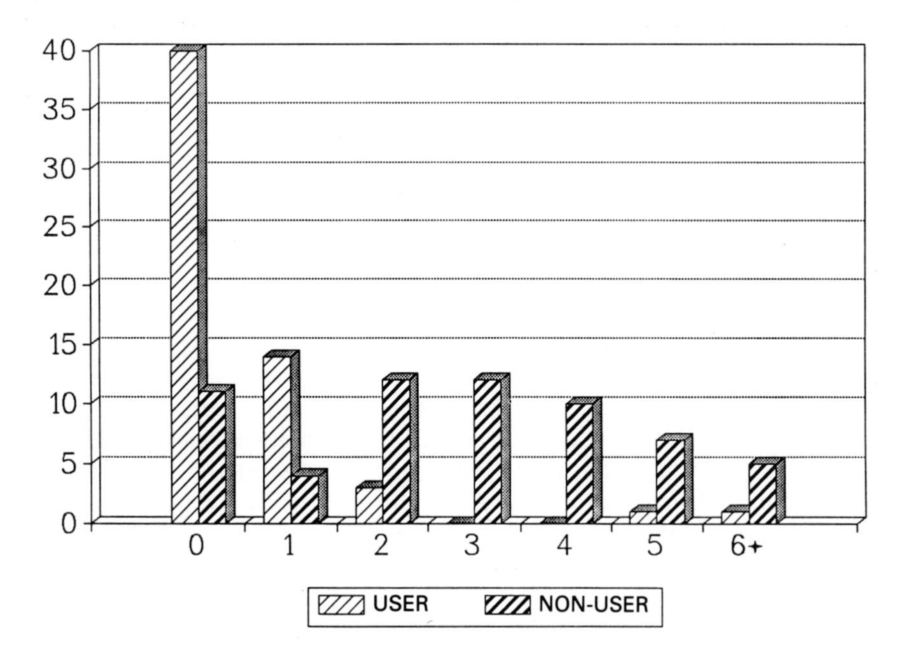

Figure 3.5–4: Diagram showing distribution of inadequate prothrombin levels among 'users' and 'non-users' of patient-regulated anticoagulation regimen.

replacement (2.3 vs. 1.1 per patient, $p<0.001$). Neither age nor the type of prosthesis had any significant effect on the outcome measures examined.

Our experiences show that the vast majority of patients (99%) were aware of the importance of anticoagulant treatment and control of their anticoagulation therapy. Therefore, it is surprising that, according to the above random sample, only about half the patients complied fully with the recommended regimen of anticoagulant self-control, despite its availability and the benefit that it should have conferred on them in preventing complications. However, this disappointing finding enabled us to make a retrospective comparison between 'users' and 'non-users' of the system under discussion.

In this random sample, less than 10% of the 59 patients using the self-controlled anticoagulation system properly had more than one abnormal prothrombin result during the past year, whereas in the 61 'non-users' the corresponding rate was significantly higher (75%).

The rate of haemorrhagic complications in this randomly selected group was higher than in other series[4,8–14]. However, by omitting the mild episodes, the rate falls to 3.1% per patient-year. By using the self-control system, the rates of thromboembolic and haemorrhage complications decreased to 1.1% and 2.2% (mild episodes excluded) per patient-year, respectively. These data show that the self-controlled anticoagulation system reduces the rate of these complications significantly. The difference is particularly striking for thromboembolic complications, in which the incidence is four times greater among the 'non-users' of the system.

Since patients were not randomly assigned to 'user' and 'non-user' groups, there inevitably exists a potential for bias in this type of retrospective assessment. It could easily be argued that the 'users' were those who were particularly concerned about their longevity and quality of life and who were well enough to participate. One may assume that, were they treated under different conditions as 'non-users', they would still achieve a significantly better outcome by following the doctors' orders meticulously. The converse is also likely to be true: those who could not be persuaded to contribute with their own effort are most likely to neglect the regular medication or to ignore relevant medical advice. Nonetheless, the fact remains that the long term outcome has been significantly better among the 'users'of the patient-control system.

In conclusion, it is suggested that patient-regulated anticoagulation is feasible in clinical practice. It enables the patient to be responsible for his own anticoagulant management and increases awareness of the importance of proper anticoagulation in preventing life-threatening complications. The method also serves to strengthen and maintain contact between the patient and the cardiovascular surgical department after prosthetic valve replacement and upgrades the patient-physician relationship by enhancing the patient's self-esteem. Full compliance with the method appears to ensure adequate anticoagulation, thereby reducing the risk of thromboembolic and haemorrhagic complications.

REFERENCES

1. Harken DE, Soroff HS, Taylor WJ, Lefemine AA, Gupta SK, Lunzer S. Partial and complete prostheses in aortic insufficiency. J Thorac Cardiovasc Surg 1960;40:744–762.
2. Forfar JC. A 7 year analysis of haemorrhage in patients on long-term anticoagulant treatment. Br Heart J 1979;42:128–132.
3. Edmunds LH Jr. Thromboembolic complications of current cardiac valvular prostheses. Ann Thorac Surg 1982;34:96–106.
4. Edmunds LH Jr. Thrombotic and bleeding complications of prosthetic heart valves. Ann Thorac Surg 1987;44:430–445.
5. McGoon DC. The risk of thromboembolism following valvular operations: How does one know. J Thorac Cardiovasc Surg 1984;88:782–786.
6. Erdman S, Vidne B, Levy MJ. A self control method for long term anticoagulation therapy. J Cardiovasc Surg 1974;15:454–457.
7. Edmunds LH, Clark RE, Cohn LH, Miller DC, Weisel RD. Guidelines for reporting morbidity and mortality after cardiac valvular operations. J Thorac Cardiovasc Surg 1988;96:351–353.
8. Miller DC, Oyer PE, Mitchell RS, et al. Performance characteristics of the Starr-Edwards model 1260 aortic valve prosthesis beyond ten years. J Thorac Cardiovasc Surg 1984;88:193–207.
9. Farah E, Enriquez-Sarano M, Vahanian A, et al. Thromboembolic and haemorrhagic risk in mechanical and biological aortic prostheses. Eur Heart J 1984;5(suppl D):43–47.
10. Miller DC, Oyer PE, Stinson EB, et al. Ten to fifteen years reassessment of the performance characteristics of the Starr-Edwards model 6120 mitral valve prosthesis. J Thorac Cardiovasc Surg 1983;85:1–20.
11. Soyer R, Redonnet M, Brunet A, et al. Long term results with Starr-Edwards mitral valve prosthesis 6120, with particular reference to thromboembolic incidence. J Cardiovasc Surg 1983;24:389–394.
12. Borkon AM, Soule L, Baughman KL, et al. Ten-year analysis of the Bjørk-Shiley standard aortic valve. Ann Thorac Surg 1987;43:39–51.
13. Marshall WG, Kouchoukos NT, Karp RB, Williams JB. Late results after mitral valve replacement with the Bjørk-Shiley and porcine prostheses. J Thorac Cardiovasc Surg 1983;85:902–910.
14. Butchart EG, Lewis PA, Grunkemeier GL, Kulatilake N, Breckenridge IM. Low risk of thrombosis and serious embolic events despite low-intensity anticoagulation. Experience with 1,004 Medtronic Hall valves. Circulation 1988;78(Suppl I):66–77.

Chapter 3.6

Home Prothrombin Estimation

Angelika Bernardo, Carola Halhuber and Dieter Horstkotte

In spite of ongoing development and the introduction of improved design and materials, mechanical valves are still thrombogenic and require life-long anticoagulation. Bioprostheses are significantly less thrombogenic, but their haemodynamic performance is restricted and their durability remains limited[1]. Furthermore, anticoagulation is necessary in a considerable proportion of patients with heart valve disease even without the presence of a mechanical prosthesis (Table 3.6–1).

For this reason any improvement in anticoagulant control and/or management can be expected to have far reaching consequences in extending longevity and decreasing complications before and after heart valve surgery[2,3]. In addition, efforts are currently being directed to reducing the substantial cost of regular laboratory controls[4]. Home prothrombin estimation has a major potential in this respect.

RATIONALE FOR HOME PROTHROMBIN ESTIMATION

A random study in Düsseldorf has demonstrated that more than 50% of patients on long term anticoagulation stay outside the target INR range at any given point in time, in spite of rigorous implementation of current anticoagulant management practice (Fig. 3.6–1, see also Chapter 3.3). This fifty percent proportion coincides with reports of other series, in which anticoagulation was found inadequate in more than 50% of the cases[5–10]. It seems logical to assume that a more efficient adjustment of oral anticoagulation would not only result in the reduction of embolic and bleeding complica-

Table: 3.6–1
Indication for anticoagulant therapy following mitral or aortic valve replacement (1976–1990)[1]
– Device vs. primary cardiac indication –

Valve replacement for		*Postoperative*	
		No need for anticoagulation without a prosthetic device[3]	*Need for anticoagulation irrespective of prosthetic device*[3]
mitral stenosis[2]	(n=806)	133 (0.14)	693 (0.86)
mitral regurgitation[2]	(n=491)	206 (0.42)	285 (0.58)
aortic stenosis[2]	(n=918)	847 (0.92)	71 (0.08)
aortic regurgitation[2]	(n=285)	233 (0.82)	52 (0.18)
	(n=2,500)	1,399 (0.56)	1,101 (0.44)

[1] Retrospective breakdown of prospectively followed patients discharged from hospital (Heinrich-Heine University, Düsseldorf)
[2] Pure or predominant stenosis or regurgitation, respectively
[3] According to Chesebro et al (1986)[12] and Horstkotte et al (1987)[5]

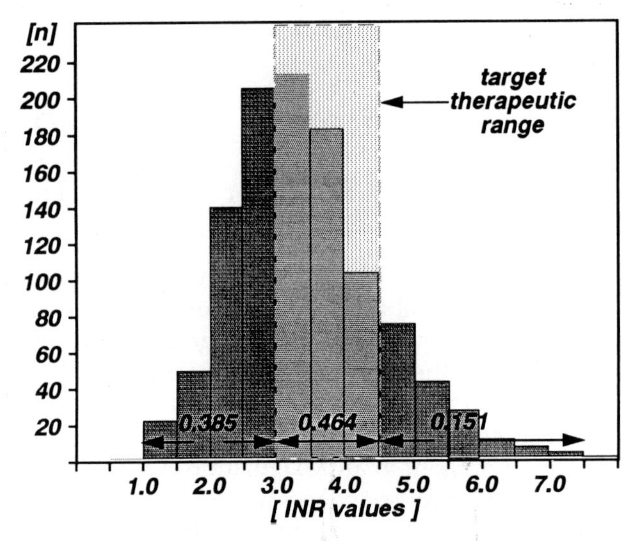

Figure 3.6–1 Measured International Normalised Ratios (INR) in 1,069 consecutive patients with heart valve prostheses (Outpatient Department, University of Düsseldorf 1991)

tions but would also allow a reduction in the target therapeutic INR range without increasing the thrombotic and embolic hazard.

The concept of home prothrombin estimation is also expected to contribute to the evolution of patient-specific anticoagulation because of its potential in the assessment of temporary changes in the prothrombin level, which may be due to diet, medication or other factors. Appropriate corrections could easily be made through frequent estimations, which could be carried out without increasing the number of out-patient visits, thereby reducing the burden on both the patient and the hospital service.

EQUIPMENT

Several coagulometers have been evaluated for home prothrombin estimation. All are currently available.

Coagulometer KC 1A (Amelung, Inc., FRG)

The Coagulometer KC employs the WHO approved standard method. Twenty μl capillary blood and 100 μl citrate-buffer solution are transferred with a micropipette into a cuvette containing small, precious metal spheres, and the contents are mixed thoroughly. The mixture is then placed in the Coagulometer KC, further mixed with 200μl Hepato-Quick reagent (Boehringer, Mannheim), and its temperature is raised to 37° within two minutes. Calcium chloride is added next with a 'starter' pipette, which starts a stop-watch automatically. As blood clotting commences, the precious metal balls are pulled together and the metal contact stops the watch automatically. The elapsed time (seconds) corresponds with the relevant Quick value on a table supplied with the instrument.

Coumatrac Protime Monitor (Du Pont Pharmaceuticals, USA)

This battery-powered, portable, laser photometer was first introduced by Biotrack, Inc. It measures the prothrombin time based on a principle similar to that used for standard prothrombin time determination using rabbit brain thromboplastin. Before application of the blood sample, a disposable plastic reagent cartridge is inserted into the monitor for warming to 37°C. The wafer-like plastic cartridge contains a capillary channel which leads to a chamber containing dry thromboplastin. Capillary blood (25μl) is allowed to drop into a well at one end of the capillary channel of the cartridge. From there, capillary action moves the blood to mix with the thromboplastin. As the blood clots, the cessation of flow is detected photometrically from the light scatter of the red blood cells. The elapsed time is then converted into prothrombin time. A multicentre validation study for this equipment with more than 500 patients demonstrated a correlation coefficient of 0.96 between capillary blood and reference plasma prothrombin time[11].

CoaguChek System (Boehringer Mannheim, USA/FRG)

This instrument distinguishes itself through the ease and speed of prothrombin time determination. The CoaguChek Meter warms the inserted test strip to the necessary temperature of 37°C. A fresh drop of fingerstick capillary blood (25 μl) is applied from the finger to a marked recipient well on the test strip. The blood is drawn into the reaction chamber and mixed with iron particles and reagents promoting the coagulation process. A pulsed electric magnet moves the iron particles and the movement rhythm is monitored photometrically. The cessation of movement, due to full development of the blood clot, is detected and constitutes the measurement endpoint.

The elapsed time is converted to reference plasma prothrombin times and the results are displayed. Additionally, the results can be expressed as a ratio to reference plasma normal values or in % Quick readings or optionally in International Normalized Ratio (INR) values. This instrument is currently undergoing clinical evaluation.

CLINICAL EXPERIENCE WITH HOME PROTHROMBIN ESTIMATION IN GERMANY

A clinical trial was started in 1986 at the Cardiac Rehabilitation Center Bad Berleburg with patients after heart valve replacement with St. Jude Medical prosthesis to evaluate the Coagulometer KC 1A instrument. The patients were trained to measure Quick's percentage, which is used in German practice, for historical reasons, instead of INR. By January 1990, 260 patients were enrolled, and 126 of them (48.5%) still continue with home prothrombin estimation. The mean age of these 126 patients at enrollment was 50.9 years ranging from 19 to 74 years and the mean duration of oral anticoagulation 36.5 months at the time of enrolment in the study. The mean duration of home prothrombin estimation was 14.1 months, range 3–54 months.

The target Quick's percentage was 10–20% (Hepato-Quick), equivalent to an INR 3.0–4.5. The results were within the therapeutic range in 81.5% of the measurements taken by the patients themselves, although the maintenance dose was temporarily lowered in some cases, mainly because of dental procedures. Of the out-of-range

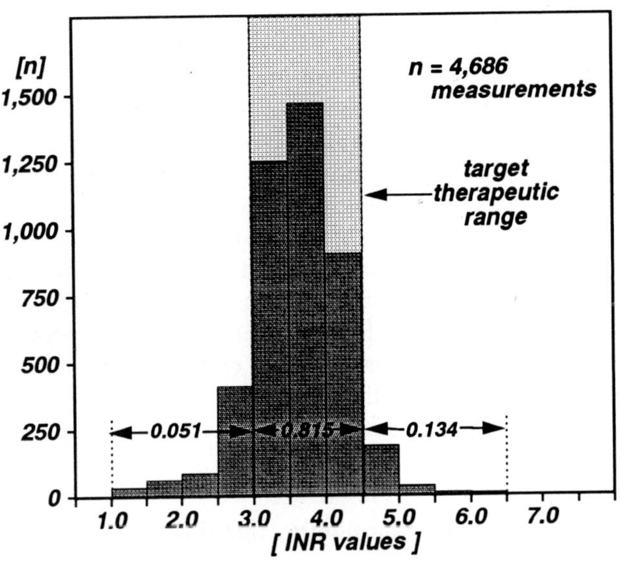

Figure 3.6–2 Home measured International Normalized Ratios (INR) in 101 consecutive patients with heart valve prostheses. Cardiac Rehabilitation Center, Bad Berleburg.

prothrombin times, 5.1% were below and 13.4% above the target range (Fig. 3.6–2). This compares very favourably with the high proportion of inaccuracy with the traditional anticoagulation management (Fig. 3.6–1).

Complication rates

Scientifically sound, valid comparison between traditional prothrombin control, that is, regular assessment carried out by the patient's general practitioner, and the home-based, frequent assessments by the patients themselves has not been completed yet. Such an evaluation requires prospective randomised trials. Nonetheless, the currently available experience permits non-randomised, retrospective comparison of complication rates with St. Jude Medical prostheses in 317 patients under traditional and 92 patients with home controlled anticoagulation management. The available total follow up information for the two groups was 4,942 months and 1,421 months, respectively.

Home control appears to reduce the rate of anticoagulant-induced bleeding (4.38% per patient year in the traditional and 3.38% per patient year in the home control group Table 3.6–2). These relatively high bleeding incidences reflect the relatively high target range (see Chapters 3.4 and 5.4). The difference in embolic events was even more remarkable. In the conventional group there were two embolic episodes causing permanent impairment and six causing transient symptoms, the linearised rates being 0.49% per patient year and 1.46% per patient year, respectively. There was no embolic episode reported in the home control group.

Although these data are not the results of a prospective, randomised trial, they correlate well with the high percentage of INR levels found to be within the therapeutic, target 3.0–4.5 range in the home control group. It seems to be logical to

Table 3.6–2
Usual Anticoagulation Management vs. Home Prothombin Estimation (1986–1990)
– Non-randomized Comparison of Complications –

		Usual *n=317* *FUM = 4,942*	*HPE* *n=92* *FUM = 1,421*
Bleeding	– mild	n=16 (3.89)	n=4 (3.38)
	– severe	n=2 (0.49)	n=0
Thromboembolism	– transient	n=6 (1.46)	n=0
	– permanent deficit	n=2 (0.49)	n=0
All complications		n=25[1] (6.07)	n=4 (3.38)
Severe complications		n=4 (0.97)	n=0

( ) % per patient year [1]two episodes in the same patient

conclude that both bleeding and embolic risks can be reduced if the patients are kept within the target INR range. Home prothrombin estimation looks promising and has a considerable potential to achieving this goal.

PRACTICAL APPROACH AND EDUCATIONAL CONSIDERATIONS

Though all three methods of home prothrombin estimation currently in clinical use are fairly simple to manage, specific training is necessary for the patients to achieve reliable and reproducible results. The training scheme is based in many respects on experiences with similar training courses for home control and management of diabetes and asthma[13–17]; it relies on the advantages of having group sessions for eight to ten persons at a time. These sessions are conducted by specialised medical/technical assistants, and normally not more than four to five 'class-room lessons' of 90 minutes duration are sufficient. Refresher courses do seem to be necessary.

The relative ease of using the Coag-I-System in particular makes it possible to complete the training within about four hours, having separate groups for beginners and for advanced 'students'. The first two lessons give basic information on the coagulometer itself, on the principles of coagulation measurement and on the questions regarding quality control. The second two lessons encompass reiteration of the practical knowledge already acquired and provide necessary, additional information on

- need for anticoagulation after heart valve replacement,
- potential interaction between coumarin-type drugs and other medication,
- potential interaction between oral anticoagulants and dietary factors,
- accurate recording of the measured prothrombin (INR) results,
- techniques of prospective determination of the necessary amount of anti–coagulant,

- calculation of the individual doses from the INR value,
- potential pitfalls and mistakes,
- corrections in case of over- or under-dosage, and
- early recognition of thromboembolic and/or bleeding complications.

An alternative is a full-day intensive course which can be held during the weekend for highly motivated well educated patients.

Although some of the benefit from home prothrombin control may derive from better understanding and compliance on the part of the patient following detailed classroom instruction, the preliminary results already warrant careful consideration of its inherent potential. Experiences with patient contribution in the home management of diabetes and asthma, and the good results that can be achieved in both cases encourage further technical development and clinical research. A properly designed, prospective clinical trial is now required.

REFERENCES

1. Horstkotte D. Prosthetic valves or mechanical valves: a vote for mechanical prostheses. Z Kardiol 1985;74(suppl 6): 19–37.
2. Ansell JE, Holden A, Knopic N. Patient self-management of oral anticoagulation guided by capillary (fingerstick) whole blood prothrombin times. Arch Intern Med 1989;149:2509–2511.
3. White RH, McCurdy StA, v Marensdorff H. Woodruff De, Leftgott L. Home prothrombin time monitoring after the initiation of warfarin therapy. A randomized, prosthetic study. Ann Intern Med 1989;111:730–737.
4. Ansell J, Hamke K, Holden A, Unupic N. Cort effectiveness of monitoring warfarin therapy: standard versus capillary prothrombin times. Am J Clin Pathol 1989;91:587–589.
5. Horstkotte D, Loogen F. Erworbene Herzklappenfehler. München-Wien-Baltimore: Urban & Schwarzenberg, 1987 49–50.
6. Moschos CB, Wong PC, Siso HS. Controlled study of the effective level of long-term anticoagulation. JAMA 1959;201:981–982.
7. Roos J, van Joost HE. The cause of bleeding during anticoagulant treatment. Acta Med Scand 1965, 178:129–131.
8. Hasted S, Andreasen F. Problems encountered in long-term treatment with anticoagulants. Acta Med Scand 1976;200:379–384.
9. Davis FB, Estruch MT, Samson-Covera EB, Voigt GC, Tobin JD. Management of anticoagulation in outpatients: experience with an anticoagulation service in a municipal hospital setting. Arch Intern Med 1977;137:197–202.
10. Errichetti AM, Holden A, Ansell J. Management of oral anticoagulant therapy. Experience with an anticoagulation clinic. Arch Intern Med 1984;144:1966–1968.
11. Lucas FV, Duncan A, Jay R, et al. A novel whole blood capillary technique for measuring the prothrombin time. Am J Clin Pathol 1987;88:442–446.
12. Chesebro J, Adams PC, Fuster V. Antithrombotic therapy in patients with valvular heart disease and prosthetic heart valves. JACC 1980;8:41-B–56-B.
13. Assal JP, Mühlhauser I, Pernet A. Geller R, Jörgens V, Berger M. Patient education as basis for diabetes care in clinical practice and research. Diabetologia 1985;28:602–613.
14. Kronsbein P, Jörgens V, Mühlhauser I, Scholz V, Venhaus A, Berger M. Evaluation of a structured treatment and teaching programme on non-insulin-dependent diabetes. Lancet 1988;2:1407–1411.
15. Maiman LA, Green LW, Gibson G. MacKenzie EJ. Education for self-treatment by adult asthmatics. JAMA 1979;214:1919–1922.
16. Tattersall R, Gale E. Patient self-monitoring of blood glucose and refinements of conventional insulin treatment. Am J Med 1981;70:177–182.
17. Fairclough PK, Clements RS, Filer DV, Bell DSH. An evaluation of patient performance of and their satisfaction with various rapid blood glucose measurement systems. Diabetes Care 1983;6:45–49.

Chapter 3.7

The Use of Computers in Anticoagulation Management

Hamsaraj G. M. Shetty and Philip A. Routledge

Anticoagulants have a narrow therapeutic index (Chapters 3.2 and 5.4) and increasing duration of anticoagulant therapy results in an increase in the risk of bleeding[1]. With conventional anticoagulant control, patients on long-term anticoagulation often remain within the therapeutic range no more than 55–65% of the time[2]. Anticoagulation clinics have resulted in better control but are resource-intensive and not available in all hospitals (Chapter 3.3). In addition, clinics in some countries (United Kingdom, for example) are often run by inexperienced junior doctors[3]. There is obviously a need for the development of a method, which is not resource intensive, relatively cheap and achieves optimum anticoagulation in the majority of patients. Computer assisted anticoagulation systems were introduced with the aim of accomplishing these goals.

Computer-managed databases have evolved from the simple filing techniques of the 1950's into extremely versatile systems. It is now possible to store and readily retrieve large amounts of information. With the introduction of portable computers and networking facilities, it is also possible to transmit enormous amounts of data with ease. Computers have been used to assist anticoagulant therapy since the late 1970's. They can be used to store and retrieve patient information, flag situations affecting anticoagulant therapy like drug interactions, and aid dose prediction for both initiation and maintenance of anticoagulant therapy.

STORING BACKGROUND INFORMATION

Many anticoagulant clinics monitor patients on behalf of physicians and surgeons who devolve the responsibility of day-to-day anticoagulation management to the clinic. In the case of patients with prosthetic heart valves, the patient's local anticoagulant clinic may be a great distance away from the cardiac surgical centre. In such a situation, it may be difficult to obtain accurate background information about a given patient at short notice. Patient details such as age, concurrent illness such as liver disease or cardiac failure, excessive sensitivity or resistance to anticoagulant therapy and target level of anticoagulation can all be incorporated into computer databases. Availability of this information in a readily retrievable format greatly assists optimal monitoring of patients on anticoagulants. In addition, computer databases can be used to reduce the administrative burden of the clinic by giving appropriate appointment dates automatically and reminding doctors about the date of discontinuation of anticoagulation. They can also facilitate audit.

Database on drug interactions.

Several drugs interact with warfarin either to enhance or diminish its anticoagulant effect[4] (see also Chapter 3.2). Many patients, especially the elderly, are receiving multiple drug therapy and may have to take additional drugs, for example antibiotics, for intercurrent illnesses. In such patients alterations in concurrent drug therapy can have important effects on anticoagulant control. Although some interactions between warfarin and other drugs are well recognised, it is a difficult task to remember all of them, especially with the ever increasing number of new drugs[5]. Computer databases can be used to list all the clinically relevant drug interactions, and this information can be used in modifying the anticoagulant dose. Availability of such information can also be very helpful in explaining sudden changes in the patient's response to anticoagulation.

COMPUTER ASSISTED DOSE PREDICTION

Due to a number of pharmacokinetic and pharmacodynamic factors, there is considerable variation between patients in the response to warfarin therapy[6]. Individual warfarin dosage is therefore essential. Attempts have been made to develop methods which quantitate warfarin effects by using mathematical models that describe the time course of its action. Since these models are complicated, computers have been used for their application.

Initiation of warfarin therapy

As it is difficult to predict prospectively a given patient's response to initial doses of warfarin, there is always a risk of over- or under-anticoagulation during the first few days of treatment. An optimum method should reduce the number of days required for attaining the therapeutic INR level, and should not produce over- or under-anticoagulation. A certain amount of empiricism is necessary since the use of historical knowledge is the only method available to select the initial dose of warfarin. Several empirical induction methods have been described (Table 3.7–1)[7]. More recently, Bayesian techniques which combine the population pharmacokinetic parameters with the actual observations in individual patients have been used to initiate warfarin therapy[8,9].

In a prospective randomised study, White and associates evaluated a computer program, which used a pharmacokinetic/pharmacodynamic model proposed by Theofanous and Barile together with Bayesian forecasting methods to predict warfarin dose for initiation of warfarin therapy[9,10,11]. They found that the program predicted warfarin dose significantly more accurately than housestaff physicians who did not routinely manage warfarin therapy. The time required for achievement of stable anticoagulation was 3.7 days shorter ($p=0.002$) using computer assisted dosing than could be achieved by the housestaff.

Abbrecht and associates evaluated a computer program based on a maximum drug-induced effect (E max) pharmacodynamic model to initiate warfarin therapy[12]. A retrospective evaluation of the program revealed that it was able to predict successfully the prothrombin complex activity (PCA) responses for three different groups of subjects. The ability of the program to predict PCA values in 10 patients was evaluated prospectively and compared with a control group of 10 patients who did not receive

Table: 3.7–1
Warfarin Induction Schedule
(For further details see reference 7)

Warfarin Day	*International normalised ratio preferably 9–10 am*	*Warfarin dose preferably given at 5–6 pm*
1	<1.4	10mg
2	<1.8	10mg
	1.8	1mg
	>1.8	0.5mg
3	<2.0	10mg
	2–2.1	5mg
	2.2–2.3	4.5mg
	2.4–2.5	4mg
	2.6–2.7	3.5mg
	2.8–2.9	3mg
	3.0–3.1	2.5mg
	3.2–3.3	2mg
	3.4	1.5mg
	3.5	1mg
	3.6–4.0	0.5mg
	>4.0	0mg
		Predicted maintenance dose
4	<1.4	>8mg
	1.4	8mg
	1.5	7.5mg
	1.6–1.7	7mg
	1.8	6.5mg
	1.9	6mg
	2–2.1	5.5mg
	2.2–2.3	5mg
	2.4–2.6	4.5mg
	2.7–3.0	4mg
	3.1–3.5	3.5mg
	3.6–4.0	3mg
	4.1–4.5	Miss out next day's dose then give 2mg
	>4.5	Miss out 2 days doses then give 1mg

1. Caution in patients with heart failure or liver disease and in post-operative patients since their sensitivity to warfarin may vary with time.
2. If the INR on day 1 is 1.4 or greater, the inital doses of warfarin should be reduced and the schedule is no longer relevant.

computer assistance. The computer assisted patients required 6.8 days as compared with 4.8 days in control patients to reach PCA values in the 20 to 30% therapeutic range. The very conservative upper limits for warfarin dosage in the first few days of therapy were thought to be the cause of initial delay in achieving therapeutic ranges in the computer assisted patients. However, after the desired PCA had been achieved, these patients remained within the therapeutic range for 83% of the time compared to only 60% of the time in the case of the control group. Interestingly, the computer assisted patients were much less over-anticoagulated.

A prospective, randomised comparison of these model-based computer methods with the simpler empirical dose induction methods has not been made to our knowledge. The latter are considerably simpler and require no sophisticated technology.

Prediction of Maintenance Dose of Warfarin

Several computer programs for prediction of steady-state warfarin doses have been clinically evaluated. Sawyer and Finn described comparative clinical evaluation of models developed by Theofanous and Barile (log-linear pharmacodynamic model) and Barr (linear pharmacodynamic model)[10,13,14]. They found that in 12 hospitalised patients a stable dose prediction could be achieved within 6.1 doses when the log-linear method was used, compared with 8 doses when the linear pharmacodynamic model was used. The mean of the average prediction error for maintenance dose was 0.25mg for both the models (percentage error + 12%).

Mungall and associates described the population pharmacokinetics of warfarin in 163 subjects and these have been used in part in the development of a Bayesian computer program to predict warfarin pharmacokinetics, pharmacodynamics and prothrombin response (WARFDA)[11,15]. Svec and associates compared the predictive performance of the program when given from zero to five measured prothrombin ratios[11]. They found that the predictions based on population parameters and one prothrombin ratio feedback were significantly biased, but when four and five prothrombin ratio feedbacks were provided the predictive performance improved sufficiently to enable them to provide clinically useful dosage guidelines early in the course of warfarin therapy. It is apparent from this study that the initial parameter estimates do not accurately represent the study population and that there is a need for further delineation of the true population parameter estimates.

The computer program based on a pharmacokinetic/pharmacodynamic model proposed by Theofanous and Smolen together with Bayesian forecasting methods (vide supra), has also been evaluated for prediction of steady state warfarin dosage. White and Mungall in a prospective, randomised clinical trial evaluated the program's ability to predict the steady state warfarin dose required to achieve the target INR in 50 patients. They found that the accuracy of warfarin dosage adjustments made using the computer program was comparable to that of an experienced anticoagulation nurse-specialist[17].

Several systems using semi-empirical methods to adjust warfarin dose have also been described. Wilson and James have described microcomputer assisted management of an anticoagulation clinic by using a program which a) provides recommended dose of warfarin in terms of the previous dose and the current prothrombin time, b) recommends the interval before the next visit, c) maintains and updates a data file on each patient, d) produces clinic and ambulance lists, e) alerts the doctors about the need to make decisions with regard to the continuation or stoppage of treatment and f) produces an updated weekly file of all patients[18]. After using the system for 16 months they claimed that anticoagulation control was as good as could be achieved manually. Wyld and associates used the program of Wilson and James with minor alterations and found that the number of under-anticoagulated patients decreased from 14% to 6% in the first 13 months whilst the number of over-anticoagulated patients did not increase in the same period[19].

Ryan and associates have described the use of a computer program similar to that of Wilson and James. After a period of 6 months, the mean INR rose from 2.98 to 3.46[20]. The number of patients in the therapeutic range increased from 45.3% to 62.9% while the number of patients below the therapeutic range decreased from 42.5% to 25.8% and those who were above it fell by 1% (12.3 to 11.3%). The systems of Wilson and James and Ryan and associates use simple dose adjustment factors which could be used to adjust warfarin dose using simple calculators.

As with systems used for initiation of anticoagulant therapy, no comparisons have been made between the more sophisticated model-based methods for long-term control and the simpler semi-empirical methods, but both appear to be reasonably effective in the clinical setting[21].

CONCLUSION

Computer assisted anticoagulation has been shown to aid control of warfarin therapy. No existing program is ideal however and, perhaps because most are presently relatively expensive to buy, no formal randomised comparison of the major programs has yet been made. It is also unclear whether the sophisticated model-based programmes provide better estimates of dose than the empirical or semi-empirical methods. Nevertheless, given the versatility of computers there is scope for development of even more comprehensive programmes fro providing optimal anticoagulant therapy. This approach can free physicians to fulfil the important educational and development roles which are still performed better by people than by machines.

REFERENCES.

1. Petitti DB, Strom BL, Melmon KL. Duration of warfarin anticoagulant therapy and the probabilities of recurrent thromboembolism and haemorrhage. Am J Med 1986;81:255–259.
2. Brotman I. Anticoagulation in myocardial infarction. Am J Cardiol 1958;1:260–270.
3. Mclnnes GT. Efficacy of anticoagulation in the UK. Lancet 1981;2:88.
4. Serlin MJ, Breckenridge AM. Drug interactions with warfarin. Drugs 1983;25:610–620.
5. Jolson HM, Tanner A, Green L, Grasela TH. Adverse reaction reporting of interaction between warfarin and fluoroquinolones. Arch Intern Med 1991;151:1003–1004.
6. Shetty HGM, Fennerty AG, Routledge PA. Clinical pharmacokinetic considerations in the control of oral anticoagulant therapy. Clin Pharmacokinet 1989;16:238–253.
7. Fennerty A, Dolbern J, Thomas P, Backhouse G, Bentley DP, Campbell IA, Routledge PA. Flexible induction dose regimen for warfarin and prediction of maintenance dose. Br Med J 1984; 188:1268–1270.
8. Sheiner LB, Beal SL. Bayesian individualisation of pharmacokinetics: simple implementation and comparison with non-Bayesian methods. J Pharmaceut Sci 1982;71:1344–1348.
9. White RH, Homg R, Venook AP, Daschbach MM, Murray W, Mungall DR, Coleman RW. Initiation of

warfarin therapy: comparison of physician dosing with computer-assisted dosing. J Gen Intern Med 1987;2:141–148.
10. Theofanous TG, Barile RG. Multiple-dose kinetics of oral anticoagulants: methods of analysis and optimised dosing. J Pharmacol Sci 1973;62:261–266.
11. Svec JM, Coleman RW, Mungall DR, Ludden TM. Bayesian pharmacokinetic/pharmacodynamic forecasting of prothombin response to warfarin therpay: preliminary evaluation. Ther Drug Monit 1985;7:174–180.
12. Abbrecht PH, O'Leary TJ, Behrendt DM. Evalution of a computer-assisted method for individualised anticoagulation: retrospective and prospective studies with a pharmacodynamic model. Clin Pharmacol Ther 1982;32:129–136.
13. Sawyer WT, Finn AL. Digital computer-assisted warfarin therapy: comparison of two models. Comp Biomed Res 1979;12:221–231.
14. Barr W. Presented at the ASHP Institute on Advanced Pharmacokinetics. Lexington, Kentucky 1975.
15. Mungall DA, Marshall J, Ludden TM, Hawkins DW, Crawford MH. Population kinetics of warfarin. Paper presented to second World Conference on Clinical Pharmacology, Washington DC, August 9 1983.
16. Theofanous TG, Smolen VF. Multiple-dose kinetics of pharmacological effects of indirect anticoagulants. J Pharm Sci 1972;61:980–982.
17. White RH, Mungall D. Outpatient management of warfarin therapy: comparison of computer-predicted dosage adjustment to skilled professional care. Ther Drug Monit 1991;13:46–50.
18. Wilson R, James AH. Computer-assisted management of warfarin treatment. Br Med J 1984; 289:422–424.
19. Wyld PJ, West D, Wilson TH. Computer dosing in anticoagulant clinics - the way forward? Clin Lab Haematol 1988;10:235–236.
20. Ryan PJ, Gilbert M, Rose PE. Computer control of anticoagulant dose for therapeutic management. Br Med J 1989;299:1207–1209.
21. Holford NHG. Clinical pharmacokinetics and pharmacodynamics of warfarin. Understanding the dose-effect relationship. Clin Pharmacokinet 1986;11:483–504.

Part 4

Anticoagulation in special circumstances

Chapter 4.1

Anticoagulation during Pregnancy

Celia M. Oakley

THROMBOEMBOLIC RISK IN PREGNANCY

Pregnancy induces a hypercoagulable state with an increased concentration of circulating clotting factors, increased platelet turnover and reduced fibrinolytic activity[1,2] (Table 4.1–1). The theoretically increased tendency to thrombosis engendered by these changes is countered to some extent by an increased cardiac output and accelerated circulation time. However, there remains an increased risk of leg vein thrombosis, left atrial thrombus formation in mitral stenosis and thrombosis on artificial heart valves.

Venous return from the legs is slowed because the veins participate in the smooth muscle relaxation that takes place in pregnancy. In addition, there is compression of the inferior vena cava by the uterus in the last trimester. This inferior vena caval obstruction reduces venous return and consequently cardiac output in the supine position. It contributes to the development of varicose veins and pedal oedema in later pregnancy, even though the cardiac output continues to rise until term when inferior vena caval flow is restored in the lateral or semi-prone position. This increased risk of venous thrombosis persists into the immediate post-partum period, since the circulatory changes take a week or more to return to normal. The risk is further increased if delivery has been by Caesarean section.

Venous thrombosis

Superficial venous thrombosis may extend into the calf veins and every calf vein thrombosis carries a risk of pulmonary embolism through extension into the large proximal veins. In one report, maternal mortality from pulmonary embolism was 15% when calf vein thrombosis was not treated with anticoagulants[3]. While calf vein thrombosis may be treated with short term heparin, recurrent deep vein thromboses, ileofemoral thrombosis or pulmonary embolism need longer term

Table 4.1–1
Changes in the blood in pregnancy

- Increase in concentration of clotting factors II, VII, VIII, IX and X.
- Increase in concentration of fibrinogen
- Increased blood viscosity
- Decreased deformability of erythrocytes
- No change in platelet count but increase in platelet turnover.

Increased risk of thromboembolism remains for the first four weeks of the puerperium.

anticoagulant treatment. Patients with a history of previous leg vein thrombosis or pulmonary embolism were estimated to have a 12% risk of thrombosis or embolism in pregnancy in one retrospective study[4].

Rheumatic heart disease

Most patients with rheumatic valve disease who become pregnant are still in sinus rhythm but some may be in atrial fibrillation with large left atria. They require long-term anticoagulants because of the otherwise serious risk of systemic embolism. Even patients with mitral stenosis who are in stable sinus rhythm with no history of previous atrial fibrillation, may develop systemic thromboembolic complications during pregnancy from left atrial thrombus caused by stasis coupled with increased coagulability.

Replacement valves

Patients with heart valve prostheses have an increased risk of thromboembolic complications in pregnancy compared with the non-pregnant state[5–22]. While the risk is greater for mechanical valves, those with bioprostheses are also at risk particularly if they are in atrial fibrillation, have large left atria or a history of previous thromboembolism.

Anticoagulant drugs are essential in pregnancy for the prevention of potentially fatal maternal thromboembolic events and the indications must therefore be the same in pregnancy as they are outside it despite possible risks to the foetus. Controversy continues concerning the magnitude of these risks, on the use of anticoagulants in pregnancy [23–26] and on the choice of prostheses for young women who will probably want to have children. It is striking how many of the reports on the complications of anticoagulant treatment have come from North America[27–29] where anticoagulation levels used for patients with prosthetic heart valves have been high for many years (see Chapter 3.4). The reported high foetal loss rates in these series are fortunately not seen in British series[30], in which lower levels of anticoagulation have been used.

HEPARIN

Heparin is a natural substance and a large molecule (Chapter 3.2). It does not reach the foetus to harm it directly but can still cause placental separation, abortion, prematurity or still birth[23–26]. Its major defect is the difficulty in maintaining an antithrombotic effect without haemorrhagic complications. The dose of heparin needed to treat existing venous thrombosis is greater than that needed to prevent it. Where short term anticoagulant use is envisaged for the treatment of acute deep vein thrombosis, carefully supervised intravenous treatment in hospital is to be preferred. When longer term prophylaxis of recurrence is the aim, subcutaneous low dose heparin, self-administered at home, is suitable (Table 4.1–2).

The dose of heparin required to prevent arterial thrombosis or prosthetic valve thrombosis is much higher than that needed to prevent venous thromboembolism. With the long-term treatment required, maternal haemorrhage is a real risk and side effects are likely. *Moreover, efficacy has not been proved.* Therefore, for the prevention of systemic thromboembolism, oral anticoagulation is a safer choice. Heparin given

Table 4.1–2
Indications for heparin usage

Prophylaxis Subcutaneous self administered 10,000 U b.d.	Prevention of venous thromboembolism
Full anticoagulation Continuous intravenous 30–40,000 U/24 hour infusion in hospital	Treatment of leg vein thrombosis Pulmonary embolism
Control by: partial thromboplastin time (1.5–2.0) heparin level clotting time	

intravenously or subcutaneously is neither safe nor effective in preventing arterial thromboembolism. It has been shown to be ineffective in sub-anticoagulant doses[7,15,16] and to be unsafe with a risk of maternal cerebral haemorrhage and retroplacental haemorrhage when higher dosage is used[29]. In addition, heparin administration is inconvenient and associated with other side effects, such as thrombocytopenia, osteopenia, alopecia and infection (if the intravenous route is chosen), although these are relatively unimportant in comparison. A major problem with heparin, which greatly limits its usefulness is the route and mode of administration. Furthermore one of three tests must be chosen in order to regulate dosage: partial thromboplastin time, clotting time or heparin level. Even then the frequency of testing in relation to the mode of administration has to be determined, and regular blood counts are required to detect thrombocytopenia which further increases the bleeding hazard and paradoxically the risk of thrombosis (see Chapter 3.2).

ORAL ANTICOAGULANTS

The coumarin oral anticoagulants have a bad reputation in pregnancy arising from the observation of skeletal abnormalities and central nervous system defects in infants born to mothers who had been given such drugs during pregnancy[27]. Oral anticoagulants cross the placenta to the foetus where their anticoagulant effect is very much greater than in the mother. This is because of the immature foetal liver and the inability of maternal liver enzymes to cross the placental barrier due to their large molecular size. This enhanced anticoagulant effect may cause haemorrhage in developing vascular cartilaginous bone and gives rise to the so-called warfarin embryopathy. The risk is greatest towards the end of the first trimester and its magnitude is dose dependent. After the first trimester cartilaginous bone is less vascular but the central nervous system remains vulnerable.

The skeletal deformity, chondro-dysplasia punctata, in its worst form comprises deafness, optic atrophy, a hypoplastic nose with upper airway obstruction and short-limbed dwarfism due to punctate dysplasia of the epiphyses. Most such foetuses are aborted, but less severe examples of the syndrome may be seen in survivors. Together with a dwindling risk of the skeletal embryopathy as pregnancy proceeds, is a continuing risk of foetal cerebral haemorrhage because the developing brain is also very vascular. Even a small haemorrhage may have a profound effect. Neurological deficits and spasticity may occur.

The risk of foetal damage by coumarin drugs given in pregnancy has probably been exaggerated (Table 4.1–3). In anecdotal cases it is likely that disaster rather than success determined reporting[7,19,22,29]. Historically, anticoagulation levels have been higher in the United States than in Europe, with a higher incidence of major bleeding complications in patients with prosthetic valves than has been reported from the UK or Europe[29,30] (see Chapters 3.3 and 3.4). Most personal series come from countries that still have a high incidence of rheumatic heart disease and therefore large numbers of young women with (mainly mitral) prostheses[8,9,11–13,15–20,31]. In developing countries, anticoagulant control is often difficult with a high incidence of both haemorrhagic and thromboembolic events in the mothers.

Reporting from the National Institute of Cardiology in Mexico and following up their previous work, Salazar's group looked at the risk of coumarin embryopathy according to the gestation time when the drug was administered, and at the maternal and foetal complications of subcutaneous heparin in the first trimester and last two weeks of pregnancy[15,16]. They used a fixed dose of 5,000 units of heparin given subcutaneously every 12 hours. Three patients suffered massive thrombosis of the prosthetic valve, two in the first trimester and one in the immediate post-partum period after receiving heparin during the last two weeks. Comparing the outcome in a) 23 patients transferred to heparin from the 6th to the 12th week (12 only from the 7th week) and b) 37 pregnancies continued on coumarin throughout, there was no difference in the high

Table 4.1–3
Foetal and neonatal complications following maternal anticoagulants in pregnancy. Pooled data from the review by Hall et al[29]

	Coumarin Drugs	*Heparin**
Number	418	135
Live born with problems	57 (14%)	30 (22%)
Embryopathy	16 (4%)	0
CNS defects	6 (1%)	0
Premature deaths	4 (1%)	10 (7%)
Spontaneous abortions	36 (9%)	2 (1%)
Still births	32 (8%)	17 (13%)
Premature normal	8 (2%)	19 (14%)
Live born, **no** problems	293 (70%)	86 (64%)

NB
These figures probably represent maximal figures for complications since most of the reports come from the USA where higher levels of anticoagulants were used.

* Various routes and regimes

incidence of spontaneous abortion. No coumarin embryopathies were seen in the infants of patients on heparin from the 6th to 12th week, but two out of eight live-born who whose mothers had received heparin from the 7th to the 12th week were affected, and eight out of 27 live-born from the group in which coumarin was continued until the last two weeks. The children were assessed by a clinical geneticist who found only facial defects such as slight hypoplasia of the nasal bones, and no children had epiphyseal stippling, central nervous system abnormalities or optic atrophy.

Ben Ismail reported the difficulties of achieving accurate anticoagulation in Tunisia[11]. Two out of five women given heparin had thromboembolic episodes and three had spontaneous abortions. Oral anticoagulants were given during 53 pregnancies with eight spontaneous abortions. They found that heparin was less effective than oral anticoagulants in preventing maternal thromboembolism and there were no embryopathies in their series. These authors did not find the use of heparin in the first trimester to be justified.

Forty seven pregnancies in 37 patients with prosthetic valves were reported from India(20). Forty infants were born at full-term and there were three premature births. There were only two spontaneous abortions, one still birth and one ectopic pregnancy giving a foetal mortality of 8.5%. Oral anticoagulants were continued throughout pregnancy with heparin substitution before labour. Valve thrombosis developed in two patients but surgical intervention was successful in both and one of the pregnancies continued to term. No embryopathies were encountered.

From South Africa, Sareli and associates reported no maternal thromboembolic complications or deaths among 49 patients with 60 mechanical valves treated with warfarin[31]. Because of late presentation, no patient had received heparin in the first trimester but heparin was substituted at 36 weeks in 23. There was one still birth amongst these. In the remaining 18 the onset of labour was premature, while the patient was still on warfarin, and there were six still births. Two warfarin embryopathies were seen (4%) with nasal hypoplasia in both and stippled epiphyses in one. There were two neonatal deaths due to intracranial haemorrhage in premature babies whose mothers were still taking warfarin (INR 4.2 and 3.2 respectively). The high incidence of premature labour (53%) and low birth weights were similar to those reported previously in valve disease. Six of eleven pregnancies in which dipyridamole was added were unsuccessful. There was no relation between haemodynamic status and foetal outcome. The authors of this important study concluded that with new generation mechanical valves (Medtronic Hall and St. Jude Medical) the maternal risk is low and that, although foetal wastage is high, the risk of a malformed liveborn is low.

Transfer from oral anticoagulants to heparin in pregnancy has been widely advocated but a literature search has revealed no published series to justify this practise and numerous reports of problems. High doses over a prolonged period, when the patient cannot be retained for observation in hospital, carry a risk not only of serious maternal haemorrhage but a considerable risk of foetal death or premature delivery due to retro-placental haemorrhage. Maternal bleeding was a major problem in 14 cases with three deaths in one series[29].

In order to avoid the need for anticoagulant treatment in pregnancy, the use of bioprostheses has been advocated for young women who may later wish to raise a family. Unfortunately, bioprostheses show very much diminished durability in children and young adults, and this rapid deterioration is likely to be accelerated during pregnancy when there is increased calcium turnover. Moreover, bioprostheses are not immune from thromboembolism or indeed valve thrombosis (Chapter 2.4) and should atrial fibrillation develop, anticoagulation is mandatory.

The author's practice is to recommend mechanical prostheses for children and young people regardless of sex. Oral anticoagulants are continued throughout pregnancy until an estimated two weeks before delivery when the patient is admitted to hospital and transferred to heparin in full anticoagulant doses. While mother and foetus are under continued observation, any problems can be immediately recognised and delivery if necessary expedited. There is no need to reverse heparin before vaginal delivery, because the contracting uterus reduces blood loss, the heparin effect wanes quickly, and it is most important to ensure that there is minimal break in the continuity of anticoagulation for the mother. Once the baby is delivered, oral anticoagulants can be restarted and heparin continued until the INR is back in the therapeutic range. In the case of surgical delivery, heparin can be briefly reversed immediately before Caesarean section, then restarted and continued until warfarin takeover is completed.

No major cardiac centre in the western world sees a sufficient number of young women with prosthetic valves to be able to gain a large experience of the use of oral anticoagulants in pregnancy. Reports from the developing world have been most encouraging, and results are likely to be even better with improved anticoagulation management (see Chapter 3.4). In the past, experience with mechanical valves in pregnancy has been reduced in Europe and North America by selection of bioprostheses in young women and by cautioning against pregnancy in women with mechanical heart valves[10]. However, risks are minimised when patient co-operation is maximal and anticoagulant control is precise. The risks of thromboembolic events in pregnant women treated with anticoagulation are no greater than reported in the non-pregnant population with mechanical heart valves[32]. If the INR is maintained between 2.0 to 2.5, the chance of oral anticoagulants damaging the foetus is small. There is an increased risk of abortion which is perhaps 25% in women taking warfarin (compared with 15% in healthy women), but the risk of a damaged child being born is no more than 5%. Contemporary thinking on oral anticoagulation is admirably epitomised by the view recently expressed by Elkayam and Gleicher, that in asymptomatic or mildly symptomatic patients with prosthetic heart valves who are willing and able to follow a strict regimen of medical care, pregnancy is not associated with an increased morbidity in the mother or foetus[33]. No such approbation exists for heparin as an anticoagulant for use in pregnancy and there is no justification for its use except for a short period prior to delivery, as outlined above.

REFERENCES

1. Todd ME, Thompson JH Jr, Bowie ETJ, Owen LA. Changes in blood coagulation during pregnancy. Mayo Clin Proc 1965;40:370–383.
2. Shaper AG. The hypercoagulable states. Ann Intern Med 1985;102:814–828.
3. Ullery JC. Thromboembolic disease complicating pregnancy and the puerperium. Am J Obstet Gynaecol 1954;68:1243–1260.
4. Badaracco MA, Vessey M. Recurrence of venous thromboembolic disease and use of oral contraceptives. Br Med J 1974;1:215–217.
5. Oakley C, Doherty P. Pregnancy in patients after valve replacement. Br Heart J 1976;38:1140–1148.
6. McLeod AA, Jennings KP, Townsend ER. Near fatal puerperal thrombosis on Bjørk-Shiley mitral valve prosthesis. Br Heart J 1978;40:934–937.

7. Bennett GG, Oakley CM. Pregnancy in a patient with a mitral valve prosthesis. Lancet 1968;1:616–619.
8. Casanegra P, Aviles G, Maturana G, Dubernet J. Cardiovascular management of pregnant women with a heart valve prosthesis. Am J Cardiol 1975;36:802–806.
9. Ibarra-Perez C, Aravalo-Toledo N, Alvarez-de la Cadena O, Noriega-Guerra L. The course of pregnancy in patients with artificial heart valves. Am J Med 1976;61:504–512.
10. Lutz DJ, Nollar KL, Spittal JA Jr, Danielson GK, Fish CR. Pregnancy and its complications following cardiac valve prostheses. Am J Obstet Gynecol 1978;131:460–468.
11. Ben Ismail M, Fekih M, Taktak M et al. Prostheses valvulaires cardiaques et grossesse. Arch Mal Coeur 1979;2:192–194.
12. Chen WWC, Chan CS, Lee PK, Wang RYC, Wong VCW. Pregnancy in patients with prosthetic heart valves: an experience with 45 pregnancies. Quart J Med 1982;51:358–365.
13. Larrea JL, Nunez L, Reque JA, Gil Aguardo M, Matarros R, Mingues JA. Pregnancy and mechanical valve prostheses in a high risk situation for the mother and the fetus. Ann Thorac Surg 1983;36:459–463.
14. Guidozzi F. Pregnancy in patients with prosthetic cardiac valves. S Afr Med J 1984;65:961–963.
15. Salazar E, Zajarias A, Guitarrazn Iturbe I. The problem of cardiac valve prostheses: anticoagulants and pregnancy. Circulation 1984;70(Suppl 1):169–177.
16. Iturbe-Alessio I, Delcarmen Fonesca M, Mutchinik D, Santos MA, Zajarias A, Salazar E. Risks of anticoagulant therapy in pregnant women with artificial heart valves. N Eng J Med 1986;27:1390–1393.
17. Lee PK, Wang RYC, Chow JSF, Cheung KL, Wong UCW, Chan TK. Combined use of warfarin and adjusted subcutaneous heparin during pregnancy in patients with artificial heart valves. JACC 1986;8:221–224.
18. Vitali E, Donatelli F, Quaini E, Gropelli G, Pellegrini A. Pregnancy in patients with mechanical prosthetic heart valves: our experiences regarding 98 pregnancies in 57 patients. J Cardiovasc Surg 1986;27:221–227.
19. Gonzalez-Santos JM, Vallejo JL, Rico MJ, Gonzales-Santos ML, Horno R, Garcia-Dorado D. Thrombosis of a mechanical valve prosthesis late in pregnancy. Case report and review of the literature. Thorac Cardiovasc Surg 1986;34:335–337.
20. Pavunkumar P, Venugopal P, Kaul U, et al. Pregnancy in patients with prosthetic cardiac valve. A 10 year experience. Scand J Thorac Cardiovasc Surg 1988;22:19–22.
21. McColgin S. Pregnant women with prosthetic heart valves. Clin Obstet Gynaecol 1989;32:76–89.
22. Tapanainen J, Ikaheimo M, Jouppila P, Kortelainen ML, Salmela P. Thrombosis in a mechanical aortic valve prosthesis during subcutaneous heparin therapy in pregnancy. A case report. Eur J Obstet Gynaecol Reprod Biol 1990;36:175–177.
23. Howie PW. Anticoagulants in pregnancy. Clin Obstet Gynaecol 1986;13:349–364.
24. Ginsberg JS, Hirsh J. Optimum use of anticoagulants in pregnancy. Drugs 1988;34:505–512.
25. Ginsberg JS, Hirsh J. Anticoagulants during pregnancy. Annu Rev Med 1989;40:79–86.
26. Wehrmacher WH, Messmore HL. Thromboembolic disease during pregnancy: Problems with anticoagulant therapy. Compr Ther 1990;16:31–35.
27. Villasanta V. Thromboembolic disease in pregnancy. Am J Obstet Gynecol 1965;93:142–160.
28. Hirsh J, Cade JF, O'Sullivan EF. Clinical experience with anticoagulant therapy during pregnancy. Br Med J 1970;1:270–273.
29. Hall JG, Pauli RM, Wilson KM. Maternal and fetal sequelae of anticoagulation during pregnancy. Am J Med 1980;68:122–140.
30. Hawkins DF. Drug treatment of medical disorders in pregnancy. In Hawkins DF (Ed): Drugs and Pregnancy. 2nd Ed. Edinburgh, Churchill Livingstone, 1987:90–114.
31. Sareli P, England MJ, Berk MR et al. Maternal and fetal sequelae of anticoagulation during pregnancy in patients with mechanical heart valve prostheses. JACC 1989;63:1462–1465.
32. Morris DC. Management of patients with prosthetic heart valves. Curr Probl Cardiol 1982;7:1–56.
33. Elkayam U and Gleicher N. Letter. N Engl J Med 1987;316:1664.

Chapter 4.2

Anticoagulation in Children

Martin J. Elliott and Christopher Young

Despite thirty years of experience with prostheses in paediatric cardiac surgery, the use of anticoagulation remains contentious for several reasons. These are summarised in the form of questions which must be answered before any firm recommendations can be made:-

a) What are the indications for antithrombotic treatment?
   - is it necessary after valve replacement?
   - is it necessary after the use of any other intracardiac prostheses?
   - is it necessary after other specific procedures or events, for example, Fontan procedure, arrhythmia?

b) If indicated, which type of antithrombotic treatment should be used and for how long?
   - warfarin
   - anti-platelet agents
   - combination therapy

c) If anticoagulation is used, how should it be monitored?
   - with what frequency?
   - at what level of INR?

d) What unwanted side-effects should be specifically sought in this age group?

e) Can we rely on children to take the drugs?

THE SPECIFIC PROBLEMS OF CHILDREN

The paediatric population clearly differs from its adult equivalent in a number of ways, and care must be exercised when extrapolating policy from data obtained in adult studies. Some differences are obvious. Others perhaps are less so.

Scale

Not only are children usually smaller than adults, but the prostheses required are usually much smaller also. As confidence has grown with surgery in infancy and the neonatal period, a rising number of children in this age group have undergone valve replacement and other cardiac surgical procedures involving prostheses. For example, 16 or 18mm prostheses are often required in the atrioventricular valve sites in infancy. Valve dynamics are different also in this age group, with more frequent valve excursions and wide variations in flow.

Complexity

Valve replacement or the insertion of prosthetic material often takes place as part of the repair of a complex congenital defect, or as a later consequence of it, for example mitral valve replacement during a Fontan procedure, or systemic atrioventricular valve replacement after earlier atrial repair of one of the forms of transposition of the great arteries. The intracardiac repair of some lesions may involve tunnels or tubes of prosthetic material. The wide variation in associated flow patterns and haemodynamics may have implications for anticoagulant regimens.

Growth

Children grow, and the younger they are the more rapidly they grow. Thus they may quickly outgrow their prostheses, changing flow rates and turbulence patterns considerably. Upstream stasis may develop, increasing the risk of thrombosis. Frequent adjustments to their therapeutic regimen may be necessary. The possible side effects of the drugs in growing children must also be considered.

Trauma risk

Anyone who has either watched children play, or worse, tried to supervise their own children's faltering beginnings on the sports field, will recall the risks to which children put themselves. Daily minor trauma is the norm and usually associated with bleeding. The process begins as a toddler with frequent coffee table collisions and the consequences of grabbing a passing pet's genitalia. Older children have sibling rivalry to contend with, and the discovery of the effects of gravity, usually made from a tree. The skateboard and bicycle present the next major challenge. Injuries to joints and head are unfortunately all too frequent with these diversions. Finally the motor-bike and the loan of the family car complete a frightening but exciting cycle of risk. The child on anticoagulants may be excluded from all these marvellous aspects of childhood by instruction, parental pressure, or fear but social isolation can be a terrible thing in adolescence.

Rebellion/compliance

The pressures for peer group conformity in adolescence are very important. Children with any serious illness are often reluctant to take their therapy if it makes them seem in any way different from their peers. This is certainly the case with anticoagulant therapy[1], which, because of a perceived risk of bleeding, can inhibit children from taking part in normal activity.

Sexuality

The problems of adolescence are not, of course, limited to those of conformity, but also include the beginnings of sexual awareness. This is a special problem for the young girl commencing menstruation whilst on anticoagulation and careful supportive counselling is vital. Expert and thorough contraceptive advice should be offered, involving both physician and family. In view of the risks described below, this time will not be wasted.

Needle phobia

Many children likely to need anticoagulation have become terrified of doctors, nurses and the sharp 'weapons' they wield. Frequent hospitalisation and even a single careless, brutal or unsympathetic blood sampling can have serious consequences for later compliance. Warfarin therapy still requires 'invasive' monitoring.

INDICATIONS FOR ANTICOAGULATION

Since the use of anticoagulation in children has so many apparent arguments against it, what are the current indications for its use in cardiac practice?

Heart valve replacement

It is widely agreed that, wherever possible, an abnormal cardiac valve in a child should be repaired rather than replaced[2–5]. If valve replacement is required, the first important decision is which prosthesis to use. Following the definition in 1976 by Braunwald and associates[6] of an ideal valve for use in children (Table 4.2–1), a number of different types of substitute valves have been tried. Initial enthusiasm for mechanical prostheses waned as their limitations in terms of size and risk of thromboembolism became apparent. The xenograft bioprostheses enjoyed a brief period of popularity, largely because they did not require anticoagulation. Unfortunately, within only a few years, it became clear that these prostheses underwent rapid, progressive and severe calcification in the paediatric population, irrespective of additional therapies such as anticoagulation[2]. Homograft valves have been used with considerably more success[7], but currently they are not applicable to all valve sites, nor are they universally available.

Wherever possible in paediatric practice, an abnormal heart valve should be repaired. If this is not possible, a homograft valve should be considered, since anticoagulation will not be required. If a homograft valve cannot be used then a mechanical prosthesis should be employed. Figure 4.2–1 summarises the changing pattern of valve usage at Great Ormond Street over the last 20 years.

Table 4.2–1
The ideal valve prosthesis for use in children

★ The valve should adequately relieve the haemodynamic abnormality

★ It should allow for growth of the child

★ It should not produce obstruction on its own account

★ It should not be prone to structural failure

★ It should be free from the risk of thromboembolism

★ It should have a low risk of infection

as defined by Braunwald et al 1976[6]

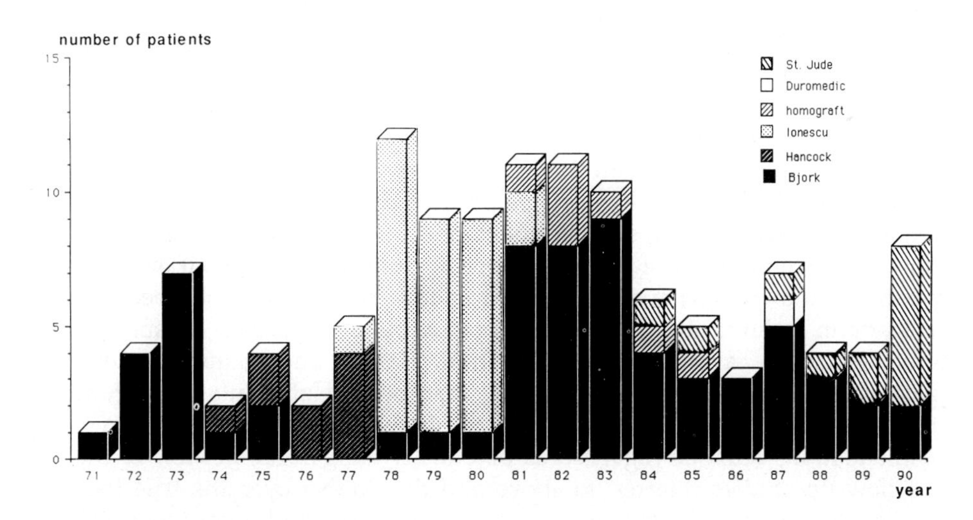

Figure 4.2–1: The changing pattern of prosthetic valve usage at The Hospital for Sick Children, Great Ormond Street, London, 1971-1990.

There has been considerable debate over the last few years as to whether the latest generation of mechanical prostheses require anticoagulation with warfarin when used in children. No anticoagulation at all, or the use of antiplatelet agents such as dipyridamole or aspirin represent the alternatives. The controversy began when Chen and associates[8] and then Weinstein, Mavroudis and Ebert[9] challenged traditional teaching by suggesting that aspirin provided adequate protection against thromboembolism in children with Bjørk-Shiley prostheses. Reviewing the available literature (on 177 children) Weinstein and his colleagues[9] concluded that warfarin did not 'dependably' protect children against thromboembolism and, in addition, haemorrhagic episodes were frequent. Earlier, Rufilinchas and colleagues[10] reported no thromboembolic complications in 22 children who underwent Bjørk-Shiley valve replacement and were subsequently managed without warfarin. Pass and associates[11] reported 31 children up to 2 years after St. Jude prosthesis insertion with no complications after receiving no anticoagulant therapy at all. Verrier and associates[12] treated 51 young patients with aspirin only after aortic valve replacement and reported no thromboembolic events up to a mean of 36 months postoperatively. Cornish and colleagues[13] did not observe any difference between the incidence of thromboembolism in unmatched groups of patients (total 81) who had either warfarin or aspirin in a period of up to 5 years follow up.

Although the idea of avoiding warfarin in children is attractive and the results described above appear encouraging, there are major problems in interpreting these data. These difficulties have been well summed up by Sade and co-authors[14] (early protagonists of no anticoagulation in children), who stated in the opening lines of their paper, that "in surgery, long term follow up often modifies beliefs based on short or medium-term follow up. Nowhere has this effect been more manifest than in the field of cardiac valve replacement with prostheses." In other words, all the enthusiastic claims for either antiplatelet therapy only or no anticoagulation at all, were based on insufficient follow up of too few patients. Subsequent reports, with longer follow up, have unfortunately exposed the illusion of safety. Thromboembolic rates in children in the absence of full anticoagulation have been unacceptably high.

Sade's group[14] in 1988 reversed their earlier (1985)[11] view on the basis of a thromboembolic rate of 5.7±2.1 events per 100 patient years (7 out of 48 patients) after left sided valve replacement with the St. Jude prosthesis. They now recommend full anticoagulation. McGrath and associates[15] reported a 24% incidence of thromboembolism in 29 survivors of valve replacement, and came to the same conclusion. There are now many studies in the literature supporting this view[16–22]. In our own series[2], the only patients known to have developed thromboembolism either stopped or reduced their warfarin voluntarily, or had it stopped by a physician. Despite the very convincing data in favour of anticoagulation, Harada and co-authors continue to suggest, on the basis of very short follow up, that antiplatelet agents alone are adequate after aortic valve replacement with the St. Jude prosthesis in children[23]. These recommendations must be regarded as potentially dangerous, in view of the longer term follow up studies referred to above and the doubts over the true therapeutic activity of dipyridamole[24] (see also Chapter 3.1). Ilbawi and associates[25] reported a mean of 6 years follow up of 162 valves (104 porcine heterografts, 40 St. Jude and 18 Bjørk-Shiley) implanted in 159 patients. Aspirin and dipyridamole were used in patients with St. Jude valves but 8 of 14 valves in the tricuspid position thrombosed on this regime; thrombosis was thought to be secondary to fibrous ingrowth, but this phenomenon may represent organisation of previous thrombus deposition (see Chapter 2.4). Three of 26 St. Jude valves on the left side of the heart developed thromboembolism, compared to none of 18 patients with a Bjørk-Shiley valve who were treated with warfarin. Despite the authors' conclusions that antiplatelet agents were adequate therapy for St. Jude valves on the left side of the heart, these data appear to support the use of warfarin rather than the use of dipyridamole and aspirin.

Despite full anticoagulation, haemorrhage has not been a problem in our own series[2,5] with up to 20 years follow up, or in the other series which advocate warfarin[17–22]. Stewart and co-authors[1] report an incidence of one major and four minor bleeding episodes in 211 patient years of warfarin therapy (2.3%/pty). The bleeding episodes were associated with excessive anticoagulation or what they describe as 'inappropriate' physical activity. Robbins and associates(26) report a single episode of gastrointestinal haemorrhage in 94 children. This was the only bleeding complication, whereas seven of 11 patients who received mechanical valves and no anticoagulation experienced major thromboembolic events. Bradley and colleagues[27] describe a similar incidence of minor haemorrhage, never life-threatening. Thus in the paediatric population, provided that appropriate control is maintained, warfarin anticoagulation does not appear to pose a significant increase in the risk of major bleeding.

There are, however, weaknesses in the pro-warfarin studies. The number of patients are still relatively small, the studies are uncontrolled and retrospective and the intensity of anticoagulation is unclear.

Other indications

There is a variety of other circumstances in which anticoagulation might be necessary in children. Some, such as dilated cardiomyopathy and severe arrhythmia are shared with the adult population; others, such as the failing Senning or Mustard procedure and primary pulmonary hypertension are less well known. However, perhaps the most controversial indication is in relation to the Fontan procedure or its various modifications.

Fontan procedure

In the Fontan family of operations the venous blood is transmitted more or less directly from the right atrium to the pulmonary artery missing out the right ventricle. The operations are used for the treatment of tricuspid atresia, pulmonary atresia with intact septum and for complex double inlet ventricles. Many authors have commented on the relatively high right atrial pressures after this operation[29,30] and, amongst several other consequences, right atrial thrombi have been reported[31]. It has been suggested that an acquired deficiency of protein C, protein S, antithrombin III or plasminogen may be the cause of this coagulopathy, but there is little published work to support this. Nor is it clear whether a tendency to thrombosis develops in the early

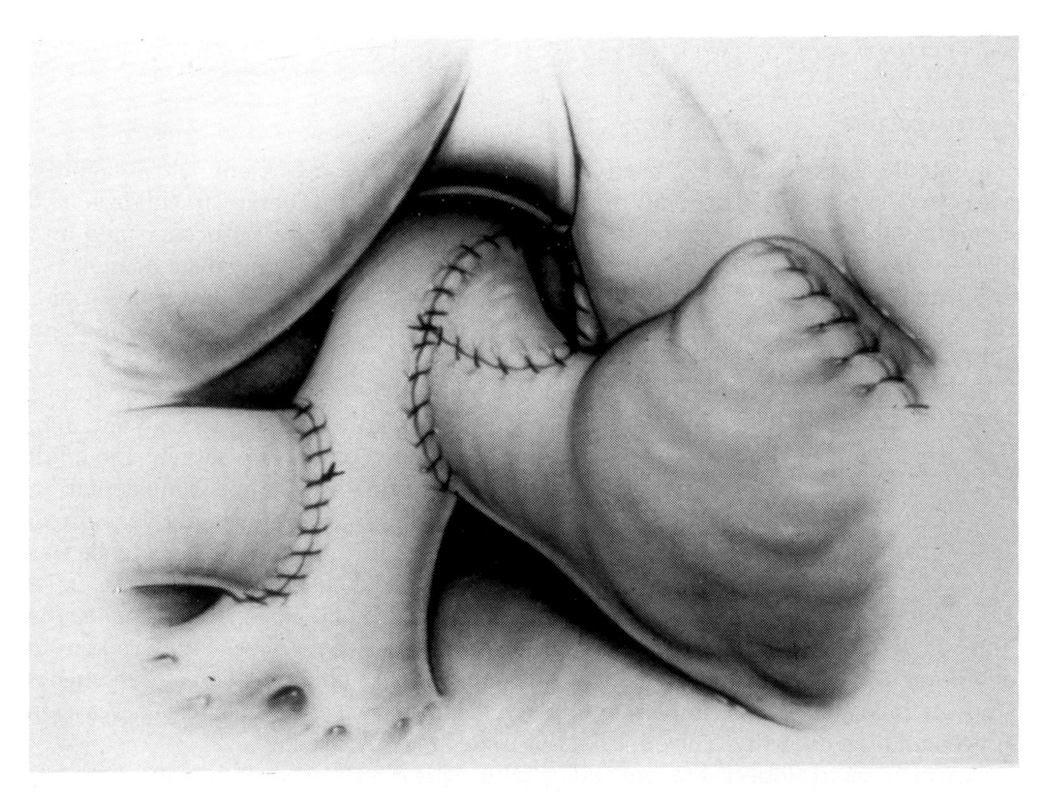

Figure 4.2–1: This figure shows the completed anastomosis for total cavopulmonary connection with the SVC having been transected and anastomosed superiorly to the upper part of the right pulmonary artery and inferiorly to the lower part of the right pulmonary artery. A Gore-Tex half tube has been inserted within the right atrium to divert the IVC blood to the inferior part of the SVC.

postoperative period as a consequence of the haemodynamics, or only later as a consequence of hepatic congestion.

Recently at Great Ormond Street[32], as at some other institutions, the policy has been to perform the total cavopulmonary connection (TCPC – Figure 4.2–2) instead of the classical or modified Fontan procedure. In most TCPCs there is less stasis than in traditional Fontan connections, but low-flow venous blood still passes across a Gore-Tex surface within the right atrium. In our first 100 TCPCs, one patient developed early right atrial pathway thrombus requiring surgery and three others were noted to have fresh clot on their intra-atrial patch at the time of reoperation to perforate the TCPC patch. It is likely that these patients represent a high risk subset with low venous flow for various reasons. However, since the Fontan operation or its TCPC equivalent depend for their viability on a low pulmonary vascular resistance, it does not make much sense to permit any potential embolic source to exist. Accordingly, it is now our policy to anticoagulate with warfarin all TCPC patients for at least 3 months and then to continue with antiplatelet therapy thereafter. Not all paediatric cardiac units adopt this policy, however. Indeed, there is wide variability in management. The nature, aetiology and management of possible post-Fontan hypercoagulability require detailed study to determine the optimum INR range for this group of patients.

ANTITHROMBOTIC DRUGS FOR USE IN CHILDREN

Anticoagulants

By far the most frequently used anticoagulant drug is the vitamin K antagonist warfarin (Chapter 3.2). The main problem with oral warfarin therapy in children is to determine the level of anticoagulation that is appropriate for a particular child and his/her clinical condition, balancing the prevention of thromboembolism against the prevention of haemorrhage. As in adults, each child needs a different dose, and laboratory testing of the anticoagulant effect of warfarin is necessary at frequent intervals.

Following the introduction of the INR in the mid 1980s[33,34], a largely arbitrary range of 3.0 – 4.5 was recommended for 'all mechanical valves'[35] (see Chapters 3.3 and 3.4). However, prior to the introduction of this guideline, drawn up largely for adult practice, many paediatric units had kept the INR in children in a range equivalent to an INR of 2.0 – 3.5. This was the practice at Great Ormond Street for many years in all children with prosthetic valves, and in this population thromboembolic incidence was minimal[2] and there were no episodes of bleeding. Hence when the new range (3.0 – 4.5) was introduced, many physicians were unconvinced of the need to change. At the time of writing, no prospective randomised studies have been undertaken to determine the optimum INR level for children. Many paediatricians feel that such a study is indicated before implementing what is otherwise an arbitrary increase in anticoagulation intensity. The ethics of this issue are complex.

Skin rashes and alopecia are rare and irritating side effects of warfarin but not serious complications. Cutaneous necrosis, associated in some cases with heterozygous protein C or S deficiency, is due to capillary thrombosis during induction of therapy which must, therefore, be performed slowly[34]. More specifically, demineralisation of bone can occur in growing children after prolonged therapy[34]. This may be of considerable importance. Conversely, Taybi and Capitanio[28] recently reported three children on warfarin after valve replacement who developed tracheobronchial calcification, similar to that seen in warfarin embryopathy. Clearly this complication must be sought during long term warfarin therapy.

Dipyridamole

Dipyridamole is given orally in doses of 5–10 mg/kg/24 hours in three divided doses. It is relatively safe. Headache, gastrointestinal upset and bruising are the main reported unwanted effects. Another disadvantage is the fact that it needs to be taken three times per day.

Aspirin

Aspirin is usually given in a dose of 2 mg/kg on alternate days but doses of up to 6mg/kg/24hrs may be used. It is safe in the tiny doses used, although for many paediatricians there is a background, but unproven, fear of its association in other circumstances with the development of Reye's syndrome. Reye's syndrome[36] is an acute illness that occurs almost exclusively in children. It is characterised clinically by profuse vomiting and neurological dysfunction, sometimes progressing to delirium, coma and death. A wide variety of causes has been implicated, including a virus, various toxins and salicylates. Aspirin was first suggested as a cause in 1965[37] but in 1982 an editorial in the Lancet concluded that there was insufficient evidence from the existing three retrospective case control studies to call into question the use of aspirin in the treatment of benign viral infections in children[38]. Only one prospective study has been published which revealed a strong association between Reye's syndrome and salicylate ingestion during the prodromal illness[39]. The United States Food and Drug Administration subsequently advised the avoidance of salicylate ingestion in previously healthy children during varicella or influenza outbreaks.

The inhibition of platelet aggregation has been shown to occur in humans at a dose of 2 mg/kg and to last for 72 hours[40]. Thus Jaklitsch and Leyland[41] suggested that the dose of aspirin given to children for antithrombotic purposes should be reduced to 2 mg/kg/72 hours during varicella and influenza outbreaks. If neurological symptoms or signs occur, the aspirin should be stopped and low-dose heparin substituted. After resolution of viral symptoms, aspirin in a dose of 6 mg/kg/24 hours can be resumed.

There are no published data to suggest that Reye's syndrome has occurred during the use of aspirin for antithrombotic treatment in children following valve replacement or other cardiac procedures.

COMPLIANCE

In view of the unwanted effects of warfarin, the need for frequent blood sampling and the psychology of the growing child, it is not surprising that it can be difficult to persuade some patients to continue their treatment. Non-compliance, or the voluntary cessation of warfarin is associated with a very high incidence of serious thromboembolic events, some fatal[1,2]. Much effort must be devoted to supporting not only the patient but parents, siblings and peers also, in order to sustain vital anticoagulation treatment. Frightening them may merely provoke bravado and great care must be exercised in dealing with the 'prickly' adolescent.

Compliance is also a problem in non-urban or underdeveloped communities. This has been clearly expressed by Kalke and associates[42] from India and Abid and colleagues[43] from Tunis, who report thromboembolism in association with poor anticoagulation compliance. Distance from hospital, cost and drug availability have all been listed as causes (see also Chapter 4.4).

CONCLUSION

Anticoagulation in children presents certain specific problems and risks. However, until prospective randomised studies of different anticoagulation levels have been conducted in children, anticoagulation with warfarin to an INR of 3.0 to 4.5 should probably be used in all children receiving mechanical cardiac prostheses.

The data to define the appropriate method or level of anticoagulation in other circumstances do not yet exist and the ground for further clinical research in this area is fertile. It may well be that an INR of 3.0 to 4.5 is too high for children with some types of mechanical valve and this must also be addressed in due course. Prosthesis-specific, or procedure-specific INR ranges must be sought, although the study design will be challenging (see Chapter 3.4).

REFERENCES

1. Stewart S, Cianciotta D, Alexson C, Manning J. The long term risk of warfarin sodium therapy and the incidence of thromboembolism in children after prosthetic cardiac valve replacement. J Thorac Cardiovasc Surg 1987; 93: 551–554.
2. Elliott MJ, de Leval MR. Valve replacement in children. World J Surg 1985; 9: 568–578.
3. Williams WG. Valve surgery in children. Can J Cardiol 1988; 4: 311–313.
4. Borman JB, Shimon DV, Deed M, Simcha A. Valve replacement in children. J Cardiac Surg 1989; 4: 260–275.
5. Almeida RS, Elliott MJ, Robinson PJ, Wyse RKH, Taylor JFN, Stark J, de Leval MR. Surgery for congenital abnormalities of the mitral valve at the Hospital for Sick Children, London from 1969–1983. J Cardiovasc Surg 1988; 29: 95–99.
6. Braunwald NS, Brais M, Castaneda A. Considerations in the development of artificial heart valve substitutes for use in infants and small children. J Thorac Cardiovasc Surg 1976; 72: 539.
7. Panel discussion. Current concepts on the use of aortic and pulmonary allografts for heart valve substitutes. In Yankah AC, Hetzer R, Miller DC, Ross DN, Somerville J, Yacoub MH (Eds.). Cardiac Valve Allografts 1962–1987. Darmstadt, Steinkopff Verlag, 1988: 371–384.
8. Chen SC, Laks H, Fagan L et al. Valve replacement in children. Circulation 1977; 56(Suppl II): 11–17.
9. Weinstein GS, Mavroudis C, Ebert PA. Preliminary experience with aspirin for anticoagulation in children with prosthetic cardiac valves. Ann Thorac Surg 1981; 102: 1022.
10. Rufilinchas JJ, Jeffe A, Miranda AL. Cardiac valve replacement with Bjørk Shiley prosthesis in young patients. Scand J Thorac Cardiovasc Surg 1977; 73: 872.
11. Pass HI, Sade RM, Crawford FA, Hohn AR. Cardiac valve prostheses in children without anticoagulation. J Thorac Cardiovac Surg 1984; 87: 832–835.
12. Verrier ED, Tranbaugh RF, Soifer SJ, Yee ES, Turley K, Ebert PA. Aspirin anticoagulation in children with mechanical aortic valves. J Thorac Cardiovasc Surg 1986; 92: 1913–1920.
13. Cornish EM, Human DG, de Moor MM, Hassoulas J, Sanchez HE, Sprenger KJ, Reichart BA. Valve replacement in children. J Thorac Cardiovasc Surg 1987; 35: 176–179.
14. Sade RM, Crawford FA Jr., Fyfe DA, Stroud MR. Valve prostheses in children: A reassessment of anticoagulation. J Thorac Cardiovac Surg 1988; 95: 553–561.
15. McGrath LB, Gonzales-Lavin L, Eldredge WI, Colombi M, Restrepo D. Thromboemboli and other events following valve replacement in a paediatric population treated with anti-platelet agents. Ann Thorac Surg 1987; 43: 285–287.
16. Sharma A, Johnson DC, Cartmill TB. Entrapment of both leaflets of St. Jude Medical aortic valve prostheses in a child. J Thorac Cardiovasc Surg 1983; 86: 453.

17. Schaffer MS, Clarke Dr, Campbell DN, Madigan CK, Wiggins JW Jr., Wolfe RR. The St. Jude Medical cardiac valve in infants and children: role of anticoagulant therapy. J Am Coll Cardiol 1987; 9: 235–239.
18. Serra AJ, McNicholas KW, Olivier HF Jr., Boe SL, Lemole GM. The choice of anticoagulation in paediatric patients with the St. Jude Medical valve prostheses. J Cardiovasc Surg 1987; 28: 588–591.
19. Rubino M, Stellin G, Mazzucco A et al. Valve replacement in children: early and late results. Thorac Cardiovasc Surg 1989; 37: 42–46.
20. Engelhardt W, Muhler E, von Bernuth G. Anticoagulation with phenprocoumon in early childhood: dosage, complications, effectiveness. Klin Padiatr 1989; 201: 21–27.
21. Rao PS, Solymar L, Mardini MK, Fawzy ME, Guinn G. Anticoagulant therapy in children with prosthetic valves. Ann Thorac Surg 1989; 47: 589–592.
22. Antunes MJ, Vanderdonck KM, Sussman MJ. Mechanical valve replacement in children and teenagers. Eur J Cardiothorac Surg 1989; 3: 222- 228.
23. Harada Y, Imai Y, Kurosawa H, Ishihara K, Kawada M, Fukuchi S. Ten year follow up after valve replacement with the St. Jude Medical prosthesis in children. J Thorac Cardiovasc Surg 1990; 100: 175–180.
24. Anon. Doubt about dipyridamole as an antithrombotic drug. Drug Therap Bull 1984; 22: 25.
25. Ilbawi MN, Idriss FS, De Leon SY et al. Valve replacement in children: guidelines for selection of prosthesis and timing of surgical intervention. Ann Thorac Surg 1987; 44: 398–403.
26. Robbins RC, Bowman FO Jr., Malm JR. Cardiac valve replacement in children: a twenty-year series. Ann Thorac Surg 1988; 45: 56–61.
27. Bradley LM, Midgley FM, Watson DC, Getson PR, Scott LP., Anticoagulation therapy in children with mechanical prosthetic cardiac valves. Am J Cardiol 1985; 56: 533–535.
28. Taybi H, Capitanio MA. Tracheobronchial calcification: an observation in three children after mitral valve replacement and warfarin sodium therapy. Radiology 1990; 176: 728–730.
29. de Vivie ER, Rushchewski W, Koveker G, Risch D, Weber H, Beuren AJ. Fontan procedure – indications and clinical results. J Thorac Cardiovasc Surg 1981; 29: 348–354.
30. Girod AD, Fontan F, Deville C, Ottenkamp J, Choussat A. Long-term results after the Fontan operation for tricuspid atresia. Circulation 1987; 75: 605–610.
31. Dobell ARC, Trusler GA, Smallhorn JF, Williams WG. Atrial thrombi after the Fontan operation. Ann Thorac Surg 1986; 42: 664–667.
32. de Leval MR, Kilner P, Gewillig M, Bull C. Total cavo-pulmonary connection: a logical alternative to atrio-pulmonary connection for complex Fontan operations. J Thorac Cardiovasc Surg 1986; 96: 682- 695.
33. Loeliger EA, Poller L, Samama M et al. Questions and answers on prothrombin time standardisation in oral anticoagulant control. Thromb Haemostas 1985; 54: 515–517.
34. BCSH Haemostasis and Thrombosis Task Force. Guidelines on oral anticoalgulation: second edition. J Clin Pathol 1990; 43: 177–183.
35. Hirsh J, Poller L, Deykin D et al. Optimal therapeutic range for oral anticoagulants. Chest 1989; 95(Suppl): 5S–11S.
36. Reye RDK, Morgan G, Baral J. Encephalopathy and fatty degeneration of the viscera: a disease entity in children. Lancet 1963; : 749- 752.
37. Giles HM. Encephalopathy and fatty degeneration of the viscera. Lancet 1965; 1: 1075.
38. Editorial. Reye's syndrome – epidemiological considerations. Lancet 1982; 1: 943–945.
39. Hurwitz ES, Barratt MJ, Bergman D et al. Public health service study of Reye's syndrome – medications. JAMA 1987; 257: 1905–1911.
40. Patrono C, Cinbattoni G, Pinca E et al. Low dose aspirin and inhibition of thromboxane B2 production in healthy subjects. Thromb Res 1980; 17: 317–327.
41. Jaklitsch M, Leyland S. Aspirin anticoagulation for mechanical heart valves and Reye's syndrome. J Thorac Cardiovasc Surg 1988; 95: 146–147.
42. Kalke BR, Desai JM, Magotra R. Mitral valve surgery in children. J Thorac Cardiovasc Surg 1989; 98: 994–998.
43. Abid F, Mzah N, el Euch F, Ben-Ismail M. Valve replacement in children under 15 years with rheumatic heart disease. Pediatr Cardiol 1989; 10: 199–204.

Chapter 4.3

Anticoagulants in the Elderly

Marc Verstraete, Raymond Verhaeghe and Philip A. Routledge

As the population of developed countries grows older, it is increasingly likely that anticoagulant therapy will be considered in a greater number of elderly patients. The potential toxicity of oral anticoagulants has been known for many years but as with other drugs, a decision to use them must be made after consideration of the risk/benefit ratio. The benefits which may be achieved from oral anticoagulants and the risks involved in their use will be considered before discussing the optimisation of the risk/benefit relationship and the role of oral anticoagulants in the treatment of thrombotic disease in the elderly.

THE BENEFITS

It is clear that the elderly are more prone to arterial, as well as venous thromboembolism, and thrombotic disease is the commonest cause of admission, disability and death in patients over 50 years of age in the developed countries. The increased risk may be related partly to an increase in clotting factor concentrations in the elderly, to an increase in platelet and clotting factor activation and to a decline in fibrinolytic activity[1]. In the case of pulmonary embolism, not only does the incidence increase with age (over 50 years) but the diagnosis is more often missed in life[2]. Non-valvular atrial fibrillation is much more common in the elderly and carries a five-fold increased risk of stroke. Any effective treatment or prophylaxis of thromboembolic disease is therefore worthy of consideration in the elderly.

There is an increasing body of evidence that oral anticoagulant therapy is effective in elderly as well as young subjects. They are commonly used in venous thromboembolism, where increasing age is a risk factor for events after surgery, and in cardiogenic embolism (eg. associated with myocardial infarction, rheumatic valvular disease, prosthetic valves and atrial fibrillation) which is commoner with increasing age. There is no evidence of decreased effectiveness of oral anticoagulants in elderly subjects with these conditions. Two recent studies of oral anticoagulation in the prevention of thromboembolic events in patients with non-valvular atrial fibrillation, have shown a reduction in events in patients from a wide age-range, for example. The Danish AFASAK study included subjects with lone atrial fibrillation who were aged between 38 and 91 years and in whom anticoagulant therapy significantly reduced thromboembolic events by 75%[3]. The Boston Area Anticoagulation Trial showed a greater than 80% reduction in stroke in an elderly population (mean age 68 years)[4]. The results of such studies are likely to encourage the increasing use of warfarin for prophylaxis of thromboembolism in the elderly (see also Chapter 1.2).

THE RISKS

Several studies have confirmed the original observation of Eccles that anticoagulant requirements decline with age[5,6,7,8]. In one study, Routledge and co-workers showed that warfarin requirements fell with increasing age so that patients aged less than 35 required more than twice as much warfarin to maintain the INR at an equivalent degree of anticoagulation than patients older than 75 (Figure 4.3–1)[7]. The correlation between age and warfarin requirements was rather weak however, indicating that other factors may be more important in determining warfarin dose than age itself. The reason for the increased sensitivity is still not fully known, although most studies indicate a pharmacodynamic sensitivity rather than any major change in the pharmacokinetics of racemic warfarin[9,10,11]. This appears also to be the case when S and R warfarin enantiomers are separately administered chronically to young and elderly individuals (Shetty, HGM – personal communication), when although steady state S and R warfarin concentrations are similar, the area under the curve for vitamin K epoxide after concomitant intravenous vitamin K_1 is greater in the elderly than in the young, indicating increased sensitivity to both enantiomers.

The most important question is whether age itself is a factor associated with an increased risk of bleeding and thus whether chronological age should be taken into account when anticoagulant therapy is being considered. There are several studies which have failed to show that age was an independent risk factor for bleeding[11–16]. The total number of patients involved in all these studies was approximately 2,000. It is

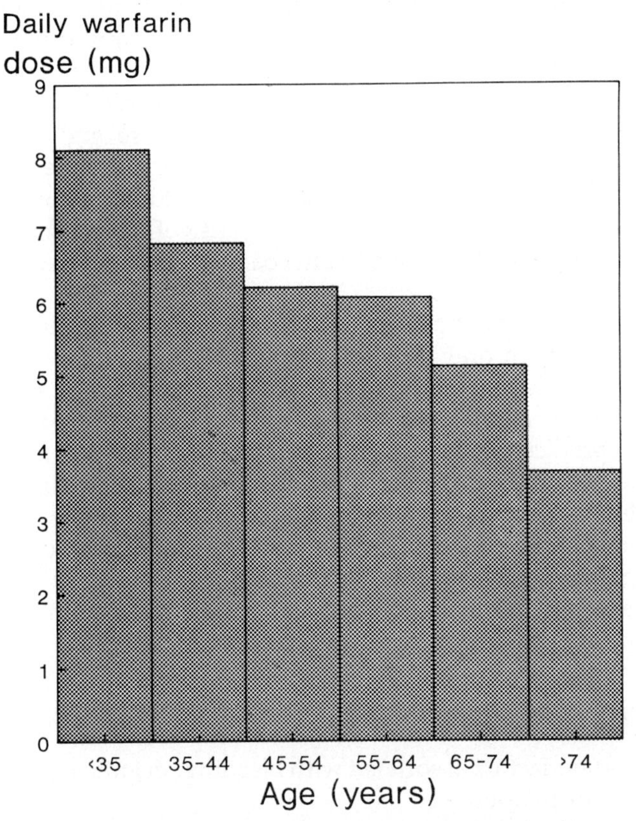

Fig. 4.3–1 Relationship between age and anticoagulant requirements in 228 subjects aged between 19 and 90 years. From the data of reference 7, with permission.

therefore unlikely that a large effect of age was missed. In the largest of these studies, (the double-blind Sixty-Plus Reinfarction Study)[11] the mean age was 67 years. Major extracranial bleeding (defined as bleeding necessitating breaking the treatment code) was observed once in 165 years at risk in the placebo group and once in 25 years in the anticoagulant group but none was fatal (28 events versus 4 events). Metastatic malignancy or other specific pathology as the source of major bleeding was found in 40% of the cases; early diagnosis of symptomatic bleeding which reveals a previously occult pathology may be looked upon as a benefit, however. Minor extracranial bleeding (mostly skin haematoma, nose bleeds or subconjunctival bleeding) occurred in the Sixty-Plus Reinfarction Study about once in nine years at risk in the anticoagulant group[11] and once in 111.5 years of observation in the control group. There was no relationship between the incidence of bleeding and the patient's age or the duration of anticoagulant therapy.

The incidence of fatal intracranial bleeding in the Sixty-Plus Reinfarction Study was 1 in 100 years of anticoagulation[11]. Intracerebral bleeding in the absence of anticoagulant therapy is closely associated with age and hypertension. In a large retrospective study utilising the centralised organisation of ambulatory long-term anticoagulant therapy in the Netherlands, Wintzen and associates concluded that the risk of intracerebral bleeding in patients over 50 years was ten times greater in those receiving anti-coagulants than in untreated individuals, irrespective of age or sex[17]. Because the two patient groups were not randomised, their comparability is limited. The groups exhibited about the same incidence of hypertension but it is not known whether the severity of the hypertension was truly comparable. The similarity among the odds ratios for all age groups in this retrospective study strongly suggests that the anticoagulant-related risk of intracerebral haemorrhage follows the trend of the natural risk, (i.e. increasing with age but at a constantly, ten-fold higher level). Whisnant and associates[18] calculated an eight-fold increase in the risk of cerebral bleeding for patients between 55 to 77 years on long-term oral anticoagulation compared to a control group of the same age range.

In one retrospective study, however, a 12% rate of major bleeding was observed in 565 patients on long-term oral anticoagulation with a cumulative risk of 22% at 48 months by life-table analysis[19,20]. In more than one-third of cases, major bleeding was fatal or life-threatening. Age over 65 years was one of the five factors known at the start of therapy which predicted independently for bleeding; the other four predictors were history of stroke, previous gastro-intestinal bleeding, atrial fibrillation and a serious comorbid condition. Intracranial bleeding accounted for seven of the 10 fatalities however and, since there was no control group, it is difficult to understand how the effects of the age-related increase in intracranial bleeding risk in non-anticoagulated subjects were allowed for in calculating the factors determining bleeding risk in patients receiving anticoagulants (see also Chapter 5.4).

REDUCING THE RISKS

The most important factors associated with bleeding on anticoagulants are:

i) Degree of anticoagulation
ii) The presence of an organic lesion, and
iii) Duration of anticoagulant therapy

i) Degree of anticoagulation

With respect to the incidence of bleeding during long-term out-patient oral anticoagulation at different intensities, the experience of the Dutch Thrombosis Service is by far the most substantial and reliable source of information[21]. In Fig. 4.3–2 the incidence of macroscopic haematuria is shown in relation to the intensity of anticoagulation. The figures of individual Thrombosis Units, indicated by the town where they are located, are retrospective data covering more than 30,000 years at risk annually; the information of the Sixty-Plus Study is provided in a prospective manner for approximately 6,000 patient-years[11]. Macro-haematuria is a form of bleeding which rarely escapes observation and is almost always reported to the doctor. Fig. 4.3–2 shows that the incidence of macro-haematuria varies between 1 per 20 and 1 per 100 years at risk, depending on the intensity of anticoagulation, and there is evidence that other bleeding episodes have a similar relationship to the degree of anticoagulation[22].

As can also be seen, the risk of bleeding appears to be *log-linearly* related to the degree of anticoagulation rather than linearly related[21,22]. Therefore it is even more important that the lowest effective level of anticoagulation should be chosen for any particular indication and the British Society of Haematology guidelines are helpful in this respect[23]. A discussion of the optimal ranges for patients with prosthetic heart valves appears in Chapter 3.4.

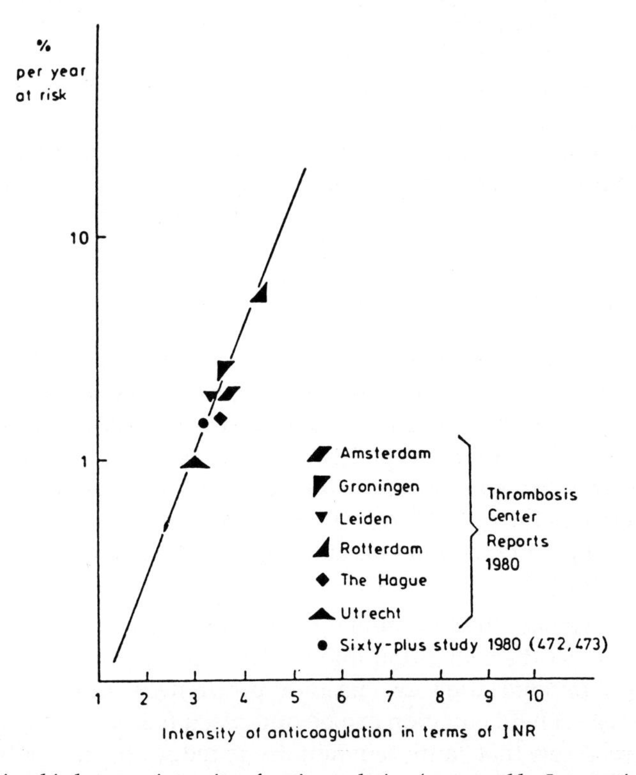

Fig. 4.3–2 Relationship between intensity of anticoagulation (expressed by International Normalised Ratio: INR) and incidence of macro-haematuria as an expression of bleeding tendency reported by several Dutch centres and by the Sixty-Plus Study. Reproduced from ref. 31 with permission.

ii) Duration of anticoagulation

The Sixty-Plus Reinfarction Study gave no indication that the risk of bleeding with long-term anticoagulant prophylaxis changed as a function of time, duration of treatment, either with respect to the period before the patient's entry to the study (six months to longer than 10 years), (mean six years) or with respect to the study period itself (two years double-blind)[217]. Nevertheless, the risk of bleeding due to anticoagulants lasts as long as the patient receives them and it is thus important to keep courses of anticoagulation as short as possible consistent with protection against risk of thromboembolism. Unfortunately, many of the conditions for which warfarin is indicated in the elderly are life-long or long-term.

iii) Presence of an organic lesion

When bleeding occurs, it is usually from an organic lesion, often in the bladder or bowel, or from an abnormal vessel (e.g. an abnormal intra-cranial vessel resulting in intracerebral haemorrhage). Fortunately the mortality from extracranial bleeding is low in most cases. Although the AFASAK study showed an increase in major bleeding, no events were fatal[3], and as has been mentioned earlier, such events may result in the discovery of potentially remediable lesions at an earlier stage than would have otherwise occurred. Certainly all patients who bleed should be investigated for underlying pathology, even if the bleeding episode occurred when the INR was excessive. This includes patients with macro-haematuria. The mortality from intracranial bleeding is high (> 60% of incidents), but the observation of Landefeld and Goldman that the incidence of such events is related to the degree of anticoagulation at discharge suggests that careful and conservative control in elderly patients may reduce the risk[19,20].

CONCLUSIONS

It has been suggested that warfarin is a potentially lethal drug and that old people are not good at taking drugs reliably or accurately[24]. However a study of compliance (using small doses of phenobarbitone added to warfarin tablets) showed no decline in compliance in elderly ambulant patients[25], and as long as mental function is unimpaired, elderly subjects appear to be reliable takers of warfarin. Indeed, the Steering Committee of the recent Stroke Prevention in Atrial Fibrillation (SPAF) Study abandoned the ineligibility criterion for anticoagulant therapy of "age > 75 years" half way through the study[26].

Although anticoagulant therapy should not be undertaken lightly in any patient, the evidence is against Scott's contention that "in the elderly, the risks usually outweigh the benefits"[27]. Provided they are used appropriately and carefully with good monitoring the risk-benefit equation can be optimised (see also Chapters 3.4 and 5.4), supporting Lowe's view that "anticoagulant drugs reduce the morbidity and mortality from venous and arterial thrombotic disease especially in older patients who have the highest risk; and that these benefits are not offset by an increased risk of bleeding due to the anticoagulant therapy"[28].

REFERENCES

1. Dodds WJ, Moynihan AC, Benson RE and Hall CA (1975). The value of age- and sex-matched controls for coagulation studies. J Haematol 29:305–317.
2. Mangion DM. Pulmonary embolism – incidence and prognosis in hospitalised elderly. Postgrad Med J 1989;65:814–817.
3. Petersen P, Godtfredsen J, Boysen G, Andersen ED and Andersen B. Placebo-controlled, randomised trial of warfarin and aspirin for prevention of thromboembolic complications in chronic atrial fibrillation. Lancet 1989;1:175–179.
4. The Boston Area Anticoagulation Trial for Atrial Fibrillation Investigators (1990). The effect of low-dose warfarin on the risk of stroke in patients with non-rheumatic atrial fibrillation. New Engl J Med 323:1505–1516.
5. Eccles JT. Control of warfarin therapy in the elderly. Age and Ageing 1975;4:161–165.
6. O'Malley K, Stevenson IH, Ward CA, Wood AJJ and Crooks J (1977). Determinants of anticoagulant control in patients receiving warfarin, Br J Clin Pharmac 4:309–314.
7. Routledge PA, Chapman PH, Davies DM and Rawlins MD (1979). Factors affecting warfarin requirements. Eur J Clin Pharmacol 15:319–322.
8. Redwood M, Taylor C, Bain BJ and Matthews JH (1991). The association of age with dosage requirement for warfarin. Age and Ageing 20:217–220.
9. Shepherd AMM, Hewick DS, Moreland TA and Stevenson IH (1977). Age as a determinant of sensitivity to warfarin. Br J Clin Pharmac 4:315–320.
10. Routledge P A, Chapman P H, Davies D M, Rawlins M D (1979). Pharmacokinetics and pharmacodynamics of warfarin at steady state. Br J Clin Pharmacol 8:243–247.
11. Sixty-Plus Reinfarction Study Research Group, Second Report (1982). Risk of 37 long-term anticoagulant therapy in elderly patients after myocardial infarction. Lancet i:64–68.
12. Forfar J C (1979). A 7-year analysis of haemorrhage in patients on long-term anticoagulant treatment. Br Heart J 42:128–132.
13. Gurwitz J H, Goldberg R J, Holden A, Knapic N and Ansell J (1988). Age-related risks of long-term oral anticoagulant therapy. Arch Intern Med 148:1733–1736.
14. Pett G W, Lennihan L, Mohr J P, Mausser W A, Weitz J et al (1988). Complications of long-term anticoagulation. Ann Neurol 23:570–574.
15. Joglekar M, Mohanaruban K, Bayer A J and Pathy M S J (1988). Can old people on oral anticoagulants be safely managed as out-patients? Postgrad Med J 64:775–777.
16. Wickramasinghe L S P, Basu S K and Bansal S K (1988). Long-term oral anticoagulant therapy in elderly patients. Age and Ageing 17:388–396.
17. Wintzen A R, De Jonge H, Loeliger and Bots T Th A M (1984). The risk of intracerebral haemorrhage during oral anticoagulant treatment: a population study. Ann Neurol 16:553–558.
18. Whisnant J P, Cartlidge N E F and Elveback L R (1978). Carotid and vertebral-basilar transient ischemic attacks: effect of anticoagulants, hypertension and cardiac disorders on survival and stroke occurrence – a population study. Ann Neurol 3:107–115.
19. Landefeld C S and Goldman L (1989). Major bleeding in outpatients treated with warfarin: incidence and prediction by factors known at the start of outpatient therapy. Am J Med 87:144–152.
20. Landefeld C S and Rosenblatt M V (1989). Bleeding in outpatients treated with warfarin: relation to the prothrombin time and important remediable lesions. Am J Med 87:153–159.
21. Loeliger E A and Broekmans A W (1988). Drug affecting blood clotting, fibrinolysis and hemostasis. In: Meyler's Side Effects of Drugs. Ed: Dukes M N G. Elsevier Science Publishers, Amsterdam, 733–775.
22. Loeliger E A, Van Dijk-Wierfda C A, Van Den Besselaar A M H P, Brockmans A W and Roos J (1984). Anticoagulant control and the risk of bleeding. In: Anticoagulants and Myocardial Infarction: A Reappraisal. Ed: Meade T W. London, John Wiley and Sons 135–137.
23. British Society for Haematology, British Committee for Standards in Haematology. Haemostasis and Thrombosis Task Force (1990). Guidelines on oral anticoagulation. 2nd edition. J Clin Pathol 43:177–183.
24. Rubin P (1988). Controversies in therapeutics. Br Med J 297:1260.
25. Kumar s, Peakers, Davies J A, Roberts B E and Feely M. Increased response to warfarin with age. Clinical Science 1989; 77:11–12.
26. Stroke Prevention in Atrial Fibrillation Investigators (1991). Stroke prevention atrial fibrillation study: final results. Circulation 84:527–539.
27. Scott P J W (1988). Anticoagulant drugs in the elderly: the risks usually outweigh the benefits. Br Med J 297:1261–1263.
28. Lowe G D O (1988). Anticoagulant drugs in the elderly: valuable in selected patients. Br Med J 197:1260–1262.

Chapter 4.4

Anticoagulation in Developing Countries

M. A. Williams

Valve replacement policy in the first world has evolved gradually over the last 30 years in response to the development of replacement devices. The early models were found to have a high incidence of thromboembolism[1]. Although subsequently modified by the use of anticoagulants[2], thrombosis and embolism have remained major problems, and the main thrust of development has been directed at lowering the incidence of these often catastrophic complications.

In the early sixties the aortic homograft was introduced[3,4]. This valve virtually eliminated the problem of valve-related thromboembolism[5] but the logistics of collection and sterilisation have restricted its use. In the early seventies the glutaraldehyde preserved porcine valve was made available commercially and was found to have a low incidence of thromboembolism without the need for anticoagulation. However, the initial enthusiasm waned when it became obvious that the valve was subject to degeneration, especially calcification in young patients, the very group in which its main application lay[6,7,8].

Further development of mechanical valves using new design concepts and materials has resulted in the presently available single and bileaflet valves that have a low incidence of thromboembolism provided that the patient is properly anticoagulated. Many surgeons practising in sophisticated communities currently insert mechanical valves in all patients, except women wishing to have children and the elderly, porcine valve degeneration being rare in patients over the age of 70[9]. This chapter will examine those factors in developing communities that make this policy difficult to apply and will suggest strategies aimed at diminishing the incidence of thromboembolism in a group of patients in whom the control of anticoagulation is difficult and often impossible.

VALVE REPLACEMENT IN DEVELOPING COUNTRIES

The undeveloped and developing countries of Asia, Africa and Latin America, not politically aligned with communist or western nations, are generally grouped together as the 'third world'. In the majority of countries with third world populations, limited resources make open heart surgery impossible and only those with a significant wealthy component are able to afford such treatment. The Ivory Coast and the Republic of South Africa are the only countries in subsaharan Africa where open heart surgery is carried out regularly[10]. The population of South Africa is ethnically complex and most of its population of 40 million are socio-economically poorly developed. There is, however, a large first world population and open heart surgery is practised at 20 institutions in six major cities. At these centres open heart surgery is available to all sectors of the population, and surgeons practising cardiac surgery have an almost unique opportunity to assess the impact of first world technology on a third world community.

In the field of valve replacement surgery, the opportunity exists to compare valve performance in different population groups. Since durability and the incidence of thromboembolism are the most important determinants of valve function, measurements of these parameters will determine the choice of a device. However, it must be remembered that the very factors which result in a population belonging to a third world community make the results very difficult to assess. Poor people are unable to travel long distances to follow-up clinics; an unsophisticated patient who is in good clinical condition after valve replacement does not understand the need to attend a clinic, nor does he understand the need to take anticoagulants, since the taking of such medication makes no apparent difference to his health. If he takes anticoagulants at all, he is likely to take them erratically. Minor thromboembolic phenomena, such as transient cerebral ischaemic episodes, are hardly ever reported and only major haemorrhages will be recorded. As a result, the true incidences of valve thrombosis, embolism and bleeding are unknown. Postmortem examinations are seldom secured and the causes of death are often conjectural.

Compared to the virtual avalanche of reports relating to valve replacement in the first world, reports from developing countries are relatively rare and often flawed by inaccurate data collection and poor follow up. In units where great efforts have been made to trace patients, a loss to follow up of between 13% and 25% has been documented[11,12]. From this is will be understood that the choice of a replacement device is not simple and the various cardiac units in South Africa have adopted different approaches at various times, as follows:

- Mechanical valves are used in all patients without anticoagulation[13].
- Mechanical valves are used in most patients and an attempt is made to anticoagulate everybody[14].
- Tissue valves are used in most patients[12].
- Tissue valves are used in older patients and mechanical valves in the young[15].

EXPERIENCE IN PORT ELIZABETH.

The cardiac unit in Port Elizabeth is situated on the Eastern seaboard of South Africa and serves an estimated population of one and a half million. When the unit was established, it was accepted that anticoagulation would be difficult to control in the third world section of the population. A broad policy of inserting porcine valves in adults was adopted, restricting the use of mechanical valves to children and adolescents. However, this policy was not strictly adhered to and a new generation tissue valve (Intact) that was claimed to resist calcification was inserted in a small number of young patients. In some older patients mechanical valves were inserted when it was judged that a porcine valve would be unacceptably stenotic.

Between 1983 and 1988 315 valves were implanted in 285 patients[15]. A variety of porcine valves was inserted in 184 patients and the Medtronic Hall valve in 101 patients. Follow up is 97% complete, which is unusual in a third world community. Good follow-up information has been achieved by several means. During the patient's stay in hospital the importance of regular attendance at follow-up clinics is repeatedly stressed and detailed information on all relatives, friends and employers is collected.

This data is updated at the follow-up clinics. Financial assistance is made available to patients who are unable to afford travelling expenses. A determined effort is made to contact any patient who has not appeared within a month of a missed appointment. Such patients are invariably found and this is due entirely to the unusual enthusiasm, tenacity and often highly imaginative detective techniques of the research workers responsible for the follow-up of patients.

Anticoagulation was attempted in all patients in whom mechanical valves were implanted and in those with porcine valves who were in chronic atrial fibrillation. Although nearly half of the patients receiving mechanical valves were given anticoagulants, only 12% were regarded as being satisfactorily anticoagulated. Anticoagulation was successful in only 15 of the 55 patients in the tissue valve group in whom it was attempted. The results are summarised in Tables 4.4–1 and 4.4–2.

Porcine valves have performed satisfactorily in the older patients; 94% are predicted to be free from valve related complications at six years (Fig. 4.4–1). This is comparable to series reported in first world populations[16,17]. In the small group of young patients in whom the Intact porcine bioprosthesis was used, the antimineralisation treatment was found to be ineffective and at four years only 11 of 26 recipients were clinically well with the original valve, demonstrating once more the unsuitability of tissue valves in young patients. If this group is included in the statistics with the adults, the freedom from valve related complications at six years drops to 79% (Fig. 4.4–1). The incidence of embolism has been 0.43% per patient year. It is accepted that the price to be paid for this low incidence is that most patients will require reoperation for valve degeneration and some may well undergo a number of reoperations. We regard this as preferable to the high rate of thrombotic complications when mechanical valves are used.

Experience from the third world, in large series with predominantly adult patients, shows a high incidence of valve thrombosis and systemic embolism. Kinsley and co-authors[13] reported an incidence of 6.8% per patient year in a group of patients in whom the Medtronic Hall valve was inserted. Stevens [14] reported an incidence of 13%

Table 4.4–1
Results of Valve Replacement Surgery

*Porcine Valves**		*Medtronic Hall Valves*	
MVR	133	MVR	63
AVR	36	AVR	23
DVR	15	DVR	15
	184		101
Hospital mortality – 3.2%		Hospital mortality – 3%	
6 year actuarial survival – 82±4.8%		6 year actuarial survival – 88±4.3%	
Cumulative follow up – 465 patient years		Cumulative follow up – 301 patient years	

MVR = Mitral valve replacement.
AVR = Aortic valve replacement.
DVR = Double valve replacement.
* 144 Intact valves, 27 Hancock valves and 13 Bioimplant valves
Reproduced from Williams et al[15] with permission.

Table 4.4–2
Thromboembolic Complications

	Porcine valves		*Medtronic Hall valves*	
	number	*%/pty*	*number*	*%/pty*
Emboli	2 (1)	0.43	2 (1)	0.65
Anticoagulant haemorrhage	2 (1)	0.43	2 (1)	0.65
Valve occlusion	0		3 (2)	1.0
	4 (2)	0.86	7 (4)	2.3

The figures in brackets represent deaths.
Reproduced from Williams et al[15] with permission

per patient year in a similar cohort with St. Jude valves. We feel that these rates are prohibitive and lend weight to our approach of using tissue valves in the adult population.

Mitral valve repair has been found to be unsatisfactory in the young[18,19] and since tissue valves are clearly unsuitable, there is currently no alternative to using mechanical valves in this group of patients. We elected to use the Medtronic Hall valve because we anticipated that the improved haemodynamics arising from its unique engineering[20] would result in a low incidence of thrombosis and embolism. Although

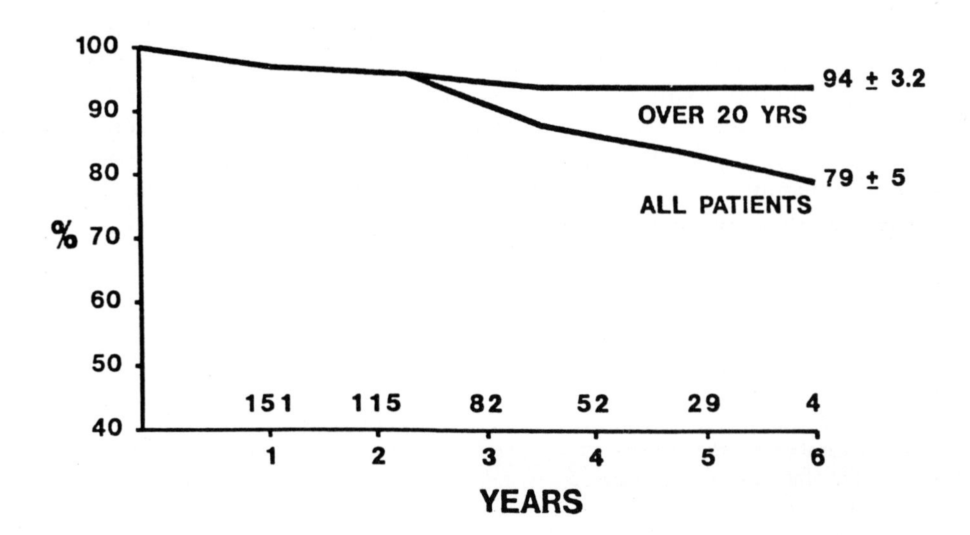

Figure 4.4–1: Porcine valves. Actuarial freedom from valve related complications. Reproduced from Williams et al[15] with permission.

only 12% of our patients were adequately anticoagulated, the incidence of embolism with this prosthesis was only 0.65% per patient year, which accords with the results of others[21,22]. However, the incidence of valve thrombosis was 1% per patient year.

Embolism and valve thrombosis are different pathological processes and should be separated when discussing thrombotic complications (Chapter 2.4). In those patients in whom valve occlusion occurred, valve thrombosis was the final event and was precipitated by the ingrowth of pannus, producing valve malfunction. The 1% per patient year incidence is almost identical to that in another group of third world patients receiving the Medtronic Hall valve (1.06%) reported by Deviri and associates[23]. The same group reported an incidence of 1.96% per patient year when the St. Jude valve was implanted. Pass and co-authors[24] reported a group of 34 children undergoing valve replacement with the St. Jude valve without anticoagulation. No thromboembolic phenomena were recorded, but the follow-up period was very short (1 – 50 months). In a series of 134 children reported from New Delhi by Iyer and associates[25], the Bjørk-Shiley valve was used and all patients were anticoagulated, a considerable feat in a third world population. In this series only one non-fatal thromboembolic episode and one anticoagulant-related haemorrhage were reported. This experience and that of our own suggest that valve thrombosis and embolism in young patients is less common than in the elderly, whether or not the patient is anticoagulated (see also Chapter 4.2). The reasons for this are conjectural but are probably related to three contributing factors; (a) most patients are in sinus rhythm, (b) most hearts return to normal size following valve replacement and (c) the greater physical activity results in a higher cardiac index with blood crossing the valve at a higher velocity, producing a greater washing effect.

Pregnancy

There were 18 pregnancies in this series (Table 4.4–3). In the porcine group all six pregnancies were successful, as were nine of twelve pregnancies in the Medtronic Hall group. None of the anticoagulated patients received heparin in the first and third trimesters. Vallejo and co-authors[26] recorded nine pregnancies in seven anticoagulated patients with no foetal wastage and no maternal deaths, although one patient required urgent surgery for a clotted valve at the time of delivery. Deviri and co-authors[27] reviewed the literature and found that the lowest thrombotic rate and the lowest incidence of spontaneous abortion occurred in those patients in whom anticoagulants

Table 4.4–3
Pregnancy and Valve Replacement

	Porcine Valves	Medtronic Hall Valves
Number of pregnancies	6	12
Satisfactorily anticoagulated	2	2
Abortions	0	3
Normal birth	6	9
Thromboemboli	0	0
Maternal mortality	0	0

were not used. In a later report[28] they recorded nine pregnancies in patients with mechanical valves with only two normal births, and compared this with 15 pregnancies in patients with bioprostheses not receiving warfarin resulting in nine normal births. They concluded that tissue valves should be inserted in patients wanting to have children. However, the appalling results associated with tissue valves in the young should contraindicate this approach in patients younger than 20 years. All of our patients with mechanical valves in whom pregnancy occurred were less than 20 years of age. The absence of thromboembolic phenomena in this group is probably related to the factors already discussed. It would also appear from these data that the hazards of pregnancy in young patients with mechanical valves may have been exaggerated (see also Chapter 4.1).

Summary and recommendations

One of the major concerns of the cardiac surgeon working in the third world is the control of anticoagulation. To diminish the incidence of thrombosis, embolism and anticoagulant-related bleeding to an acceptable level, the use of anticoagulants has been minimised by using tissue valves in as many patients as possible and a policy of using tissues valves in older patients and mechanical valves in children and young adults has evolved. This strategy has eliminated entirely the hazards of anticoagulation in a large number of patients.

Nevertheless, there remains a group with mechanical valves and a further group with tissue valves in chronic atrial fibrillation where anticoagulation is mandatory. Long-term anticoagulation has been attemped in such cases, but on many occasions this therapy was abandoned either because the patient did not take the tablets or took them erratically producing wide and often alarming variations in the INR. Where consistent anticoagulation has been possible, an INR in the range of 1.5 to 2.5 has been recommended. This low level of anticoagulation was deliberately selected to mitigate the risk of haemorrhage (see Chapter 3.4).

Antiplatelet drugs have not been prescribed in our population, on the basis that non-compliant patients who will not take anticoagulants will not take these agents either. The series reported from Saudi Arabia by Solymar and associates[29] suggests that, with some prostheses, antiplatelet agents can be as effective as anticoagulants in controlling embolism in children and should be considered as an alternative, thus eliminating the hazard of bleeding. However, although antiplatelet therapy may well be capable of diminishing embolic complications with some prostheses in young patients, it may not provide adequate protection against valve thrombosis[30].

In our series, all of the thrombosed valves were related to pannus ingrowth. This was noted as a common cause of valve thrombosis in the series reported by Deviri and associates[23] in a similar population group. This phenomenon of aggressive pannus ingrowth may be related to ethnic factors. Other ethnic factors may also contribute to the low incidence of thrombosis and embolism (see Chapter 2.4).

REFERENCES

1. Starr A, Edwards ML. Mitral replacement: Clinical experience with ball valve prosthesis. Ann Surg 1961;154:726–740.
2. Starr A, Herr RH, Wood JA. Mitral replacement: review of 6 years' experience. J Thorac Cardiovasc Surg 1967;54:333–358.

3. Barratt-Boyes BG. Homograft aortic valve replacement in aortic incompetence and stenosis. Thorax 1964;19:131–150.
4. Ross DN. Homograft replacement of the aortic valve. Lancet 1962;2:487.
5. Barratt-Boyes BG. Long-term follow up of patients receiving a free-hand antibiotic sterilized homograft aortic valve. In Rabago G & Cooley DA (Eds.). Heart Valve Replacement and Future Trends in Cardiac Surgery. Mount Kisco, NY, Futura Publishing, 1987;167–179.
6. Antunes MJ, Santos LP. Performance of gluteraldehyde preserved bioprosthesis as a mitral valve substitute in a young population group. Ann Thorac Surg 1984;37:387–392.
7. Williams MA. The Intact bioprosthesis – early results. J Cardiac Surg 1988;3(Suppl):347–351.
8. Thaneroyen FT, Whitton ID, Pirie D, Rogers MA, Mitha AS. Severe calcification of gluteraldehyde preserved porcine xenografts in children. Am J Cardiol 1980;45:690–696.
9 Jamesion WRE, Rosado LJ, Munro AL et al. Carpentier-Edwards porcine bioprosthesis – primary tissue failure (structural valve deterioration) by age groups. Ann Thorac Surg 1988;46:155–162.
10. Bertrand E. Cardiovascular diseases in Abidjan, Ivory Coast. Cardiovasc J South Africa 1990;1:208–210.
11. Antunes MS, Wessels A, Sadowski RG, et al. Medtronic-Hall valve replacement in a third world population group: a review of the performance of 1000 prostheses. J Thorac Cardiovasc Surg 1988;95:980–993.
12. Odell JA, Mitha AS, Vanker A, Whitton ID. Experience with tissue and mechanical valves in the pediatric age group. In Rabago G and Cooley DA (Eds.). Heart Valve Replacement and Future Trends in Cardiac Surgery. Mount Kisco, NY, Futura Publishing, 1987;185–208.
13. Kinsley RH, Colsen PR, Antunes MJ. Medtronic Hall valve replacement in a third world population group. Thorac Cardiovasc Surg 1983;31(Suppl II):69–72.
14. Stevens JE. The Cape Town experience with the St. Jude prosthetic valve. Abstract. XIIIth Southern Africa Cardiac Congress, 6–8th September, 1982.
15. Williams MA, Bosman AR, Crause LA, Spilkin SP. The selection of a satisfactory prosthesis for valve replacement in a third world community. In Bodnar E (Ed.). Surgery for Heart Valve Disease. London, ICR Publishers, 1990;244–248.
16. Jamieson WRE, Gerein AN, Tyers GFO et al. Carpentier-Edwards supra-annular porcine bioprosthesis: clinical experience and implantation characteristics. J Thorac Cardiovasc Surg 1986;91:555–565.
17. Gallucci V, Mazzucco A, Bortolotti U, et al. The standard Hancock porcine bioprosthesis: overall experience at the University of Padova. J Cardiac Surg 1988;3(Suppl):337–345.
18. Essop R, Tweedie G, Chun R, Middlemost S, Sareli P. Surgical results in active rheumatic carditis: comparison of mitral valve repair versus replacement. Abstract. International Symposium on Surgery for Heart Valve Disease. Westminster, London, 12–16 June 1989.
19. Antunes MJ, Kinsley RH. Mitral valve annuloplasty: results in an undeveloped population. Thorax 1983;38:730–736.
20. Hall KV, Kaster RL, Woien A. An improved pivotal disc-type prosthetic heart valve. J Oslo City Hosp 1979;29:3–21.
21. Hall KV, Nitter-Hauger S, Abdelnoor M. Seven and one half years' experience with the Medtronic Hall valve. J Am Coll Cardiol 1985;6:1417–1421.
22. Beaudet RL, Poirier NL, Doyle D, Nakhle G, Gauvin C. The Medtronic Hall valve: 7 years' clinical experience. Ann Thorac Surg 1986;42:644–650.
23. Deviri E, Sareli P, Wisenbaugh T, Cronje SL. Obstruction of mechanical heart valve prostheses: clinical aspects and surgical management. J Am Coll Cardiol. 1991;17:646–650.
24. Pass HI, Sade RM, Crawford FA, Hohn AR. Cardiac valve prostheses in children without anticagulation. J Thorac Cardiovasc Surg 1984;87:832–835.
25. Iyer RS, Reddy KS, Rao IM, Venugopal P, Bhatia ML, Gopinath N. Valve replacement in children under twenty years of age. J Thorac Cardiovasc Surg 1984;88:217–224.
26. Vallejo JL, Gonzales-Santos JM, Albertos J, et al. Eight year experience with the Medtronic Hall valve prosthesis. Ann Thorac Surg 1990;50:429–436.
27. Deviri E, Levinsky L, Yechezkel M, Levy MJ. Pregnancy after valve replacement with porcine xenograft prosthesis. Surg Gynecol Obstet 1985;160:437–443.
28. Deviri E, Levinsky L, Schachner A, Nili M, Levy MJ. Thromboembolism and anticoagulant treatment in patients with heart valve prostheses. In Rabago G & Cooley DA (Eds.). Heart Valve Replacement and Future Trends in Cardiac Surgery. Mount Kisco, NY, Futura Publishing, 1987;285–296.
29. Solymar L, Rao PS, Fawzy E, Galal O, Wilson N, Guinn G. Late results of aortic valve replacement using the Smeloff valve in children and adolescents. In: Bodnar E (Ed.). Surgery for Heart Valve Disease. ICR Publishers, London, 1990;582–589.
30. Ribeiro PA, Al Zaibag M, Idris M et al. Antiplatelet drugs and the incidence of thromboembolic complications of the St. Jude Medical aortic prosthesis in patients with rheumatic heart disease. J Thorac Cardiovasc Surg 1986;91:92–98.

Chapter 4.5

Anticoagulation During Non-Cardiac Surgical Operations in Patients with Prosthetic Valves

Mark H. Eckman

This chapter is written from a perspective of clinical decision analysis and presents a logical, objective and provocative account of this type of approach to clinical problem solving as applied to patients with mechanical prosthetic heart valves about to undergo other forms of surgery. It represents an American viewpoint, based on cost-effectiveness analysis of various forms of treatment at current US costs and on the risk of anticoagulant-related haemorrhage in patients anticoagulated at the relatively high intensities used for many years in the USA (INR 5.0 – 10.0, see Chapters 3.3, 3.4 and 5.4). It makes the assumption, with which many surgeons would disagree, that the best course of action preoperatively is to discontinue warfarin and switch to intravenous heparin. In countries where lower intensities of anticoagulation are used, many non-cardiac surgeons perform minor and intermediate operations without discontinuing warfarin at all, simply maintaining the INR in the range 2.0 to 2.5. Most surgeons find that an INR in this range has a barely discernible effect on surgical bleeding. For postoperative patients unable to take warfarin orally, for example after gastrointestinal surgery, it should not be forgotten that warfarin can be given intravenously, using exactly the same dose as the oral preparation (see Chapter 3.2). (Editors' comment)

From a cost-effectiveness perspective, decisions regarding the management of anticoagulation in patients with prosthetic heart valves undergoing non-cardiac surgery must consider the trade-off between the risks of thromboembolism if anticoagulation is stopped and the cost of prevention. As the rate of embolic events is quite low, in the order of 10^{-4} per day, and the period of increased risk is very short, one might anticipate that the cost of preventing these rare events would be great.

Having discontinued warfarin, should we admit such patients prior to planned surgery for treatment with intravenous heparin, awaiting a normal prothrombin time; if so, for how many days? What should we do postoperatively? Should we again heparinise them, as inpatients, until they are adequately anticoagulated with oral agents? While numerous opinions exist, many authors in the USA recommend the discontinuation of oral anticoagulants from one to five days before surgery, with reinstitution as soon as the patient is able to take oral medications postoperatively[1–6]. During the preoperative and postoperative periods of increased risk, while the patient is not receiving oral anticoagulant therapy, infusions of heparin are recommended to maintain adequate anticoagulation[7].

There are many diverse approaches. At one extreme, the patient is admitted shortly after discontinuing warfarin, to start an intravenous infusion of heparin. Shortly before surgery, generally the fourth hospital day, the heparin infusion is discontinued and then restarted postoperatively as soon as possible. Warfarin is also restarted when the patient can take medications by mouth. The patient is then kept in the hospital, receiving heparin until the prothrombin time is once more in the therapeutic range. For a minor surgical procedure, such as an excisional breast biopsy or a polypectomy, this will require prolonging the hospital stay.

At the other extreme, a minimalist strategy consists of discontinuing warfarin on an out-patient basis, bringing the patient into the hospital the morning of surgery, and restarting warfarin as the sole anticoagulant in the postoperative period as soon as feasible. In this case, the hospitalisation is not prolonged by waiting for a therapeutic prothrombin time.

Another strategy is to have a visiting nurse administer subcutaneous heparin postoperatively on an out-patient basis while the patient is concurrently taking warfarin over the period during which the prothrombin time is returning to the therapeutic range.

Clinicians must consider the trade-off between the financial costs and inconvenience of lengthening the hospitalisation beyond that necessitated by the surgical procedure and the risks of thromboembolic events while oral anticoagulants are discontinued. Decision analysis can be used to examine the cost/effectiveness of such strategies for managing anticoagulation during the perioperative period in patients with prosthetic valves undergoing non-cardiac surgery. In a previously developed model we considered the marginal cost/effectiveness of additional days of preoperative hospitalisation and additional days of postoperative hospitalisation for the administration of heparin therapy[8].

The central issues in both preoperative and postoperative strategies are: (1) how long is the hospitalisation prolonged solely for the administration of intravenous heparin and (2) how many days of heparin therapy does the patient receive? All strategies consider the same adverse events. These consist of (1) embolism and its complications, death, major morbidity, or resolution with minor morbidity, (2) prosthetic valve thrombosis leading to either survival or death and (3) haemorrhage with its attendant complications of death, major morbidity, or resolution.

DECISION ANALYSIS

The process of clinical decision analysis[9–11] involves seven steps. First, the clinical question is framed in an explicit and concise manner. Second, the alternative decisions (choices) and their consequences (chance events) are explicitly structured in a decision model, often represented as a decision tree. Third, the probability of each event is determined. Fourth, all outcomes are assigned a value (utility) on a consistent scale. Fifth, the tree is evaluated by folding back and averaging out the value of each outcome weighted by the likelihood of its occurrence. The strategy with the greatest expected or average utility is selected as the best. Sixth, sensitivity analyses are performed on each of the parameters in the decision tree. Seventh, the results are interpreted.

Assumptions

In formulating our model we made several assumptions. First, we described changes in the efficacy of anticoagulation as a simple process in which the probability of embolism and valve thrombosis rises (or falls) linearly as a function of time during which warfarin is being discontinued (or restarted).

Second, we assumed that it takes three days from the time warfarin is discontinued for the prothrombin time to return to normal and that once restarted, it takes another 3 days for the prothrombin time to return to the therapeutic range.

Third, we assumed that the patient would be able to resume oral medications on the day after surgery.

The probability of thromboembolic complications varies greatly depending upon the location and type of valve. The likelihood of such events is greater in patients with prosthetic valves in the mitral position than in those with aortic valves. While some investigators feel that the adequacy of anticoagulation is the most important factor affecting the rate of thromboembolic complications, overshadowing the importance of other phenomena, such as atrial fibrillation and left atrial thrombus[12], others have found a history of previous emboli[3], thrombus in the left atrium[14], atrial fibrillation[15,16], and operation before the mid–1970s[17] to be independent risk factors for thromboembolic events (see also Chapters 1.3, 2.4 and 3.4). On a daily basis, the likelihood of such events is quite small for any valve, all being in the order of 10^{-4}. The probability of death from embolism varies from a low of zero to as high as 0.28. Consequently, the marginal cost/effectiveness of additional days of hospitalisation varies from patient to patient, depending upon the location and type of valve, the presence of atrial fibrillation, a history of previous embolic events, the patient's age, co-morbid disease processes, and the nature of the surgical procedure under consideration.

The following two cases demonstrate some of this variability:

Case 1. On routine mammography a 64-year-old woman was found to have developed new microcalcifications in her left breast. Her past medical history included a mitral valve replacement with a Bjørk-Shiley standard valve for rheumatic heart disease six years previously. Her course had already been complicated by supraventricular tachycardias (other than atrial fibrillation), pulmonary oedema, congestive heart failure, and a craniotomy for a subdural haematoma while receiving oral anticoagulant therapy. Echocardiographic examination did not reveal left atrial thrombus. She had no history of previous embolic events. Because the microcalcifications could be markers for malignancy, an excisional breast biopsy was planned.

Case 2. A 75-year-old woman complaining of recurrent right upper quadrant abdominal pain with radiation to her back, nausea, and vomiting was found to have multiple gallstones and a thickened gallbladder wall on a right upper quadrant ultrasound. Her past medical history was unremarkable except for a St. Jude aortic valve replacement. She had been receiving anticoagulation therapy with warfarin since the valve replacement eight years previously and had suffered no complications. An elective cholecystectomy was planned.

Decision tree

The decision tree depicted in Figure 4.5–1 begins at the left margin with a square decision node having four alternative strategies, each entailing an additional day of hospitalisation from zero to three. These may refer to either preoperative or postoperative days. The curly brace signifies subtree notation, indicating that the same tree structure applies to all of the strategies although the probabilities and utilities for each of the strategies may be different. The first circular chance node represents the possibility that the patient may experience an embolic event, valve thrombosis, or neither. Following the topmost branch, an embolic event may result in death,

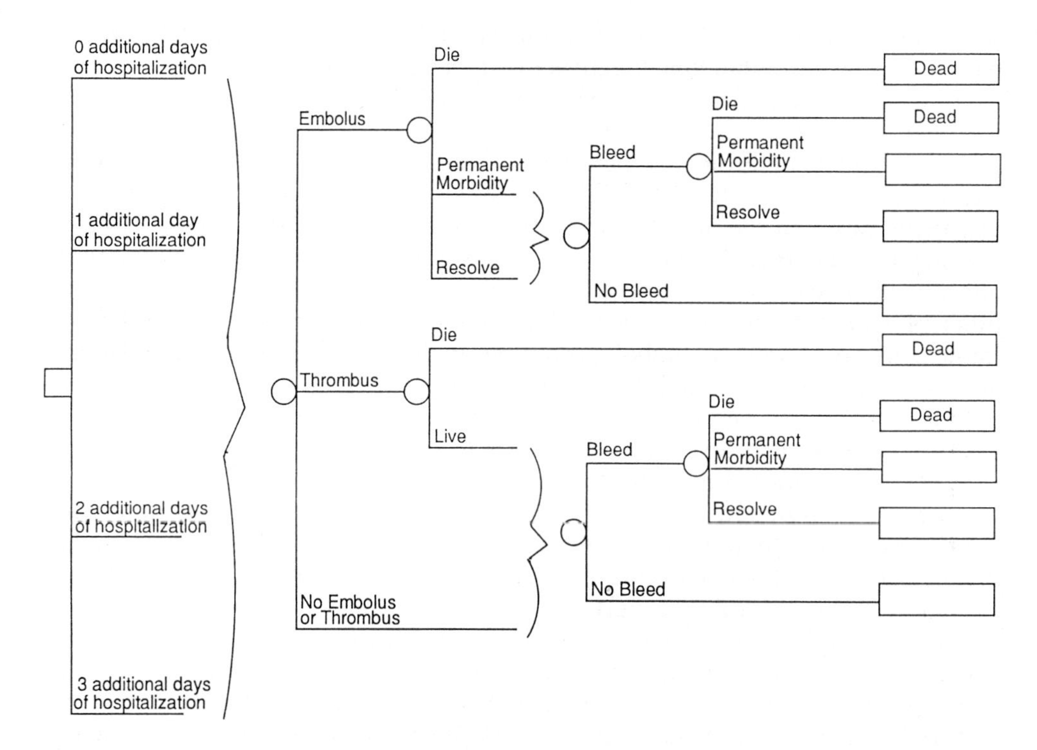

Figure 4.5–1

permanent morbidity or may resolve without any permanent deficits. Similarly for the middle branch, valve thrombosis may result in death or the patient may survive. If the patient survives or does not experience a complication, he/she may then develop a bleeding complication from heparin therapy as depicted in the remaining subtree. The haemorrhagic event may result in death, permanent morbidity, or resolve without any permanent residual effects. The rectangles at the end of each branch are terminal nodes and reflect the value of the respective outcomes. As our decision only relates to the perioperative management of anticoagulation therapy, we have not modelled any events specific to the surgical procedures planned.

Probabilities

Thromboembolic complications in patients receiving anticoagulant therapy

We performed an extensive review of the literature to obtain data for thromboembolic events and valve thrombosis in patients with a wide variety of prosthetic heart valves. Studies were rejected from the analysis for a variety of reasons. These included failure to state the total duration of patient follow-up, that is patient-years or patient-months, failure to present complete results on the basis of valve position whether aortic or mitral, failure to stratify results on the basis of anticoagulation status, in other words, receiving warfarin, antiplatelet therapy, or nothing, and failure to report valve thrombosis separate from other thromboembolic events. Using weighted averages from a series of studies, we calculated the daily probability of such events in

Table 4.5–1
Thromboembolic Complications of Prosthetic Valves

		Incidence of Thromboemboli per 100 Patient-Years			
		Emboli Patients Receiving Anticoagulant Therapy		*Valve Thrombosis*	
Valve Position	*Valve Type*	*Fatal*	*Nonfatal*	*Anticoagulant Therapy*	*No Anticoagulant Therapy*
Aortic	Ball	0.61	2.75	0.03	1.32
	Bjørk-Shiley	0.65	1.64	0.33	3.14
	Lillehei-Kaster	0.11	2.30	0.48	3.40
	St. Jude	0.46	1.42	0.11	1.64
Mitral	Ball	1.11	7.59	0.55	. . .
	Bjørk-Shiley	0.80	3.69	0.70	5.74
	Lillehei-Kaster	1.04	3.27	2.26	10.40
	St. Jude	0.55	2.46	0.31	1.64

both anticoagulated and non-anticoagulated patients. Table 4.5–1 describes the incidence of thromboemboli per 100 patient-years for four types of valves in both the aortic and mitral position[17–43]. Yearly rates (*r*) from Table 4.5–1 were converted to daily probabilities by the relation $(1 - e^{-rt})$, where *t* is equal to one day, that is 1/365 year. Multiplying these probabilities times 10^5 yielded events per 100,000 patient days, as shown in Table 4.5–2. Table 4.5–2 illustrates the differences between valve-specific events that might be applied to the two patients. The rate of thromboembolic events and valve thrombosis might be expected to be significantly greater in the first case of the patient with a Bjørk-Shiley valve in the mitral position. The incidence of thromboembolism is reported to increases some three- to six-fold when anticoagulant therapy is discontinued[5,6,44–48]. This is well described for older valves, such as the ball

Table 4.5–2
Probabilities and Rates for Valve-Specific Events

		Case 1	*Case 2*
Valve Position		Mitral	Aortic
Type		Bjørk-Shiley	St. Jude
Thromboembolism:	With anticoagulation	12.3	3.9
	Without anticoagulation	36.9	11.7
Valve thrombosis:	With anticoagulation	1.92	0.30
	Without anticoagulation	15.72	4.49
Death from embolism (%)		18	24

Event rates are per 100,000 patient-days.

and Bjørk-Shiley valves. However, few data exist for patients with either Lillehei-Kaster or St. Jude valves not receiving anticoagulant therapy.

In addition, there are few well-reported trials describing the rate of prosthetic valve thrombosis in patients not receiving anticoagulation therapy. Many reports are case-based and retrospective. Others, while documenting the cumulative prevalence of valve thrombosis, do not provide information describing the number of years of patient follow-up, making it difficult to calculate event rates[49–58]. The mortality associated with valve thrombosis ranges between 25% and 90%, with a mean of 50%[15,40,59–65].

Bleeding complications of anticoagulant therapy

Using data for bleeding risks of long-term anticoagulant therapy from randomised, controlled trials examining the use of anticoagulants in patients following myocardial infarction[66–70], we calculated a bleeding rate of 10 events per 100 patient-years, or 27.4 bleeding events per 100,000 patient-days. The probability of death given a major bleeding event was 0.062. Intracerebral haemorrhage accounts for most fatalities and long-term neurological impairment in the survivors accounts for most of the morbidity. Most other bleeds do not result in long term morbidity. Using data from the Sixty Plus Re-infarction Study[71], approximately 1% of all bleeds result in long-term neurological sequelae.

Utilities

Effectiveness

Quality-adjusted life expectancy was used as the measure of effectiveness. It considers both the quality and the quantity of life. A declining exponential approximation[72,73] was used to calculate average life expectancy as the reciprocal of the sum of all mortality rates effecting the patient[74]. As shown in Table 4.5–3, describing the life expectancy calculations for the two cases, the demographic, age-sex-race related annual mortality rate is 0.051/y for a 64 year and 0.085/y for a 75 year old woman. Both have an excess annual mortality associated with having a prosthetic valve. The magnitude of this risk is highly dependent upon the clinical status of the patient at the time of valve replacement. Patients with prosthetic mitral valves, classified as New York Heart Association (NYHA) classes III and IV have an average excess annual mortality rate of roughly 0.03/y[75,76]. Long term follow up data on patients

Table 4.5–3
Life Expectancy Calculations

	Case 1	*Case 2*
Age:	64	75
age-sex-race related annual mortality rate:	0.051/y	0.085/y
Excess annual mortality rate for prosthetic valve:	0.03/y	0.01/y
Life expectancy:	12.3 yrs	10.5 yrs
Surgical procedure:	breast biopsy	cholecystectomy
average length of stay:	1 day	5 days

with prosthetic aortic valves reveal annual excess mortality rates of approximately 0.01/y for patients with good preoperative cardiac function, in NYHA functional class II[77].

All health outcomes modelled in the decision tree have their own excess mortalities and long-term morbidities. The average annual excess mortality following a major thromboembolic or haemorrhagic event can be calculated as a weighted average of mortality rates for their long-term sequelae, for example major neurological impairment or a cardiovascular event. These patients have an additional annual excess mortality rate of roughly 0.5/y[78,79].

Quality of life

To adjust life expectancy for the quality of life, we multiply the life expectancy by a quality of life factor, where full health is equal to one and death equals zero. To adjust for temporary or short term morbidity, we deduct the number of days by which the hospitalisation is prolonged from the quality adjusted life expectancy. A weighted average of the quality adjustments for long-term sequelae of non-fatal embolic events, like permanent neurological impairment, limb amputation and bowel resection, yields a quality adjustment factor (QAF) of 0.5. Long-term morbidity associated with haemorrhagic events usually follows intracerebral bleeds. The QAF associated with permanent neurological impairment is also 0.5.

Costs

Costs are described as variable costs in American dollars, not charges. From a social perspective, variable cost assumes that the institutional superstructure is already in place and that additional laboratory facilities or hospital beds need not be built to accommodate the intervention(s) under consideration. The cost of additional hospital days for the sole purpose of intravenous anticoagulation includes the costs of heparin therapy and laboratory tests ($21.97/day) and the daily cost of a hospital bed (the largest portion of which is for nursing care), resulting in a total daily cost of $377.97. In addition, thromboembolic or haemorrhagic events increase lengths of stay and costs.

RESULTS

In our analysis, we examine the outcomes of costs, quality-adjusted life expectancy, embolic events and deaths. Table 4.5–4 displays results for the patient in Case 1 in terms of costs and quality-adjusted life expectancy. We calculate the marginal cost-effectiveness for this patient undergoing a minor procedure, in whom heparin therapy prolongs the hospital stay by one to three days during the preoperative period. In the first column are the additional days of hospitalisation. The remaining columns show the predicted costs, quality-adjusted life expectancy and the marginal costs and life expectancy gained for each strategy. The last column shows the marginal cost-effectiveness ratio for each strategy, found by dividing the marginal cost by the marginal effectiveness.

While quality-adjusted life expectancy improves with each additional day of hospitalisation, the marginal cost of each hospital day increases. As a result, each

Table 4.5–4
Calculation of Marginal Cost-effectiveness for Case 1

Additional Days of Hospitalization	*Cost, $*	*Effectiveness (Quality-Adjusted Life Expectancy), y*	*Marginal Cost (Additional Cost Beyond Next-Cheapest Strategy), $*	*Marginal Effectiveness (Additional Quality-Adjusted Life Expectancy)*	*Marginal Cost-Effectiveness Ratio, Thousands of $ per Additional Quality-Adjusted Year of Life Expectancy**
0	1484	12.2945	...	...	...
1	1856	12.2970	372	0.0025	152,272
2	2231	12.2981	375	0.0011	332,225
3	2608	12.2985	377	0.0004	997,280

* Discrepancies between the marginal cost-effectiveness ratios given in the table and values computed using the figures for marginal cost and marginal effectiveness are due to rounding errors.

additional day in the hospital is progressively less cost-effective with the third day costing 997 thousand dollars per quality-adjusted life year gained.

We also performed the analysis examining the cost in dollars per embolic event averted and per death averted. Since these events are quite rare in the few days patients are at increased risk, the marginal cost/effectiveness is exceptionally high. Table 4.5–5 summarises the marginal cost-effectiveness ratios for both cases as a function of additional days of hospitalisation. As shown in the second column, the cost of preventing a single embolic event can be as great as 16 million dollars for a third day of hospitalisation, while the cost of preventing a single death, as shown in the third column, can be as great as 50 million dollars.

Since the patient described in Case 1 may have a higher risk of thromboembolic

Table 4.5–5
Marginal Cost-effectiveness ratios:
$/QALY, $/thromboembolic event averted, and $/death averted

Additional Days of Hospitalization		*Thousands of $ per* Additional Quality-Adjusted Year of Life Expectancy*	*Thromboembolic Event Averted*	*Death Averted*
Case 1	1 day	152	894	3,035
	2 days	332	1,951	6,624
	3 days	997	5,855	19,913
Case 2	1 day	443	2,395	7,607
	2 days	962	5,199	16,519
	3 days	2,885	15,592	49,562

complications compared with the patient in Case 2, the marginal cost-effectiveness ratios are less in each category for the first case.

As yet, we have made no mention of whether these additional days of hospitalisation are preoperative or postoperative. However, the real issues are: 1) how long the hospitalisation is prolonged and 2) how many days of heparin the patient receives. The results presented in Table 4.5–4 and Table 4.5–5 are relevant to prolonging the hospital stay, be they preoperative or postoperative days. We have also examined the number of days of heparin therapy where no additional days of hospitalisation are required. This would be the situation if major surgery were performed, requiring a more prolonged hospitalisation, as in Case 2, in which a cholecystectomy was being performed. The marginal cost-effectiveness ratios in this setting are predictably lower since we only consider costs of additional intravenous heparin therapy and not additional hospital days. The marginal cost-effectiveness ratios are reasonable for the first and second postoperative days of heparin therapy; $31 thousand and $54 thousand per additional quality-adjusted life year (QALY), respectively. The third additional day of heparin therapy costs $166 thousand for the same.

Sensitivity analyses

Hypercoagulable state

Sensitivity analyses were done on all parameters in the model. The one variable having the greatest influence upon results was the relative risk of thromboembolic events in non-anticoagulated patients as compared to those receiving anticoagulant therapy. In the base case, we assumed that a hypercoagulable state would not exist during the few days surrounding the discontinuation of warfarin[2,80,81]. In this sensitivity analysis we have relaxed that assumption. In Figure 4.5–2, examining the Bjørk-Shiley mitral valve in patient 1, we have varied the relative risk of thromboembolic events on the horizontal axis, between 1.0 and 6.0, where 3.0 is the baseline. The vertical axis depicts the marginal cost/effectiveness ratio on a logarithmic scale between $100,000 and ten million dollars per QALY. The three strategies involve either one, two or three additional days of hospitalisation. Even if we assume that a hypercoagulable state exists, in which the risk of thromboembolic events in non-anticoagulated patients is twice the baseline risk (a relative risk six times that of patients receiving anticoagulant therapy), with this particular valve, the cost of a single additional hospital day is greater than $63,000 per QALY. For the patient in case 2 with the St. Jude valve the cost of a single additional hospital day is roughly $185,000 per QALY.

Postoperative use of subcutaneous heparin

In response to the current pressures for early hospital discharge, we also examined a strategy of discharging the patient as soon as possible postoperatively, while providing home therapy with subcutaneous heparin twice daily until the prothrombin time returns to the therapeutic range. Given the short duration of therapy, it was not felt that self-administration was a practical alternative. Therefore, the costs associated with such treatment include professional assistance with home administration of subcutaneous heparin. Visiting nurse charges are $220 per day for two visits in the Boston area. This was used as the best proxy for actual costs. Since the 64 year old woman in

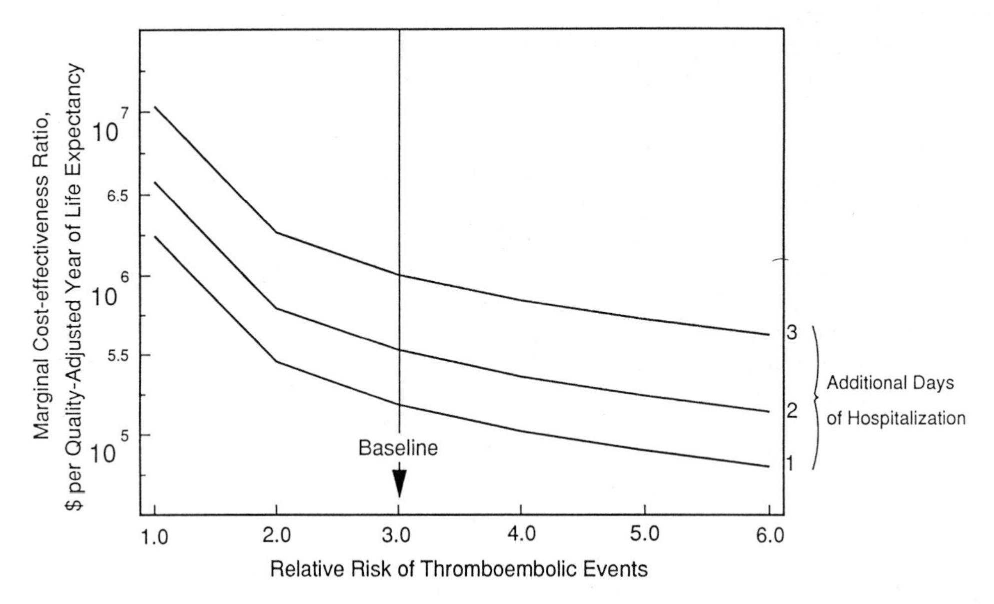

Figure 4.5–2 Relationship between cost-effectiveness and relative risk of thrombo-embolic events.

Case 1, admitted for breast biopsy, could otherwise have been discharged the next day, we considered home administration of subcutaneous heparin as opposed to prolonging the hospitalisation for the sole purpose of intravenous heparin therapy. As expected, this strategy has a lower marginal cost-effectiveness ratio than strategies requiring hospitalisation, but the cost per year of life saved is still substantial, $201,616 per QALY for one additional day of home therapy and $609,394 for a second additional day. Furthermore, this assumes that subcutaneous heparin is equally efficacious as intravenous heparin. As shown in Figure 4.5–3, when the relative efficacy of subcutaneous heparin becomes less than 0.62 times that of intravenous heparin, the marginal cost-effectiveness ratio of home heparin administration exceeds that of keeping the patient hospitalised.

Continuing the anticoagulation therapy

Up to this point the analyses performed have all assumed the cessation of oral anticoagulation therapy during the perioperative period. In anticoagulated patients at low risk for haemorrhage due to the minor nature of the surgical procedure, one might consider a strategy of continuing oral anticoagulant therapy throughout the perioperative period. Unfortunately, sufficient data are not available to quantify the risks of oral anticoagulant therapy in various surgical settings. After a MEDLINE search of the literature between 1966 and 1991, using medical subject headings (MESH) of *anticoagulants* and (*postoperative-complications* or *surgery*) and *haemorrhage*, only a limited number of articles could be found. Of these, most discussed the management during dental surgery of patients receiving anticoagulant therapy[82–87], and one discussed continuation of anticoagulants in patients undergoing ophthalmological surgery[88]. This is clearly an area which requires further investigation.

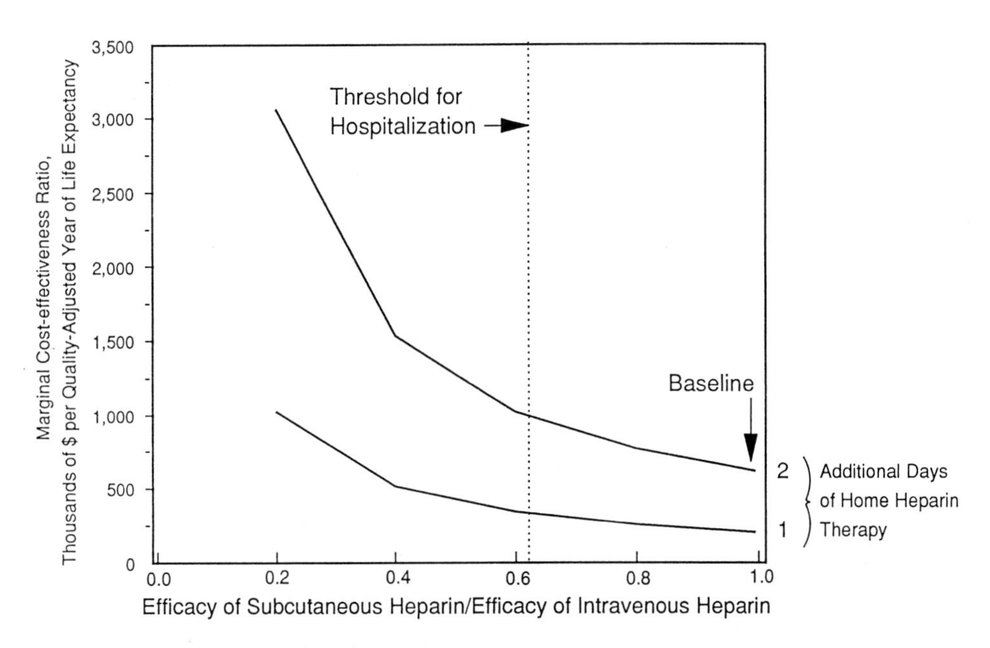

Figure 4.5–3 Relationship between cost-effectiveness and heparin treatment.

Figure 4.5–4 explores the strategy of continuing oral anticoagulant therapy through the perioperative period. In this strategy, no additional days of hospitalisation are required to address the management of anticoagulant therapy. The 64 year old woman in case 1 is admitted on the day of surgery for an excisional breast biopsy and discharged the next day. Since no data are available to quantify the risks of oral anticoagulant therapy in women undergoing excision breast biopsies, we performed a sensitivity analysis examining the relative risk of bleeding complications during the month surrounding the perioperative period. Quality adjusted life expectancy is shown on the horizontal axis while cost in American dollars is shown on the vertical axis. The open squares describe the cost-effectiveness frontier for the previously examined strategies in which oral anticoagulants are discontinued and the hospitalisation is prolonged for an additional zero to three days for intravenous heparin therapy. The slope in the interval between each square is the marginal cost-effectiveness ratio ($152,000/QALY for one additional day of hospitalisation) previously detailed in Table 4.5–5. The open triangles represent the strategy of continuing oral anticoagulant therapy while varying the relative risk of bleeding complications.

Different relative risks would be appropriate for different surgical procedures. At the far right, if the relative risk of major bleeding complications were unity, that is no increased risk due to the surgical procedure, as might be the case in a subset of patients undergoing dental extractions[82], the strategy of continuing oral anticoagulants would dominate all others, being both most effective and least expensive. As the relative risk increases beyond 1.3, continuing oral anticoagulants is no longer the most effective strategy. If the relative risk of bleeding complications exceeds approximately 1.5, continuing oral anticoagulant therapy becomes both less effective and more expensive than any of the strategies in which anticoagulants are discontinued before surgery. The

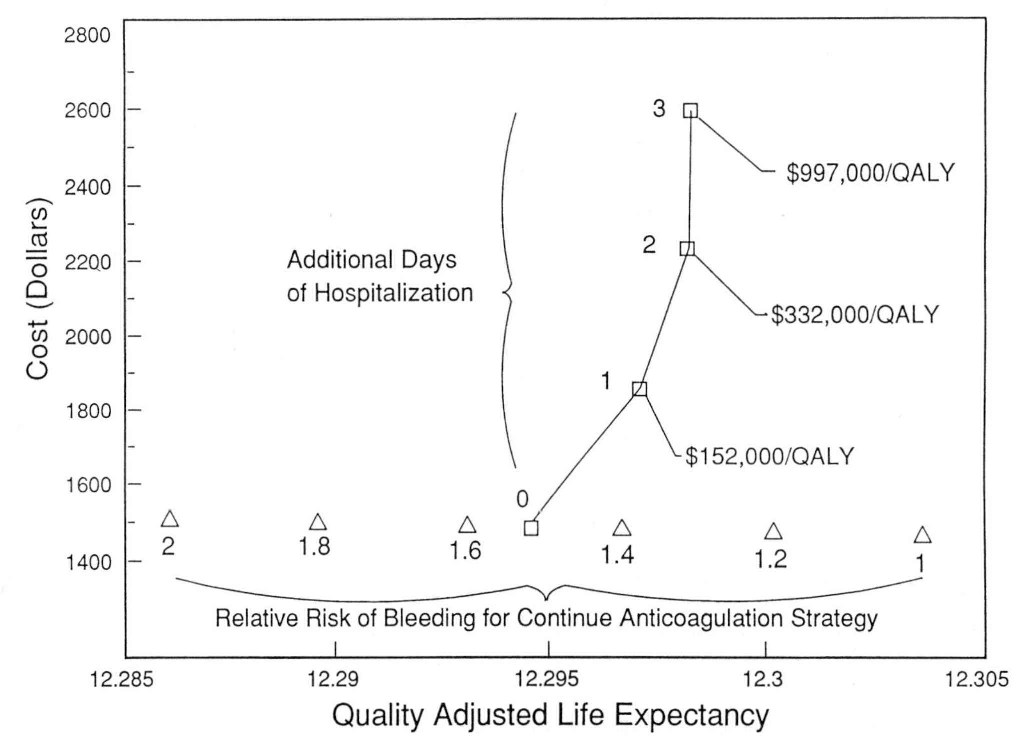

Figure 4.5–4 Relationship between cost and life expectancy.

slight increase in cost as the relative risk of bleeding complications increases from unity to two is due to induced costs of treating patients with major haemorrhages.

CONCLUSION

In both cases discussed, our analysis suggests that by continuing intravenous heparin therapy for 3 days, until their prothrombin times were therapeutic, the patients received the care that would yield the highest quality-adjusted life expectancy, the least number of embolic events and the fewest deaths. However, compared to most medical therapies, that strategy has a very high marginal cost-effectiveness ratio. This result is not surprising as the duration of time at increased risk is short and the daily rate of thromboembolic events is small. The marginal cost-effectiveness of prolonging hospitalisation for intravenous anticoagulation beyond a day is roughly 10 to 100 times more than even very expensive forms of treatment such as haemodialysis ($22,000 per additional year of life)[89], renal transplantation ($12,500 to $18,000 per additional year of life)[71], screening for and treating hypertension ($7,000 to $15,000 per additional year of life)[90], or the diagnostic evaluation of chest pain ($10,000 to $50,000 per additional year of life)[91].

How then should cost be incorporated into medical decision making? "The standard of care is a moving target, evolving to reflect considerations such as cost-effectiveness. Evolution in the standard of care is dependent upon clinical trials published in the medical literature, consensus statements of policy setting organisations, detailed analyses examining strategies of practice, and the reactions of clinicians and their institutions working hard to incorporate new information and ways of thinking into their daily practice"[8]. Cost-effectiveness "analyses should be *one* factor (not the only factor) in establishing the standard of care"[8].

In summary, decisions regarding anticoagulation during non-cardiac surgical operations in patients with prosthetic valves must be made in a highly individualised manner. In general, if the postoperative administration of intravenous heparin for an additional *one* or *two* days does not result in a prolongation of the hospital stay, the marginal cost/effectiveness is within the range of that described for presently accepted health technologies, for any type of valve. A *third* day of heparin therapy is reasonable in patients or valves that have a higher risk of valve thrombosis or thromboembolism. When the administration of heparin results in a prolongation of the hospital stay, the marginal cost/effectiveness becomes great for any type of valve. Even if a putative hypercoagulable state were to increase the rate of thromboembolic events in non-anticoagulated patients to twice the baseline rate, the marginal cost-effectiveness of even one additional day of hospitalisation would be prohibitive for all but the most thrombogenic valves.

REFERENCES

1. Stein PD, Collins JJ, Kantrowitz A. Antithrombotic therapy in mechanical and biological prosthetic heart valves and saphenous vein bypass grafts. Chest 1986;89(suppl):46S–51S.
2. Stein PD, Kantrowitz A. Antithrombotic therapy in mechanical and biological prosthetic heart valves and saphenous vein bypass grafts. Chest 1989;95(suppl):107S–117S.
3. Tinker JH, Tarhan S. Discontinuing anticoagulant therapy in surgical patients with cardiac valve prostheses. JAMA 1978;239:738–739.
4. Grady RF. Non-cardiac surgery in the elderly patient with heart disease. Mt Sinai J Med 1985;52:634–642.
5. Chesebro JH, Adams PC, Fuster V. Antithrombotic therapy in patients with valvular heart disease and prosthetic heart valves. JACC 1986;8(suppl):41B–56B.
6. Bodnar AG, Hutter AM. Anticoagulation in valvular heart disease preoperatively and postoperatively. Cardiovascular Clinics 1984;14:247–264.
7. Katholi RE, Nolan SP, McGuire LB. Living with prosthetic heart valves: Subsequent non-cardiac operations and the risk of thromboembolism or haemorrhage. Am Heart J 1976:92:162–167.
8. Eckman MH, Beshansky JR, Durand-Zaleski I, Levine H, Pauker SG. Anticoagulation for non-cardiac procedures in patients with prosthetic heart valves: Does low risk mean high cost? JAMA 1990;263:1513–1521.
9. Pauker SG, Kassirer JP. Decision Analysis. N Engl J Med 1987;316:250.
10. Sox HC, Blatt MA, Higgins MC, Marton KI. Medical Decision Making. Boston, Butterworths, 1988.
11. Kassirer JP, Moskowitz AK, Lau J. Decision analysis: A progress report. Ann Intern Med 1987;106:275–291.
12. Edmunds LH. Thrombotic and bleeding complications of prosthetic heart valves. Ann Thorac Surg 1987;44:430–445.
13. Acar J, Enriquez-Sarano M, Farah E, et al. Recurrence of systemic embolic events with valve prosthesis. Eur Heart J 1984;5(suppl D):33–38.
14. Gonzalez-Lavin L, Tandon AP, Chi S. et al. The risk of thromboembolism and haemorrhage following mitral valve replacement. A comparative analysis between the porcine xenograft valve and Ionescu-Shiley bovine pericardial valve. J Thorac Cardiovasc Surg 1984;87:340–351.
15. Barnhorst DA, Oxman HA, Connolly DC, et al. Long-term follow-up of isolated replacement of the aortic or mitral valve with the Starr-Edwards prosthesis. Am J Cardiol 1975;35:228–233.
16. Cohn LH, Allred EN, DiSesa VJ, Sawtelle K. Shemin RJ, Collins JJ. Early and late risk of aortic valve replacement. A 12-year concomitant comparison of the porcine bioprosthetic valve and tilting disc prosthetic aortic valves. J Thorac Cardiovasc Surg 1980;80:834–841.
17. Macmanus Q, Grunkemeier GL, Lambert LE, Teply JF, Harlan BJ, Starr A. Year of operation as a risk factor in the late results of valve replacement. J Thorac Cardiovasc Surg 1984;88:695–705.
18. Lee SJ, Barr C, Callaghan JC, Rosall RF. Long-term survival after aortic valve replacement using Smeloff-Cutter prosthesis. Circulation 1975;52:1132–1137.

19. Starr A, Grunkemeier GL. Lambert LE, et al. Aortic valve replacement: a ten year follow-up of non-cloth vs cloth-covered caged-ball prostheses. Circulation 1977;56(Supplement II):133.
20. Limet R, Lepage G, Grondin CM. Thromboembolic complications with the cloth-covered Starr-Edwards aortic prosthesis in patients not receiving anticoagulants. Ann Thorac Surg 1977;23;529–533.
21. McHenry MM, Smeloff Ea, Mattlof HJ, et al. Long-term survival after single aortic or mitral valve replacement with the present model of Smeloff-Cutter valves. J Thorac Cardiovasc Surg 1978;75:709–715.
22. Bloodwell RD, Okies JE, Hallman GL. Cooley DA. Aortic valve replacement. Long term results. J Thorac Cardiovasc Surg 1969;58:457–466.
23. Cheung D, Flemma RJ, Mullen DC, et al. Ten-year follow-up in aortic valve replacement using the Bjørk-Shiley prosthesis. Ann Thorac Surg 1981;32:138–145.
24. Starek PJK, McLaurin LP, Wilcox BR, Murray GF. Clinical evaluation of the Lillehei-Kaster pivoting-disc valve. Ann Thorac Surg 1976;22:362–368.
25. Zwart HHJ, Hicks G, Schuster B, et al. Clinical experience with the Lillehei-Kaster valve prosthesis. Ann Thorac Surg 1979;28:158–165.
26. Marvasti MA, Markowitz AH, Eich RH, Parker FB. Late results of Lillehei-Kaster valve. Circulation 1980;62(Suppl III):328.
27. Nicoloff DM, Emery RW, Arom KV, et al. Clinical and haemodynamic results with the St. Jude Medical cardiac valve prosthesis: a three-year experience. J Thorac Cardiovas Surg 1981;82:674–683.
28. Fishman NH, Edmunds LH, Hutchinson JC, Roe BB. Five-year experience with the Smeloff-Cutter mitral prosthesis. J Thorac Cardiovasc Surg 1971;62:345–356.
29. Oxman HA, Connolly DC, Ellis FR. Mitral valve replacement with the Smeloff-Cutter prosthesis. J Thorac Cardiovasc Surg 1975;69:247–254.
30. Starr A, Grunkemeier GL, Lambert L, et al. Mitral valve replacment: a 10-year follow-up of non-cloth covered vs cloth-covered cage-ball prostheses. Circulation 1976;54(Suppl III):47–56.
31. Macmanus Q, Grunkemeier GL, Thomas D, et al. The Starr-Edwards Model 6000 valve. Circulation 1977;56:623–625.
32. Bjørk VO, Henze A. Ten years' experience with the Bjørk-Shiley tilting disc valve. J Thorac Cardiovasc Surg. 1979;78:331–342.
33. Lepley D, Flemma RJ, Mullen DC, et al. Long-term follow-up of the Bjørk-Shiley prosthetic valve used in the mitral position. Ann Thorac Surg 1980;30:164–172.
34. Sutton J, Miller GAH, Oldershaw PJ, Paneth M. Anticoagulants and the Bjørk-Shiley prosthesis: Experience of 390 patients. Br Heart J 1978;40:558–562.
35. Starr A, Bonchek LI, Anderson RP, Wood JA, Chapman RD. Late complications of aortic valve replacement with cloth-covered, composite-seat prostheses. Ann Thorac Surg 1975;19:289–300.
36. Mitha AS, Matisonn RE, le Roux BT, Chesler E. Clinical experience with the Lillehei-Kaster cardiac valve prosthesis. J Thorac Cardiovasc Surg 1976;72:401–407.
37. Hartz RS, LoCicero J, Kucich V, DeBoer A, O'Mara S, Meyers SN, Michaelis LL. Comparative study of warfarin versus antiplatelet therapy in patients with a St. Jude medical valve in the aortic position. J Thorac Cardiovasc Surg 1986;92:684–690.
38. Myers ML, Lawrie GM, Crawford ES, Howell JF, Morris GC, Glaeser DH, DeBakey ME. The St. Jude valve prosthesis: Analysis of the clinical results in 815 implants and the need for systemic anticoagulation. JACC 1989;13:57–62.
39. Czer LSC, Matloff JM, Chaux A, DeRobertius MA, Gray RJ. Comparative clinical experience with porcine bioprosthetic and St. Jude valve replacement. Chest 1987;91:503–514.
40. Arom KV, Nicoloff DM, Kersten TE, et al. Six years experience with the St. Jude Medical valve prosthesis. Circulation 1985;72(Suppl II):153–158.
41. Baudet EM, Oca CC, Roques XF, et al. A 5½ year experience with the St. Jude cardiac valve prosthesis. J Thorac Cardiovasc Surg 1985;90:137–144.
42. Kinsley RH, Antunes MJ, Colsen PR. St. Jude medical valve replacement: An evaluation of valve performance. J Thorac Cardiovasc Surg 1986;92:349–360.
43. Sade RM, Crawford FA, Fyfe DA, Stroud MR. Valve prostheses in children: a reassessment of anticoagulation. J Thorac Cardiovasc Surg 1988;95:553–561.
44. Edmunds LH. Thromboembolic complications of current cardiac valvular prostheses. Ann Thorac Surg 1982; 34:96–111.
45. Vidne B, Levy MJ. Incidence of thromboembolic complications using totally cloth-covered Starr-Edwards prostheses. Israel J Med Sci 1974;10:586–589.
46. Moggio RA, Hammond GL, Stansel HC, Glenn WWL. Incidence of emboli with cloth-covered Starr-Edwards valve without anticoagulation and with varying forms of anticoagulation. J Thorac Cardiovasc Surg 1978;75:296–299.
47. Larsen GL, Alexander JA, Stanford W. Thromboembolic phenomena in patients with prosthetic aortic valves who did not receive anticoagulants. Ann Thorac Surg 1977;23:323–326.

48. Bjørk VO, Henze A. Management of thromboembolism after aortic valve replacement with the Bjørk-Shiley tilting disc valve. Scand J Thorac Cardiovasc Surg 1975;9:183–191.
49. Stein DW, Rahimtoola SH, Kloster FE, Selden R, Starr A. Thrombotic phenomena with non-anticoagulated, composite-strut aortic prostheses. J Thorac Cardiovasc Surg 1976;71:680–684.
50. Wright JO, Hiratzka LF, Brandt B, Doty DB. Thrombosis of the Bjørk-Shiley prosthesis. Illustrative cases and review of the literature. J Thorac Cardiovasc Surg 1982;84:138–144.
51. Copans H, Lakier JB, Kinsley RH, Colsen PR, Fritz VU, Barlow JB. Thrombosed Bjørk-Shiley mitral prostheses. Circulation 1980;61:169–174.
52. Kontos GJ, Schaff HV. Thrombotic occlusion of a prosthetic heart valve: diagnosis and management. Mayo Clin Proc 1985;60:118–122.
53. McGoon MD, Fuster V, McGoon DC, Pumphrey CW, Pluth JR, Elveback LR. Aortic and mitral valve incompetence: long-term follow-up of patients treated with the Starr-Edwards prosthesis. JACC 1984;3:930–937.
54. Effler DB, Favaloro R, Groves LK. Heart valve replacement: clinical experience. Ann Thorac Surg 1965;1:4–24.
55. Barnhorst DA, Oxman HA, Connolly DC, Pluth JR, Danielson GK, Wallace RB, McGoon DC. Isolated replacement of the mitral valve with the Starr-Edwards prosthesis: An eleven year review. J Thorac Cardiovasc Surg 1976;71:230–237.
56. Gadboys HL, Litwak RS, Niemetz J, Wisch N. Role of anticoagulants in preventing embolization from prosthetic heart valves. JAMA 1967;202:282–286.
57. Messmer BJ, Okies JE, Hallman GL, Cooley DA. Mitral valve replacement with the Bjørk-Shiley tilting-disc prosthesis. J Thorac Cardiovasc Surg 1971;62:938–946.
58. Stanford W, Lindberg EF, Armstrong RA. Implantation of heart valve prostheses without anticoagulants. J Thorac Cardiovasc Surg 1972;63:648–651.
59. Fernandez J, Yang SS, Maranhao V, Goldberg H. Late thrombosis of the aortic Bjørk-Shiley prosthesis. Chest 1976;70:12–16.
60. Gray LA, Fulton RL, Srivastava TN, Flowers NC. Surgical treatment of thrombosed Bjørk-Shiley aortic valve prosthesis. J Thorac Cardiovasc Surg 1976;71:429–432.
61. Moreno-Cabral RJ, McNamara JJ, Mamiya RT, Brainard SC, Chung GKT. Acute thrombotic obstruction with Bjørk-Shiley valves. J Thorac Cardiovasc Surg 1978;75:321–330.
62. Ayuso LA, Juffe A, Rufilanchas JJ, Babin F, Burgos R, Figuera D. Thrombectomy: surgical treatment of the thrombosed Bjørk-Shiley prosthesis. J Thorac Cardiovasc Surg 1982;84:906–910.
63. Hylen JC. Mechanical malfunction and thrombosis of prosthetic heart valves. Am J Cardiol 1972;30:396–424.
64. Lytle BW, Cosgrove DM, Taylor PC, Gill CC, Goormastic M, Golding LR, Stewart RW, Loop RD. Reoperations for valve surgery: perioperative mortality and determinants of risk for 1,000 Patients, 1958–1984. Ann Thorac Surg 1986;42:632–643.
65. Winters WL, Samuels DA. Long-term prognosis following valvular heart surgery. Cardiovasc Clin 1986;16:437–505.
66. Sullivan JM, Harken DE, Gorlin R. Pharmacologic control of thromboembolic complications of cardiac valve replacement. N Engl J Med 1971;284:1391–1394.
67. Meuwissen O, Vervoorn AC, Cohen O, et al. Double blind trial of long-term anticoagulant treatment after myocardial infarction. Acta Med Scand 1969;186:361–368.
68. Harvald B, Hilden T, Lund E. Long-term anticoagulant therapy after myocardial infarction. Lancet 1962;2:626–630.
69. Loeliger EA, Hensen A, Kroes F, et al. A double blind trial of long-term anticoagulant treatment after myocardial infarction. Acta Med Scand 1967;182:549–566.
70. Bjerkelund CG. Therapeutic level in long-term anticoagulant therapy after myocardial infarction: its relation to recurrent infarction and sudden death. Am J Cardiol 1963;1:158–163.
71. Sixty Plus Reinfarction Study Group: Risks of long-term oral anticoagulant therapy in elderly patients after myocardial infarction. Lancet 1982;1:64–68.
72. Beck JR, Kassirez JP, Pauker SG. A convenient approximation of life expectancy (The "DEALE"): I. Validation of the method. Am J Med 1982;73:883–888.
73. Beck JR, Pauker SG, Gottlieb JE, Klein K, Kassirer JP. A convenient approximation of life expectancy (The "DEALE"): II. Use in medical decision making. Am J Med 1982;73:889–897.
74. National Center for Health Statistics: Vital statistics in the United States. 1981, Vol II, Mortality, Part A. DHSS Pub. No. (PHS) 86–1101. Public Health Service, Washington, U.S. Government Printing Office, 1986; section 6, pp. 10–11.
75. Rackley CE, Edwards JE, Karp RB. Mitral valve disease. In Hurst JW (ed.): The Heart. 6th ed. New York, McGraw-Hill Book Company, 1985:754.
76. Singer RB, Levinson L. Medical Risks. Lexington. Lexington Books, D.C. Heath and Company. 1976:3–120.

77. Copeland JG, Griepp RB, Stinson BB, Shumway NE. Long-term follow-up after isolated aortic valve replacement. J Thorac Cardiovasc Surg 1977;74:875–885.
78. Singer RB, Levinson L. Medical Risks. Lexington. Lexington Books, D.C. Heath and Company. 1976:2–15.
79. Kannel WB, Abbott RD. Incidence and prognosis of unrecognized myocardial infarction: An update on the Framingham study. N Engl J Med 1984;311:1144–1147.
80. Evans RW, O'Rourke RA, McGranahan MC. Thromboembolic complications of anticoagulant withdrawal. Circulation 1968;37(Suppl VI):74–77.
81. Michaels L. Incidence of thromboembolism after stopping anticoagulant therapy. JAMA 1971;215:595–599.
82. McIntyre H. Management during dental surgery of patients on anticoagulants. Lancet 1966;2:99–100.
83. Debernadi C, Catpano F, Bulla A. Dental extractions in patients treated with anticoagulants. The preoperative assessment. Minerva Stomatologica 1986;35:1043–1047.
84. Blomback M, Hohnsson H, Ramstrom G. Oral surgery procedures for patients under anticoagulant therapy. Tandlakartindningen 1976;68:654–657.
85. Horejs J, Sochmanova L. Patients under anticoagulant therapy in dental practice. Ceskoslovensak Stomatologie 1971;71:135–139.
86. Catapano B, Bertera F. Problems of dental surgery in patients with haemorrhagic diathesis, or patients subjected to anticoagulant therapy. Rivista Italiana di Stomatologia 1969;24:1182–1196.
87. Pawlikowski W. Some dental surgical procedures during long-term treatment with anticoagulant agents. Wiadomosci Lekarskie 1965;18:1007–1011.
88. Mellin KB, Waubke TN. Surgery on the eye under anticoagulative therapy. Klin Mntsbl Augenheilkunde. 1979;174:1–4.
89. Strange PB, Sumner AT. Predicting treatment costs and life expectancy for end-stage renal disease. N Engl J Med 1978;298:372–378.
90. Weinstein MC, Stason WB. Hypertension. A Policy Perspective. Cambridge, Harvard Univ. Press, 1976.
91. Doubilet P, McNeil BJ, Weinstein MC. The decision concerning coronary angiography in patients with chest pain. Med Decis Making 1985;5:293–309.

Part 5

Management of thromboembolic and bleeding complications

Chapter 5.1

Valve Thrombosis: Diagnosis and Management

Dirk Hausmann, Andreas Mügge and Werner G. Daniel

Depending on the thrombogenicity of the prosthesis used (Chapter 2.4), up to 6% of patients may experience valve thrombosis[1–3]. Valve thrombosis often presents as an emergency, and in those cases the mortality approaches 50%[1,2,4]. Immediate recognition and management are therefore essential if this mortality is to be reduced.

The risk of thromboembolism in patients with prosthetic valves is affected by the intensity and quality of anticoagulation (Chapter 3.4) as well as by additional factors, like the presence of atrial fibrillation and/or large left atrium[1,2,5] (Chapter 1.3). The risk of prosthetic valve thrombosis is greatest in the tricuspid position (in one reported series 20% of tricuspid prostheses thrombosed[6]), intermediate in the mitral and lowest in the aortic position. The risk of valve thrombosis is also influenced by surgical technique and by the type of prosthesis[7,8] (see also Chapters 1.6 and 2.4).

Since the clinical features of prosthetic thrombosis are usually non-specific, confirmation of the diagnosis requires echocardiography or fluoroscopy. As soon as the diagnosis is established, urgent thrombolytic or surgical treatment is mandatory.

DIAGNOSIS

Symptomatology (Table 5.1–1)

Any significant clinical deterioration in a patient after prosthetic valve replacement should raise the suspicion of valve thrombosis. Although more likely to occur in non-anticoagulated or inadequately anticoagulated patients[9], the diagnosis of valve thrombosis should be considered even in patients with good anticoagulation control[1–3,10].

In most cases, symptoms develop over several hours or a few days[9] and the patient presents with acute congestive heart failure, cardiogenic shock, pulmonary oedema,

Table 5.1–1
Clinical Findings in Patients with Prosthetic Valve Thrombosis

Clinical Symptoms (non-specific)
- development of symptoms usually within hours-days
- left/right heart failure, pulmonary oedema, shock
- arrhythmias, syncope, cardiac arrest
- angina pectoris, myocardial infarction
- embolisation (pulmonary/systemic)

Auscultatory Findings
- absent/"muffled" valve sounds
- new systolic or diastolic murmurs

syncope or arrhythmia [1,2,9,11]. However, sometimes clinical deterioration occurs slowly and insidiously over a period of several weeks[9]; this course is usually accompanied by symptoms of increasing dyspnoea, angina pectoris or fatigue[12]. The time course over which clinical symptoms develop does not necessarily reflect the rapidity of thrombus accumulation, the early stages of which may be asymptomatic. The development of symptoms and physical signs may represent only the final stage of the process. On the other hand, it should not be forgotten that valve thrombosis can occur even in the early postoperative period[13].

Occasionally, prosthetic valve thrombosis may cause systemic or pulmonary embolism, which may be the presenting feature[11]. In the case of tricuspid prosthetic valve thrombosis, repeated minor pulmonary emboli may lead to atypical symptoms. Emboli from thrombosed left sided prosthetic valves become symptomatic most frequently when they reach the brain. Rarely, left sided valve thrombosis leads to coronary artery embolism or even direct obstruction of the ostium of a coronary artery, resulting in acute myocardial infarction or sudden death[14]. However, it must be stressed that most embolism arises not from thrombosed prostheses but from other sources within the heart and from small platelet thrombi on the sewing ring[15–19] (see also Chapter 2.4).

Auscultation (Table 5.1–1)

The physical examination may reveal more specific signs. A thrombus attached to a prosthetic valve usually interferes with the free movement of the occluder(s), causing changes in opening and closing sounds[20].

Under normal conditions, ball valves produce the loudest sound on both opening and closure, tilting disk valves create a loud closing but only a faint opening sound, and biological valves are associated with auscultatory findings similar to those of normal native valves[21]. The intensity of the sound generally depends on the site of the replaced valve. Analysis of the quality and timing of the sound can provide important diagnostic information[12,13,23–25]. In patients with prosthetic valve thrombosis, the most frequent finding on auscultation is absence or muffling of the opening or closing sounds. New systolic or diastolic murmurs may also be audible due to incomplete opening and closing of the prosthesis.

Phonocardiography

The time interval for opening of a prosthesis may be changed by valve thrombosis. This time interval can be measured by phonocardiography. In patients with normally functioning mitral prostheses and normal left ventricular function, the interval between aortic valve closure and mitral valve opening (A2-MO) ranges between 55–150 msec[21,26,27]. In mitral prosthetic thrombosis, the A2-MO interval may either be prolonged due to thrombus-induced restriction of the occluder movement[13] or shortened as a result of obstruction to mitral flow[26,27]. In patients with aortic prostheses, the interval between mitral closure (or Q-wave in the electrocardiogram) and aortic opening (Q-AO) normally ranges between 98 and 109 msec. In the presence of aortic thrombotic obstruction, the Q-AO interval may remain normal or show variation from beat to beat[28].

In modern cardiological practice, phonocardiography has been largely superceded by echocardiography for the diagnosis of valve thrombosis.

Table 5.1–2
Laboratory Findings in Patients with Prosthetic Valve Thrombosis

Echocardiography
- abnormal time intervals (e.g. reduced or prolonged interval between aortic valve closure and peak opening)
- reduced prosthetic movement
- assessment of pressure gradients and valve area by Doppler
- direct visualisation of thrombus
- detection of thrombi and spontaneous echo contrast.

Fluoroscopy
- reduced excursion of the prosthetic valve occluder

Cardiac Catherisation
- assessment of haemodynamic severity (pressure gradients and valve area)

111-Indium-Labelled Autologous Platelet Imaging
- detection of thrombotic material (differentiation old/fresh thrombus)

Echocardiography (Table 5.1–2)

The rapid development of new echocardiographic techniques during the last three decades has enormously increased the role of cardiac ultrasound in the diagnosis of prosthetic valve malfunction in general and valve thrombosis in particular. The ease of application, low cost and safety of the techniques make them ideal for bedside diagnosis of acute valve thrombosis in most patients. Furthermore, echocardiography can be used to monitor morphological and functional changes during and after thrombolytic therapy[23,28–30].

Initial observations in patients with prosthetic valve thrombosis were reported in the early 1970s using M-mode echocardiography (Figure 5.1–1 and 5.1–2), demonstrating shortening of the time interval from aortic valve closure to peak opening of the mitral prosthesis in obstructed mitral prostheses[26]. Impaired disc motion and thrombotic material were also visualised[31]. M-mode echocardiography has also been used to monitor reversal of valve motion abnormalities during thrombolytic therapy in acute prosthetic valve thrombosis[23].

The introduction of two-dimensional echocardiography has significantly improved the ultrasound evaluation of prosthetic valves and in particular the capacity to diagnose valve thrombosis. Two-dimensional echocardiography images may provide visualisation of attached thrombotic material and abnormal valve motion[12]. The combination of these images with spectral or colour Doppler allows qualitative and quantitative analysis of normal and abnormal blood flow across the prosthesis and assessment of the degree of obstruction or regurgitation[29,32]. Thus, while two-dimensional echocardiography demonstrates the anatomical abnormality, Doppler provides important additional information about its functional consequences. Doppler techniques have been validated by simultaneous Doppler and catheter haemodynamic studies which have shown close correlation between the two methods for estimating prosthetic valve pressure gradients and valve areas[32].

It is important to remember that there is considerable variation in the 'normal' value of valve area depending on the type of prosthesis and its size. Even in normally

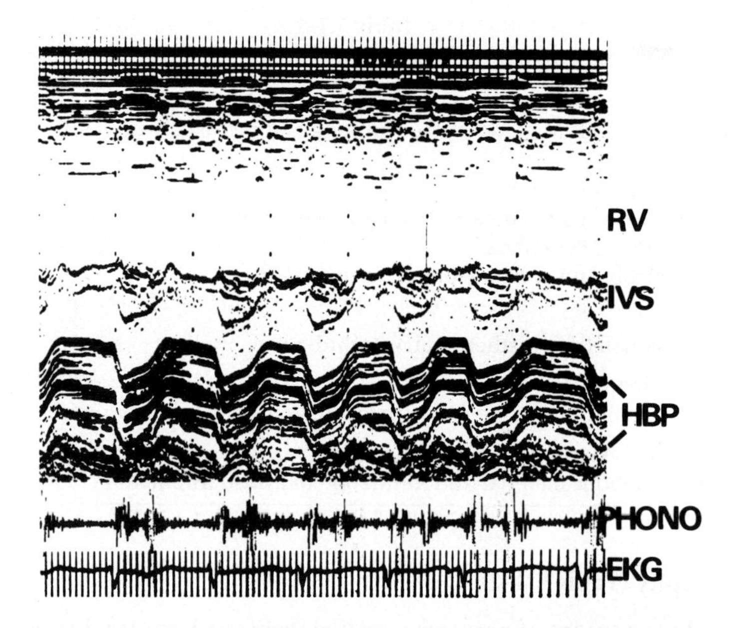

Figure 5.1–1: Transthoracic M-mode echocardiogram in a patient with a thrombosed Hancock bioprosthesis in the mitral position. Multiple heavy echos instead of the thin leaflets are seen within the prosthesis. Thrombosis of all three leaflets of the prosthesis were subsequently proven at surgery (see also Figure 2). EKG = electrocardiogram,) IVS = interventricular septum; HBP = Hancock bioprosthesis; PHONO = phonocardiogram. (Reference 63).

functioning mitral prostheses, the mean values for mitral valve area have been reported to range between 1.8±0.6 sq cm (Lillehei-Kaster) and 2.9±0.6 sq cm (St. Jude Medical). Doppler derived mean mitral valve gradients may range between 2.3±1.1 mm Hg (St. Jude Medical) and 4.5±2.4 mm Hg (Starr Edwards)[33,34]. In the presence of valve thrombosis, the valve area may be less than that expected for the size and type of prosthesis and the valve gradient may be higher than expected. However, these findings alone are insufficient to make a diagnosis of prosthetic valve thrombosis, since many factors influence these measurements, including for example the presence of atrial fibrillation.

Mechanical prosthetic valves are sometimes difficult to evaluate by transthoracic echocardiography, because they are composed of highly reflective material which creates artefacts. These may obscure the image of the prosthetic valve mechanism, for example the interior of a ball valve cage. For the same reason, the atrial surface of a mitral prosthesis may be difficult to visualise[35–37].

Fortunately, transoesophageal echocardiography has overcome these problems by providing a new window into the heart and the great vessels. Several studies have shown that the transoesophageal approach, when compared with conventional transthoracic echocardiography, has increased diagnostic accuracy in the detection of a variety of cardiovascular diseases, including prosthetic valve malfunction[36–38]. Although transoesophageal echocardiography is associated with some minor discomfort to the patient, it almost always provides high quality images[39]. This is due to the proximity of the heart to the oesophagus and to the higher-frequency transducers used

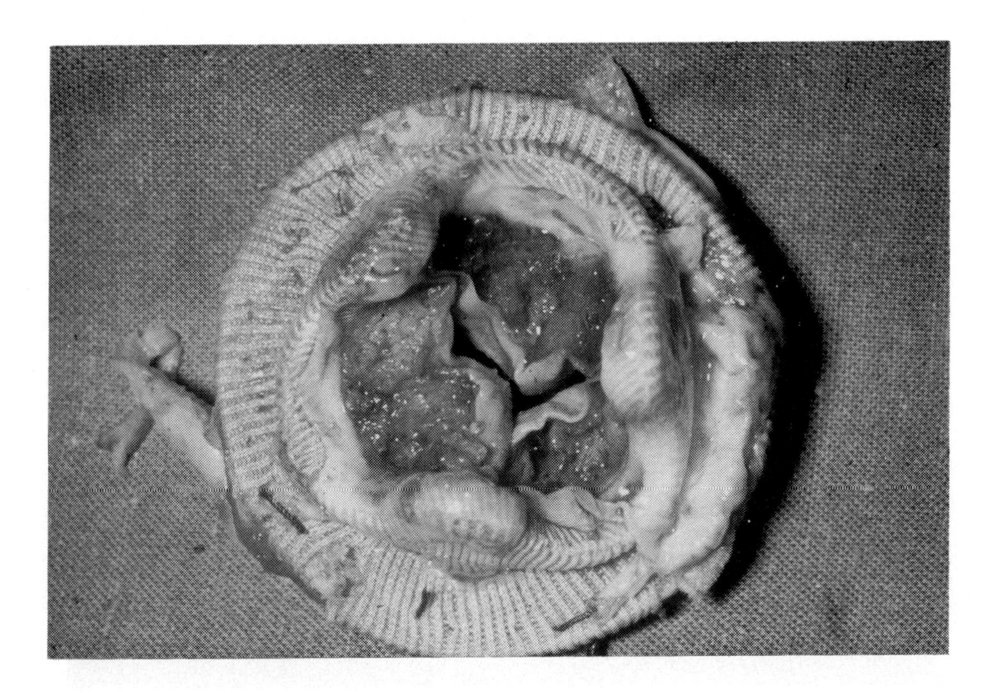

Figure 5.1–2: Explanted Hancock bioprosthesis (same patient as in Figure 5.1–1). Severe thrombosis of all three leaflets of the prosthesis is shown.

in transoesophageal echocardiography which improve image resolution. The technique is particularly useful when transthoracic echocardiography fails to provide an adequate image quality because of advanced obesity, chest deformity, emphysema, artificial ventilation or recent cardiac surgery.

In a series of 100 prosthetic valves examined by surgery or autopsy, Mügge and associates reported that transoesophageal echocardiography increased the percentage of correct morphological diagnoses (endocarditis, bioprosthetic degeneration or valve thrombosis) from 56% to 84% when compared to transthoracic echocardiography[36]. In particular, mechanical devices and prostheses in the mitral position could be more successfully evaluated by transoesophageal echocardiography. In this series, all six thrombosed prostheses were correctly diagnosed by transoesophageal echocardiography (Figures 5.1–3 – 5.1–6) compared to only one out of six by the precordial examination[36]. Similar findings have been reported by Guéret and co-authors[40] who detected prosthetic thrombi in 13 of 68 patients by transoesophageal echocardiography but none using the transthoracic approach. Mechanical devices in the aortic position are somewhat more difficult to evaluate than those in the mitral position, if monoplane transoesophageal echocardiography is used.

Transoesophageal echocardiography also allows the detection of mural thrombus[16,17,41] and spontaneous echo contrast in the left atrium. The latter phenomenon is associated with slow blood flow and an increased thromboembolic risk (see Chapter 2.6). When used by experienced operators with appropriate safety precautions, transoesophageal echocardiography is associated with an acceptably low

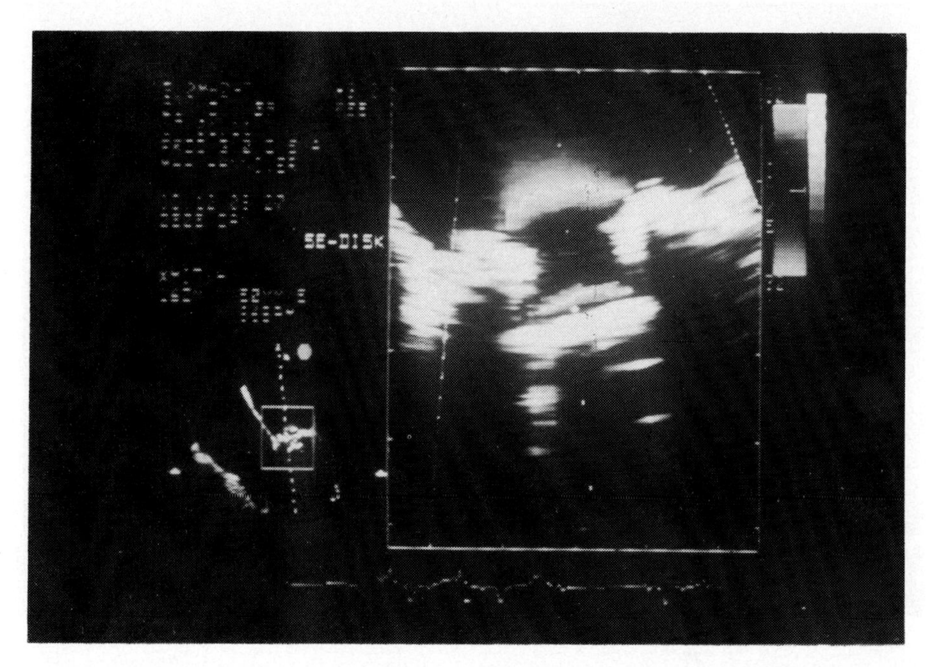

Figure 5.1–3: Transoesophageal colour Doppler echocardiogram in a patient with a Starr-Edwards disc prosthesis in the mitral position. Normal diastolic opening and normal diastolic flow through the valve.

risk[39]. It should be performed whenever praecordial echocardiography fails to document a clinically suspected prosthetic valve malfunction.

Radiology and cardiac catheterisation (Table 5.1–2)

In patients with radiopaque prostheses, the motion of the disc or leaflets as well as that of the prosthetic ring may be studied by fluoroscopy and cineradiography[42]. These studies are usually performed with an X-ray tube which can be rotated 360 degrees around the patient and angled in cranial and caudal directions. The prosthesis should be viewed in different projections during several cardiac cycles. In particular, a beam direction corresponding to the axis of the motion of the disc should be sought.

Thrombosis of the valve (Figure 5.1–7) should be suspected if the opening angle is much below the normal range (vide infra) or if the occluder is immobilised in an intermediate position or exhibits reduced movement around this position. Using these criteria, Ledain and associates diagnosed 15 of 16 cases of prosthetic valve thrombosis by cineradiography[11]. During thrombolysis, incremental increase in the opening angle may be used as an additional indication of successful treatment.

Before using this method for the diagnosis of valve thrombosis, a knowledge of the normal opening angle of the prosthesis under investigation is essential. It is important to appreciate that many prostheses fail to open completely under low flow conditions, especially in the mitral position, and that some have smaller opening angles in vivo than in vitro. Among the various models of Bjørk-Shiley prostheses, normal opening angles range between 60 and 70 degrees[43,44,45]. When the prosthesis becomes

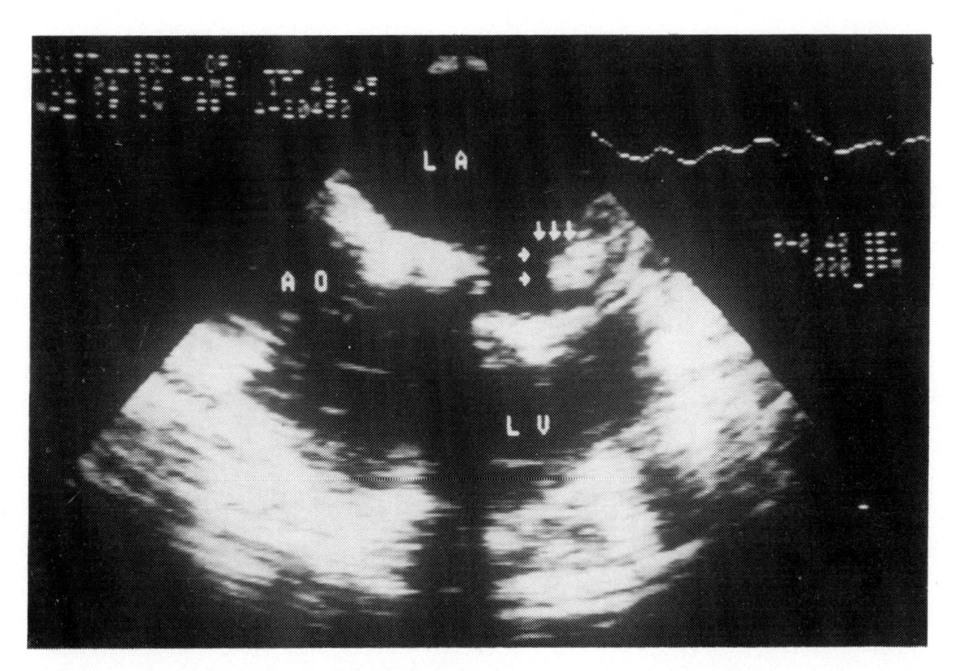

Figure 5.1–4: Transoesophageal echocardiogram in a patient with a thrombosed Starr-Edwards disc prosthesis in the mitral position. A thrombus is attached to the prosthesis (arrows). AO = aortic valve; LA = left atrium; LV = left ventricle.

thrombosed, the opening angle decreases to between zero and 39 degrees[30]. Although possibly influenced by the orientation of the larger orifice, especially in the mitral position[46], the Omniscience valve appears prone to incomplete opening. The in vitro opening angle of this prosthesis is 80 degrees, but in one study the opening angles of 'normal' prostheses in the mitral and aortic positions ranged between 38 and 80 degrees, whilst two thrombosed valves had opening angles of 15 and 31 degrees respectively[47]. Similarly, the Lillehei-Kaster valve, the predecessor of the Omniscience valve, also has an in vitro opening angle of 80 degrees but often fails to achieve full opening in vivo. Sigwart and associates found opening angles in non-thrombosed valves of this type between 57 and 74 degrees[48]. The Medtronic Hall valve opens to 75 degrees in the aortic models and 70 degrees in the mitral models.

The various bileaflet valves differ in both their opening and closing angles, so that a detailed knowledge of the normal angles for each prosthesis is essential for fluoroscopic evaluation. In the closed position, the leaflets of the Edwards-Duromedics valve meet the housing in the horizontal plane, whereas the leaflets of the Carbomedics and larger sized St. Jude valves make an angle of 130 degrees on closure (sizes 25 mm and less have a closing angle of 120 degrees). The opening angles of the three bileaflet valves are: St. Jude 85 degrees; Edwards-Duromedics aortic 77 degrees, and mitral 73 degrees; Carbomedics 78 degrees[49].

Cardiac catheterisation has only limited value for assessment of acute prosthetic valve thrombosis. Pressure recordings allow the measurement of the gradient across an obstructed valve and the valve area can be calculated[12,42], but these haemodynamic

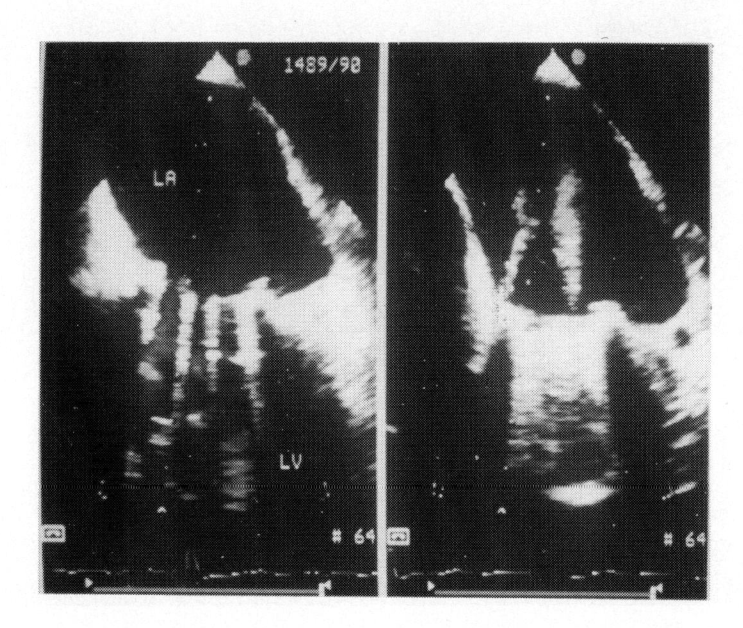

Figure 5.1–5: Transoesophageal colour Doppler echocardiogram in a patient with a Carbomedics prosthesis in the mitral position. Left: Normal diastolic opening of both leaflets of the prosthesis and normal diastolic flow. Right: In systole, visualisation of two small systolic regurgitant jets. LA = left atrium; LV = left ventricle.

data can also be obtained by non-invasive Doppler echocardiography. Furthermore the arterial puncture may increase the risk of bleeding if thrombolytic therapy is used.

Scintigraphy

Recently, a new technique for detection of prosthetic valve thrombosis has been proposed by Acar and associates[50], using 111-indium-labelled autologous platelets to image thrombus attached to the prosthesis. This method detected thrombosis in 24 of 41 patients with recent thromboembolic events after prosthetic valve replacement and in 8 of 10 patients with anatomically confirmed valve thrombosis the test was abnormal. The method may also provide information about the haematological activity of the thrombus and hence its age[50](see also Chapter 2.5). Its major limitation is the fact that it is too time-consuming to perform in a critically ill patient.

A stepwise approach to diagnosis

Based on evaluation of the foregoing diagnostic methods, the following diagnostic strategy is suggested in clinically suspected prosthetic valve thrombosis. After a detailed history and careful physical examination, a transthoracic two-dimensional Doppler echocardiogram should be performed in the emergency room or at the patient's bedside. Echo data should be compared with previous echocardiographic studies if these are available. If transthoracic echocardiography is inconclusive, a transoesophageal examination should be performed. In most instances, these simple

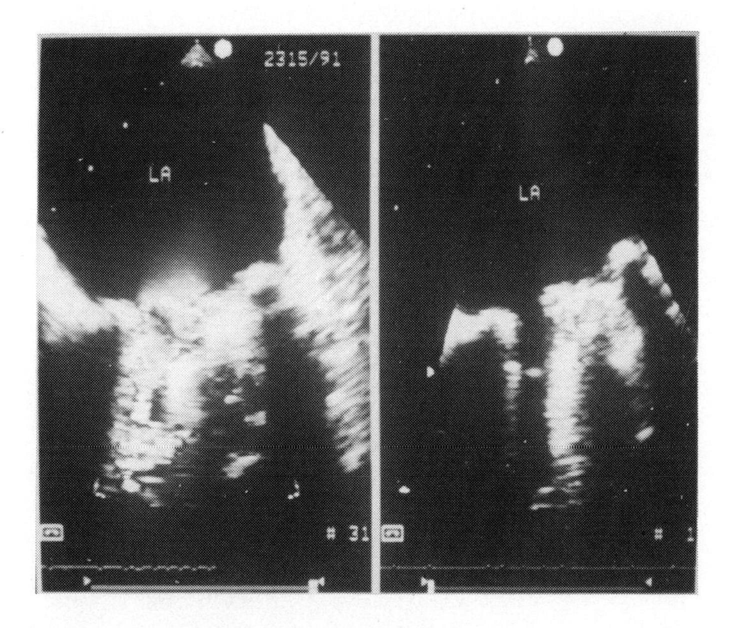

Figure 5.1–6: Transoesophageal echocardiogram in a patient with a thrombosed Carbomedics prosthesis in the mitral position. Right: In contrast to Figure 5, only one leaflet shows diastolic opening (the left leaflet). Left: Correspondingly, colour Doppler shows high turbulence diastolic inflow through the same orifice. Thrombotic obstruction of the posterior leaflet of the prosthesis was subsequently proven by surgery (see also Figure 7).

diagnostic steps in combination with the clinical features should lead to the correct diagnosis.

In patients with mechanical prostheses who are not in a critical condition, fluoroscopic evaluation of occluder motion may provide additional information if the echocardiographic examination remains inconclusive. However, fluoroscopy alone is insufficient for unequivocal diagnosis of valve thrombosis since this method does not distinguish between the various causes of incomplete occluder movement. Nuclear studies should rarely be required, but in any case are only suitable for patients who are not in a critical condition.

MANAGEMENT

Thrombolysis

As soon as the diagnosis of acute valve thrombosis is established, urgent treatment is necessary and a choice must be made between thrombolysis and reoperation. The best clinical results from thrombolysis have been reported in patients with a short history of symptoms. Although thrombolytic therapy has been successful in some cases of chronic prosthetic valve thrombosis of up to three months duration, the recurrence rate is higher under these circumstances[25].

In patients with haemodynamically significant valve thrombosis, thrombolysis should be considered only if there is no absolute necessity for immediate reoperation.

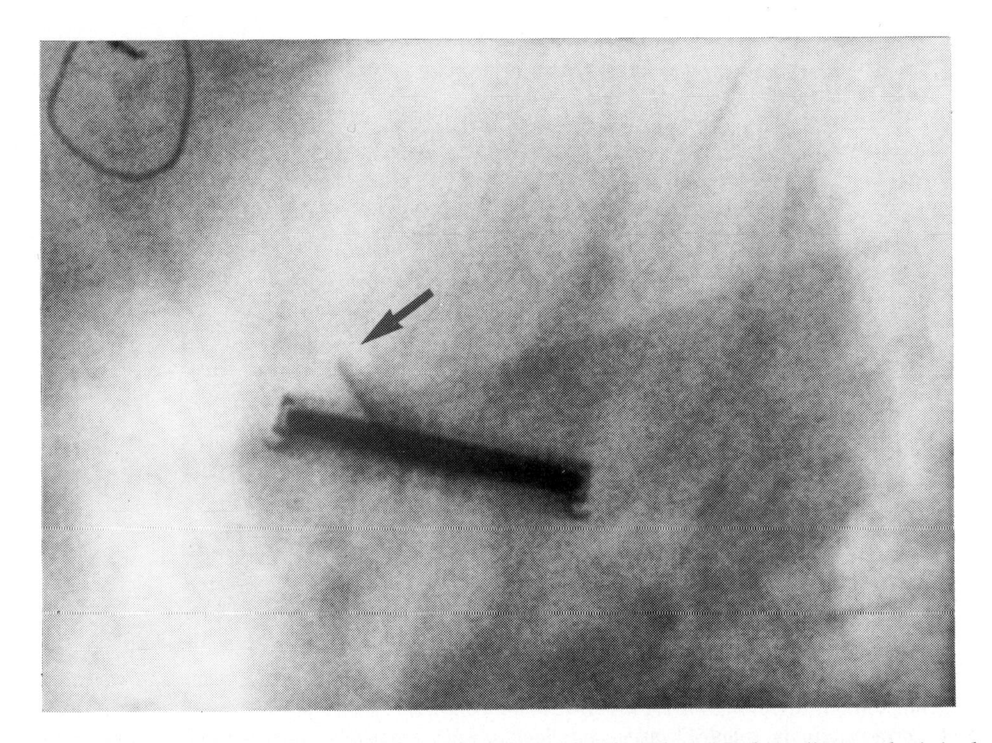

Figure 5.1–7: Cineradiographic examination of a patient with a thrombosed Carbomedics prosthesis in the mitral position (same patient as in Figure 6). Diastolic opening of only one leaflet can be demonstrated (arrow). Thrombotic obstruction of the second leaflet of the prosthesis was subsequently proven at surgery.

In patients with acute valve thrombosis associated with cardiogenic shock and pulmonary oedema, immediate surgery is preferable. At the other extreme, in patients with non-critical valve obstruction or those suffering from systemic embolism alone, the benefits of thrombolytic therapy may outweigh the risks of this intervention[51].

The major risks of systemic thrombolysis in patients with prosthetic valve thrombosis consist of bleeding complications, thromboembolism and allergic reactions. In particular, thrombolysis of left-sided prostheses is complicated by a considerable risk of systemic embolism. During in vitro thrombolysis in explanted thrombosed prosthetic valves, Karagoz and associates[52] have shown that fragments of organised thrombus may be released into the medium. Overall, the rate of thromboembolic complications caused by thrombolytic therapy in patients with prosthetic valve thrombosis may reach 10%[53]. Because of this considerable risk of embolism, thrombolytic therapy was initially used for right-sided prostheses only. Thrombolytic therapy in tricuspid valve thrombosis was first performed successfully in 1971 by Luluaga and associates[54]. Three years later, Baille and associates used fibrinolysis for treatment of a left-sided prosthesis[55]. Since then, many reports on thrombolysis of left-sided prostheses have been published[11,24,28,34,51,56,57]. Reviewing the literature in 1988, Graver and co-authors found only one death due to embolic stroke during thrombolytic therapy in 58 reported cases[51]. However, non-fatal systemic embolism continues to be a major problem associated with thrombolytic therapy in left-sided prostheses[11,56].

In the early years of thrombolysis, streptokinase was used exclusively as the thrombolytic agent, usually in a dose of 100,000 units/hour following initial neutralisation[11,24,28,57,58]. Recently, other fibrinolytic agents such as urokinase[11,23] and tissue plasminogen activator[29,59] have been used, but so far experience with these newer agents has been limited to right-sided prostheses[23,29,59]. Overall, attempts to treat acute prosthetic valve thrombosis with thrombolysis have only been described in small series or case reports. Larger controlled studies are not available and the optimal thrombolytic agent in this condition has therefore not yet been determined. Moreover, the optimal dosage and the duration of therapy also remain unclear. Although clinical and haemodynamic improvement is usually achieved within six to 12 hours when streptokinase therapy is successful, some studies have continued the treatment up to 72 hours[24].

Substantial differences in the therapeutic regimen, patient population, anatomical site and type of thrombosed prosthetic valve preclude a reliable comparison between the different therapeutic strategies, and the overall results of thrombolytic therapy are difficult to summarise. The previously mentioned review of the literature by Graver and co-authors[51] analysed 58 cases of left sided prosthetic valve thrombosis. The initial success rate of thrombolytic therapy was 62% (67% when patients with success after repeated thrombolysis were included) and the mortality rate was 10%.

Successful thrombolytic therapy should lead to rapid improvement in clinical and haemodynamic parameters. Echocardiographic monitoring of the size of thrombotic material and repeat assessment of the degree of valve obstruction by Doppler are mandatory[28,29,34]. Fibrinolytic therapy should be stopped if there is no clinical or haemodynamic improvement within 12 hours or if the haemodynamic state continues to deteriorate[24]. This latter situation occurs in about 20% of patients, in whom immediate surgery becomes necessary even though it is associated with a high mortality rate[51]. Patients who rethrombose their prostheses after initial successful thrombolysis also require urgent surgery.

If a prosthesis is obstructed by already organised thrombotic material or by pannus (tissue ingrowth), fibrinolytic therapy may have little or no impact on the thrombus. In 100 patients with prosthetic valve obstruction, Deviri and associates found pannus formation alone in 7% and a combination of both pannus and thrombus in 44%[9]. Because of the high percentage of pannus formation as a contributing factor to valve obstruction they concluded that surgery was superior to fibrinolysis in their population.

A new method has been described as an adjunct to thrombolysis for right-sided prosthetic valve thrombosis, involving the use of a balloon catheter. The technique was used successfully to free the immobile disc of a Bjørk-Shiley prosthesis in a RV-PA conduit in a child with tetralogy of Fallot. Manipulations of the balloon catheter were combined with selective ventricular streptokinase infusion[58].

In summary, thrombolytic therapy may offer a relatively safe and effective form of treatment in selected patients with early valve thrombosis. Surgical treatment is necessary a) in chronic thrombosis, b) when the obstruction is caused by pannus, c) when the patient's haemodynamic and clinical condition deteriorates during thrombolytic therapy and d) when significant improvement cannot be achieved after 6 – 12 hours of thrombolysis.

Surgical treatment

When the haemodynamic situation of the patient cannot be improved by thrombolytic therapy or when the clinical condition is deteriorating, there is no question that immediate reoperation is necessary. In patients with relatively stable haemodynamic conditions, the indication for surgical treatment of prosthetic valve thrombosis without a preliminary trial of thrombolytic therapy is still controversial.

In centres preferring not to use thrombolysis, surgical treatment is usually performed within hours or a few days after the diagnosis has been established. In the series of Kontos and associates, 73% of patients with prosthetic valve thrombosis underwent surgery within one week[12].

Once the thrombosed valve has been exposed at reoperation, a decision must be made either to replace it or to simply remove the thrombus and/or pannus. The technique of choice remains a matter of ongoing discussion, but is influenced by such factors as the anticoagulation history, the accessability of the thrombus, contributing technical factors (e.g. oversized prosthesis or suture technique) and the thrombogenicity of the prosthesis. If cessation of anticoagulation or very poorly controlled anticoagulation has led to valve thrombosis, thrombectomy alone should be considered providing that good quality anticoagulation can be assured postoperatively. If, on the other hand, valve thrombosis has occurred despite good anticoagulation control, simple thrombectomy is likely to be followed by recurrence of the problem and the valve should be replaced either by a less thrombogenic mechanical valve or a bioprosthesis, paying attention to any technical factors at the first operation which may have contributed to valve thrombosis (see Chapter 1.6). It should be added that in this respect thrombolysis should be regarded as equivalent to thrombectomy and subject to the same caveats. If thrombectomy is to be undertaken, it is important that all thrombus is removed. In the case of mitral tilting disc valves particularly, much of the thrombus may be hidden from the surgeon's view and relatively inaccessible because it is 'behind' the disc on its ventricular aspect. This problem is magnified in small sized prostheses. If there is any doubt concerning the completeness of removal, it is much safer to replace the valve. It is probable that some cases of 'recurrence' after thrombectomy are in fact due to incomplete removal of thrombus. Aortic prosthesis thrombectomy is easier to perform and is reported to be associated with low mortality[60,61]. Non-randomised studies comparing thrombectomy with valve replacement have been carried out. In a non-randomised study, Martinell and associates reported a hospital mortality of 16% (six of 37) following valve replacement and 15% (four of 27) following thrombectomy. Rethrombosis occurred in 3% (one of 34) of patients following valve replacement and in 22% (five of 23) following thrombectomy[61]. The authors of this study concluded that valve replacement was preferable to thrombectomy. Other authors have reported similar findings and conclusions[62].

If successful thrombectomy has been possible, normal prosthetic function may be restored on serial evaluation of valve function by cinefluoroscopy and echocardiography[30]. It is possible that thrombectomy may have a place in selected patients whose primary problem has been failure of anticoagulation rather than failure of implantation technique or failure of the prosthesis. Each case should therefore be assessed individually.

REFERENCES

1. Edmunds LH, Jr. Thrombotic and bleeding complications of prosthetic heart valves. Ann Thorac Surg 1987;44:430–445.
2. Edmunds LH, Jr. Thromboembolic complications of current cardiac valvular prostheses. Ann Thorac Surg 1982;34:96–106.
3. Moreno-Cabral RJ, McNamara JJ, Mamiya RT, Brainard SC, Chung GKT. Acute thrombotic obstruction with Bjørk-Shiley valves. J Thorac Cardiovasc Surg 1978;75:321–329.
4. Acar J, Enriquez-Sarano M, Farah E, Kassab R, Tubiana P, Roger V. Recurrent systemic embolic events with valve prosthesis. Eur Heart J 1984;5(suppl D):33–38.
5. Horstkotte D, Haerten K, Herzer JA, Loogen F, Scheibling R, Schulte HD. Five-year results after randomized mitral valve replacement with Bjørk-Shiley, Lillehei-Kaster, and Starr-Edwards prostheses. Thoracic Cardiovasc Surgeon 1983;31:206–214.
6. Thorburn CW, Morgan JJ, Shanahan MX, Chang VP. Long-term results of tricuspid valve replacement and the problem of prosthetic valve thrombosis. Am J Cardiol 1983;51:1128–1132.
7. Butchart EG, Lewis PA, Grunkemeier GL, Kulatilake N, Breckenridge IM. Low risk of thrombosis and serious embolic events despite low-intensity anticoagulation. Experience with 1004 Medtronic Hall valves. Circulation 1988;78(suppl I):66–77.
8. Kuntze CEE, Ebels T, Eijgelaar A, Homan van der Heide JN. Rates of thromboembolism with three different mechanical heart valve prostheses: Randomised study. Lancet 1989;1:514–517.
9. Deviri E, Sareli P, Wisenbaugh T, Cronje SL. Obstruction of mechanical heart valve prostheses: Clinical aspects and surgical management. J Am Coll Cardiol 1991;17:646–650.
10. Copans H, Lakier JB, Kinsley RH, Colsen PR, Fritz VU, Barlow JB. Thrombosed Bjørk-Shiley mitral prostheses. Circulation 1980;61:169–174.
11. Ledain LD, Ohayon JP, Colle JP, Lorient-Roudaut FM, Roudaut RP, Besse PM. Acute thrombotic obstruction with disc valve prostheses: Diagnostic considerations and fibrinolytic treatment. J Am Coll Cardiol 1986;7:743–751.
12. Kontos GJ, Schaff HV, Orszulak TA, Puga FJ, Pluth JR, Danielson GK. Thrombotic obstruction of disc valves: Clinical recognition and surgical management. Ann Thorac Surg 1989;48:60–65.
13. Craige E, Hutchin P, Sutton R. Impaired function of cloth covered Starr-Edwards mitral valve prosthesis. Detection by phonocardiography. Circulation 1970;41:141–148.
14. Quintanilla MA, Haque AK. Thrombotic obstruction of prosthetic aortic valve presenting as acute myocardial infarction. Am Heart J 1987;117:1378–1379.
15. Dollar AL, Pierre-Louis ML, McIntosh CL, Roberts WC. Extensive multifocal myocardial infarcts from cloth emboli after replacement of mitral and aortic valves with cloth-covered, caged-ball prostheses. Am J Cardiol 1989;64:410–411.
16. Daniel WG, Nellessen U, Schröder E, Nonnast-Daniel B, Bednarski P, Nikutta P, Lichtlen PR. Left atrial spontaneous echo contrast in mitral valve disease: An indicator for increased thromboembolic risk. J Am Coll Cardiol 1988;11:1204–1211.
17. Mügge A, Daniel WG, Hausmann D, Gödke J, Wagenbreth I, Lichtlen PR. Diagnosis of left atrial appendage thrombi by transesophageal echocardiography: Clinical implications and follow-up. Am J Cardiac Imag 1990;4:173–179.
18. Pop G, Sutherland GR, Koudstaal PJ, Sit TW, deJong G, Roelandt JRTC. Transesophageal echocardiography in the detection of intracardiac embolic sources in patients with transient ischemic attacks. Stroke 1990;21:560–565.
19. Zenker G, Erbel R, Krämer G, Mohr-Kahaly S, Drexler M, Harnoncourt K, Meyer J. Transesophageal two-dimensional echocardiography in young patients with cerebral ischemic events. Stroke 1988;19:345–348.
20. Kupari M, Tötterman KJ, Ventilä M, Harjula A, Mattila S. Auscultatory and echophonocardiographic characteristics of the normally functioning Medtronic-Hall aortic valve prosthesis. Eur Heart J 1985;6:779–785.
21. Najmi M, Segal BL. Auscultatory and phonocardiographic findings in patients with prosthetic ball-valves. Am J Cardiol 1965;16:794–799.
22. Smith ND, Raizada V, Abrams J. Ausculatation of the normally functioning prosthetic valve. Ann Intern Med 1981;95:594.
23. Joyce LD, Boucek M, McGough EC. Urokinase therapy for thrombosis of tricuspid prosthetic valve. J Thorac Cardiovasc Surg 1983;85:935–937.
24. Wilkinson GAL, Williams WG. Fibrinolytic treatment of acute prosthetic heart valve thrombosis. 5 cases and a review. Eur J Cardiothorac Surg 1989;3:178–183.
25. Boskovic D, Elezovic I, Boskovic D, Simin N, Rolovic Z, Josipovic V. Late thrombosis of the Bjørk-Shiley tilting disc valve in the tricuspid position. Thrombolytic treatment with streptokinase. J Thorac Cardiovasc Surg 1986;91:1–8.

26. Brodie BR, Grossman W, McLaurin L, Starek PJK, Craige E. Diagnosis of prosthetic mitral valve malfunction with combined echo-phonocardiography. Circulation 1976;53:93–100.
27. Wise JR, Webb-Peploe M, Oakley CM. Detection of prosthetic mitral valve obstruction by phonocardiography. Am J Cardiol 1971;28:107–110.
28. Cunha CLP, Giuliani ER, Callahan JA, Pluth JR. Echophonocardiographic findings in patients with prosthetic heart valve malfunction. Mayo Clin Proc 1980;55:231–242.
29. Cambier P, Mombaerts P, DeGeest H, Collen D, Van de Werf F. Treatment of prosthetic tricuspid valve thrombosis with recombinant tissue-type plasminogen activator. Eur Heart J 1987;8:906–909.
30. Venugopal P, Kaul U, Iyer KS, et al. Fate of thromboectomized Bjørk-Shiley valves. A long-term cinefluoroscopic, echocardiographic, and haemodynamic evaluation. J Thorac Cardiovasc Surg 1986; 91:168–173.
31. Chandraratna PAN, Lopez JM, Hildner FJ, Samet P, Ben-Zvi J. Diagnosis of Bjørk-Shiley aortic valve dysfunction by echocardiography. Am Heart J 1976;91:318–324.
32. Hatle L, Angelsen B. Doppler Ultrasound in Cardiology: Physical Principles and Clinical Applications, 2nd edition. Philadelphia, Lea & Febiger, 1985.
33. Koblic M, Carey C, Webb-Peploe MM, Braimbridge MV. Streptokinase treatment of thrombosed mitral valve prosthesis monitored by Doppler ultrasound. Thorac Cardiovasc Surgeon 1986;34:333–334.
34. Curtius JM, Pawelzik H, Mittmann B, Breuer HWM, Loogen F. Normal Doppler echocardiographic values of different types of prosthetic mitral valves. Z Kardiol 1987;76:25–29.
35. Nellessen U, Schnittger I, Appleton CP, et al. Transesophageal two-dimensional echocardiography and color Doppler flow velocity mapping in the evaluation of cardiac valve prostheses. Circulation 1988;78:848–855.
36. Mügge A, Daniel WG, Grote J, Frank G, Lichtlen PR. Morphological assessment of prosthetic valve degeneration, endocarditis, and thrombosis by precordial and transesophageal echocardiography. In: Bodnar E (ed.). Surgery for Heart Valve Disease. London, ICR Publishers, 1990;84–90.
37. Daniel LB, Grigg LE, Weisel RD, Rakowski H. Comparison of transthoracic and transesophageal assessment of prosthetic valve dysfunction. Echocardiography 1990;7:83–95.
38. Daniel WG, Mügge A, Martin RP, et al. Improvement in the diagnosis of abscesses associated with endocarditis by transesophageal echocardiography. N Engl J Med 1991;324:795–800.
39. Daniel WG, Erbel R, Kasper W, et al. Safety of transesophageal echocardiography: A mulicenter survey of 10,419 examinations. Circulation 1991;83:817–821.
40. Guéret P, Fournier P, Chabernaud JM, Lacroix P, Bensaid J. Normal transthoracic echo-Doppler parameters cannot rule out thrombosis of mitral mechanical prosthesis. Demonstration by transesophageal echocardiography. Eur Heart J 1991;12 (suppl. 1): 404 (Abstract).
41. Mügge A, Daniel WG, Frank G, Lichtlen PR. Echocardiography in infective endocarditis: Reassessment of prognostic implications of vegetation size determined by the transthoracic and the transesophageal approach. J Am Coll Cardiol 1989;14:631–638.
42. Huhmann W, Lichtlen PR, Rickards AF, Yacoub M, Borst HG. Hämodynamischer Vegleich von Starr-Edwards-, Lillehei- Kaster- und Homograft-Klappen in Mitralposition. Z Kardiol 1978;67:667–671 (English abstract).
43. Bjørk VO, Henze A, Hindmarsh T. Radiopaque marker in the tilting disc of the Bjørk-Shiley heart valve. Evaluation of in vivo prosthetic valve function by cineradiography. J Thorac Cardiovasc Surg 1977;73:563–569.
44. Godwin RJ. Cineradiographic assessment of Bjørk-Shiley aortic and mitral prosthetic heart valves. Clin Radiol 1977;28:355–360.
45. Albrechtsson UG, Thulin LI, Olin CL. Cineradiographic functional evaluation of the Bjørk-Shiley monostrut prosthesis. Scand J Thorac Cardiovasc Surg 1987;21:91–95.
46. De Wall RA. Thrombotic complications with the Omniscience valve: A current review. J Thorac Cardiovasc Surg 1989;98:298–299.
47. Ohlmeier H, Mannebach H, Greitemeier A. Clinical follow-up of patients after valve replacement with Omniscience cardiac valves: Can this valve be recommended? Z Kardiol 1982;71:350–356.
48. Sigwart U, Schmidt H, Gleichmann U, Borst HG. In vivo evaluation of the Lillehei-Kaster heart valve prosthesis. Ann Thorac Surg 1976;22:213–220.
49. Horstkotte D, Bodnar E. Bileaflet valves. In Bodnar E, Frater RWM (Eds.) Replacement Cardiac Valves. New York, Pergamon Press, 1991;201–228.
50. Acar J, Vahanian A, Dorent R, et al. Detection of prosthetic valve thrombosis using ^{111}-indium platelet imaging. Eur Heart J 1990;11:389–398.
51. Graver LM, Gelber PM, Tyras DH. The risks and benefits of thrombolytic therapy in acute aortic and mitral prosthetic valve dysfunction: Report of a case and review of the literature. Ann Thorac Surg 1988;46:85–88.
52. Karagoz HY, Babacan KM, Zorlutuna YI, Tasdemir O, Yakut C, Bayazit K. In vitro thrombolysis of

thrombosed valve prostheses: Therapeutic considerations of left sided thrombotic lesions. Eur J Cardiothorac Surg 1989;3:87–88.
53. Kurzrock S, Singh AK, Most AS, Williams DO. Thrombolytic therapy for prosthetic cardiac valve thrombosis. J Am Coll Cardiol 1987;9:592–598.
54. Luluaga IT, Carrera D, D'Oliveira J, et al. Successful thrombolytic therapy after acute tricuspid valve obstruction. Lancet 1971;1:1067–1068.
55. Baille Y, Choffel J, Sicard MP, et al. Traitement thrombolytique des thromboses de prothèse valvulaire. Nouv Presse Med 1974;11:1233–1236.
56. Witchitz S, Veyrat C, Moisson P, Scheinman N, Rozenstajn L. Fibrinolytic treatment of thrombus on prosthetic heart valves. Br Heart J 1980;44:545–554.
57. Draur RA. Successful streptokinase therapy of prosthetic aortic valve thrombosis. Am Heart J 1984;108:605–606.
58. Hartzler GO, Diehl AM, Reed WA. Non-surgical correction of a 'frozen' disc valve prosthesis using a catheter technique and intracardiac streptokinase infusion. J Am Coll Cardiol 1984;4:779–783.
59. Prieto-Palomino MA, Ruiz de Elvira MJ, Sanchez-Llorente F. Successful thrombolysis on a mechanical tricuspid prosthesis. Eur Heart J 1989;10:1115–1117.
60. Ayuso LA, Juffe A, Rufilanchas JJ, Babin F, Burgos R, Figuera D. Thrombectomy: Surgical treatment of the thrombosed Bjørk-Shiley prosthesis. J Thorac Cardiovasc Surg 1982;84:906–910.
61. Martinell J, Jimenez A, Rabago G, Artiz V, Fraile J, Farre J. Mechanical cardiac valve thrombosis. Is thrombectomy justified? Circulation 1991;84(Suppl III):70–75.
62. Antunes MJ. Fate of the thrombectomized Bjørk-Shiley valve (letter). J Thorac Cardiovasc Surg 1986;92:956–957.
63. Daniel W, Klein H, Oelert H, Gahl K, Lichtlen P. Echocardiographic diagnosis of thrombus on a Hancock bioprosthesis in mitral position following endocarditis. Thoraxchirurgie 1978;26:413–417.

Chapter 5.2

Recurrent Thromboembolism: Significance and Management

Albert Starr and Gary L. Grunkemeier

This review of our thromboembolism (TE) experience with isolated caged ball valve replacement examines the risks and consequences of recurrent TE. The assumption of constant hazard implied in the use of 'linearised' rates to summarise TE risk is not valid for a series with heterogeneous risk. Rather, the *population* risk of TE decreases with time, which is most reasonably explained by a mixture of constant, but different, individual *patient* risks. The population TE-free curve can be inverted mathematically to reveal the distribution of these individual risks. Risk factor analysis shows that the time to a second TE is related to the severity, but not the timing, of the first. The risk of TE in double valve replacement is less than predicted from an additive risk of the two individual valves. These findings are consistent with the theory that the majority of 'valve-related' TE can be ascribed to patient-related factors, or factors other than the particular type of prosthesis (see Chapter 2.4).

THE PORTLAND EXPERIENCE

A total of 1,593 aortic and 1,032 mitral Starr-Edwards caged ball valves were implanted between 1965 and 1988. These have been followed continuously since implant (Table 5.2–1). This series includes the early cloth-covered and composite-strut 'track' valves, and the current silastic ball valves. In the analysis which follows, TE is defined according to the published guidelines for reporting[1]: valve thrombosis, embolic events secondary to endocarditis, and events occurring within one day of surgery are excluded. However, cerebrovascular events occurring in patients with known cerebrovascular disease, including a history of preoperative stroke, are included. The severity of each event is coded as transient, reversible, permanent, fatal or peripheral.

Statistical methods

For TE-free analysis, both the (non-parametric) actuarial method and the parametric (modelling) method of fitting standard probability distributions to the data are used.

The exponential distribution, the simplest (parametric) lifetime distribution, has only one (scale) parameter, R, and the event-free curve has the equation

$$e^{-R\times t} = \exp(-R\times t),$$

where t is postoperative time. The scale factor R serves to stretch out or compress the curve as it extends through time (horizontally).

Usually only the first embolic event is analysed in a TE-free curve. Embolic events subsequent to the first are evaluated using 'linearised' rates, the total number of TE

Table 5.2–1
Clinical material

	AORTIC		*MITRAL*	
Model	Cloth[1]	Current[2]	Cloth[3]	Current
Implant Years	1967–80	1965–88	1967–80	1965–88
Total Valves	728	865	517	515
Mean Age (years)	55	59	52	57
Male Gender	80%	69%	39%	38%
Followup (years)				
Total	5,704	5,476	4,463	2,856
Mean	7.8	6.3	8.6	5.5
Maximum	22.1	24.5	23.0	25.1
Number of TE				
1	114	114	90	86
2	23	26	26	30
3	6	9	5	6
4+	4	3	4	6
Total TE Patients	147	152	125	128
Total TE Events	196	207	174	188

Starr-Edwards valve models included:
1. 2300, 2310, 2320, 2400
2. 1200, 1260
3. 6300, 6310, 6320, 6400
4. 6120

divided by the total number of valve-years of follow-up. The linearised rate is an appropriate summary statistic only if an event has a constant risk, and if the risk of recurrence is equal to the risk of an original event. It is an estimate of the scale parameter for an exponential TE-free curve.

The Weibull distribution is an extension of the exponential curve that adds an additional (shape) parameter A, which may be regarded as an ageing factor, to accommodate risks that change over time. The Weibull distribution follows the equation

$$\exp(-(R \times t)^A).$$

When A is greater than 1, the risk increases with time (detrimental ageing), and when A is less than 1 the risk diminishes with time (advantageous ageing). When A equals one, the Weibull curve becomes exponential (constant risk through time). In all cases, the event-free curve eventually goes to zero, although it takes an infinite amount of time to do so.

To examine the relationship of certain risk factors with initial TE and recurrent TE, proportional hazards regression is used, in both the (non-parametric) Cox[2] and the (parametric) Weibull[3] models.

Thromboembolism-free curves

Freedom from subsequent TE may be constructed by considering the events 'second TE' and 'third TE' (Fig. 5.2–1). Another approach is to take each TE to be the start of a

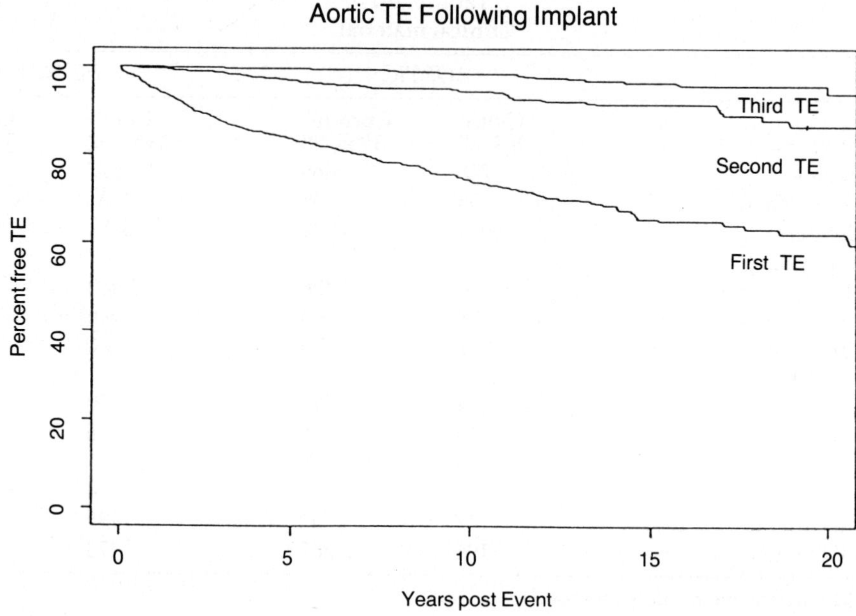

Figure 1A

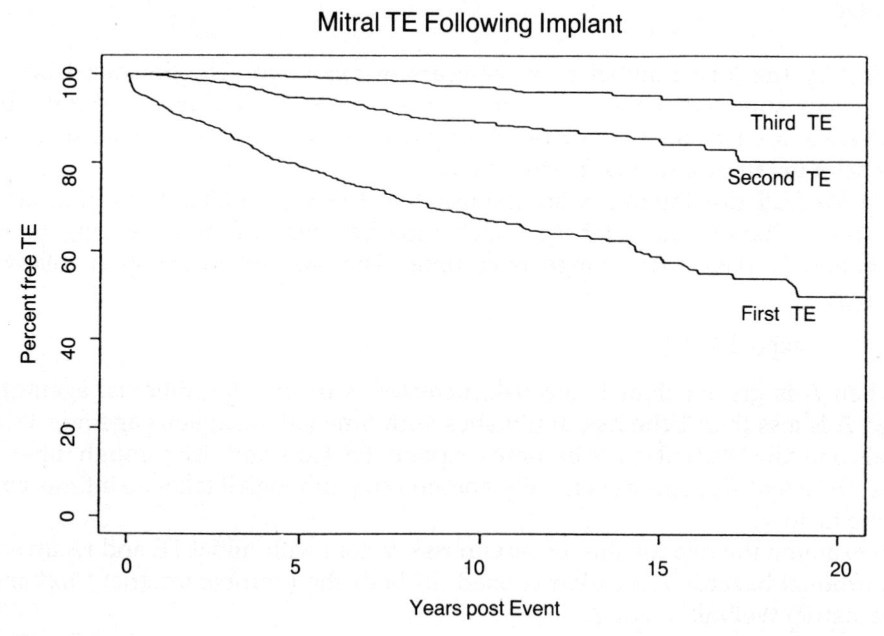

Figure 1B

Figure 5.2–1: Freedom from the first, second and third TE for aortic (A) and mitral (B) valve replacement, starting from the time of surgery. The lower curve is the usual freedom from first TE. The area below the curve represents those free from any TE, and the area above represents those who have had one or more.

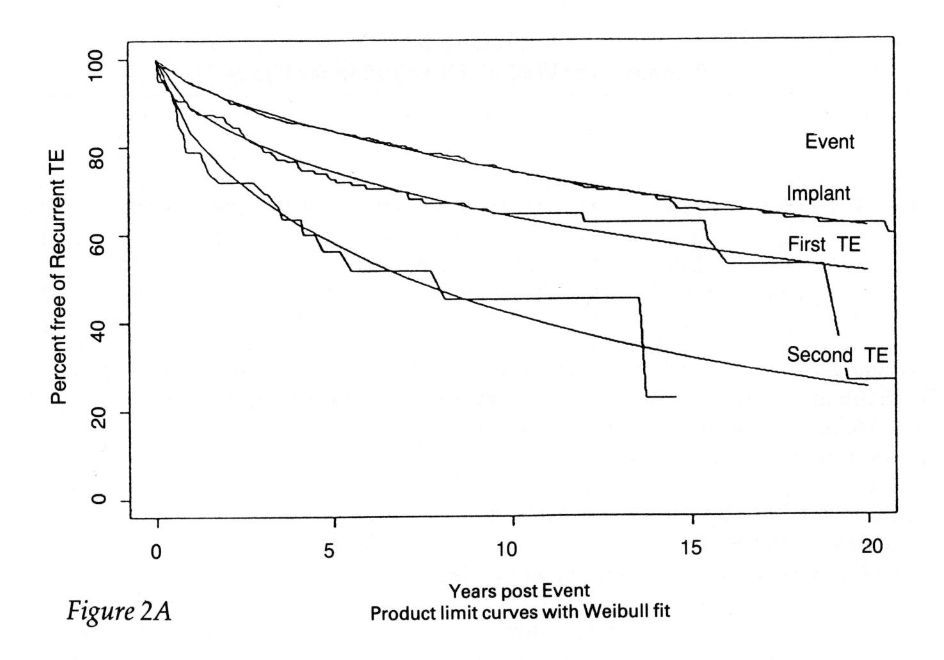

Figure 2A

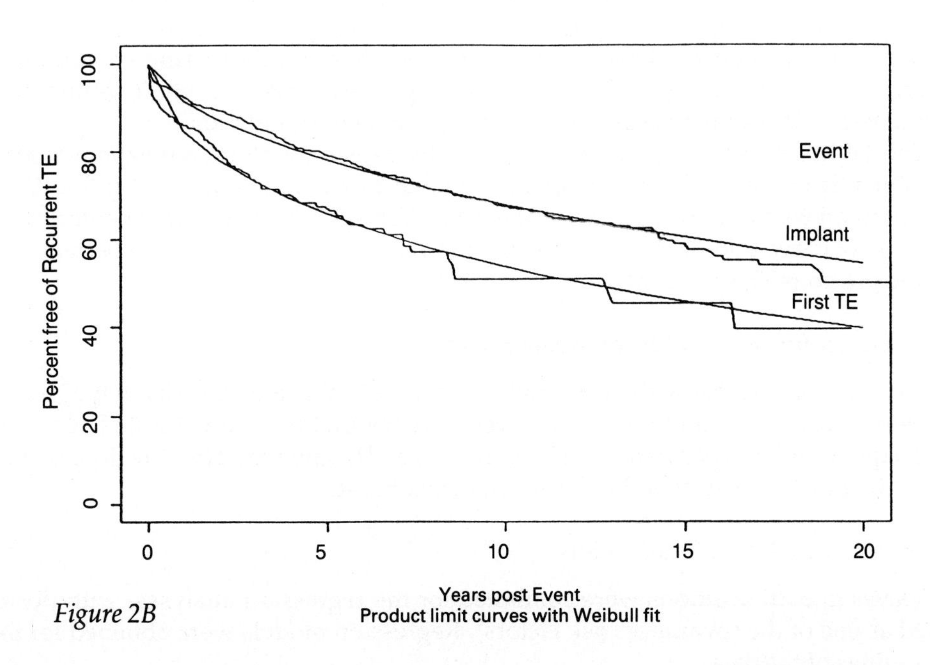

Figure 2B

Figure 5.5–2: Freedom from first and recurrent TE for aortic (A) and mitral (B) valve replacement, starting from the time of surgery or from the time of the previous TE. The curves depict freedom from the first TE after surgery, freedom from a second TE after a first, and (for aortic valve replacement) freedom from a third TE after a second.

Table 5.2–2
Parameters of Weibull Distribution for Figure 2

POS	*TE*	*Valves*	*Valve Years*	*No. TE*	*Coefficients (SE)* *A = Shape*	*R = Scale*	*Years to TE** *Mean*	*SD*	*Median*
AVR	1	1545	9516	295	0.71 (0.035)	0.018 (0.002)	69	100	33
	2	259	1372	70	0.59 (0.061)	0.025 (0.007)	61	111	21
	3	59	206	22	0.68 (0.120)	0.081 (0.029)	16	24	7
MVR	1	1008	5983	248	0.64 (0.036)	0.023 (0.003)	60	97	25
	2	225	977	75	0.57 (0.057)	0.044 (0.011)	37	70	12

SE = Standard error (a measure of the precision with which the coefficient is estimated)
SD = Standard deviation (a measure of the intrinsic variability in the population)
* With Weibull TE-free function in the form $\exp(-(R^*t)^A)$,
the formulas for these statistics are:
Mean $= \Gamma(1 + 1/A)/R$
SD $= [\Gamma(1 + 2/A) - (\Gamma(1 + 1/A))^2]^{1/2}/R$
Median $= [\ln(2)]^{1/A}/R$
where Γ() represents the gamma function (ref. 17).

new experience or 'epoch' and measure freedom from subsequent TE (Fig. 5.2–2). This shows that the risk of a second TE, given the occurrence of a first, is greater than the risk of the first, and sets the stage for a regression analysis of recurrent TE. The pattern for third TE in the mitral position is similar to that for a second, and is not shown. The representations in Figure 5.2–2 are somewhat artificial because patients with lower risk will eventually enter the lower curves and raise them by decreasing or diluting the overall risk; however, the differences among these curves even if temporal, do demonstrate that a mixture of risks exists in the patient population.

The TE-free curves for aortic and mitral valve replacement are not exponential, but exhibit a decreasing hazard. Adequate fits in all cases were found using the Weibull distribution with a shape parameter of 0.6–0.7 (Table 5.2–2). The number entering each successive curve is lower than the number of TE's in the previous curve because some of the previous TE's were fatal.

Risk factors for recurrent thromboembolism

For valves associated with more than one TE, the timing and severity of the second is shown according to the timing and severity of the first in Figure 5.2–3. The risk of a subsequent serious (permanent or fatal) recurrent TE, any time after the first, is shown according to the severity of the first TE in Figure 5.2–4.

Regression analysis of risk factors

Valves in both positions were combined for the regression analyses, with position used as one of the covariates (risk factors). Regression models were obtained for three groupings of the data.

Group 1. Initial TE. All 2553 patients with follow-up times greater than zero (543 with at least one TE after day zero) were used to identify risk factors for initial TE. Risk factors considered were: age, sex, year of implant, valve position, model (silastic or

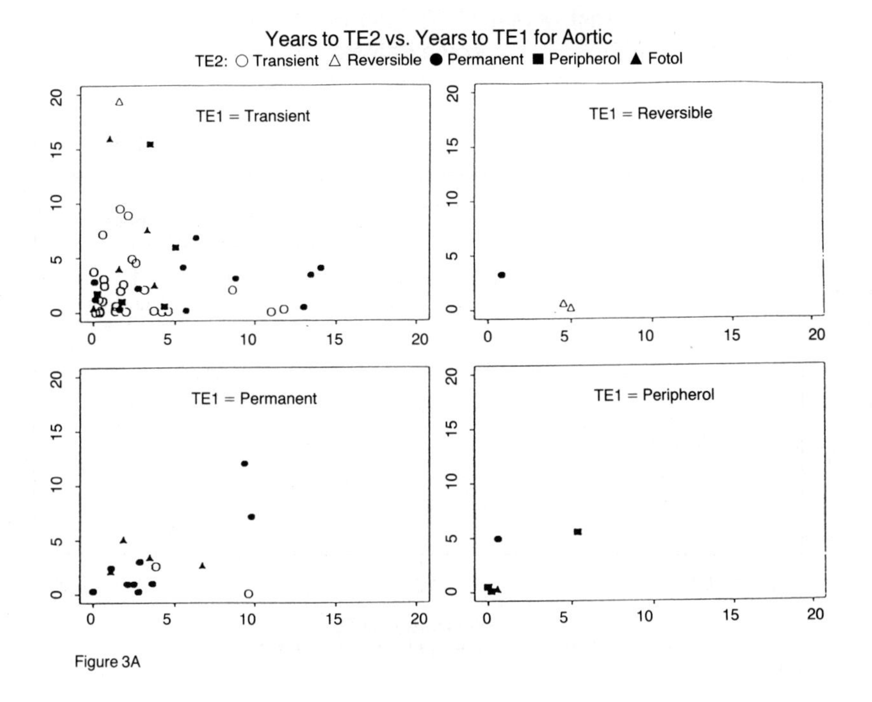

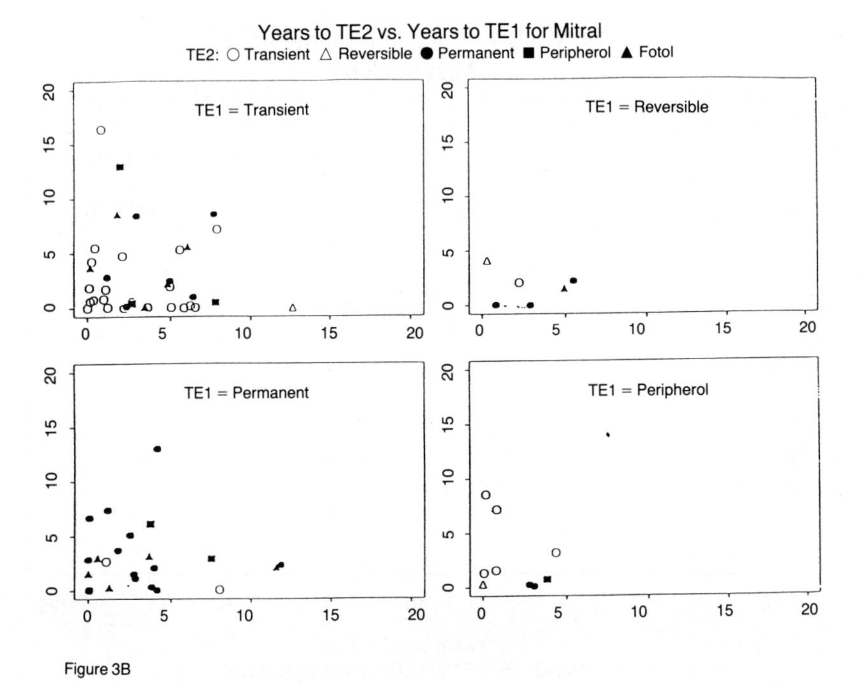

Figure 5.2–3: Years from first to second TE (vertical axis) vs. years from surgery to first TE (horizontal axis) for aortic (A) and mitral (B) valves. The plots are separated according to the severity of the first TE, and the plotted symbols indicate the severity of the second TE.

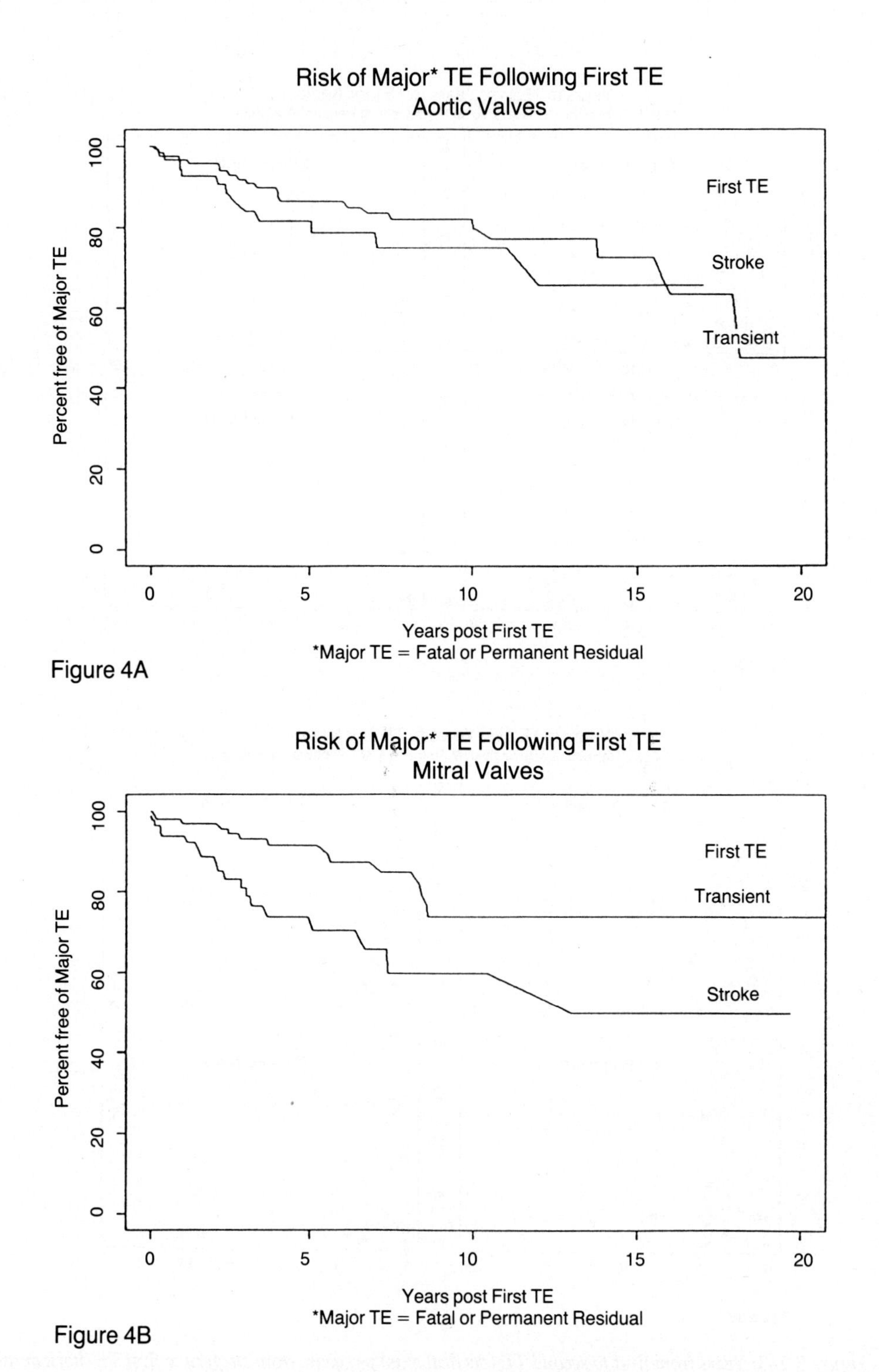

Figure 5.2–4: Risk of ever having a serious TE following a first TE, according to the severity of the first TE for aortic (A) and mitral (B) valve replacement.

cloth), valve size, reoperation, coronary artery surgery and hospital. A univariate analysis identified four significant factors: mitral position, original implant, large valve size and female gender (Table 5.2–3). Only mitral position and original implant were significant in the Cox regression. A proportional hazards Weibull regression was performed using these two factors, resulting in similar coefficients (Table 5.2–3).

Group 2. All TE. In the above analysis, each valve contributed once, up until the time of the first TE, or most recent status. Another Cox regression was run with each valve contributing up to four records, or 'epochs', based on the number of TE's experienced[4,5]. For each of the 484 valves that had a (first) non-fatal TE, the experience was restarted at time zero, and continued until a second TE, death or most recent follow-up. For each of these which had a second TE, the experience was restarted at time zero again, for the third time. For each of those who had a third TE, a fourth record was begun at time zero. Thus up to four TE's were considered for each valve, resulting in 3368 epochs, of which 760 ended in a TE event. A Cox regression was done using the two risk factors identified in step one plus the number of previous TE's (0–3) for each epoch, all of which were significant (Table 5.2–3). This formal test of the effect of number of previous TE's confirmed what is visually obvious from Figure 5.2–2.

Group 3. Recurrent TE. The original epochs, which started at implant (N=2553 in Group 1), were removed from Group 2, leaving only the 743 epochs beginning with a TE, of which 208 ended in a recurrent TE. A Cox regression was done with the three

Table 5.2–3
Risk analysis using Cox and Weibull models

Group 1. All valves, from surgery to first TE

				Multivariate					
	Univariate			*Cox model*			*Weibull Model*		
	coeff.	*se*	*p*	*coeff.*	*se*	*p*	*coeff.*	*se*	*p*
Mitral position	0.286	0.085	0.001	0.285	0.085	0.001	0.282	0.086	0.001
Previous valve	−0.607	0.190	0.001	−0.606	0.190	0.001	−0.633	0.192	0.001
Big valve size	0.030	0.013	0.017						
Female gender	0.187	0.085	0.029						
Constant							−2.382	0.248	0.000
Shape							0.676	0.025	0.000

Group 2. All TE-epochs: from implant to first TE, from each TE to next TE (Cox model)

	coefficient	*se*	*p*
Number of previous TE's	0.404	0.052	0.000
Mitral position	0.270	0.073	0.000
Previous valve	−0.536	0.167	0.001

Group 3. Recurrent TE epochs only: Group 2 minus Group 1 (Cox model)

	coefficient	*se*	*p*
Number of previous TE's	0.333	0.112	0.003
Severity of previous TE	−0.392	0.141	0.005

TE, of which 208 ended in a recurrent TE. A Cox regression was done with the three risk factors from Group 2, plus the time to the most recent previous TE, and the severity of the most recent previous TE. Only the number of previous TE's, and the severity (recoded to a dichotomy: transient/reversible vs. permanent/peripheral) of the most recent TE were significant (Table 5.2–3). The coefficient associated with severity was negative, indicating that a more severe previous TE was associated with a lower risk of subsequent TE.

Individual versus population risk

The decreasing risk of first or recurrent TE (Fig. 5.2–2) is the 'population' risk for the entire series, and may not apply to any individual. The decreasing risk could be explained in two ways: (a) the risk is decreasing with time for each patient, or (b) the risk is constant for each patient, but individual patients have different risks; a combination of (a) and (b) is also possible. The increased risk demonstrated by patients who have more than one TE is consistent with explanation (b).

A mixture of subpopulations with constant, but different, hazard rates will always result in a decreasing population hazard, due to early elimination of patients with relatively high risk. In particular, a Weibull event-free curve with a shape parameter less than 1 (advantageous ageing) can arise from a mixture of exponentials[6,7], and an inversion formula can be used to determine the mixing distribution[8]. Figure 5.2–5 contains the mixing distributions obtained by inverting the initial TE-free Weibull curves in Figure 5.2–2.

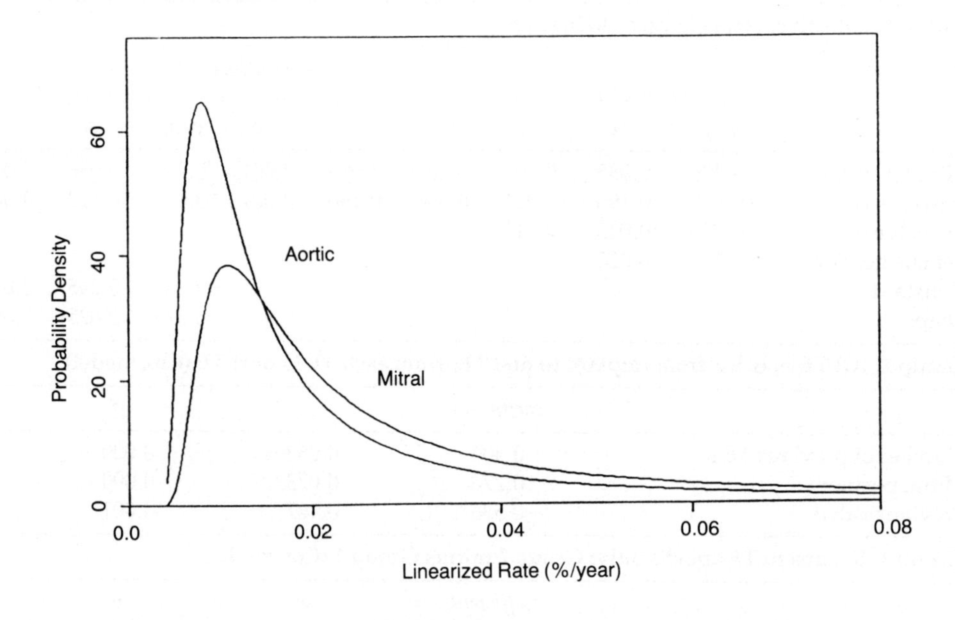

Figure 5.2–5: Risk distribution for initial TE, constructed by an inverse transformation of the Weibull distribution which fits the TE-free curve.

Double valve replacement

Double valve replacement was performed in 267 patients using combinations of the valve models for which the Weibull regression was performed. The empirical TE-free curve for these double valves was compared to that estimated on additive TE risks for the aortic and mitral valves, using the Weibull coefficients for initial TE from Table 5.2–3. The observed risk of TE was less than that predicted by adding the risk for each position (Fig. 5.2–6), consistent with the concept that most of the risk is patient-specific.

Reoperation for multiple thromboembolism

Valve removal was performed for recurrent TE in 17 of the valves in this series, at a mean of 7.5 years (range 3.3 to 23.1 years) post-implant. In 15 cases a porcine valve was used as a replacement device, and in two cases another ball valve. Three patients were reoperated elsewhere and no subsequent follow up was available. The remaining 14 have been followed for a total of 56 patient/years subsequent to their reoperation (93% follow up). There was one non-fatal stroke and one late death, attributed to cerebral haemorrhage. In addition, five patients with various models of the cloth-covered valves underwent thrombectomy, all within two years of implant. Three of these patients, all of whom had received a briefly introduced close-clearance design prone to thrombosis, subsequently died. The other two are alive and well at 11 and 21 years

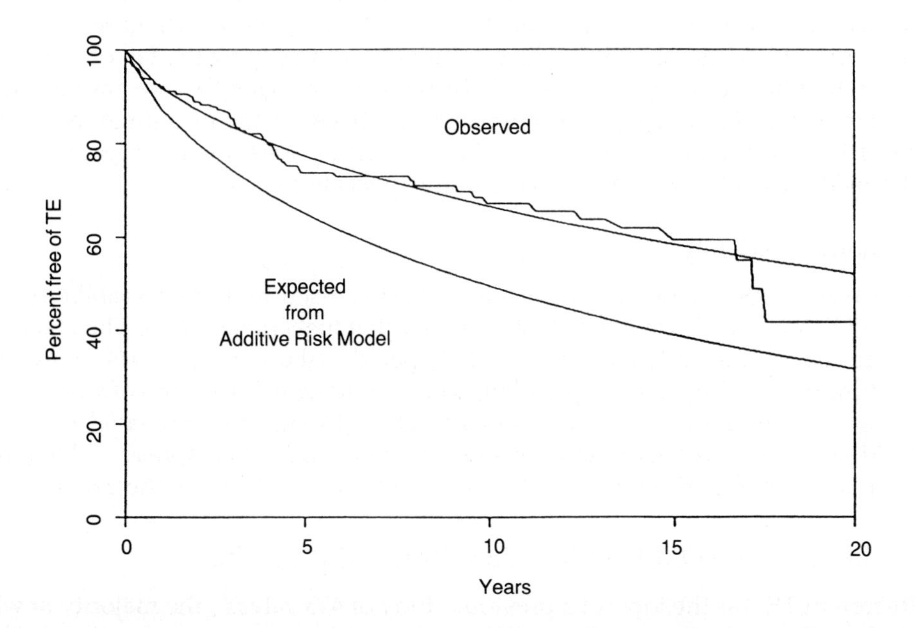

Figure 5.2–6: Freedom from TE for 267 patients undergoing double valve replacement with valve models used in the present series. Stepped line segments represent observed TE-free rates using product-limit method, and smooth line represents the expected TE-free rates based on a model of additive and independent risks.

post-implant, with no further TE. Thus the total experience following surgery for recurrent TE in 16 patients is 88 patient/years, with one stroke.

THE UTILITY OF THROMBOEMBOLISM RISK ANALYSIS

Parametric models

The Cox regression determines which risk factors are important, and provides measures of the risk relative to the underlying risk, but leaves the basic risk unspecified. The parametric method completely specifies the risk, so that an actual estimate or prediction can be given. It provides a smooth, continuous risk model, rather than the discontinuous empirical fit of a particular data set. It allows the calculation of the mean and median times to failure (Table 5.2–2), which otherwise would have to wait until the TE-free curve had dropped to 0% and 50%, respectively. It allows mathematical derivation of other probability functions, such as the inversion transformation which provides the risk mixture distribution, and the expected TE curves for double valves based on the risk of each.

Heterogeneity of TE risk in the Portland experience was expected, since it included several models of the ball valve and spanned a 25 year implant period. The TE curve for a more time-homogeneous group of patients with the same model valve may have a Weibull shape parameter closer to unity, especially if the patients were not followed long enough for the decreasing hazard phenomenon to be demonstrated.

There are also distributions other than the Weibull that could fit these data well and give rise to somewhat different risk distributions than those in Figure 5.2–5. The behaviour of those curves close to zero is influenced mostly by the tail of the TE-free curve, which has not yet been observed. Thus we do not claim that we have found the exact model for TE, but pragmatism encourages its use in the meantime. Newtonian physics is known to be inexact since it does not incorporate quantum features, but it still provides useful approximations for many applications.

Individual uncertainty

The Weibull risk model unfortunately is characterised by large variability (SD) in time to TE, implying low predictability for an individual (Table 5.2–2). The mean does not measure central tendency as for a bell-shaped distribution. The SD is a measure of the intrinsic variability in the population, while the standard error (SE) of an estimate is a measure of the precision of the estimate. Thus, though the estimated risk for an individual may have very good precision (small SE), the spread (SD) among individuals is inherently large, and seems to defy summarisation in the usual sense.

RECURRENT THROMBOEMBOLISM IN OTHER STUDIES

Recurrent TE was the topic of a previous study of 453 valves[9], the majority of which were Starr-Edwards silastic ball prostheses. This study reported results very similar to the Portland experience, including the decreasing risk over time for both initial and recurrent TE. By Cox regression, four variables significantly affected the risk of a first TE: mitral position, atrial fibrillation, left atrial enlargement and poor anticoagulation, but only poor anticoagulation was found to increase the risk of recurrence. The experience following reoperation in 27 of 1436 patients was described as "encouraging", with one TE and four non-TE deaths in 86 patient/years.

A combined series of Starr-Edwards ball valves and porcine valves was examined using Cox regression to evaluate the patient-related factors contributing to the risk of TE[10]. Valve type and previous TE were significant in both aortic and mitral valves, together with age and previous operation for the aortic position and endocarditis and congestive heart failure for the mitral position. Reoperation was associated with a greater risk of TE, in contrast to the Portland experience, in which reoperation was a negative risk factor for TE. This unexpected result in the Portland series may be due to selection; patients who underwent reoperation clearly could not have experienced a fatal TE with their original valve and, since they received a mechanical valve as their second or subsequent prosthesis, they probably had no particular factors predisposing to TE.

A recent series consisting mainly of Starr-Edwards aortic valves, including both cloth-covered and silastic ball models[11], described clinical material and mean follow-up very similar to the Portland series, but with somewhat better TE-free rates of 85% at 10 years and 82% at 15 years. At a mean follow-up of 6.5 years, there were 69 embolic events in 55 patients (1.25 TE per TE-patient), while the Portland aortic series had 1.35 TE per TE-patient at a mean of 7.0 years. Only kidney failure was a significant factor for TE by Cox regression.

A Cox regression analysis of TE and thrombosis in 839 Medtronic Hall valves found age and preoperative regurgitation in the aortic position and female sex in the mitral position to be significant[12]. Cumulative hazard curves for TE in this series appear to be markedly concave downward, supporting our contention that TE risk decreases with time.

A recent publication[5], which evaluated experience after mitral commissurotomy, but included a comprehensive analysis of recurrent TE, strongly influenced our choice of analytical methods. Corresponding to our Cox analysis of Group 2, the number of previous TE's was an extremely significant risk factor for recurrent TE. This is confirmatory evidence of the heterogeneity of risk, and implicates non-valve factors, since the patients in this series did not receive a prosthesis.

These published studies support the concepts (a) that patient factors have a considerable influence on thromboembolism, and (b) that the population risk diminishes over time. These are related concepts, since a mixture of different, but constant, individual risks produces a declining population risk. There is much current research on describing heterogeneity of risk in biological populations[8,13–15]. However, the challenge is to identify the particular risk factors responsible for the heterogeneity, and measure their relative importance.

PATIENT MANAGEMENT AFTER RECURRENT THROMBOEMBOLISM

The overall strategy in managing recurrent TE must be based on the premise that there is a broad spectrum of patient-related susceptibility to TE. Unless a detailed preoperative risk factor profile has been performed, the location of a particular patient within this spectrum is unknown; a postoperative TE declares a patient to be at higher risk and helps refine his treatment options. The optimal response to the occurrence of TE varies according to the number of events, the valve position, any patient-related risk factors and the anticoagulation status. Although very satisfactory results have been achieved with valve re-replacement for recurrent TE, the need to resort to reoperation is relatively rare unless recurrent TE is associated with valve thrombosis.

As seen from this review, the occurrence of a first event marks the patient as being in a high risk group for subsequent TE, and therefore must be taken very seriously. If anticoagulation control has been poor, efforts must be made to improve it. If the patient is already well controlled, dipyridamole should be added (see also Chapter 3.4). A baseline CT scan of the brain, to look for scars from previous silent events, and a review of the preoperative clinical history should be carried out. The occurrence of preoperative neurological events increases the likelihood that the TE was caused by conditions other than the prosthesis.

With a second TE the patient assumes an even higher location along the risk spectrum. The evidence implicating the valve versus the patient as the most likely cause of the TE must be weighed. Before considering a change of prosthesis, it is vital to exclude patient factors, which would not be altered by changing the prosthesis, as being responsible for the TE. A CT scan of the brain and carotid Doppler studies should be carried out and a search made for possible causes of hypercoagulabilty which may be remediable (Chapter 1.5). Stopping dipyridamole and adding aspirin increases the risk of bleeding (Chapter 3.1) but may be justified in certain high risk patients.

With a mitral patient in atrial fibrillation, there is a strong probability that the valve itself is not at fault, unless it is obstructive and failing to relieve conditions of stagnation within the left atrium (Chapters 2.4 and 2.6); if there is no significant mitral prosthetic gradient and no evidence of thrombus on the prosthesis, one should be reluctant to reoperate. With an aortic patient in sinus rhythm, the presence of carotid disease would similarly inhibit reoperation.

If it seems that the valve is at fault and that reoperation is the best therapy, the patient should be evaluated with respect to the risk of reoperation. It is justifiable to be more aggressive with aortic than mitral patients, since there are fewer non-valve related factors to be considered. One should be reluctant to explant an aortic valve after two minor embolic events, but if the CT scan reveals additional scars in comparison to a baseline scan, one should be correspondingly more aggressive. However, if a preoperative CT scan is not available, it should not be forgotten that untreated calcific aortic stenosis is associated with the presence of silent cerebral infarcts on CT scan in a significant percentage of patients[16]. In our own practice, we would almost certainly operate on an aortic Starr Edwards valve after a third TE.

If thrombus is found on the valve, simple debridement should be considered, depending on the operative findings (see Chapter 5.1). When re-replacement is performed, a heterograft bioprosthesis should not be an automatic choice, but the usual age threshold for using a tissue valve should be lower in this situation. A homograft valve, depending on availability, would be an attractive option.

REFERENCES

1. Edmunds LH, Clark RE, Cohn LH, Miller DC, Weisel RD. Guidelines for reporting morbidity and mortality after cardiac valvular operations. Ann Thorac Surg 1988;46:257–259.
2. Cox DR. Regression methods and life tables. J Roy Stat Soc 1972;34:187- 220.
3. Aitkin M, Clayton D. The fitting of exponential, Weibull, and extreme value distributions to complex censored survival data using GLIM. Appl Statist 1990;29:156–163.

4. Prentice RJ. Williams BJ, Peterson AV. On the regression analysis of multivariate failure time data. Biometrika 1981;68:373–379.
5. Hickey MSJ, Blackstone EH, Kirklin JW, Dean LS. Outcome probabilities and life history after surgical mitral commissurotomy: implications for balloon commissurotomy. JACC 1991;17:29–42.
6. Jewell NP. Mixtures of exponential distributions. Ann Stat 1982;10:479- 484.
7. McNolty F, Doyle J, Hansen E. Properties of the mixed exponential failure process. Technometrics 1980;22:555–565.
8 Hougard P. Survival models for heterogeneous populations derived from stable distributions. Biometrika 1986;73:387–396.
9. Acar J, Enriques-Sarano M, Farah E, Kassab R, Tubiana P, Roger V. Recurrent systemic embolic events with valve prosthesis. Eur Heart J 1984;5(Suppl D):33–38.
10. Mitchell RS, Miller DC, Stinson EB, Oyer PE, Jamieson SW, Baldwin JC, Shumway NE. Significant patient-related determinants of prosthetic valve performance. J Thorac Cardiovasc Surg 1986;91:807–817.
11. Lund O, Pilegaard HK, Magnussen K, Knudsen MA, Nielsen TT, Albrechtsen OK. Long-term prostheses-related and sudden cardiac-related complications after valve replacement for aortic stenosis. Ann Thorac Surg 1990;50:396-406.
12. Abdelnoor M, Hall JK, Nitter-Hauge S, Rostad H, Risum O. Morbidity in valvular heart repacement: risk factors of systemic emboli and thrombotic obstruction. Int J Artif Organs 1988;11:303–307.
13. Manton KG, Stallard E, Vaupel JW. Alternative models for the heterogeneity of mortality risks among the aged. J Am Stat Assoc 1986;81:635–644.
14. Aalen OO. Heterogeneity in survival analysis. Stat Med 1988;7:1121–1137.
15. Clayton D. The analysis of event history data: a review of progress and outstanding problems. Stat Med 1988;7:819–841.
16. Davidson CJ, Skelton TN, Kisslo KB et al. The risk of systemic embolization associated with percutaneous balloon valvuloplasty in adults. Ann Intern Med 1988;108:557–560.
17. Cohen AC, Whitten BJ. Parameter Estimation in Reliability and Life Span Models. New York, Marcel Dekker, 1988:26.

Chapter 5.3

Management of Cerebral Haemorrhage in Patients with Prosthetic Heart Valves: The Place of Surgical Treatment

A. David Mendelow

The neurosurgical view of stroke in patients with prosthetic heart valves is necessarily narrow. There are many more strokes that occur in these patients than are referred for neurosurgical care. This is because a percentage of patients will die rapidly of the initial ictus. A further percentage develop cerebral infarction that is not amenable to surgical treatment. Although cerebral infarction is the commonest cause of stroke in these patients, it will not be considered in any further detail here, because embolectomy is rarely performed and even less frequently successful. Some guidelines for management based on the CT scan appearance are proposed in Table 5.3–1.

The neurosurgical problem therefore is confined to those patients with intracerebral haemorrhage (ICH) and subarachnoid haemorrhage (SAH) who survive the initial event. This group should also be considered in the context of the many other causes of ICH seen in neurosurgical departments. Probably the commonest cause is hypertension, but anticoagulant-associated haemorrhage now accounts for about a quarter of all

Table 5.3–1
Management plan for stroke patients based on CT scan

CT finding	*Initial action*	*Response*	*Subsequent action*
Infarction:	Continue anticoagulants	– Improve	– Continue anticoagulants
		– Deteriorate	– Repeat CT – if haemorrhagic transformation then proceed as for haemorrhage
Haemorrhage:	Stop anticoagulants	– Surgery considered	– Factors II, VII, IX and X – Consider vitamin K (Chapter 5.4)
		– Identify cause	– Treat cause (eg aneurysm, AVM)
		– Improve	– Reintroduce anticoagulants when stable

cases of spontaneous ICH admitted to neurosurgical wards. This includes patients on warfarin for venous thrombosis and pulmonary embolism as well as patients on heparin for a variety of indications. Ruptured berry aneurysms and arteriovenous malformations are also common and sometimes are the underlying cause of an anticoagulant related bleed. Other causes of haemorrhage include blood dyscrasias, vasculitides, cerebral amyloid angiopathy and alcoholism[1].

DIAGNOSIS

The first priority in any patient presenting with a cerebral episode is to confirm the diagnosis. The initial presentation may take the form of a sudden headache with or without loss of consciousness. One of the first signs of haemorrhage may be a focal epileptic seizure. Alternatively, the patient may present with a focal neurological deficit or coma. In any of these situations, it may be impossible to differentiate an infarct from a haemorrhage on clinical grounds alone. Imaging techniques are therefore essential and either computer tomographic (CT) or magnetic resonance (MR) imaging will clarify the cause. CT is usually reliable, but on occasions an isodense ICH may appear very similar to an infarct (Fig. 5.3–1). Although infarction is often correctly diagnosed on CT (Fig. 5.3–2), only haemorrhage is considered in detail in this chapter. CT will usually be the first investigation and will clarify the nature of the haemorrhage, which may be subarachnoid (Fig. 5.3–3), intracerebral (Fig. 5.3–4), intraventricular (Fig. 5.3–5) or subdural (Fig. 5.3–6).

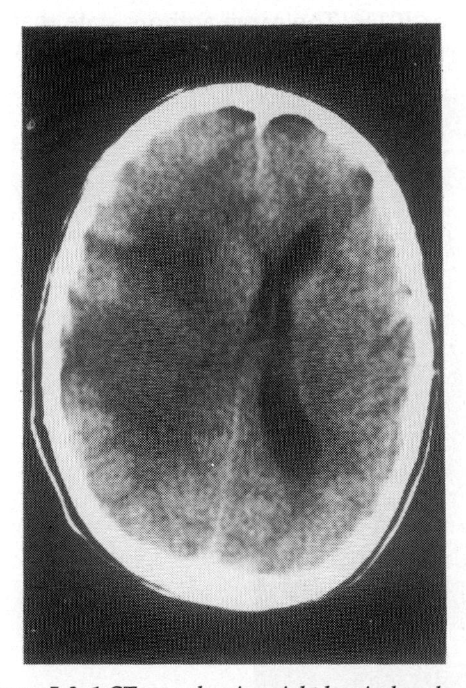

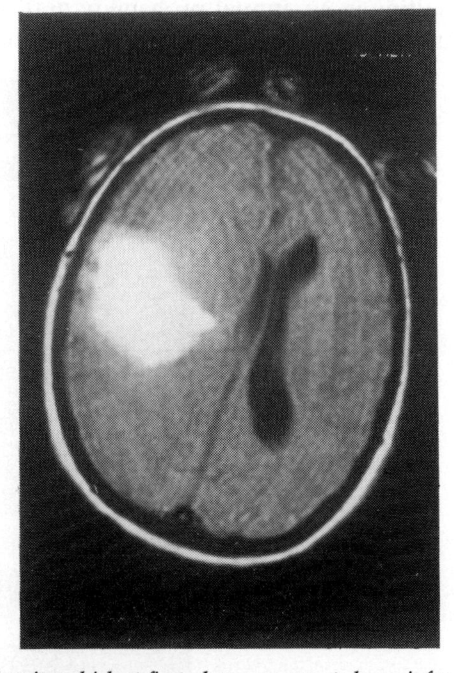

Figure 5.3–1 CT scan showing right hemisphere low density which at first glance appears to be an infarct: subsequent MR scan (right) showed that this in fact was an isodense intracerebral haematoma with surrounding oedema.

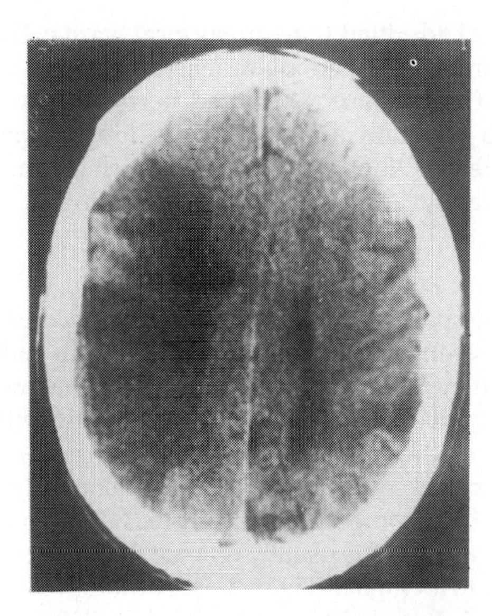

Figure 5.3–2 CT scan showing large intra-cerebral infarction.

INCIDENCE

The annual probability of haemorrhage in patients on anticoagulants with prosthetic heart valves was quoted as 0.043 in one risk analysis with 12% being intracerebral, resulting in an annual probability of 0.005 for ICH[2]. The same authors state that the annual probability of subdural haemorrhage (SDH) is somewhere between 0.00043 and

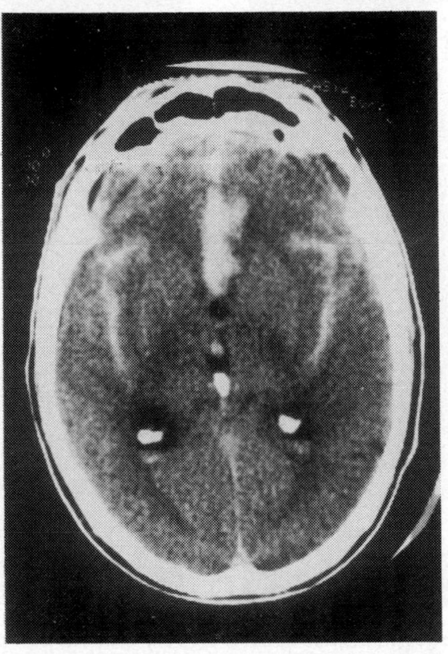

Figure 5.3–3 CT scan showing typical subarachnoid haemorrhage with blood in the Sylvian fissure and interhemispherically.

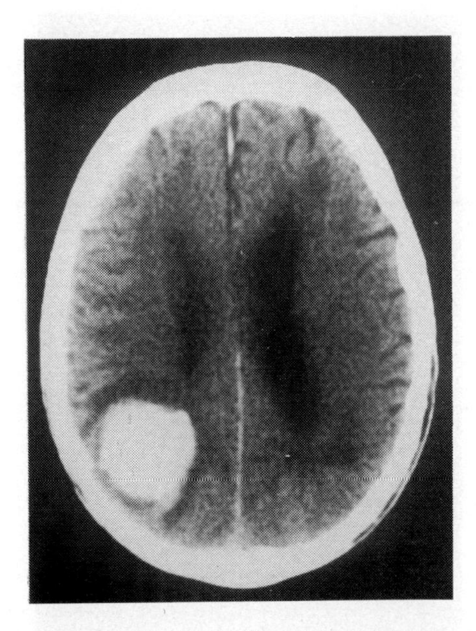

Figure 5.3–4 CT scan showing large intracerebral haematoma.

0.0083. The combined probability of ICH and subdural haemorrhage therefore should be less than 0.013 (see also Chapter 5.4). However, because such a small percentage of intracranial haemorrhages (ICH + SDH) are in anticoagulated patients with prosthetic heart valves, accurate epidemiological data are sparse and have not been well documented. Data from neurosurgical and neurological units are flawed because of the selection criteria that have resulted in these patients being referred. In a recent study[1]

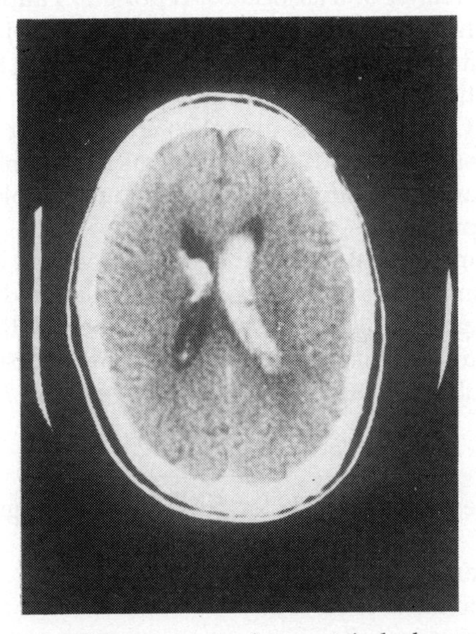

Figure 5.3–5 CT scan showing intraventricular haemorrhage.

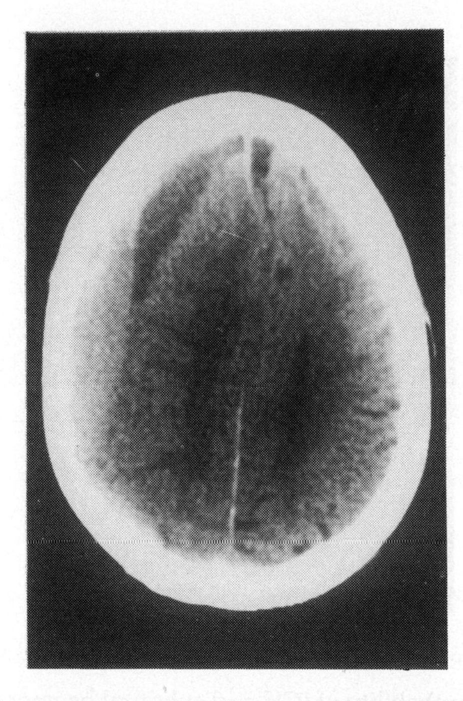

Figure 5.3–6 CT scan showing chronic subdural haematoma (anteriorly) with a separate more recent subacute subdural haematoma lying on the same side more posteriorly.

six of 100 patients with ICH were on warfarin, although it was not stated why they had been anticoagulated.

The incidence of ICH is quoted as 14 per 100,000 per annum (0.014%) in one study from the Netherlands[3]. Franke and associates[4] reported 79 anticoagulant related ICHs, also from the Netherlands, of which 38 arose from one hospital that provided 14,000 anticoagulant treatment years during the same period, giving an annual risk of ICH of 271 per 100,000 population per treated year (0.271% per year): this represents a 19-fold increase in the risk of ICH for patients on anticoagulants. For SDH, the risk has been assessed as being increased four- to 13-fold[5]. It seems reasonable, therefore, to describe the risk of ICH on anticoagulants as being about tenfold that of ICH in the non-anticoagulated population.

The duration of treatment did not appear to be as important in Franke's study as was thought previously[4]. Similarly, the degree of anticoagulation did not seem to influence the risk of haemorrhage: an all or none phenomenon with a low threshold was suggested. With subdural haematomas about one third of cases occur within the first six months of anticoagulation[5], but ICH may occur even after 10 years of treatment.

MANAGEMENT

For a patient with established ICH or SAH on anticoagulants, there are three problems:

1) Should anticoagulants be stopped? If so, for how long?
2) Should the haematoma be removed?
3) Is there an underlying cause?

Reversal of anticoagulants

Because of the often devastating consequences of ICH, all neurosurgeons would agree that anticoagulation should be reversed for patients with documented ICH. Franke and associates[4] recommend immediate intramuscular vitamin K with coagulation factors II, VII, IX and X for those with large clots or a depressed level of consciousness. By contrast, in a patient with a chronic subdural haematoma with preserved level of consciousness in whom surgery is *not* contemplated, it may be sufficient just to stop anticoagulants and watch the patient. In the patient in Fig. 5.3–6 with two densities of chronic subdural haematoma, stopping the anticoagulants for four days was sufficient to permit delayed surgery without resorting to vitamin K and factor concentrates. In general, most neurosurgeons prefer to delay the reintroduction of anticoagulation for at least 10 days after any surgical treatment. Further postponement may be necessary if there is a requirement for angiography or elective surgery for aneurysm or delayed complications like hydrocephalus (vide infra).

Should the haematoma be removed?

Formal controlled trials of the treatment of the haematoma itself have not been well evaluated because of the difficulty in finding comparative groups of well matched but untreated patients. Opinions are therefore divided about the need for surgical evacuation: some are enthusiastic[6,7] whereas others are not[8]. There is a wide spectrum of cases of ICH, and it is not possible to generalise about treatment except at the extremes. Few neurosurgeons doubt that delayed deterioration in a young patient with a subcortical haematoma is an indication for surgery, whereas most would not contemplate the evacuation of a large dominant hemisphere haematoma in an elderly patient who has been in coma with fixed dilated pupils from the outset. The dilemma lies between these two extremes.

Sakas[9] has suggested that surgical evacuation should be reserved for those with Glasgow Coma Scale scores between six and eight, although no control group was studied. McKissock's original study indicated that there was no overall benefit from surgery, with the results of the surgically treated group being slightly worse than in the non-surgical group[10]. However, that study was in the pre-CT era, and better localisation should now lead to improved results from surgery. Volpin and associates[11] related the outcome to the size of the haematoma, reporting that lesions larger than 85 ml were almost always fatal, while survival was more likely with surgical evacuation of haematomas of about 50 ml volume on CT scan.

It has been postulated that haematomas in patients on anticoagulants will be larger than those in patients not on anticoagulants, but Franke and associates[4] found that once a haematoma had occurred it was not significantly more serious than in patients who were not anticoagulated. Kanno and associates[12] reported 459 patients and showed that overall there was no difference between surgical and non-surgical patients. Results tended to be better with more laterally sited lesions and if surgical treatment was undertaken within six hours of the ictus. Juvela and associates[13] reported the results of a prospective randomised controlled study and showed no benefit from surgical treatment.

There has been an increase in the number of reports of surgical treatment with stereotaxic aspiration[14–20]. However, randomised trials have not yet identified a definite role for this surgical technique. The possibility of inducing liquefaction of the clot with intra-cavity urokinase has also been considered[21], but not evaluated. The first prospective randomised controlled study to suggest that surgical treatment is superior to medical treatment came from Auer and co-workers[22] who showed that endoscopic aspiration resulted in a mortality of 46% compared with a mortality of 70% in the medically treated group. The high mortality in the medically treated group indicates the importance of matching patients in a prospective randomised trial. Whether these results are reproducible has yet to be seen, because endoscopy is not in routine use in most neurosurgical units.

Treatment of the underlying cause

If ICH is associated with a berry aneurysm, there is a high risk of recurrent haemorrhage. For this reason, if a haematoma appears to be near the circle of Willis or its branches (Fig. 5.3–7), exclusion of an underlying structural lesion becomes a priority and angiography is often performed acutely. In other cases angiography may be delayed until the patient recovers. This may reveal an aneurysm or arteriovenous malformation. In such a situation it is advisable *not* to re-introduce anticoagulants until after definitive surgery, which may have to be delayed sometimes for months, according to the patient's condition. If angiography is negative, it is probably safe to re-introduce anticoagulation.

CONCLUSIONS

Because of the uncertainty about surgical treatment of ICH, and the almost anecdotal data about anticoagulant-related ICH, trials of surgical treatment need to be undertaken urgently. Once it is established whether or not operative treatment is

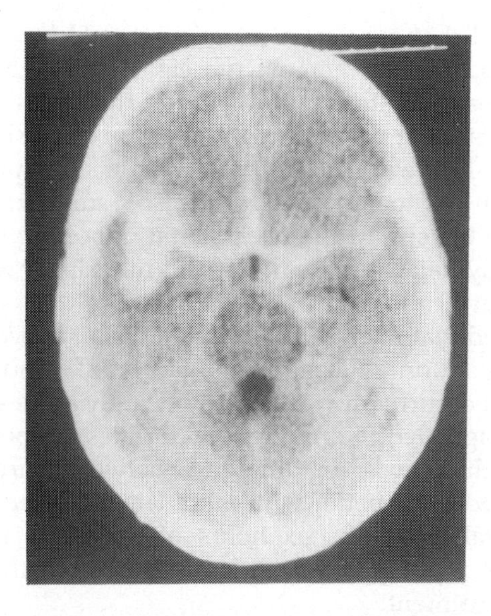

Figure 5.3–7 CT scan showing subarachnoid haemorrhage with small intracerebral haemorrhage in the Sylvian fissure from a ruptured middle cerebral artery aneurysm.

indicated in the majority of patients with ICH, it should be possible to design trials to answer the questions about the cessation and re-introduction of anticoagulants in high risk patients with prosthetic heart valves. In the meantime, measures should be taken to reduce the risk of ICH in these patients by using anticoagulation intensities no higher than necessary for their specific prosthesis and their own risk factors (see Chapter 3.4), by rigorously treating hypertension[23,24] and by giving advice about alcohol consumption[25,26].

REFERENCES:

1. Schutz H, Bodeker RH, Damian M et al. Age-related spontaneous intracerebral haematoma in a German community. Stroke 1990;21:1412–1418.
2. Wong JB, Webb RK, Pauker SG. Double-trouble: a patient with two prosthetic valves and two episodes of intracranial bleeding. Med Decis Making 1987;7:174–193.
3. Herman B, Layten ACN, Van Luyk JH et al. Epidemiology of stroke in Tilburg, the Netherlands: the population based stroke incidence register: 2. Incidence, initial clinical picture and medical care, and three week case fatality. Stroke 1982;13:629–634.
4. Franke CJ, de Jonge J, van Swieten JC et al. Intracerebral haematomas during anticoagulant treatment. Stroke 1990;21:726–730.
5. Mattle H, Kohler S, Huber P et al. Anticoagulation-related intracranial extracerebral haemorrhage. J Neurol Neurosurg Psych 1989;52:829–837.
6. Kanaya H, Yukawa H, Kanno T et al. A neurological grading for patients with hypertensive intracerebral haemorrhage and a classification for haematoma location on computed tomography. In: Proceedings of the 7th Conference on Surgical Treatment of Stroke. Tokyo, Neuron, 1978:265–270.
7. Kaneko M, Tanaka K, Shimada T et al. Long-term evaluation of ultra-early operation for hypertensive intracerebral haemorrhage in 100 cases. J Neurosurg 1983;58:838–842.
8. Dei-Anang K. Kramer G, Besser R et al. Treatment of spontaneous intracerebral haemorrhage – operative or conservative? Radiologe 1989;29:423–426.
9. Sakas DE, Singounas EG, Karvounis PC. Spontaneous intracerebral haematomas: surgical versus conservative treatment based on Glasgow Coma Scale score and computer tomography data. J Neurosurg Sci 1989;33:165–172.
10. McKissock W, Richardson A, Taylor J. Primary intracerebral haemorrhage. A controlled trial of surgical and conservative treatments in 180 unselected cases. Lancet 1961;2:221–226.
11. Volpin L. Cervellini P, Colombo F et al. Spontaneous intracerebral haematomas: a new proposal about the usefulness and limits of surgical treatment. Stroke 1984;15:663–666.
12. Kanno T, Sanno H, Shinomiya Y et al. Role of surgery in hypertensive intracerebral haematoma. J Neurosurg 1984;61:1091–1099.
13. Juvela S, Heiskanen O, Poranen A et al. The treatment of spontaneous intracerebral haemorrhage. A prospective randomized trial of surgical and conservative treatment. J Neurosurg 1989;70:755–758.
14. Hayashi M, Hasegawa T, Kobayashi H et al. Aspiration of hypertensive intracerebral haematoma by stereotactic technique. No Shinkei Geka 1981;9:1365–1371.
15. Hondo H. CT-guided stereotactic evacuation of hypertensive intracerebral haematomas. A new operative approach. Tokushima J Exp Med 1983;30:25–39.
16. Lunsford LD, Martinez AJ, Latchaw RE. Stereotaxic surgery with a magnetic resonance and computerized tomography-compatible system. J Neurosurg 1986;64:872–878.
17. Tanizaki Y, Sugita K, Toriyama T et al. New CT-guided stereotactic apparatus and clinical experience with intracerebral haematomas. Appl Neurophysiol 1985;48:11–17.
18. Tanikawa T, Amano K, Kawamura H et al. CT-guided stereotactic surgery for evacuation of hypertensive intracerebral haematoma. Appl Neurophysiol 1985;48:431–439.
19. Shiwaku T, Tanikawa T, Amano K et al. A new treatment of hypertensive intracerebral haematoma: a follow-up study on 46 patients with haematoma treated by CT guided stereotactic method. No Shinkei Geka 1986;14:751–758.
20. Honda E, Hayashi T, Shimamoto H et al. A comparison between stereotaxic operation and conservative therapy for thalamic haemorrhage. No Shinkei Geka 1988;16(Suppl 5):665–670.
21. Niizuma H, Otsuki T. Johkura H et al. CT-guided stereotactic aspiration of intracerebral haematoma: result of a haematomalysis method using urokinase. Appl Neurophysiol 1985;48:427–430.
22. Auer LM, Deinsberger W, Niderkjorn K et al. Endoscopic surgery versus medical treatment for spontaneous intracerebral haematoma: a randomised study. J Neurosurg 1989;70:530–535.
23. Feldmann E. Intracerebral hemorrhage. Stroke 1991;22:684–691.
24. MacMahon S, Peto R, Cutler J et al. Blood pressure, stroke and coronary heart disease. Part 1,

prolonged differences in blood pressure: observational studies corrected for the regression dilution bias. Lancet 1990;335:765–774.
25. Camargo CA. Moderate alcohol consumption and stroke. The epidemiologic evidence. Stroke 1989;20:1611–1626.
26. Gorelick PB. The status of alcohol as a risk factor for stroke. Stroke 1989;20:1607–1610.

Chapter 5.4

Anticoagulant-Related Bleeding

Gordon D. O. Lowe and Isobel D. Walker

BLEEDING AND THROMBOSIS IN A POPULATION CONTEXT

Throughout life, we are threatened by both bleeding and thrombosis, processes which appear to be in a state of balance. All of us bleed, especially after trauma, surgery and invasive medical procedures; 'spontaneous' bleeding also occurs commonly, sometimes from lesions shown by endoscopy or radiology, but often from no identifiable local or haematological cause. Careful necropsy studies have suggested that both arterial and venous thrombosis are also very common, and increase with age. Minimal risk of both bleeding and clotting occurs with an optimal balance of cardiovascular integrity and function of platelets, coagulation and fibrinolysis.

The balance between bleeding and thrombosis is well illustrated by congenital haemophiliacs (one in 10,000 of the population), who have a relative risk of coronary heart disease of only 20% compared to non-haemophiliacs, and consequently a longer average life expectancy if the haemophilia is mild[1]. On the other hand, the congenital haemophiliac exchanges the risk of thrombosis for a higher incidence of morbidity and mortality from bleeding, especially if the haemophilia is severe. Such excessive bleeding may be 'spontaneous' or follow trauma, surgery, invasive medical procedures or use of antihaemostatic drugs such as aspirin; intracranial, gastro-intestinal and retroperitoneal haemorrhage are the commonest causes of death[1,2].

In the general population, all major factors for thrombotic cardiovascular disease (smoking, obesity, blood pressure, cholesterol and triglyceride) are associated with increased blood coagulability (as measured by plasma levels of fibrinopeptide A, a measure of thrombin activity), as well as an imbalance of blood coagulation over fibrinolysis (as measured by the ratio of fibrinopeptide A to the fibrin fragment β15–42, a measure of plasmin activity)[3]. Such imbalances may reflect the associations of risk factors with increased levels of clotting factors (fibrinogen, factor VII, factor VIII) or inhibitors of fibrinolysis (plasminogen activator inhibitor) which are also predictors of coronary heart disease.

Long term oral anticoagulant therapy is effective in the prophylaxis of thromboembolism complicating non-valvular atrial fibrillation, venous thromboembolism and recurrent arterial thrombosis[4]; and is under evaluation (in low doses) for primary prophylaxis of arterial thrombosis in high-risk persons[5]. However, the price of long term anticoagulation is increased bleeding tendency: the 'iatrogenic haemophiliac' resembles the congenital haemophiliac in his or her increased risk of bleeding. Such bleeding may likewise be 'spontaneous', or follow trauma, surgery, invasive medical procedures or aspirin; with intracranial, gastro-intestinal and retroperitoneal bleeding being the commonest causes of death[4–9].

MANAGEMENT OF THE 'IATROGENIC HAEMOPHILIAC'

Like the congenital haemophiliac, patients on anticoagulants must be carefully educated, regularly monitored at audited, specialised clinics with experienced staff, and have easy access to hospitals with adequate diagnostic services, to include computerised tomographic (CT) scanning, endoscopy, coagulation screening and therapeutic services for management of potentially fatal or disabling haemorrhage (resuscitation, provision of blood and blood products, and provision of endoscopic and surgical haemostatic procedures including evacuation and control of intracranial haematomas).

As with the congenital haemophiliac, the first questions which should be asked when an anticoagulated patient develops a new symptom are:

- is it a bleed?
- how do I confirm or exclude a bleed?
- what local measures are required to stop bleeding?
- is reduction or reversal of the coagulation defect required?
- is replacement of blood required?

Intracranial bleeding is the most feared site of bleeding. Suspected stroke in anticoagulated patients requires rapid diagnosis of stroke type (eg. by CT scanning) for appropriate management, which is described in Chapter 5.3. Gastro-intestinal bleeding occurs in 9–22% of patients on anticoagulants, often from peptic ulcers (including ulcers induced by non-steroidal anti-inflammatory drugs) or neoplasms. In a recent series[9], 50% of bleeds occurred from the upper and 30% from the lower gastro-intestinal tract. An identifiable site of bleeding was found in 81% of patients with upper, but in only 52% with lower tract bleeding. No bleeding site was detectable in 47% of patients, even after full investigation. Haematuria is common, and related to the intensity of anticoagulant effect; it may however occur from an identifiable urinary tract lesion such as a tumour. Retroperitoneal haemorrhage requires a high index of suspicion for diagnosis, and may be fatal[8].

THE HEART VALVE PATIENT: A SPECIAL CASE

Patients with heart valve prostheses present particular problems in anticoagulation management. As discussed throughout this book, they have long been recognised to have an increased risk of fatal or disabling thromboembolism. However, because of the historical mandatory use of long term anticoagulants to reduce this risk, there is a lack of randomised placebo-controlled trials of anticoagulant prophylaxis[4,7,10]: placebo-controlled trials may not be ethically possible. As a result, we do not know accurately the balance between thromboembolic complications on the one hand, and the haemorrhagic complications of long term anticoagulation on the other. These opposing risks must be balanced in the heart valve patient, and also considered in the context of the background incidence of both bleeding and thromboembolism in the general population (as shown, for example, in the placebo groups of randomised controlled trials of oral anticoagulants in other studies[4]).

Despite the uncertain magnitudes of these risks (see Section 6 of this book), clinicians must try to minimise the risks of both bleeding and thromboembolism in patients anticoagulated because of heart valve disease or valve prostheses. This chapter reviews the risks of bleeding with long-term oral anticoagulants, and the variables which influence these risks. Recognition and monitoring of these variables are important parts of reducing the risk of bleeding in patient management. The second part of this chapter considers the management of bleeding, as well as the prevention of bleeding in patients who are over-anticoagulated, traumatised or undergo surgery or invasive procedures. Bleeding associated with the perioperative period of heart surgery has been discussed in Chapter 1.7, and will not be considered here.

OVERALL RISK OF BLEEDING ON LONG TERM ANTICOAGULANTS

The overall risk of bleeding in patients taking long term oral anticoagulants is difficult to estimate for several reasons. Firstly, definitions of bleeding severity such as 'minor', 'major' or 'life-threatening' differ between reported series. Major bleeding is what matters, and it seems reasonable to define this as that which is either fatal, intracranial, retroperitoneal, or which requires hospitalisation, blood transfusion or blood products and/or surgical intervention. Minor bleeding, such as bruising, nose-bleeds, haematuria or bleeding haemorrhoids is up to ten times commoner than major bleeding, but is much less important.

Secondly, different series vary greatly as to patient selection, duration of follow up, and especially the intensity of the anticoagulation. As regards the latter, clinicians in North America have tended to use higher intensities of anticoagulation than clinicians in Europe; they have also been slower to adopt the International Normalised Ratio (INR) for reporting prothrombin time results[4].

Thirdly, as previously stated, there is a lack of randomised, placebo-controlled trials to assess the relative risks of bleeding and thromboembolism in patients with heart valve disease or prostheses. However, an estimate can be made from the increase in bleeding risk in placebo-controlled trials of long term oral anticoagulants in other groups of patients.

Fourthly, different series have expressed the risk of bleeding in different ways: for example, percentage of patients who bled (with or without reporting the exposure time – see Chapter 6.2); cumulative incidence of bleeding with time (arguably the most important to the patient); or incidence of bleeding per 100 patient-years of follow-up (the conventional way to express risks, which is followed in this volume).

Levine and colleagues[7] calculated the overall risk of major bleeding per 100 patient-years in several groups of patients receiving long term anticoagulants. Few of the 53 descriptive studies of patients with prosthetic heart valves which they reviewed gave adequate data for reliable estimates of bleeding risk: these authors therefore concentrated on five randomised controlled trials of oral anticoagulants versus either oral anticoagulants plus antiplatelet drugs, or less intense oral anticoagulants[11–16]. However, the risk of bleeding per hundred patient-years could only be calculated for two of these studies. The bleeding risks were as follows:

Patient group	*Major bleeds/100 patient years*
Prosthetic heart valve patients	0.8
Post-myocardial infarction patients	0–7.7
Cerebrovascular disease patients	2–22

The confidence intervals for these estimates in these various patient groups are clearly wide, and also overlap. The problems in comparing series add to the uncertainty of comparisons. Whether patients with cerebrovascular disease have a greater risk of bleeding has been questioned by other authors[6].

Data from two recent randomised trials of intensity of long term anticoagulation in patients with prosthetic heart valves[17,18] are consistent with an estimated risk of major bleeding of 1–2 per 100 patient years. Based on these figures, a patient with a valve prosthesis taking long term oral anticoagulants for 30 years has about a 50% chance of a major bleeding complication. While reinforcing the need for careful monitoring to minimise bleeding risk, this increased risk of bleeding must be weighed against the protection which anticoagulants afford, not only against thromboembolism from the heart, but also against venous thromboembolism and arterial thrombosis[4]: two major health risks in western societies.

Risk factors for bleeding: The four D's

It is useful to group the variables which affect bleeding risk on long term anticoagulants into the 'four D's:

(1) *Dose* of anticoagulants, resulting in intensity of anticoagulant effect on the blood (reduction in plasma activity levels of coagulation factors II, VII and X, and hence prolongation of the prothrombin time and INR; levels of factor IX are also reduced but this does not affect the prothrombin time).
(2) *Drugs* which either interact with oral anticoagulants or vitamin K, enhancing their effect, or which interfere with other haemostatic factors (see Chapter 3.2).
(3) *Diseases*, such as peptic ulcer, neoplasms or liver disease.
(4) *Demographic* variables, such as age and sex. Other variables which influence bleeding risk include patient compliance, and the practice and performance of the anticoagulant clinic (see Chapters 3.5–3.7).

Dose of anticoagulants and intensity of anticoagulant effect

There is good evidence that the higher the dose (and therefore the anticoagulant effect), the greater the risk of bleeding. Such evidence is derived from three types of study.

1. Relation of bleeding to dose/intensity of anticoagulant effect

Loeliger and colleagues[19] summarised the largest reported experience of bleeding during out-patient anticoagulant therapy; that of the Dutch Thrombosis Centres, including the Sixty-Plus Reinfarction Study[20] and the large British clinic study of Forfar[21] (see Fig. 4.3–2). The risk of bleeding increased exponentially with the intensity of anticoagulation, as measured by the INR. The annual incidence increased from about 1.6% in the older non-anticoagulated population (as estimated by the incidence in the placebo group of the Sixty-Plus Study[20,22]), to about 5% (relative risk 3) at an INR of 2.5, and to about 50% (relative risk 30) at an INR of 4.0. Fuster and colleagues[23] reported that 50% of their bleeding complications occurred when the INR was greater than 7.5.

2. Intensity of anticoagulant effect at the time of major bleeding

Several studies have observed that in patients with major bleeding (for example intracranial bleeding), the INR was higher than in patients without such bleeding[6,7,17,18,21–25]. For example, Forfar[21] reported that the prothrombin time was prolonged beyond the therapeutic range in 23 of 24 episodes of life-threatening haemorrhage, and Petty and colleagues[6] in eight of 13 patients with life-threatening or fatal bleeding.

3. Randomised trials of higher- and lower-intensity oral anticoagulants

Four recent randomised comparative trials have each shown that higher-intensity regimens were associated with a higher risk of bleeding than lower-intensity oral anticoagulants, and with no apparent decrease in the risk of thromboembolic events (although there is a possibility of a type II statistical error with the latter conclusion in each study).

In patients with proximal deep vein thrombosis treated for three months, Hull and colleagues[26] observed 11 bleeding episodes in 49 patients given a higher-intensity regimen (target INR 2.5–4.1) and two bleeding episodes in 47 patients receiving a lower intensity regimen (target INR 2.0–2.3) (bleeding incidence 22.4% versus 4.2%, $p<0.02$).

In patients with bioprostheses, Turpie and associates[16] observed 60 bleeding episodes, 20 major, in patients receiving a higher-intensity regimen (target INR 2.5–4.0) and 24 bleeding episodes, none major, in patients receiving a lower-intensity regimen (target INR 2.0–2.25).

In patients with mechanical prosthetic valves, Saour and colleagues[17] observed 12.1 bleeding episodes per 100 patient-years, 2.1 major, in patients given a higher-intensity regimen (target INR 7.4–10.8), and 6.2 bleeding episodes per 100 patient-years, 0.95 major, in patients receiving a lower-intensity regimen (target INR 1.9–3.6).

In another recent trial in patients with mechanical prosthetic valves, Altman et al[18] observed 24.7 bleeding episodes per 100 patient-years in patients given a higher-intensity regimen (target INR 3.0–4.5), and 3.8 bleeding episodes per 100 patient-years in patients receiving a lower-intensity regimen (target INR 2.0–3.0). In this study, all patients also received aspirin and dipyridamole.

In summary, there is now substantial evidence that the intensity of oral anticoagulation is a major determinant of bleeding risk. It may therefore be appropriate to choose lower-intensity target ranges (e.g. INR 2.0–3.0) to minimise the risk of bleeding, especially in patients with additional risk factors for bleeding and/or lower risk of thromboembolism. On the other hand, higher intensity regimens (e.g. target INR 3.0–4.5) may be appropriate in patients at higher risk of thromboembolism, especially if they do not have additional risk factors for bleeding. The concept of prosthesis-specific and patient-specific anticoagulation is discussed further in Chapter 3.4.

Drug interactions and risk of bleeding

Many drugs interact with oral anticoagulants, for example by changing their plasma levels or by affecting vitamin K metabolism. Such interactions are discussed in Chapter 3.2 and in recent reviews[4,26,27]. Some drugs which interfere with platelet function, like aspirin and other non-steroidal anti-inflammatory drugs also increase the risk of bleeding in patients taking oral anticoagulants.[4,7,12-15] This effect of aspirin and other non-steroidal anti-inflammatory drugs may also reflect their ulcerogenic actions on the gastro-intestinal tract[4]. On the other hand, it is possible that the antithrombotic effects of combining lower-intensity oral anticoagulants with low doses of aspirin or newer anti-platelet agents, for example ticlopidine, may outweigh their bleeding risks. Future trials are required to assess this possibility.

The addition of dipyridamole to oral anticoagulants does not appear to increase the risk of bleeding, but reduces the risk of embolism in studies of patients with older mechanical prostheses[28] (see also Chapters 3.1 and 3.4).

Diseases increasing the risk of bleeding

It has long been recognised that co-morbid conditions increase the risk of bleeding in patients receiving anticoagulant treatment. In a large recent study, history of stroke, gastro-intestinal bleeding, atrial fibrillation, recent myocardial infarction, severe anaemia or renal failure were each associated with an increased risk of bleeding[24,25]. Other studies, but not all[6], have also suggested an increased risk of intracranial bleeding in patients with cerebrovascular disease[7,8,20,22], possibly because of a higher incidence of intracranial aneurysms associated with cerebrovascular disease or its two main risk associations: age and hypertension. However, hypertension was not associated with intracranial bleeding in the Sixty-Plus Study[22].

The increased risk of bleeding in renal failure may also reflect associated hypertension, as well as the associated impairment in primary haemostasis (low haematocrit, which reduces platelet adhesion and aggregation, and decreased intrinsic platelet function). The increased risk of bleeding in severe anaemia may also reflect impaired primary haemostasis or, alternatively, unsuspected disease (eg. malignancy or chronic blood loss from ulcerating lesions, especially in the gastro-intestinal tract). Other haemostatic disorders which increase the risk of bleeding include thrombocytopenia, von Willebrand's disease, haemophilia, liver disease and alcoholism (which as well as liver disease is associated with poor compliance with oral anticoagulant medication, low platelet counts, increased fibrinolysis and increased risk of peptic ulcer).

When considering the initiation, intensity and duration of anticoagulant therapy in patients with these conditions, clinicians should weigh the increased risk of bleeding against the risk of thromboembolism, which may also be increased in some of these diseases (eg. thromboembolic stroke, atrial fibrillation, or recent myocardial infarction). The important question is not the extent to which these conditions increase bleeding risk on anticoagulants, but to what extent the balance between thromboembolic risk and bleeding risk is affected by anticoagulation in the individual patient. For example, the reduction in risk of thromboembolic stroke by anticoagulants may outweigh the increased risk of haemorrhagic stroke, resulting in an overall reduction in morbidity and mortality[19,20,22] (see also TEB index in Chapter 6.4).

It is important to search for an underlying lesion as the cause of bleeding in patients on oral anticoagulants, because anticoagulation may unmask its presence. One series[24,25] suggested that patients who bled while their anticoagulant effect was within the target range were more likely to have such lesions than patients who bled while over-anticoagulated. However, as previously discussed, in many patients no lesion is found even after thorough investigation[9]. This is also true in congenital bleeding disorders (haemophilia and von Willebrand's disease), and in such patients the systemic bleeding disorder is presumably largely responsible for the bleeding episode.

Intercurrent trauma, surgery (including dental extraction) or invasive procedures also increase the risk of bleeding in anticoagulated patients; reduction or reversal of anticoagulant effect to prevent bleeding in such circumstances is considered below.

Demographic factors and the risk of bleeding

Age is the most important demographic factor which may affect the risk of bleeding on long term oral anticoagulants. While some series report age as a risk factor for bleeding[24,25,29,30], others have failed to find such a correlation[7,19,21,22,31,32]. Because the risk of thromboembolism also increases strongly with age, the question is not the extent to which anticoagulant-related bleeding increases with age, but rather to what extent the balance between thromboembolic risk and bleeding risk is affected by anticoagulants in the individual patient. Because of the high thromboembolic risk, anticoagulants are often positively indicated in older patients, rather than contraindicated solely because of age[33]. The special problems of anticoagulants in the elderly are considered further in Chapter 4.3.

Sex does not appear to relate to the bleeding risk in patients on long term anticoagulants[22], and there is no information on racial or national differences in bleeding rates, other than the higher intensity of anticoagulation traditionally practised in the United States[4].

CONCLUSIONS ON THE RISK OF ANTICOAGULANT-RELATED BLEEDING IN HEART VALVE PATIENTS

Both thromboembolism and bleeding are common in the general population, in whom there is evidence for a balance between haemostasis and thrombosis. Anticoagulation reduces thromboembolic risk, but increases the risk of bleeding. Both thromboembolic and bleeding risks are increased in patients with heart valve disease or heart valve prostheses, who for many years have been treated arbitrarily with high-dose, long term anticoagulants. The balance between bleeding risk and antithrombotic benefit is poorly defined because of the lack of randomised placebo-controlled trials. The risk of bleeding (as well as the anti-thrombotic effect) depends on the intensity of anticoagulant effect (which in recent years has been more precisely defined using the INR), concurrent use of other drugs, especially antiplatelet agents, concurrent diseases or trauma, and possibly old age.

Future studies of the incidences of bleeding and thromboembolism should therefore record all these variables. Future randomised trials should either stratify for these variables where practicable, or else allow for their effects in multivariate analysis. Further randomised trials are required to assess whether or not lower-intensity regimens of oral anticoagulants (with or without antiplatelet drugs) reduce bleeding risk without reducing antithrombotic efficacy. One randomised trial in patients with mechanical prosthetic valves (intensity of anticoagulation unstated) found that warfarin was more effective in prevention of thromboembolic complications than aspirin (relative risk reduction 60–79%), but carried a higher risk of bleeding[4,34]. Optimal antithrombotic prophylaxis (ie. that with the lowest risks of both thromboembolism and bleeding) in patients with heart valve disease or heart valve prostheses remains to be defined[4,10]. Perhaps the most important study would be one of four groups of patients; warfarin at a target INR of 2.0–3.0, warfarin at a target INR of 3.0–4.5, and each of these two groups with the addition of low-dose aspirin.

MANAGEMENT OF ANTICOAGULANT RELATED BLEEDING

Haemorrhage in an anticoagulated patient is a potentially life threatening emergency and medical or surgical units responsible for such patients must formulate clear guidelines for the management of patients presenting with major or minor bleeding or found at routine or chance investigation to have an excessively high INR.

At the initial institution of anticoagulant therapy patients require information and advice about the signs and symptoms of bleeding and to whom these should be reported. They must understand the potential hazards of anticoagulant therapy and the requirement of regular monitoring, and they must appreciate that changes in their general health, life-style or concomitant medication may potentiate the effect of their oral anticoagulant and require dose adjustment. Advice about analgesics which they may self-administer with relative safety (eg. those containing dextropropoxyphene hydrochloride or paracetamol) for minor aches or trauma should be offered.

Management of acute bleeding

Unexpected bleeding from any site should stimulate an immediate check of the current INR. Patients with a bleed serious enough to prompt hospital admission should in addition have blood grouping and antibody screening tests performed. If bleeding is massive, recurrent or prolonged assessment of full blood count indices is valuable.

Management of the bleeding episodes will depend on a number of factors including the site and severity of the bleeding, the INR level, the general medical condition of the patient and the reason for anticoagulation.

The following approaches may be considered either in isolation or in combination:

(a) Simply stopping anticoagulant therapy for a few days. In some patients with venous thrombotic disorders permanent cessation of therapy may be possible, but in patients with prosthetic heart valves discontinuation can only be temporary.
(b) Replacement of clotting factors by plasma products containing vitamin K dependent factors.
(c) Reversal of anticoagulation by administering vitamin K.
(d) Supportive measures including blood volume and/or red cell replacement if indicated.

Any recommendation on the reversal of anticoagulant therapy must take into account the potential risk of thrombus formation, particularly on the artificial valve in patients with prostheses, and particularly if the coagulant defect is over-corrected with vitamin K. On the other hand plasma products, and in particular fresh frozen plasma which at present is not subjected to viral inactivation procedures, carry the risk of transmitting hepatitis and/or human immunodeficiency viruses. Bearing in mind these risks, and recognising that in the average patient at least six to eight hours must be allowed for an adequate clinical response to vitamin K_1, the following recommendations are made.

If bleeding is potentially life threatening and the prothrombin time is prolonged, the anticoagulant should be withheld and the coagulation defect corrected by the infusion of plasma products. In the United Kingdom, for patients with no evidence of liver disease, a concentrate of factors II, IX and X in a dose calculated on the basis of 50 IU of factor IX/kilogram body weight is recommended[26]. Factor VII concentrate may be preferable and potentially less thrombogenic but it is not widely available. If no concentrate is readily available, or if the patient has evidence of hepatic dysfunction, fresh frozen plasma should be used (about 1 litre for an adult), but this may not be fully effective and may be problematic in patients with poor cardiac reserve, unable to tolerate the volume. Patients with massive bleeding may require supportive measures including blood transfusion.

It is generally recommended that administration of vitamin K to reverse anticoagulation should be avoided in patients with prosthetic heart valves. However, if the INR is significantly elevated and the bleeding is life threatening or persistent, some centres may consider using vitamin K_1. For life threatening haemorrhage the British Society for Haematology[26] has recommended immediate administration of 5 mgs of vitamin K_1 by slow intravenous infusion, in addition to factor II, IX and X concentrate.

In North America 5–10 mg of vitamin K_1 by subcutaneous injection is widely used. Doses of more than 10 mg of vitamin K_1 cause the patient to become refractory to further anticoagulation with vitamin K antagonists for an unpredictable period of time but for at least several days. Where haemorrhage is persistent but not life threatening, a smaller dose of 0.5–2.0 mg vitamin K_1 may be considered, but as already stressed should be used only after very careful consideration.

Less severe haemorrhage such as epistaxis or haematuria in patients with a prolonged prothrombin time may require no intervention other than local measures (such as nasal packaging) if appropriate, and withholding anticoagulation for one or more days to allow bleeding to stop and the INR to return to the therapeutic range.

Once the immediate danger is past and bleeding stopped or settling, plans for future management must be discussed. Patients with artificial heart valves require long term anticoagulation but steps must be taken to minimise the risk of recurrent bleeding. Anticoagulation must be reinstated as soon as possible. If the bleeding was associated with elevated INR levels, the patient must be questioned carefully about recent changes in medication, prescribed and self-administered, changes in life-style or changes in diet or alcohol intake. Anticoagulation therapy should be reintroduced aiming for an INR towards the lower limit of the recommended target range and carefully monitored. Advice about concomitant medication, diet and alcohol should be repeated.

All patients who bleed, whether bleeding occurred in association with an INR in the target therapeutic range or with an elevated INR, merit investigation to determine whether or not they have underlying pathology requiring treatment. Patients with gastrointestinal or urinary tract malignancy, or with non-malignant ulceration or diverticulae may first present while on oral anticoagulant therapy[24,25]. These lesions obviously require treatment in their own right but also to minimise the risk of recurrent bleeding.

If bleeding recurs in patients with no evidence of underlying pathology and while their target INR is within the therapeutic range, it may, in some instances, be necessary to accept a reduction in the intensity of anticoagulation and maintain the INR between 2.0 and 2.5.

Management of excessive anticoagulation with no bleeding

Management of a patient with a prosthetic heart valve who is not bleeding but found by chance or at routine monitoring to have an INR above the therapeutic range may be problematic. Obviously an INR deemed to be only slightly above the recommended range is usually most simply dealt with by withholding anticoagulation therapy for one or more days and rechecking the INR as it falls back into the desired range. Unfortunately, there are no clear data on which to base a recommendation about an INR limit, up to which it may be relatively safe not to actively reverse anticoagulation in a patient who is not bleeding and who may be managed by temporarily withholding anticoagulation only. Advice on the management of excessively anticoagulated patients who are not bleeding is therefore quite arbitrary.

In the UK and many other countries, the recommended INR range for patients with prosthetic heart valves is currently 3.0–4.5 for mechanical valves and 2.0–3.0 for bioprostheses[26] (see Chapter 3.4). The British Society for Haematology recommends that if the INR exceeds 7.0, consideration should be given to vitamin K_1 administration, 0.5 mg by slow intravenous injection. In North America an INR of 10 is usually held to be the threshold for active intervention. If the INR exceeds 10, vitamin K_1 in a dose of 2.5–5.0 mg may be given orally, in addition to withholding anticoagulant. Oral vitamin K_1, however, may produce a variable response. The INR should be checked after 24 hours and daily thereafter, and anticoagulation reintroduced as soon as possible. In patients with prosthetic valves, vitamin K_1 should only be given after full discussion with the cardiac surgeon concerned.

A recently published study of patients with elevated INRs (5.6–25.9), who were not bleeding and were given either 1.0 mg or 0.5 mg vitamin K_1 intravenously, showed that 0.5 mg vitamin K_1 resulted in INR values of 5.5 or less 24 hours after injection and in none did the INR fall to below 2.0[35]. The authors suggest that 0.5 mg vitamin K_1 given slowly intravenously should be effective in the majority of individuals with raised INRs who are not bleeding but who require reasonably rapid correction of excessive anticoagulation, and in whom it is important not to prejudice the timely reinstatement of adequate anticoagulant therapy.

Preparation for surgery or dental extraction

Even minor surgical procedures and dental extractions may be associated with troublesome bleeding if these are performed under high intensity anticoagulation. Randomised studies[36] have shown that the bleeding risk is relatively low if the INR on the day of the operation is between 2.0 and 2.5, but the risk and degree of bleeding clearly depends on the type and extent of the surgery. An INR in this range may usually be achieved by withholding anticoagulant for one to two days before operation. If necessary, plasma products may be used to reverse anticoagulation for surgery in an emergency situation, aiming for an INR of 2.0–2.5. A cost analytical approach to this problem based on risk/benefit assessment is discussed in Chapter 4.5.

REFERENCES

1. Rosendaal FR, Varekamp I, Smit C, et al. Mortality and causes of death in Dutch haemophiliacs, 1973–86. Br J Haematol 1989;71:71–76
2. Bloom AL. Inherited disorders of blood coagulation. In: Bloom AL, Thomas DP (eds): Haemostasis and Thrombosis, 2nd edition. Churchill Livingstone, Edinburgh 1987:393–436
3. Lowe GDO, Wood DA, Douglas JT, et al. Relationships of plasma viscosity, coagulation and fibrinolysis to coronary risk factors and angina. Thromb Haemostas 1991;65:339–343
4. Hirsh J. Oral anticoagulant drugs. N Engl J Med 1991;324:1865–1875
5. Meade TW, Wilkes HC, Stirling Y, Brennan PJ, Kelleher C, Browne W. Randomized controlled trial of low dose warfarin in the primary prevention of ischaemic heart disease in men at high risk: design and pilot study. Eur Heart J 1988;9:836–843
6. Petty GW, Lennihan L, Mohr JP, et al. Complications of long term anticoagulation. Ann Neurol 1988;23:570–574
7. Levine MN, Raskob G, Hirsh J. Hemorrhagic complications of long term anticoagulant therapy. Chest 1989;95, Suppl 2:26S–36S
8. Mackie MJ, Douglas AS. Drug-induced disorders of coagulation. In: Ratnoff OD, Forbes CD (eds): Disorders of Haemostasis, 2nd edition. WB Saunders, Philadelphia 1991:493–517
9. Wilcox CM, Truss CD. Gastrointestinal bleeding in patients receiving long term anticoagulant therapy. Am J Med 1988;84:683–690
10. Lowe GDO. Anticoagulants in cardiac thromboembolism, cardiac surgery, peripheral arterial disease and cerebrovascular disease. In: Meade TW (ed): Anticoagulants and Myocardial Infarction. A Reappraisal. Wiley, Chichester 1984:203–221
11. Sullivan JM, Harken DE, Gorlin R. Pharmacologic control of thromboembolic complications of cardiac valve replacement. N Engl J Med 1971;284:1391–94
12. Altman R, Coullon F, Rouvir JH, de la Fuente L, Favolovo R. Aspirin and prophylaxis of thromboembolic complications in patients with substitute heart valves. J Thorac Cardiovasc Surg 1976;72:127–129
13. Dale L, Myhre E, Storstein O et al. Prevention of arterial thromboembolism by acetylsalicylic acid: a controlled study in patients with aortic ball valves. Am Heart J 1977;94:101–111
14. Dale L, Myhre E, Loew D. Bleeding during acetyl-salicylic acid and anticoagulant therapy in patients with reduced platelet activity after aortic valve replacement. Am Heart J 1980;99:746–751
15. Chesbro JH, Fuster V, Elveback LR et al. Trial of combined warfarin plus dipyridamole or aspirin in prosthetic heart valve replacement: danger of aspirin compared with dipyridamole. Am J Cardiol 1983;51:1537–41
16. Turpie AGG, Gustensen J, Hirsh J, Nelson H, Gent M. Randomised comparison of two intensities of oral anticoagulant therapy after tissue heart valve replacement. Lancet 1988;i:1242–45
17. Saour JN, Sieck JO, Mamo LAR, Gallus AS. Trial of different intensities of anticoagulation in patients with prosthetic heart valves. N Engl J Med 1990;322:428–432
18. Altman R, Rouvier J, Gurfinkel E et al. Two levels of anticoagulant therapy in patients with substitute heart valves. J Thorac Cardiovasc Surg 1991;101:427–431
19. Loeliger EA, Van Dijk-Wierda CA, Van den Besselaar AMHP, Broekmans AW, Roos J. Anticoagulant control and the risk of bleeding. In: Meade TW (ed): Anticoagulants and Myocardial Infarction. A Reappraisal. Wiley, Chichester 1984:135–177
20. Sixty-Plus Reinfarction Study Research Group. A double-blind trial to assess long term anticoagulant therapy in elderly patients after myocardial infarction. Lancet 1980;2:989–984
21. Forfar JC. A 7-year analysis of haemorrhage in patients on long term anticoagulant treatment. Br Heart J 1979;42:128–132
22. Sixty-Plus Reinfarction Study Research Group. Risks of long term oral anticoagulant therapy in elderly patients after myocardial infarction. Lancet 1982;1:64–68
23. Fuster V, Badimon L, Badimon JJ, Chesebro JH. Prevention of thromboembolism induced by prosthetic heart valves. Semin Thromb Hemostas 1988;14:50–58
24. Landefeld CS, Goldman L. Major bleeding in out-patients treated with warfarin: Incidence and prediction by factors known at the start of out-patient therapy. Am J Med 1989;87:144–152
25. Landefeld CS, Rosenblatt MW. Bleeding in out-patients treated with warfarin: relation to the prothrombin time and important remediable lesions. Am J Med 1989;87:153–159
26. British Committee for Standardisation in Haematology, Haemostasis and Thrombosis Task Force. Guidelines on oral anticoagulation. J Clin Pathol 1990;43:177–183
27. British Medical Association and Royal Pharmaceutical Society of Great Britain. British National Formulary. London, Pharmaceutical Press, 1991
28. Israel DH, Fuster V, Chesebro JH, Badimon L. Antithrombotic therapy for coronary artery disease and valvular heart disease. Bailliere's Clin Haematol 1990;3:705–743

29. Coon WW, Willis PW,III. Hemorrhagic complications of anticoagulant therapy. Arch Intern Med 1974;133:386–392
30. Wintzen AR, de Jonge H, Loeliger EA, Bots GTAM. The risk of intracerebral hemorrhage during oral anticoagulation treatment: a population study. Ann Neurol 1984;16:553–558
31. Gurwitz JH, Goldberg RJ, Holden A, Knapic N, Ansell J. Age-related risks of long term oral anticoagulant therapy. Arch Intern Med 1988;148:1733–36
32. Errichete AM, Holden A, Ansell J. Management of oral anticoagulant therapy. Experience with an anticoagulant clinic. Arch Intern Med 1985;144:1966–68
33. Lowe GDO. Anticoagulant drugs in the elderly: valuable in selected patients. Br Med J 1988; 297:1260–63
34. Mok CK, Boey J, Wang R et al. Warfarin versus dipyridamole-aspirin and pentoxifylline-aspirin for the prevention of prosthetic heart valve thromboembolism: a prospective clinical trial. Circulation 1985;72:1059–1063
35. Shetty HGM, Backhouse G, Bentley DP, Routledge PA. Effective reversal of low dose warfarin induced excessive anticoagulation with low dose vitamin K. Thromb Haemostas 1992;67:13–15
36. Francis CW, Marder VJ, McColliser EC et al. Two step warfarin therapy. JAMA 1983;249:374–378

Part 6

Follow up methods and data analysis

Chapter 6.1

Data Collection and Management

Peter A. Lewis

The long-term follow-up of cohorts of heart valve replacement patients provides data which may be used for two research activities. First, data may be used as an independent set for testing hypotheses generated from other studies (providing, of course, that the relevant data has been collected). Second, the database may be used for case finding and thus aid in the design and administration of further studies in particular subsets of these patients[1].

All methods used to pursue the investigation of thromboembolism after heart valve surgery rely on a variety of analytical techniques. Each of these techniques has its own strengths and limitations. Therefore, it is necessary to have a complete understanding of them if one is to design technically realistic and clinically useful studies[2]. The remaining chapters discuss some of these techniques in detail. However, they cannot be considered in isolation, as they interact in important ways. For example, the data model used to define the structure of the data collected can actually prevent certain types of analysis being performed on that particular set of data.

MANAGEMENT OF THE DATABASE AND DATA SELECTION.

The administration of the data on a day to day basis.

This task requires a system which will be in day to day use by relatively inexperienced computer users. It needs to be capable of finding, checking and where necessary changing data in a relatively simple way and with maximum reliability. Typically, one would be considering over one million data items, any one of which should be found within a few seconds.

It is now widely accepted that straightforward administration of most complex data sets is best carried out by using a relational database management system (DBMS)[3]. Using such a system may be structured according to a set of rules. This process is called normalisation. A normalised data set may be thought of as having been broken down into its component parts. When a data set needs to be extracted from the DBMS, the appropriate component part can then be assembled and output. The process of normalisation is a stepwise procedure, the application of each step further breaking down the original data structure. After applying the first step, the data structure is then said to be in 'first normal form'. Database theorists recognise at least six normal forms, but for practical purposes the third normal form is sufficient. Such an implementation will avoid data duplication and the ensuing problems of 'update anomalies'.

A modern DBMS has a number of features which allow recovery of data if mistakes are made in an updating process. The essential elements of the system allow frequent copies of the database to be taken and electronic copies of all transactions are recorded (the journal). If a mistake is found to have been made which has propagated errors through the database, then one reverts to an earlier, error-free copy, corrects the journal and 'rolls' the database forward using the journal until the correct up-to-date version is obtained.

Manipulation of the data into the appropriate structure for analysis.

The restructuring of the raw data into a suitable form for analysis takes place only occasionally. The intervals between analyses may be measured in years. It is impossible to specify a fixed data model which would be suitable for all plausible analyses with prior processing. This processing is an irreversible process as it imposes a greater degree of structure on the relational model, and also involves the discarding of some data items which are not considered important for the particular analysis. Thus the most complete set of data is the 'unstructured' relational set, from which all data models for analysis are produced.

The long-term collection, checking and storage of clinical data is a specialised task. The ideal policy is to separate completely the workers who collect, check and store the data from the clinical staff who manage the patients. This has several advantages. The research staff never have to argue priorities with the clinical staff, they are in an environment which has appropriate career opportunities for non-clinical technical staff and they are removed from any direct involvement with factional clinical interests. The long-term employment of these research workers is then dependent on the reputation of their research group in attracting work rather than the success or failure of only one project.

The clinical staff are responsible for ensuring that the appropriate clinical data have been collected from the patient. The research staff have to find, check, code and enter the data into the database. Patients may be under the care of a number of clinicians so that clinical data may need to be collected from different sources. Also the results of tests may not be known for some time, and this may interfere with the orderly way some database management systems have to work. If the research staff finds the clinical data unclear or ambiguous, these data should be referred back to a clinician for clarification. Research staff should not make clinical judgements.

If this research group is independent, they are able to work across specialities, and thus have a number of unrelated projects running concurrently. This provides the opportunity for staff to broaden their practical and technical experience. The prospect of challenging, secure employment enables good, well motivated staff to be recruited and retained.

Clinicians with little experience of large, longitudinal studies often do not realise that the coding of the data is only one aspect of the work. The patients in the Cardiff Valve Study, although all receiving surgical treatment in one regional centre, come from a geographical region of seven thousand square miles, with a widely scattered population of over two million, and receive other aspects of their medical care from a variety of clinicians in a variety of institutions. A major task facing the data collection team lies in keeping track of the patients and knowing where to look for clinical data. Some studies have attempted to overcome some of these problems of tracking the clinical experience of patients by contacting the patient by telephone or letter to obtain a resumé of their recent experience. Even this simple approach requires an up-to-date patient register with telephone numbers. It is not always possible to get an accurate picture of a patient's clinical history from only one data source. Careful attention to detail will enable the routine follow-up data to be acquired, but potential problems may arise when patients suffer clinical events leading to hospitalisation remote from the regional centre. These data have to be collected retrospectively and it may take a number of months before such events are coded.

In Cardiff, the patient database contains details of hospitals where patients are likely to be treated, providing a basis for the start of the search if a patient appears lost to clinical follow up. Major clinical studies in the UK receive help from the Chief Statistician at the Office of Population, Censuses and Surveys (OPCS), a government organisation. One of the functions of the OPCS is to maintain the National Health Service (NHS) Central Register. This register contains, amongst other things, details of all births and deaths of UK citizens. The Chief Statistician at the OPCS will flag named cases on his register, and subsequently send to the researchers independent notification of deaths, together with cause of death and other useful data (including place of death, the name of the doctor who signed the death certificate and whether a post-mortem examination was conducted). The Cardiff Valve Study uses this facility as a back-up system. Thus while a few patients may be lost to follow-up temporarily, none of them are lost forever.

The scale of the problem of data collection can be illustrated by some recent statistics from the Cardiff Valve Study. In 1991, there were 1,200 surviving patients on active follow up. Each patient has, on average, two clinical follow up visits per year, hence 2,400 clinical assessments each year. Each patient has about nine anticoagulation tests per year (once every six weeks), hence 10,800 tests per year. Clinical data is collected from 39 different hospital locations and blood tests from 35 anticoagulation clinics. There are some 1,800 general practitioners in Wales; about half of them are responsible for one or more of these patients. A small number of patients have moved outside of Wales and these patients also need data collection. With time, some of these data collection problems will be substantially overcome. While it is technically feasible for the database on research computers to interrogate the clinical databases on service computers, there are many practical, organisational and political problems to be overcome before this becomes a reality. However, slow progress is being made, and some data are now exchanged electronically.

There are two separate and distinct approaches to the computerisation of clinical data in general, and heart valve data in particular. The first method establishes the structure of the model which will be used in the analysis and collects and stores data in a way which has an exact correspondence with this analysis model. Such a system needs to be specifically designed. The data collected can then be analysed with little or no preparation. The second method stores the data using a 'normalised' data model in a relational database management system. When the data are to be analysed, specific programs need to be written to convert the data to the required model. The reason for these problems lies in the theories used in computer science which govern the storage of data.

The relational data model, which forms the basis of all widely available database management systems, does not have the property of 'order'. Some implementations do support some elements of 'order', but as this would not be a documented feature of the system, later versions may not have this property. By removing it, major performance gains are possible. If there are patient assessments repeated over time, which are labelled with the date of the assessment, these database systems will not be able to provide the data which answers the question, "what is the first assessment of the patient following a given date or given event?" for example. The production of the programs to 'order' the data into a form suitable for analysis can be a complex and time consuming task. The reason for using this strategy is that it allows very complex questions to be asked. The complexity of such questions are illustrated by the hypothetical examples given below.

1. Suppose we wish to investigate the influence of heart rhythm on embolic rate. In particular, we wish to determine if the risk of an embolic event is greater or less in the time period immediately after the rhythm changes from sinus rhythmn (SR) to atrial fibrillation (AF). One plausible way of investigating this is to identify patients who were in stable SR postoperatively and subsequently convert to AF. The temporal nature of the embolic experience of these patients can be calculated and compared to patients who were in AF postoperatively. We might define the questions to be answered thus:

For a defined set of patients:

a) what proportion were event free at 180 days post operation;
b) of these patients how many were in SR and subsequently went into AF; and
c) was their embolic rate after they went into AF greater or less than the embolic rate of patients who were already in AF at 180 days.

2. It is widely believed that a proportion of embolic events or bleeding events are related to periods when the patient's anticoagulation is 'out of control'. We could define 'out of control', identify those patients who had a period before their events when their anticoagulation was out of control and determine whether this was associated with an 'event'.

We might define 'out of control' as any one of

(a) two successive INRs below 1.8 (b) two successive INRs above 5.0 (c) a three month period averaging less than 2.0 (d) a three month period averaging more than 4.5 (e) a sudden fall or another combination. In fact we may wish to try a number of definitions for 'out of control' to see which, if any, have a predictive value[4]. Each new definition will require a further ordering and processing of the base data set.

It is clear from the two examples quoted that for research purposes, unprocessed data needs to be stored using a flexible data model and that prior to any analysis the data will need considerable work to transform it into a suitable form. Further examples of possible analyses are available elsewhere[5].

The purpose written systems which are currently available have little use in research in the full sense of the word because they 'simplify' the data. However, they do have a use in audit and quality assurance. If they are programmed to reflect how well a patient series is meeting the agreed outcome criteria, their routine use allows heart valve replacement programs to be continuously monitored with certain caveats. For example, if the outcome criteria are not being met there is no guarantee that the data which might identify the cause of the deficiency have been collected or are available (Table 6.1–1).

Those centres wishing to start observational studies or improve existing studies face a bewildering array of options. The objectives of the study, the data to be collected and the analysis protocols to be used all need to be well formulated before any decisions are taken which might limit the range of options available. There are also the practical

Table 6.1–1
Choosing a database management system for the long-term follow-up of heart valve replacement patients. Purpose written software versus general purpose software.

Purpose written software	*General purpose software*
Share purpose written software – can have low start-up costs once first system is installed. Subsequent systems can be started quickly.	Use widely available commercial software to store data. Available 'off the shelf'.
Standardisation of data collected and method of analysis enforced by the system.	No standards other than those adopted by the researchers.
Changes to the analysis model may be inconsistent with the way data have been processed.	Can re-define analysis model to take advantage of latest issues in subject and latest ideas in analysis.
Problems of software maintenance due to having to rely on individual or small company.	Continued support, maintenance and upgrading from well established companies.
The production of the prototype system is time consuming and delays the start of the data collection.	Data collection can begin as soon as data model is defined.
Usually only available on one class of machine.	Portable across a wide range of hardware platforms often with no modifications.
Can analyse easily and frequently.	Analysis of the data is a major undertaking.
Software is application specific so expertise is not easily transferable to other applications.	The same software may be used for all applications, so staff expertise is transferable between applications and even from non-clinical applications.
No networking facilities.	Has an extensive set of communication utilities for networking to other databases.

decisions about the computer manufacturers, operating systems, database management systems and high level programming languages that are to be used on such a project. Different solutions can have very different resource implications, but in general, the cheaper the system installed the greater the risks of jeopardising the overall project due to the commercial failure of a supplier or the unavailability of software fixes when problems arise with the system. Any computing costs of such a project are only a very small part of the overall cost of the work. The ideal solution would involve using software from a multinational software house which included an extensive range of micro, mini and mainframe hardware platforms, with few, if any, modifications needed to port the code from one platform/operating system to another. After extensive investigations the solution adopted for the Cardiff Valve Study was to use the ORACLE DBMS running under the Unix operating system[6]. The manufacturers of the hardware then became of secondary importance. The high level language and the statistical packaging used are probably best determined by local circumstances, provided that it is well established and that there is a suitable pool of programmers from which to recruit.

While the study of heart valve replacement patients is a technically complex task there is now sufficient experience in data management and analysis to adequately support properly conducted clinical trials. The methodologies and techniques are well enough understood and practised to be able to produce a sound managerial, administrative and analysis protocol together with reasonable costings and schedules which should allow clinicians to take advantage of this resource to resolve the many outstanding issues in the therapy of heart valve disease. With high standards of study design, data collection and management, appropriate methods of analysis should provide the information on which clinicians can base their decision making.

REFERENCES

1. Department of Epidemiology and Biostatistics, McMaster University, Hamilton, Ont. How to read clinical journals: IV. To determine etiology or causation. Can Med Assoc J 1981; 124: 985–990.
2. Pockcock SJ. Clinical Trials. Chichester, John Wiley, 1983.
3. Deen SM. Principles and Practise of Database Systems. London, Macmillan, 1985.
4. Butchart EG, Lewis PA, Kulatilake ENP, Breckenridge IM. Anticoagulation variability between centres: implications for comparative prosthetic valve assessment. Eur J Cardiothorac Surg 1988; 2: 72–81.
5. Bodnar E, Wain WH, Haberman S. Assessment and comparison of the performance of cardiac valves. Ann Thorac Surg 1982; 34: 146–156.
6. Oracle Corporation, Belmount, California, USA.

Chapter 6.2

Analyses of Thrombosis, Thromboembolism and Bleeding after Heart Valve Replacement as Time-related Outcome Events

Eugene H. Blackstone

This chapter is written from the perspective that: a) analysing the time-relatedness of thrombotic and anticoagulation complications after heart valve replacement and identifying their correlates remain of value in optimising the clinical management of patients and in guiding scientific research and development efforts aimed at reducing the prevalence and consequences of these events; b) the milieu for most such studies is the longitudinal observational clinical study that uses rigorous scientific methods to yield helpful clinical inferences, to assist in formulating testable hypotheses, to predict expected outcome in future patients, and to compare alternative treatments; c) the analyses of greatest scientific value are those that use the available follow-up clinical data to the fullest and that generate equations that can be solved for patient-specific and group-specific (risk-prevalence adjusted) predictions and comparisons; and d) current methods in common use are inadequate for these tasks and even may be misleading. The intent of this chapter is to propose a methodological approach to the scientific investigation of these clinical events that fulfills the qualifications of a), b), and c) above, that exposes the inadequacies of d), and that exploits modern statistical developments from both academic and industrial arenas.

This intentionally provocative chapter will not propose *standardisation* of publications reporting thrombosis, thromboembolic, and bleeding events but will embrace efforts to define and characterise the nature of these events more precisely. It is recognised that a uniform publication format is cherished by regulatory agencies. Such sterile reporting, however, rarely leads to new inferences and thus adds little to the scientific advancement of the field. Admittedly, availability of standardised reports simplifies the task of performing quasi-meta-analyses of the comparative prevalences or rates of events from literature sources; however, such analyses tend to be of limited, rather circumscribed value for the purposes proposed above.

Comprehensive analysis of outcome events in a large, variable-rich, multi-institutional, high-quality heart valve data base in the manner proposed has not so far been accomplished. Yet advances in the statistical field known as 'Martingale theory', the slow, but continual development of analytical computer software incorporating this theory, and the increasing availability of the powerful, very high speed computers essential for these computationally-intensive efforts and the validation of the results, encourage one to believe that in the near future it will be possible to undertake such a project[1,2]. Enough work has been accomplished to date to demonstrate the great potential of such an analysis and to expose the inadequacies of 'routine' analyses perfunctorily performed and reported.

The price that must be paid for a more clinically satisfying analysis is, in part, complexity of the analytic process. However, the intricacies of molecular and cellular biology have not deterred us from embracing their achieved and perceived potential applicability, and a *general* understanding of that science is well within the grasp of the cardiovascular specialist. In like manner, the theory and process of a comprehensive analysis of complex thrombotic and anticoagulation events is comprehensible in a general way. Just as we are not all forced to *perform* the science of molecular biology, so we are not all forced to develop, or extend, methods and perform the analysis of the post valve replacement state. The few who do, in intensive collaboration with their clinical colleagues, should be expected to present in a comprehensible way the analyses and the clinical inferences derived therefrom so that we and our patients can reap the benefit. Admittedly, a disadvantage of many statistical methods in the past has been that the clinical applications and inferences from the models have been difficult to extract. This situation by and large has been rectified.

The proposal contains the following, clinically realistic elements: 1) the analysis of *all outcome events,* without artificial segmentation of the continuous time line into early or late events following valve implantation, 2) the recognition that the events may *repeat* in a patient, 3) the inclusion of the *severity* of the functional sequelae of these events, thus treating comprehensively minor and major events, 4) the inclusion of the *site* of the event, 5) the identification of the patient, procedure, prosthesis, and time-varying anticoagulation regimen *risk factors*. It thus permits patient-specific (risk factor adjusted) *predictions* and *comparisons*.

The proposal falls short of the ideal in several specific ways. It models the outcome events as *point processes* (occurring in an instant in time). Yet, for example, valve thrombosis may be the culmination of a time-related process, or a thromboembolic event may consist of a 'shower' of emboli, which may in some patients last for some hours or days. It is not clear how such complexities can be analysed more realistically than as point processes[3]. Thus a remaining limitation is that we propose analysing a complex event as an 'episode', and the sequelae as the cumulative effects of the complex episode. Further limitations relate to the present incomplete state of observational information, including, for example, the continuous moment-to-moment state of anticoagulation, the quantity of blood lost in a bleeding event, or the uncertainty that a reported event is truly valve-related. These limitations of the data base degrade the quality of the analysis, no matter how comprehensive it may be. Finally, the analyses lead to identification of empirical association of variables with outcome. At best they only hint at the underlying, fundamental mechanisms whose understanding may lead to a definitive solution.

CHARACTERISTICS OF THE EVENTS THAT PRESENT ANALYTICAL CHALLENGES

Occlusive valve *thrombosis* is a catastrophic outcome that is more reliably identified as a valve-related event than a thromboembolic event. However, valve thrombosis is probably a process, developing over a variable period of time from hours to days that becomes evident when acute haemodynamic compromise occurs (see Chapter 2.4). Generally, it is underestimated in clinical series without routine autopsy studies of all patients dying after a valve replacement, since valve thrombosis is often lethal and may lead to death before it is clinically diagnosed.

The analysis of valve thrombosis as a dichotomous (binary) terminating event analogous to the event death is appropriate.

Valve-related *thromboembolic* events are far more difficult to analyse. There is lack of a uniformly accepted definition of the event itself, in large part because the event is simply a presumptive diagnosis[4,5]. The majority of the events diagnosed involve the brain, probably because neurological symptoms are more apparent than those from other organ systems. But, since neurological events occur in the general, and particularly the ageing, population (Chapter 1.1), are all neurological events due to valve-related thromboemboli? And should the events include very transient neurological events since transient ischaemic attacks are both overdiagnosed and subject to the unreporting biases described in Chapter 6.4? Should they also include very early neurological symptoms clearly present at initial recovery from surgery? Should they include only neurological events?

It is my recommendation that all, even 'possibly valve-related' organ ischaemic events be classified arbitrarily as thromboembolic events. These should be characterised as to a) the time of occurrence of the event, b) the site (brain, gut, kidney, extremities, etc.) of lodgement and c) the severity of residual functional consequences of the event. The latter, for example, might use the ordinal Karnofsky performance status scale (Table 6.2–1)[6]. At times the emboli occur in 'showers', or as an intermittent succession of events over a few hours or days. Arbitrarily, this complex event should be characterised as a single thromboembolic 'episode'.

Patients often survive their thromboembolic events. Thromboembolism may,

Table 6.2–1
Estimation of Functional Impairment Using the Karnofsky Performance Status Scale

Functional Impairment (%)	*Criteria*
0	No evident impairment
10	Very minor signs or symptoms of impairment, but not affecting ability to carry out normal activities
20	Some signs or symptoms of impairment; normal activities can be carried out, but with effort
30	Unable to carry on normal activities or do active work; but patient cares for self
40	Impaired to the extent of requiring occasional assistance, although cares for most needs
50	Requires considerable assistance and frequent care
60	Disabled, requiring special care and assistance
70	Severely disabled; hospitalised (or institutionalised), but death is not imminent
80	Very ill, hospitalised, active supportive treatment required
90	Moribund; death imminent
100	Dead

therefore, recur. All episodes of thromboembolism should be recorded, and methods to analyse the data must accommodate such *repeating (non-terminating) morbid events*[7] (see also Chapter 5.2).

To place presumed valve-related thromboembolism rates and prevalences into perspective, an informal comparison might be made to such events in an age- and gender-adjusted, matched, general population. There is no clinical need, however, to 'adjust' the actual data for events occurring in the general population (or in cohorts with heart disease, etc.). Instead, risk factors can be identified and risk-adjusted prevalences and rates calculated from those analyses. In like fashion, there is no clinical need to agonise as to whether or not the event is truly valve-related or not. Rather, risk-factor adjusted analyses provide a mechanism whereby the expected occurrence of these events, as a general phenomenon of the post valve replacement state can be portrayed. From a mechanistic scientific and manufacturing point of view, of course, it would be important to know the minimum possible 'background' level of thromboembolism that would occur, were a perfectly thromboresistant prosthesis to be developed. Quite possibly the closest we can come to estimating such a level is by analysing such events in patients receiving allograft aortic valves.

Bleeding events, like thromboembolic events, may be counted incompletely. They may not easily be categorised as being anticoagulant-related. Minor bleeding from ordinary trauma may occur so often as to preclude meaningful analysis. Thus generally 'major' episodes only are recorded. Again, the site and severity of the bleeding should be recorded, the latter on a quantitative or ordinal scale. These episodes can be recurrent, and, like thromboembolic events, require methods of analysis of repeating events of variable severity.

Changing incidence of outcome events over time

The simplicity and convenience of calculating and expressing the incidence of thrombosis, thromboembolism, and bleeding events as so-called linearised rates is indisputable. Not well appreciated by all readers, however, is that the easily calculated rate implies a 'constant hazard' or incidence of events across all time (industrial terminology: a homogeneous Poisson process[8]). The facts seem to argue to the contrary; namely, that a constant hazard is uncharacteristic of these events (see Chapter 5.2). This suggests that in most situations linearised rates should be abandoned[9]. This argumentative and admittedly purist inference is based on at least a small amount of data, and is intended as a challenge to those who present linearised rates to defend them, if they can. The data seem to be as follows.

Thromboembolism: Shortly after awaking from operation, the incidence of thromboembolic phenomena appears to peak steeply, falling to low levels after a few days to weeks[10]. Is this a biological phenomenon, perhaps related to the unprotected prosthesis and sewing ring surfaces (see Chapters 2.4 and 3.1)? A similar phenomenon does occur after open or closed mitral valve commissurotomy (Fig. 6.2–1)[11]. Is the peak, instead, an artefact of observation and reporting, since trained observers are present in the initial postoperative period? Is the subsequent rapid decrease a reflection of the 'weeding out' of particularly susceptible patients (in statistical terms, a mixed population as described in Chapter 6.3)? These unresolved questions invite inquiry about the nature of the phenomenon and are perhaps the most cogent argument for

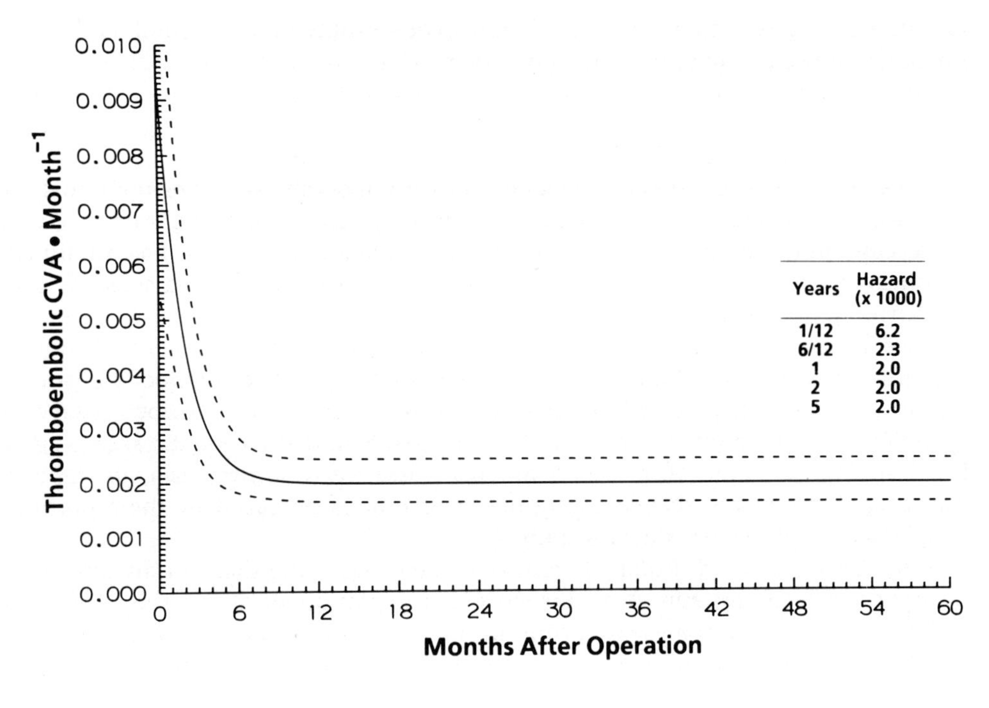

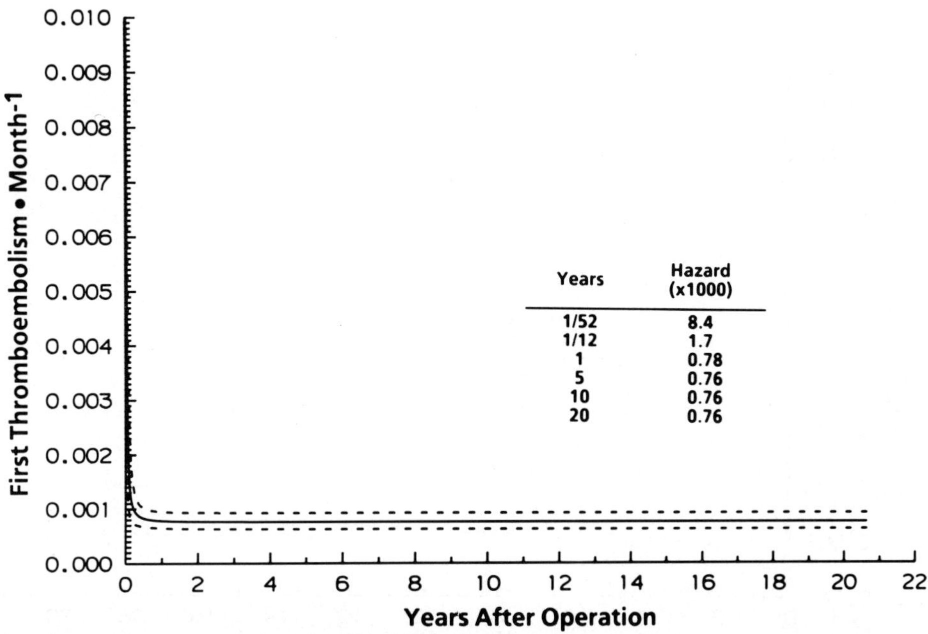

Figure 6.2–1: Hazard functions (instantaneous risk) for first thromboembolic event. (a) Hazard function for first thromboembolic event after valve replacement (3 devices, aortic and mitral positions)[10]. (b) Hazard function for first thromboembolic event after surgical mitral commissurotomy[11]. Notice that both hazard functions exhibit a rapidly falling early hazard phase that merges into a constant hazard phase.

describing the phenomenon in detail before over-simplifying to constant hazard rates, no matter how close an approximation they may be.

Another consequence of ignoring the time-related changes in the hazard function is that the calculated linearised rate will tend to decrease as the length of average follow-up increases. This is a clue to a non-constant hazard.

The shape of the time-related incidence of thromboembolism after the initial peak depends upon whether or not repeated events are considered. In the context of mitral valve commissurotomy, when all events are considered, a rising hazard function becomes apparent (Fig. 6.2–2). The reasons for this will be discussed under "Recurrence of the Events".

Valve Thrombosis: The hazard function (instantaneous risk) for valve thrombosis seems to have an importantly different shape from that for thromboembolism (Fig. 6.2–3)[12]. It appears to peak within about a year, then decline. This curious observation again invites exploration of the responsible mechanism. It also cogently argues against the lumping together of thromboembolism and valve thrombosis for reporting purposes. Once again, this changing risk over time is obscured by the reporting of simple and inappropriate linearised rates.

Anticoagulation-related bleeding: I know of no analyses of the shape of the time related incidence of bleeding episodes. But since our explorations of the shape of hazard functions in over 2000 analyses of events in clinical data sets has yielded only a few with constant hazard, it would be surprising if bleeding complications were to occur at a

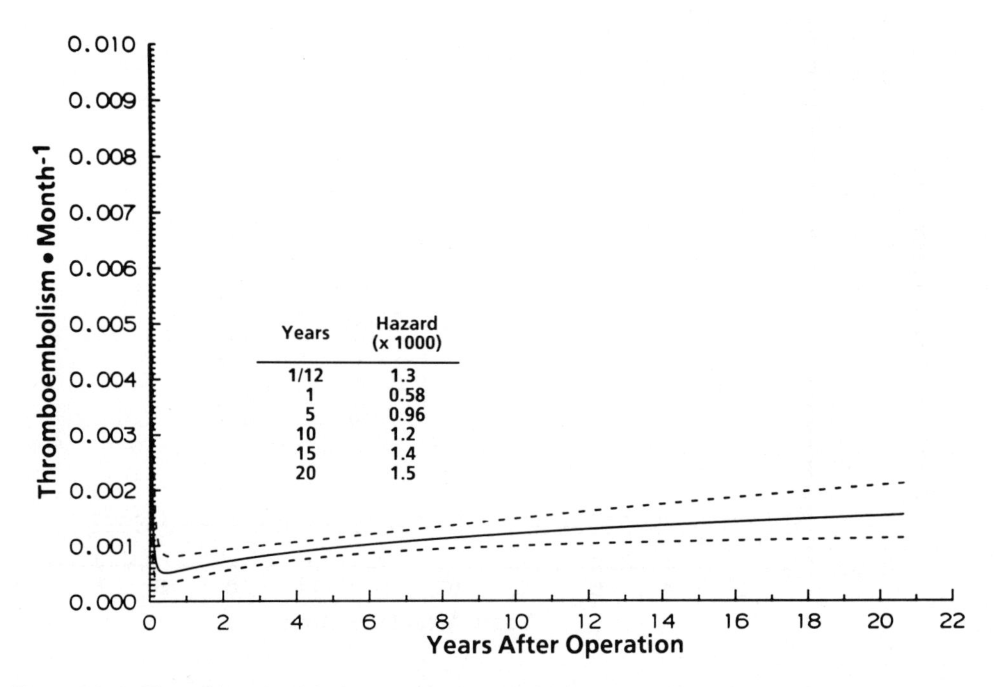

Figure 6.2–2: Hazard function (the instantaneous risk) of a first, second, or third thromboembolic event at any moment in time after time zero for any thromboembolic event after mitral commissurotomy. Notice the slowly increasing later phase of hazard for any *event, compared with the constant hazard for the* first *event as depicted in Figure 6.2–1b.*

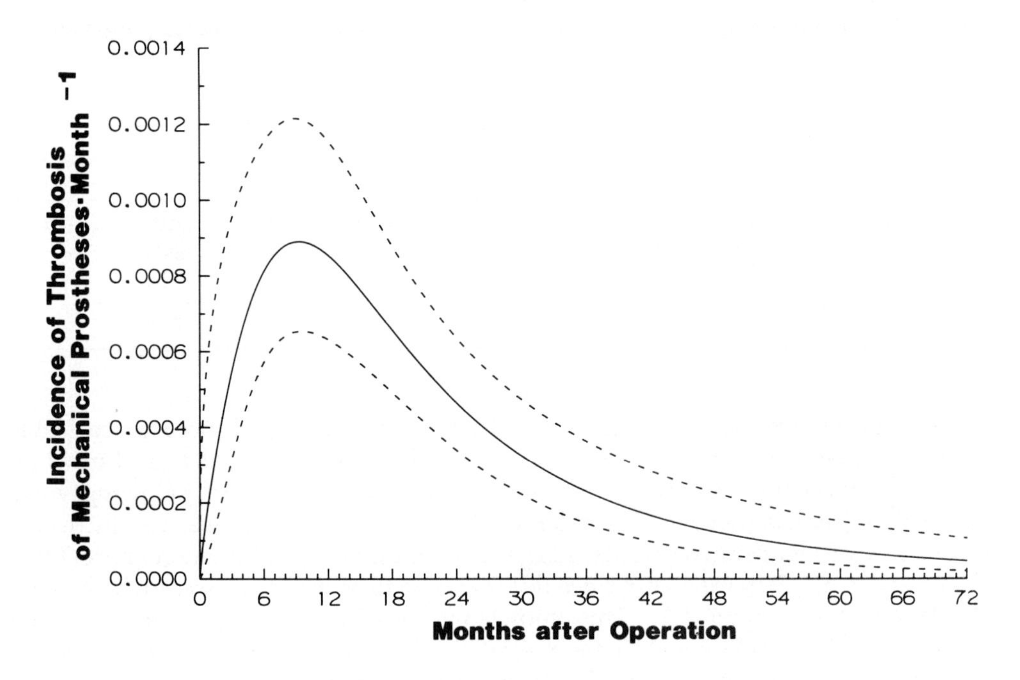

Figure 6.2–3: Hazard function for valve thrombosis (Bjørk-Shiley standard valves in aortic or mitral position) (UAB; 1975-July 1979; n=1084)[12].

constant rate over time. Indeed, the information provided in Chapter 5.4 would translate into a two-phase hazard function.

Implications for Analysis: Since the incidence of these valve complications occurs at an inconstant rate, and since the rate of occurrence varies depending on whether or not repeating episodes are counted, methods of analysis must accommodate time-varying hazard functions[13]. In the major analytical computer software packages available today, the exploration of shape is possible with, for example, PROC LIFEREG under the SAS System[14], and using our own PROC HAZARD[15]. Methods using splines[16] are available from Duke University (Dr. Frank Harrell), and non-parametric methods using the cumulative hazard function are prevalent in industry and quite easy to implement[17]. The various phases of the time-related incidence (hazard function) are influenced by different risk factors (non-proportional hazards). The implication is that either different mechanisms are involved during each phase or that the mix of patient susceptibility changes over time. This observation and inference again argues against both the use of simple linearised rates and the ordinary Cox proportional hazards regression model.

Recurrence of the events

Almost ignored, and yet of great importance for those involved in the ongoing management of patients who have a prosthetic valve in place, is the repetitive nature of thrombosis, embolism, and bleeding. In our exploration of repeating thromboembolic events after mitral valve commissurotomy, for example, we found that the risk of

Table 6.2–2
Thromboembolic events immediately postoperatively or during the followup period after surgical mitral commissurotomy

Number of Episodes of Thromboembolism	*n*	*Thromboembolism*	
		No.	*% of n*
One	339	33	10%
Two	33	8	24%
Three	8	3	38%
Total	380	44	12%

another thromboembolic event incrementally increased after each occurrence (Table 6.2–2) and that the same peaking and falling pattern of risk held true, but at an augmented level (Fig. 6.2–4)[11]. A similar pattern has been found following valve replacement (see Chapter 5.2). The risk for a thromboembolic event was also increased by a history of preoperative events, suggesting a true biological phenomenon (Table 6.2–3 and Fig. 6.2–5), particularly since this is known to be true of strokes in the general population (see Chapter 1.1). This knowledge should assist those attempting to prevent thromboembolic events in their regulation of anticoagulation in these patients. It also invites specific research to clarify the mechanism for this pattern of repeating events. Is it exceptional thrombogenicity of the prosthesis, inadequate anticoagulation, hypercoagulability or other factors affecting the patient-specific precarious balance between under and over anticoagulation? These mechanisms are discussed in detail in Chapters 1.3, 1.5, 2.4 and 3.4 and the influence of patient participation in anticoagulation control is discussed in Chapter 3.5.

Interestingly, the shape of the overall risk of thromboembolism (Fig. 6.2–2) comes about because these repeated events peak and fall to a new, and higher, constant hazard level (Fig. 6.2–4). Thus, the overall hazard (technically known as a non-homogeneous Poisson process[8]) should, in this case, be analysed as a so-called

Table 6.2–3
Increment risk factors for postcommissurotomy thromboembolic events after mitral commissurotomy (repeating event analysis)

Incremental Risk Factors for Postcommissurotomy Thromboembolism	*Hazard Phase*	
	Early	*Late*
Demographic		
Older age at commissurotomy	•	
History of precommissurotomy thromboembolism		•
Morphological		
Leaflet calcification (Grade 0-5)		•
Leaflet Immobility (Grade 0-5)		•
Number of previous postcommissurotomy thromboembolic episodes (0, 1, 2)		•

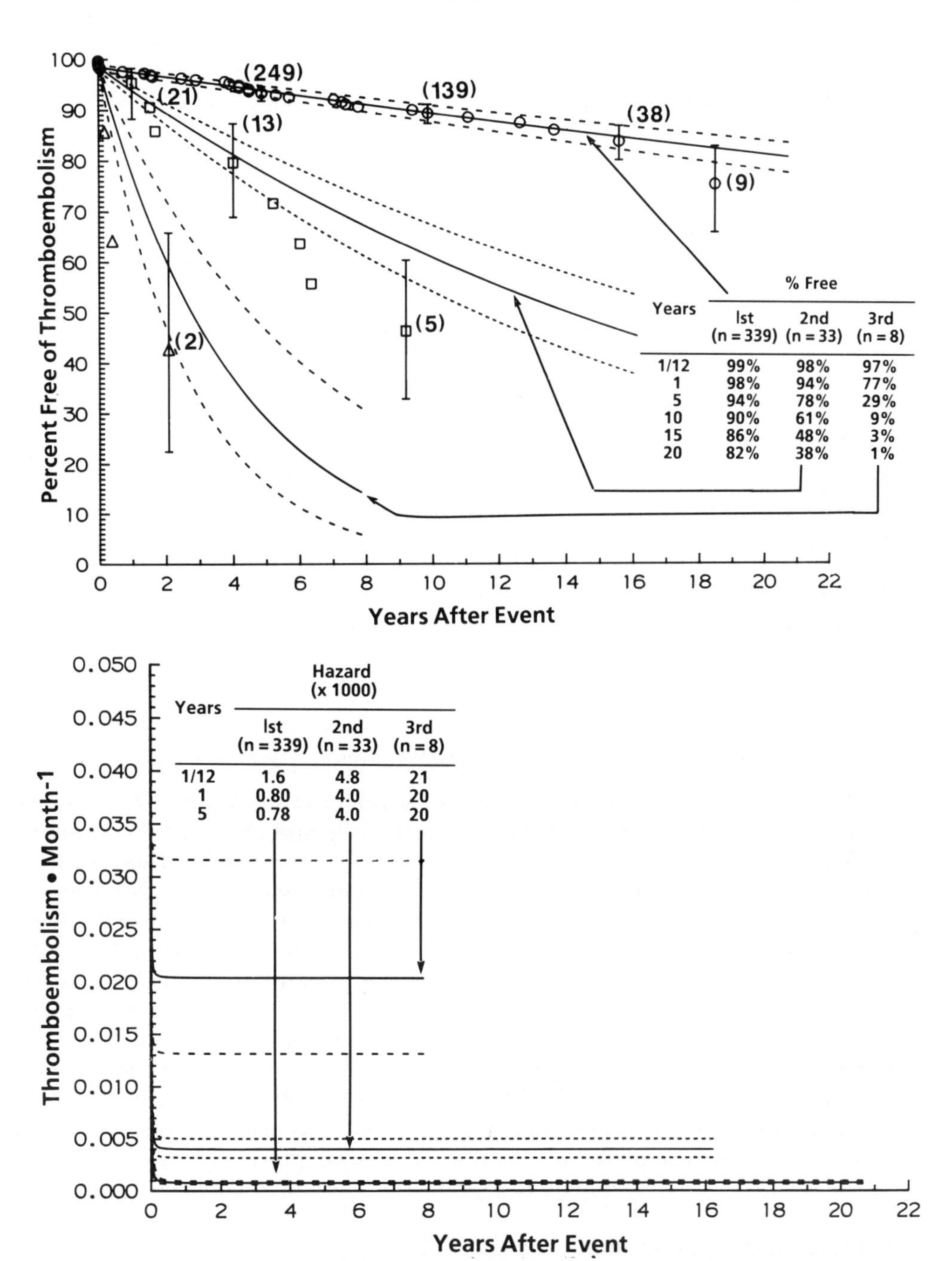

Figure 6.2–4: Postcommissurotomy thromboembolic events[11]. (a) Freedom from a postcommissurotomy thromboembolic event. Open circles represent the first postcommissurotomy thromboembolic event in terms of percent freedom from the event in the total group of 339 patients; time zero is the time of the commissurotomy. Open squares represent the second thromboembolic event in a similar fashion among the 33 patients who had a first thromboembolic event; time zero is the time of the first event. Open triangles represent the third thromboembolic event among the eight patients who had a second event; time zero is the time of the second event. (b) Hazard functions similarly presented.

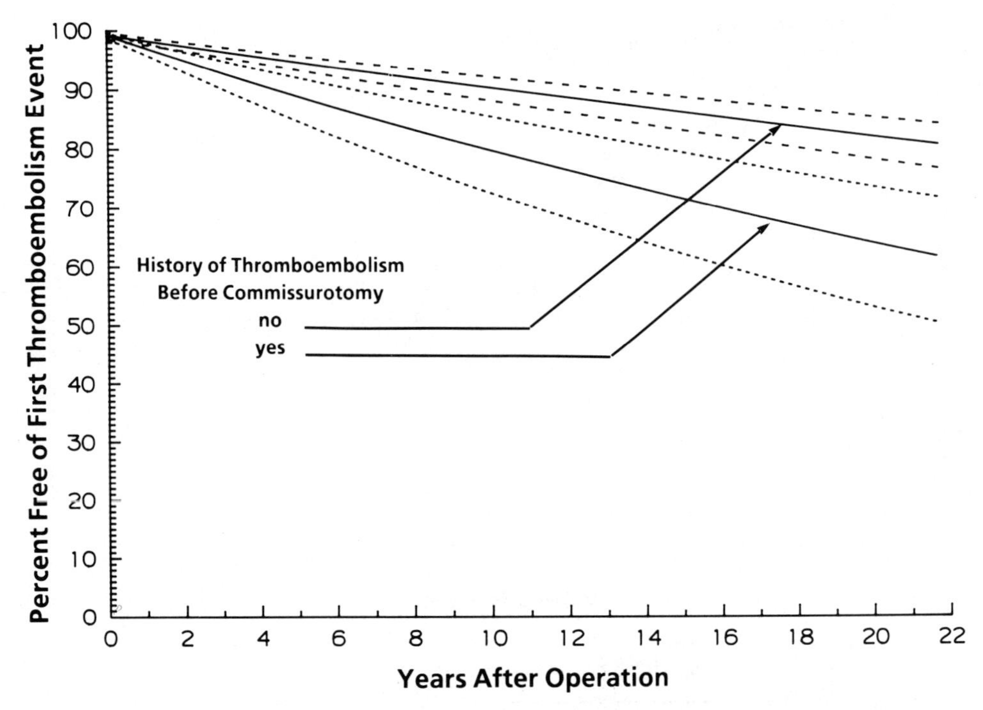

Figure 6.2–5: Influence of precommissurotomy history of thromboembolism on the risk of the first postcommissurotomy thromboembolic episode (solution of equation embodied in Table 6.2–3).

modulated renewal process[18]. The latter provides a specific avenue for the introduction of new time-related explanatory variables such as the site and nature of the event, the interval since the last event, and so forth (see appendix for details). These variables represent one form of 'time varying covariables' to be discussed more fully below.

Full exploration of the repetitive nature of thromboembolism, valve thrombosis and bleeding after valve replacement has, to my knowledge, not been accomplished. My recommendation that we explore repeated events in greater depth is, however, somewhat dampened by the possibility that if we do so, we may have to learn to deal with events in a new domain: the domain of the cumulative hazard function[19]. Conceptually, this domain is not a foreign one (Fig. 6.2–6), for on the vertical axis is simply the number of events (in the figure, expressed *per person*) accumulating in the study group over time. We are just not accustomed to viewing events this way. On the other hand, if the data suggest that a modulated renewal process is appropriate, then we can revert to the survivorship domain with which we are all familiar (Fig. 6.2–4a).

Variable sequelae of the events

Unlike the terminating event death, the morbid events thrombosis, thromboembolism and bleeding are associated with *variable* sequelae leading to functional limitation of the patient. Thus, controversy exists for conventional analyses as to whether or not 'minor' and 'major' sequelae should be allowed to co-exist[4]. The solution is to abandon the analysis of these events as yes/no (0,1) phenomena, and adopt a method of analysis that permits the event to take on any positive value. This

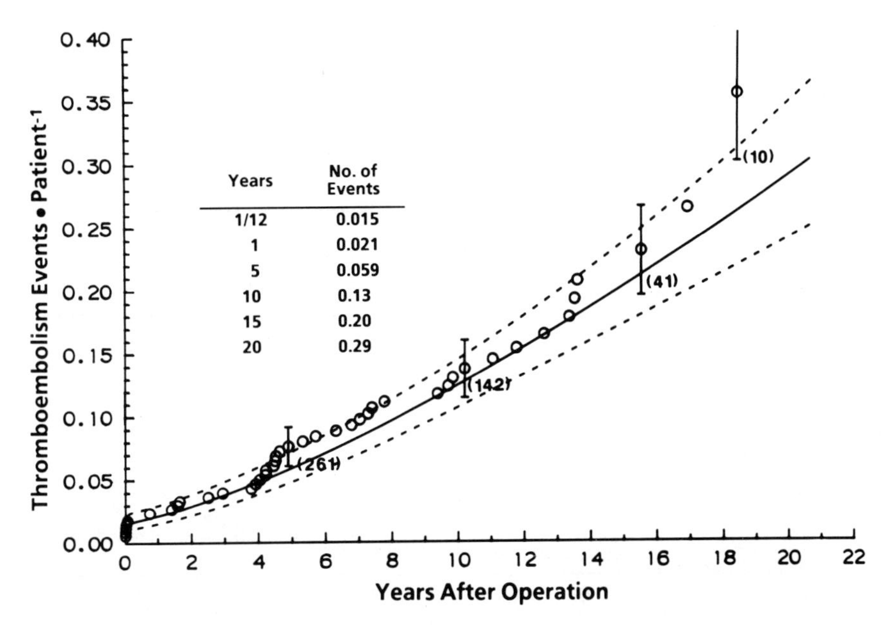

Figure 6.2–6: Cumulative event function for all thromboembolic events after mitral commissurotomy. Each circle represents a thromboembolic event, positioned on the vertical axis according to the method of Nelson[19], and on the horizontal axis at the time of the event. The vertical bars are 70% confidence limits (I)1 standard deviation) of the nonparametric estimates, and the numbers in parentheses are the number of patients remaining at risk at the time depicted. The solid line enclosed within 70% confidence limits is the parametric estimate for a nonhomogeneous Poisson process.

idea has been introduced recently in industry where the *cost* of an event, such as a repair, is of great interest[19]. The mechanism for accomplishing this is to generalise the existing concepts of event analyses in the fashion described in the appendix.

A scale for functional limitation may need to be adopted[4,11]. For one analysis, we used a very simple 5-level scale: 0 = no apparent sequelae, 1 = mild sequelae, 2 = moderate sequelae, 3 = severe sequelae, and 4 = death from the event[11]. More recently, we have used the Karnofsky performance status scale to determine if it is adaptable to valve-related events (Table 6.2–1)[6]. To date, we have not analysed that data to determine if an 11-level scale is too fine for clinical classification although we keep in mind that valve disease patients sometimes seem to fall into fractional NYHA classes. Further, it is as yet unclear whether the *increments* between intervals on that scale are at an appropriate distance one from another. For example, is the 20-point difference between no sequelae and minor sequelae equivalent to the 20-point difference between a severely impaired hospitalised individual and a dead patient?

Presentation of sequelae data is conceptually easy to grasp, but is foreign to us. Along the vertical axis is 'cost' in terms of functional limitation, accumulating in the study group over time (Fig. 6.2–7). The rate of accumulation is analogous to a hazard function. Note that events with no sequelae appear as events, but do not increment the curve. This is an appropriate way of 'weighting' the event, either because of its unimportance or because it is believed that such minor events are incompletely reported.

A risk factor analysis in this domain is no more difficult than in the domain of yes/no

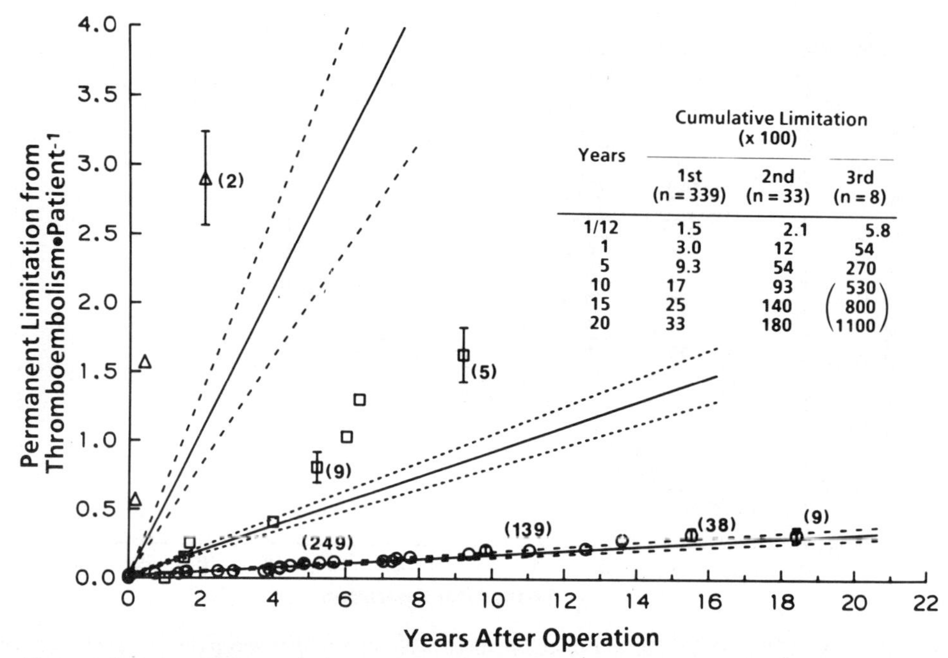

Figure 6.2–7: Stratified cumulative "permanent functional limitation from thromboembolism" after surgical mitral commissurotomy, according to whether the limitation was from the first (n=339), second (n=33), or third (n=8) postcommissurotomy thromboembolic event. The nonparametric estimates are made according to Nelson[19] and the parametric estimates from an analysis for a weighted modulated renewal process. Symbols are the same as in Fig. 6.2–4.

(0,1) events. As expected, the severity appears to increase with each repetition of the event. This may be a biological phenomenon related to loss of functional reserves. Alternatively, it may be that patients (or their families) experiencing multiple, ever more severe events, are more prone to report to the interviewer earlier, less severe events.

Apparent target organ of the event

The site of apparent thromboembolic lodgement or of bleeding is usually determined (for example, see Table 6.2–4). The prevalence of a particular target site may change with repetition of the event, as is apparent in the Table[11]. Subsequently, in an analysis of a modulated renewal process, that site can be incorporated as a risk factor (Table 6.2–5). This is a more appropriate strategy than restricting the analysis to a single site, or ignoring the site.

Risk factors for the event

In any observational clinical study or randomised trial, the prevalence of risk factors will vary. For example, in the United States, and no doubt elsewhere, the demographics of the typical valve replacement patient have shifted importantly[20]. On a global scale, the aetiology of the underlying disease differs markedly. Since all time-related depictions of events after valve replacement reflect the characteristics of the study group, these give rise to inter-institutional, era-related, and geographically-

Table 6.2–4
Relation of the Site of the Thromboembolic Event and the Thrombolic Event Number to the Severity of Permanent Functional Limitation after Mitral Commissurotomy

Severity of Permanent Functional Limitation	*Thromboembolic Event*					
	First		*Second*		*Third*	
	Brain	*Other*	*Brain*	*Other*	*Brain*	*Other*
0	9	2	1	0	0	0
1	2	2	0	0	0	0
2	1	1	3	0	0	0
3	2	0	1	0	0	0
4	8	0	0	1	3	0
Unknown	5	1	2	0	0	0
Total	27	6	7	1	3	0

$P<0.0001$ for relation of site of the event to the event number and for relation of severity of permanent functional limitation to the event number; P values were derived from the multivariable risk factor equation for permanent functional limitation from postcommissurotomy thromboembolism.

related differences in event rates. Some, perhaps most, of the variability in reported event rates described in Chapter 6.3 may relate to these differing prevalences. It is therefore proposed that risk factors be identified for each event in the form of multivariable analyses[9]. These include special risk factors for thromboembolic, bleeding and thrombosis events such as previous history of thromboembolic events, valve size, location, and type, and anticoagulant regimen.

In part, this proposal for multivariable analysis as the corner-stone for drawing scientific inferences about valve-related events runs counter to trends encouraged, particularly, by regulatory agencies and device marketing. These latter would resist the notion of 'mixing', for example, valves of different types (not only manufacturer, but specific models), location, and size. Instead, separate assessment is made for each model and location. It would be my contention that this 'stratification' leads to low power for scientific and clinical inferences, the subject of our endeavours. Better estimates arise from analyses of large and heterogeneous groups of valves, locations,

Table 6.2–5
Permanent Functional Limitation after Mitral Commissurotomy (UAB; 1967-1988; n=339)

Incremental Risk Factors for Permanent Functional Limitiation	*Hazard Phase*	
	Early	*Constant*
Demographic		
Older age at commissurotomy	•	
Morphological		
Leaflet calcification (Grade 0-5)		•
Site of thromboembolism		
Brain		•
Number of previous postcommissurotomy thromboembolic events (0, 1, 2)		•

and sizes, looking for specific risk factors. This process may involve interaction terms with specific valves and their characteristics to identify very specific valve model differences if they are more than accounted for by chance. The advantages of the risk factor approach include the increased statistical power of a large number of events and patients, better characterisation of the time-varying risk (hazard function), identification of those (probably few) true valve characteristic differences that may exist, and risk factor adjustment for all other variables. I would go so far as to contend that this type of information would allow regulatory agencies to draw meaningful inferences about valve replacement devices.

A valid criticism against combining valve types is if the hazard functions are distinctly different in a way not accounted for by prevalences of risk factors. If differences in shape can be demonstrated, then separate analyses are appropriate.

TIME-VARYING COVARIABLES

Without question the conditions of post valve replacement patients change over time, and these changes may increase or decrease the chances of outcome events. A panacea for accounting for such changes in time-related analyses is thought to be the incorporation of *time-varying* covariables[18]. Both the mathematical complexities of doing this, and the limitations of interpretability of the resulting analyses, indicate that there is misplaced hope in this panacea.

Lest we become too discouraged, however, there *is* at least a limited place for analyses incorporating time-varying covariables. For example, Figure 6.2–4 and 7 and Tables 6.2–3 and 6.2–5 depict analyses that do, in fact, incorporate time-varying covariables in a special and useful way. Specifically the modulated renewal process, without introducing any mathematical complexity, allows one in a stepwise fashion to incorporate changes in condition at the time of each event, including any change in anticoagulation strategy.[18] A limitation is that the analysis will produce only the risk for the *next* event, after which a patient 'switches' to a new curve that has the same *shape* as the previous curve, but is modulated up or down by a multiplier. Without also a model of the time sequencing of all events (as in Fig. 6.2–6) one cannot deduce from the analysis the complete life history of events expected for an individual patient.

At least for completely parametric models, with only a little increase in mathematical complexity, *stepwise* changes in time-varying covariates (such as switch to a new anticoagulation regimen) can be incorporated into either a modulated renewal process or a homogeneous or non-homogeneous Poisson process.[18] In the latter case, the hazard function can be visualised as being *shifted* directly upward or downward by these covariables, but the *shape* remains identical. This may make sense, but it may not. It is the method used in available Cox regression software. One great advantage of a completely parametric model is not only that such analyses are easier to make than using the Cox model (by simple stepwise entry of follow-up information as shown in the appendix), but also that they allow graphical depiction of the result, which may indicate to the investigator a result that is unrealistic.

Interpretation is also a problem, as illustrated by another area of cardiac surgery, the treatment of congenital heart disease. An operation may be thought of as a time-varying covariable in the life history of such patients. In a multi-institutional study of transposition of the great arteries (TGA) with entry of patients shortly after birth, a small proportion of the patients died before surgical intervention (crossover from medical to surgical therapy)[21]. Can we infer from an analysis of death before repair (censoring at crossover) the 'natural history' of medical treatment for TGA? Not at all. The percent dying before repair over a several year period is small compared to the well established and highly lethal natural history of these babies[22]. What is missing is the risk in the crossovers, and that is not discernible in the data. One might imagine that in a lethal disease, diagnosed and cured immediately at birth in all patients, *no* deaths before repair would have occurred, yet the lethality of the lesion untreated would remain, although neutralised by the treatment strategy. Time-varying covariable analyses will *not* yield any information about natural history or comparisons of therapy to it[23].

This underscores the impossibility of determining the current risk of pure medical treatment of either ischaemic or valvular heart disease from observational studies of initially medically treated persons allowing for the possibility of crossover (transition) to surgery as a time-varying covariate. One *can* assess current protocols, but that is all. These, are the reasons for being cautious about just how to interpret any analysis of time-varying covariables that behave, more or less, as a form of crossover to another mode of treatment and are thus susceptible to the general analytical problem of what is known as competing risks.

With these limitations clearly in mind, the purposes of using time-varying anticoagulation covariables can be revisited from the perspective of their importance. If their importance is to somehow determine an *optimum* anticoagulation strategy, then perhaps specific studies (ideally randomised crossover in design) can be designed and analysed in a helpful way. For example, if *weighting* of each thromboembolic and bleeding event were accomplished according to an equivalent severity scale, an optimisation problem would result. If a sufficient number of levels of anticoagulation were studied, an optimum level could be established that minimised the combined sequelae of bleeding and thromboembolism. Such a study could far outweigh the analytical imponderables we have mentioned.

PREDICTIONS

One of the purposes of multivariable analyses of events after valve replacement is to permit patient-specific predictions to be made. For reasons unclear to me, this natural outgrowth of multivariable analysis is rarely exploited. One excuse is that the analysis is not considered 'good' enough to use for serious, real-life care and decision-making for individual patients; only 'general inferences' are to be drawn as a backdrop to the informal decision-making process known as clinical judgement. Yet the interest and public awareness of risk factors, their importance to individuals and their relevance in modifying behaviour, has been around as long as the Framingham heart disease study, whose time-related risk factor equations have recently been updated[24,25].

The very real limitations of prediction must, of course, be recognised. Projection in time beyond the data is treacherous, particularly if models such as splines are employed. If follow-up is short, phases of late increasing risk may not yet be evident, and, again, predictions far in the future are, thereby, affected[13]. The data base may not be rich enough, or the number of patients too small, or the number of events too few to yield reliable predictions. These latter limitations apply not just to the predictions, however, but to all the scientific inferences from the study.

COMPARISONS

Valve studies invite comparisons because of the availability of various device types and, indeed, alternatives such as valve repair. The general comparison of prostheses is probably best done in the context of a large, multiple device-type study. Overall comparisons can then be made in the form of a multivariable analysis. However, even if this direct comparison yields a highly significant P-value, it does not imply that under all conditions that valve is demonstrably superior (or inferior) to another, or that the difference will remain the same over all time. Thus, for patient decision-making, the comparisons should be risk-adjusted (patient-specific) time-related solutions of the multivariable equation.

Less useful for patient management are the more usual comparisons done by separate analyses of valve data sets. If the variables and their definitions are congruent, however, they can yield useful comparisons on a patient-specific basis. Even less useful are comparisons from meta-analyses and quasi-meta-analyses of the medical literature. They have the advantage of large numbers, and the severe disadvantage of lack of risk-factor adjusted patient-specific comparison.

Whichever type of analysis forms the basis for the comparison, an interesting dilemma is to decide *what* feature of outcome to compare! In the Task Force Subcommittee report on coronary bypass grafting surgery, three different comparison domains were presented: the hazard function domain (relative risks), the survivorship domain (survivorship differences), and the length of life domain (duration of freedom differences), which may yield different inferences depending on patient preferences[26]. For example, one might compare the time-related ratio of hazard functions. Depending on the risk-avoidance viewpoint of the patient, he may choose a higher early risk over the potential of a long term gain, or vice versa. One would caution, however, that a large hazard ratio does not imply a large survivorship difference (although it may), and a smaller ratio a small survivorship difference. It all depends on the magnitude of the base risk. If the prevalence of the event is very small, a risk 10, 100 or 1000 times as great may yield a small difference in prevalence. However, if the prevalence of the event is high, even a small difference in hazard may greatly magnify the prevalence (see Ref. 27 for a discussion of the logit relationship of risk factors to the probability of events).

Differences in survivorship are another meaningful way to make comparisons. Such comparisons result from the integration of risks (hazard) over time. This integration will emphasise the considerable duration of time it may require for even large hazard ratios (relative risks) to result in an important difference in survivorship (freedom from events).

Differences in length of life (or freedom from the event) require yet another integration over time. To illustrate, if the risk of an event were, indeed, constant over time and resulted in a 5% prevalence at 10 years (95% freedom, a hazard rate of 0.005129 events per year per individual) for one valve type, and a 10% prevalence at 10 years for another (90% freedom, a hazard rate of 0.01054 events per patient), on the average, patients would be free of that event for 9.75 years out of 10 in the first instance and 9.49 in the second. This is a comparative average difference in length of freedom of only 3 months in 10 years of follow-up!

Thus, there are multiple types of comparison that can be made, and each has its place, depending on the question being asked.

SUMMARY

Serious, in-depth studies of the post valve replacement state quickly reveal inadequacies in routine analytical methods. More help for hypothesis generating, as well as for suggesting optimum patient management strategies, is likely to come from newer, generalised methods for analysing time-related morbid events. These methods are computer-intensive, they require the development of new presentation formats, and they are only really successful when the separate expertise of analyst and medical investigator are combined.

The methods proposed are unlikely to solve directly the problems of thrombosis, embolism, and bleeding after valve replacement. They may, however, provide valuable clues to mechanisms, means to optimise the clinical management of valve recipients, and suggest ways to neutralise some of the inherent problems of this life-saving surgery while basic research is in progress.

APPENDIX

A generalised log likelihood formulation for a generalised outcome event.

The general formulation of the likelihood function (L) for a time-related point process with right censoring is:

$$L = \prod_{i=1}^{n} f(t_i)^{di} S(t_i),^{1-di} \qquad (1)$$

where f(t) is the death (event) density function at time t, S(t) is the survivorship function:

$$S(t) = 1–F(t), \qquad (2)$$

$$F(t) = \int_o^t f(u)du, \qquad (3)$$

and d is the event indicator (d=1 if event, d=0 if no event (right censored)). The maximum of the liklihood function will be the same as that of its logarithm (LL):

$$LL = \sum_{i=1}^{n} d_i \ln [f(t_i)] + (1 - d_i) \ln [S(t_i)]. \qquad (4)$$

Equation 4 can be reformulated interms of the hazard $\lambda(t)$ and cumulative hazard $\Lambda(t)$ functions:

$$\lambda(t) = f(t)/S(t), \qquad (5)$$

$$\Lambda(t) = \int_o^t \lambda(u)du, \qquad (6)$$

$$S(t) = \exp\,[-\lambda(t)], \qquad (7)$$

and therefore,

$$LL = \sum_{i=1}^{n} d_i \ln\,[\lambda(t_i)] - \Lambda(t_i). \qquad (8)$$

We propose that the exponent d be generalised to *any (positive) value*. By this, an "event" can take on a value reflecting severity (in Nelson's cumulative cost function, d would be the monitary cost of an event[19]).

Further generalisation can be made to the *interval censored* case, in which we would suggest that $\lambda(t)$ be replaced by the first order apprioximation $\Lambda(t)-\Lambda(t_c)$, where $\Lambda(t_c)$ is the cumulative hazard function at the start of the interval t_c and $\Lambda(t)$ is the cumulative hazard at the end of the interval t. Although it is superflous in the use of the log likelihood (LL) for either optimisation or of statistical testing, we can consider stabilizing the actual value of the LL function by using $[\Lambda(t)-\Lambda(t_c)]/(t_c\text{-}t)$.

Left censoring is introduced by adjusting the second term in equation 8:

$$LL = \sum_{i=1}^{n} d_i \ln[\lambda(t_i)] - [\Lambda(t_i) - \Lambda(t_{s,i})], \qquad (9)$$

where t_s is the beginning of observation. The importance of this is that the non-homogenous Poisson process is incorporated into a parametric modelling scheme simply by segmenting individual longitudinal observations into pieces ending at each event t_k and beginning at the previous event $t_s\text{-}t_{k-1}$ ($t_s=0$ for first event).

A generalised log likelihood function, then, for any mixture of possibly weighted events, including simplifications for exact duplicate observations, would be:

$$LL = \sum_{i=1}^{n} C_{1,i}\, W_{1,i} \ln[\lambda(t_i)] + (C_{1,i} + C_{2,i} + C_{3,i}) \bullet \qquad (10)$$

$$[\Lambda(t_i) - \Lambda(t_{s,i})] + C_{3,i} W_{3,i} \ln[\Lambda(t_i) - \Lambda(t_{o,i}],$$

where C_1 is the count of identically weighted (W_1) events at t_i, C_2 is the count of right censored events at t_i, and C_3 is the count in identically weighted (W_3) interval censored events. In all cases, t_s is the left censoring time.

This generalised formulation of the log likelihood function permits analysis of a wide range of longitudinal data in a more relavent way than most current formulations because: a) it permits incorporation of both longitudinal and cross-sectional (interval censored) observations; b) it permits left censoring, essential for certain forms of repeated events and time-varying covariate analyses; and c) it permits the event to take on a continuous value, rather then simply 0 or 1.

REFERENCES

1. Gill RD. Understanding Cox's regression model: A Martingale approach. J Am Stat Assn 1984;79:441–447.
2. Therneau TM, Grambsch PM, Fleming RT. Martingale-based residuals for survival models. Biometrika 1990;77:147–160.
3. Clayton D. The analysis of event history data:A review of progress and outstanding problems. Statistics in Medicine 1988;7:819–841.

4. McGoon DC. The risk of thromboembolism following valvular operations: How does one know? J Thorac Cardiovasc Surg 1984;88:782–786.
5. Edmunds LJ Jr, Clark RE, Cohn LH, Miller DC, Weisel RD. Guidelines for reporting morbidity and mortality after cardiac valvular operations. J Thorac Cardiovasc Surg 1988;96:351–353.
6. Schag CC, Heinrich RL, Ganz PA. Karnofsky performance status revisited: Reliability, validity, and guidelines. J Clin Oncol 1984;2:187–193.
7. Blackstone EH. Research methods for decision-making in cardiac surgery: inferences from repeating morbid events. In D'Alessandro LC, ed: Heart Surgery 1989. Rome: Casa Editrice Scientifica Internazionale, 1989:301–309.
8. Ascher H, Fiengold H. Repairable Systems Reliability. New York, Marcel Decker, 1984:7–46.
9. Blackstone EH. Methods and limitations of follow up assessment (clinical studies of time-related events). In: Bodnar E and Frater RWM (Eds): Replacement Cardiac Valves. New York, Pergamon Press, 1991:391–434.
10. Kuntze CEE, Ebels T, Eijgelaar A, Homan van de Heide JN. Rates of thromboembolism with three different mechanical heart valve prostheses: randomised study. Lancet 1989;1:514–517.
11. Hickey MSJ, Blackstone EH, Kirklin JW, Dean LS. Outcome probabilities and life history after surgical mitral commisurotomy: implications for balloon commissurotomy. J Am Coll Cardiol 1991;17:29–42.
12. Blackstone EH, Kirklin JW. Death and other time-related events after valve replacement. Circulation 1985;72:753–767.
13. Blackstone EH, Naftel DC, Turner ME Jr. The decomposition of time-varying hazard into phases, each incorporating a separate stream of concomitant information. J Am Stat Assn 1986;81:615–624.
14. SAS Institute Inc. SAS[R] User's Guide:Statistics, Version 5 Edition. Cary, NC:SAS Institute Inc. 1985:507–528.
15. SAS Institute Inc. SAS[R] Technical Report:P–175. Changes and Enhancements to the SAS[R] System, Release 5.18, Under OS and CMS. Cary, NC:SAS Institute Inc. 1988:192–265.
16. Jarjoura D. Smoothing hazard rates with cubic splines. Commun Statist-Simula 1988;17:377–392.
17. Nelson W. Hazard plotting for incomplete failure data. J Qual Technol 1969;1:27–52.
18. Kalbfleisch JD, Prentice RL. The Statistical Analysis of Failure Time Data. New York, John Wiley and Sons, 1980:179–188.
19. Nelson W. Graphical analysis of system repair data. J Qual Technol 1988;20:24–35.
20. Ferrazzi P. McGiffin DC, Kirklin JW, Blackstone EH, Bourge RC. Have the results of mitral valve replacement improved? J Thorac Cardiovasc Surg 1986;92:186–197.
21. Castaneda AR, Trusler GA. Paul MH, Blackstone EH, Kirklin JW. The early results of treatment of simple transposition in the current era. J Thorac Cardiovasc Surg 1988;95:14–27.
22. Liebman J, Cullum L, Belloc NB. Natural history of transposition of the great arteries. Anatomy and birth and death characteristics. Circulation 1969;40:237–262.
23. Crowley J, Storer BE. Comment. J Am Stat Assn 1983;78:277–281.
24. Anderson KM, Odell PM, Wilson PWF, Kannel WB. Cardiovascular disease risk profiles. Am Heart J 1991;121:293–298.
25. Anderson KM, Wilson PWF, Odell PM, Kannel WB. An updated coronary risk profile: A statement for health professionals. Circulation 1991;83:356–362.
26. Kirklin JW, Akins CW, Blackstone EH, et al (ACC/AHA Task Force Subcommittee on Coronary Artery Bypasss Graft Surgery): Guidelines and indications for the coronary artery bypass graft operation. J Am Coll Cardiol 1991;17:543–589 and Circulation 1991;83:1125–1173.
27. Kirklin JW, Barratt-Boyes BG. Cardiac Surgery. New York, John Wiley and Sons, 1986:117–204.

Chapter 6.3

Reliability of Comparative Data from Different Sources

Gary L. Grunkemeier and Marla R. London

This chapter reviews the comparative literature on thromboembolism (TE), thrombosis and bleeding following heart valve replacement, with emphasis on the reliability and reproducibility of results.

Selection of series

Articles were considered that described results of valve replacement reported since 1985[1–45]. In most cases, they were found by a search of the National Library of Medicine Medline literature database using the following criteria: heart valve prosthesis, year of publication greater than 1984, and English language. Only publications that reported results separated by model and position were used. One exception is that models of porcine valves were often pooled; if the great majority of porcine valves in a series were the same model, the whole series was classified according to that valve model.

Only those articles which reported the linearised rate for TE, or sufficient data to compute it (number of TE and total follow-up) were included. When one centre had more than one report on the same series, only the most complete, usually the most recent, results were used. Only series with a minimum of 200 years of follow-up were used for analysis, employing the same criterion used by McGoon in his excellent review of the adequacy of thromboembolism reporting[46].

Selection of summary statistics

Data dealing with death, TE, thrombosis and bleeding were extracted from each report (Table 6.3–1). In some articles, cumulative follow-up years were available for valve model but not for valve position. When necessary, follow-up years were prorated according to the number of valve replacements for each position, assuming that the valves inserted into different positions were used during roughly the same time frame.

Selection of valve models

The list of valve models included in this study was not meant to be exhaustive, merely sufficient to provide an adequate data base of reports to compare. Six models were selected: four mechanical and two tissue valves, all of which yielded a relatively large amount of comparative data. Together, these valve models accounted for 45 papers containing almost 30 thousand patients and over 125 thousand patient-years of follow-up (Table 6.3–2).

Table 6.3–1
Summary data extracted from selected papers

General	**Thromboembolism**
Valve model	Total number of TE
Position	Patients with TE
Number of patients	Number of late TE
Mean age	Number of TIA
Percent males	Number of fatal TE
Follow-up	**Other events**
Total patient-years	Percent anticoagulated
Percent completeness	Number of anticoagulant related bleeds
Death	Number of thromboses
Operative deaths	
Late deaths	

STATISTICAL METHODS

The statistical methods used were based on a constant rate model. This model implies an exponential event-free curve, for which a 'linearised' rate is the scale parameter, and a Poisson distribution for the number of events occurring in a fixed number of patient-years. Although the incidence of TE in a population seems to decrease with time[9], and the clusters of events that sometimes occur no doubt exhibit extra-Poisson variation[47], constant risk models, or linearised rates, are used almost universally and may be approximately valid for making broad comparisons, especially for series with comparable mean follow-up. Despite their limitations (see Chapter 6.2), linearised rates are useful for summary and comparison since large numbers of time-related curves are awkward to compare graphically.

Two quantitative statistical methods were employed to assess the variation among reported event rates: (a) confidence intervals for individual rates and (b) hypothesis tests (p-values) of the equivalence of all rates for a given event, model and valve position.

Confidence intervals. Of the several methods available for computing confidence intervals for constant rate events, the best from a theoretical standpoint seems to be the use of the likelihood ratio statistic[48], which has good statistical properties for many sampling schemes. Nevertheless, another method based on the relationship between the Poisson and Chi-square distributions[49], was used for this analysis because of its speed and simplicity. Confidence intervals of size 70% were used[50,51].

Rate comparisons. Comparisons among multiple rates were based on a test using the likelihood ratio statistic[52].

RESULTS

Traditionally, weighted averages have been used in an attempt to obtain precise estimates from pooled data (Fig. 6.3–1), but this method obscures the inherent variation among the series.

When TE rates for individual series are plotted separately (Fig. 6.3–2) there appears to be more variability within series of the same model than between series of different

Table 6.3–2
Clinical material: grouped by valve model and position

Valve Type	*Model*	*Position*	*Reports*	*Patients*	*Pt-Years*
Mechanical	Starr-Edwards	Aortic	6	3,609	16,876
		Mitral	7	4,112	22,226
		Double	2	503	2,063
		Total	**10**	**8,224**	**41,165**
	Bjørk-Shiley Standard	Aortic	6	1,210	7,097
		Mitral	7	1,627	10,393
		Double	3	330	1,867
		Total	**10**	**3,167**	**19,357**
	Medtronic Hall	Aortic	6	2,193	8,520
		Mitral	6	2,217	8,043
		Double	5	950	3,748
		Total	**6**	**5,360**	**20,311**
	St. Jude	Aortic	9	3,373	8,313
		Mitral	9	2,071	5,289
		Double	4	377	1,156
		Total	**11**	**5,821**	**14,758**
Porcine	Hancock	Aortic	6	716	3,484
		Mitral	8	1,674	7,827
		Double	2	104	550
		Total	**9**	**2,494**	**11,861**
	Carpentier	Aortic	7	1,501	7,510
		Mitral	8	1,980	9,311
		Double	3	326	1,500
		Total	**9**	**3,807**	**18,321**

models. The overall differences among series of each model are highly significant, as shown by the p-values below the horizontal axis. This implies that pooling the raw data as in Fig. 6.3–1 is not justified. To test whether discrepancies among TE rates were due to variable reporting of minor events, similar graphs for fatal TE rates and thrombosis were produced (Fig. 6.3–3). Although the overall rates were lower, the patterns of variation were similar. Bleeding rates were similarly scattered among series of the same valve (Fig. 6.3–4), suggesting that different intensities of anticoagulation may have been used.

Relationship of TE rates to other factors

Some of the factors that might help explain the variation in TE rates are listed in Table 6.3–3. Unfortunately, the published reports did not contain enough information to distinguish the relative importance of all these factors. Some factors were missing from all reports, while others, such as fatal TE rate, transient TE rate and completeness of follow-up (Table 6.3–1), were only available in a few series.

However, it was possible to demonstrate the relationship of TE rate to some other factors, including late death rate and bleeding rate. Since late deaths include fatal TEs, we adjusted the death rate by subtracting the fatal TE rate, when given. For series that did not report fatal TE, we adjusted the death rate downward by 17%, because this was the average percentage of deaths due to TE in the series where it was available: 15% in 32 aortic, 17% in 36 mitral and 23% in 13 double valve series. The remaining, non-TE

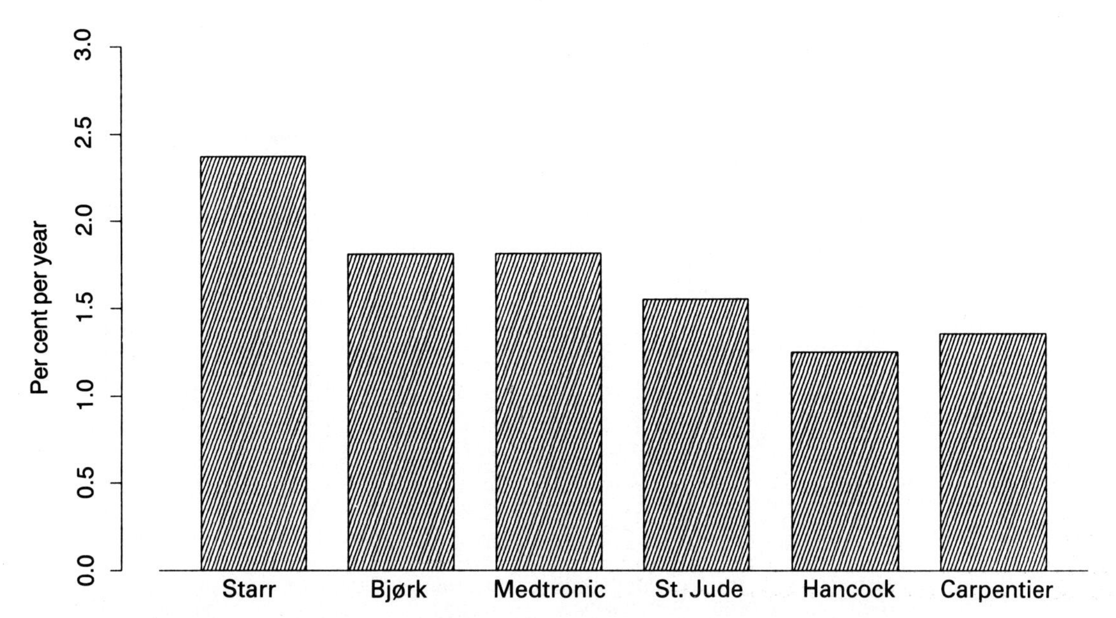

Figure 6.3–1: Summary of thromboembolism rates from published aortic valve replacement series. Traditional 'pooling' by computing weighted means disguises the variability and is misleading.

death rate was significantly related to the TE rate (Fig. 6.3–5). The bleeding rate was also significantly related to the TE rate (Fig. 6.3–6).

DISCUSSION

The traditional scientific method is based on the concept that a single study, no matter how large or well performed, cannot serve by itself to make substantial inferences without corroboration by other investigators. It is important to see to what extent results with the same valve in different centres are reproducible. Also, when an event is relatively rare, as are TE and especially thrombosis, it requires more experience than a single study may possess to determine precisely its rate of occurrence.

Sources of observed variation

The overall distribution of TE rates from series with over 500 valve-years is shown as a histogram in Fig. 6.3–7. A smooth density function is drawn to fit the histogram, and portrays a variation among series very similar to a published graph of variation in anticoagulant adequacy[53], and also to the variation ascribed to patients within a given series[9] (Chapter 5.2).

Major sources of variation among reported TE rates may be due to patient risk factors (Chapters 1.1, 1.2, 1.3 and 1.5), age and valve position, valve model, centre/series (Table 6.3–3) and differences in the intensity of anticoagulation used (Chapter 3.4).

Many patient-related factors are known to influence TE[54,55]. It is noteworthy in this respect, that TE rates in some epidemiological studies of atrial fibrillation (Chapter 1.2) and the elderly (Chapter 1.1) are equal to those observed in prosthetic valve series. The

Aortic TE Rate Comparisons

with 70% confidence intervals and comparison p-values

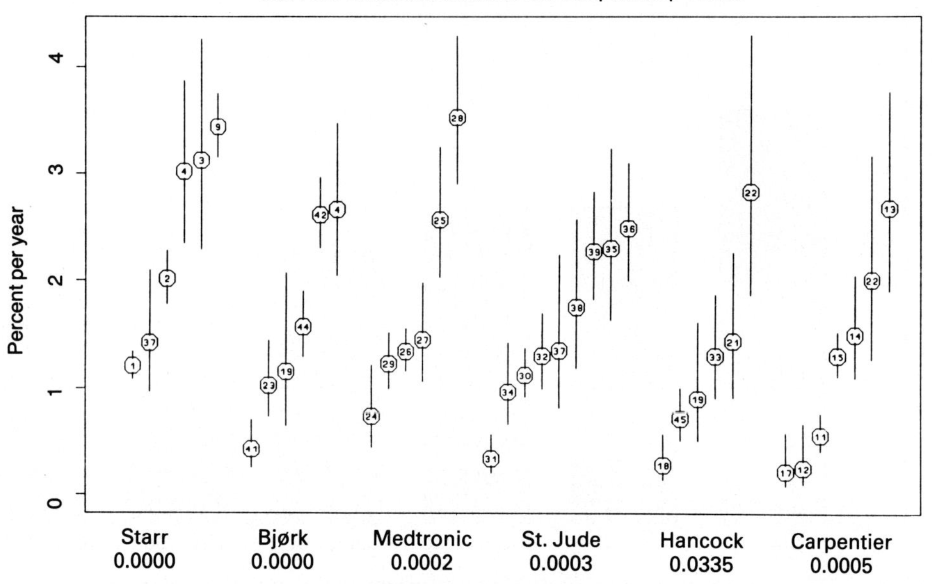

Mitral TE Rate Comparisons

with 70% confidence intervals and comparison p-values

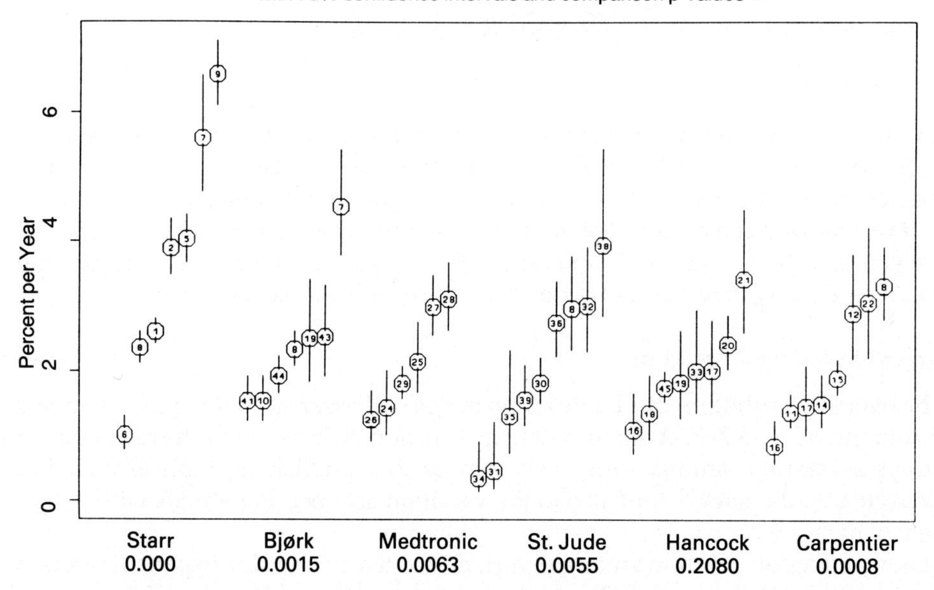

Figure 6.3–2: A. An unmixed version of the comparative aortic series which were pooled together in Figure 6.3–1. Circled (reference) numbers are plotted at mean values for each series, and vertical bars span the 70% confidence intervals. Numbers below the horizontal axis are the p-values for differences among the series with the same valve. B. Same display for the mitral valve series. Note that Ref 28 and Ref 36 comprise 'third world' patients, many of whom were not anticoagulated.

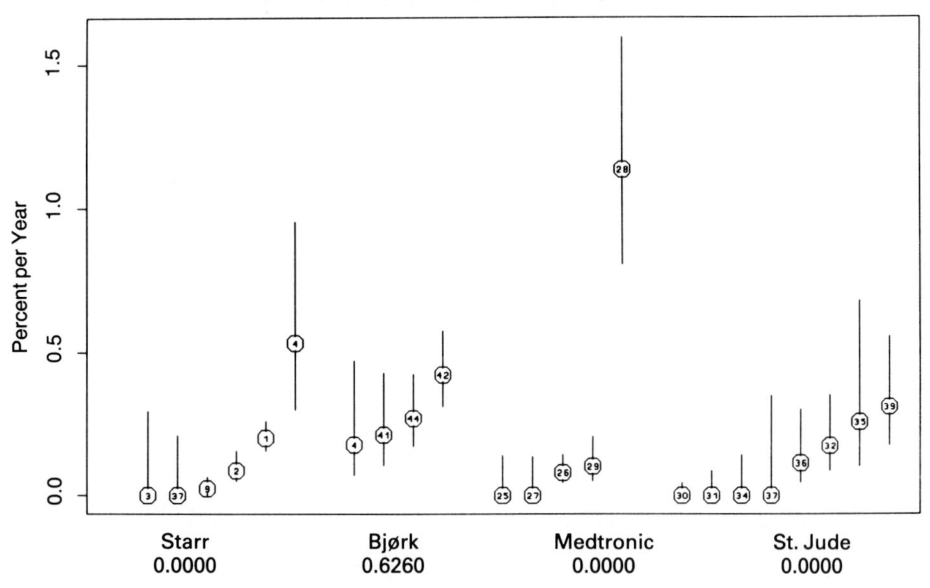

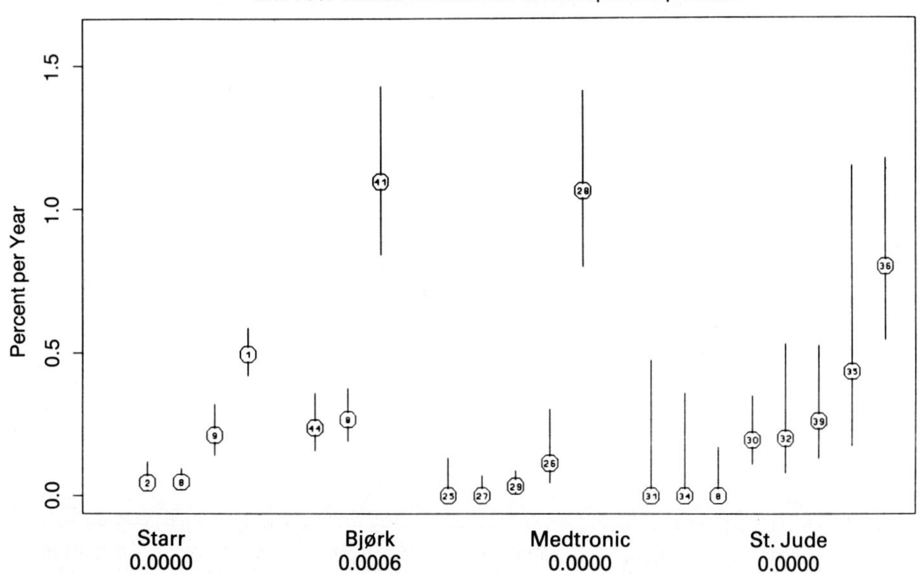

Figure 6.3–3: Comparison of reported thrombosis rates for aortic (A) and mitral (B) series. See legend to figure 6.3–2. Note that Ref 28 and Ref 36 comprise 'third world' patients, many of whom were not anticoagulated.

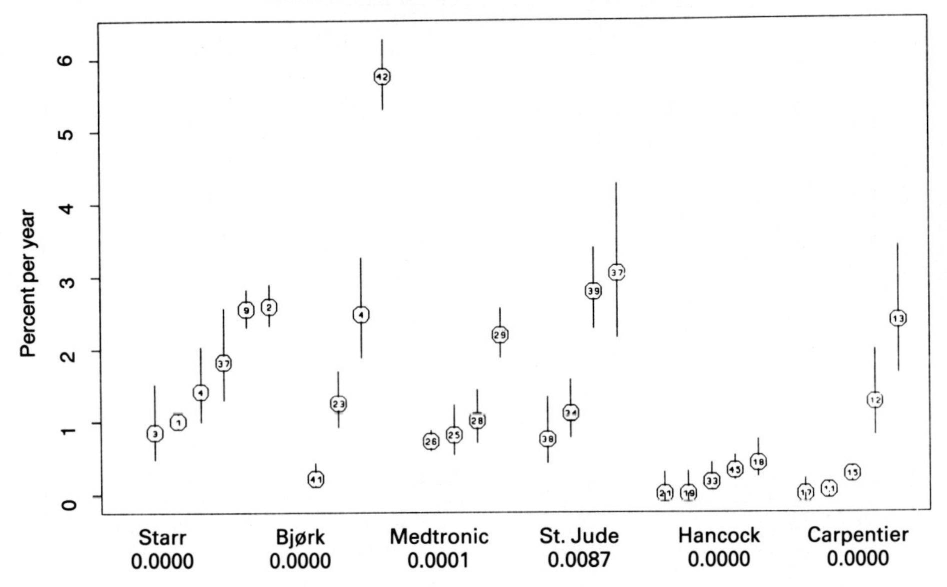

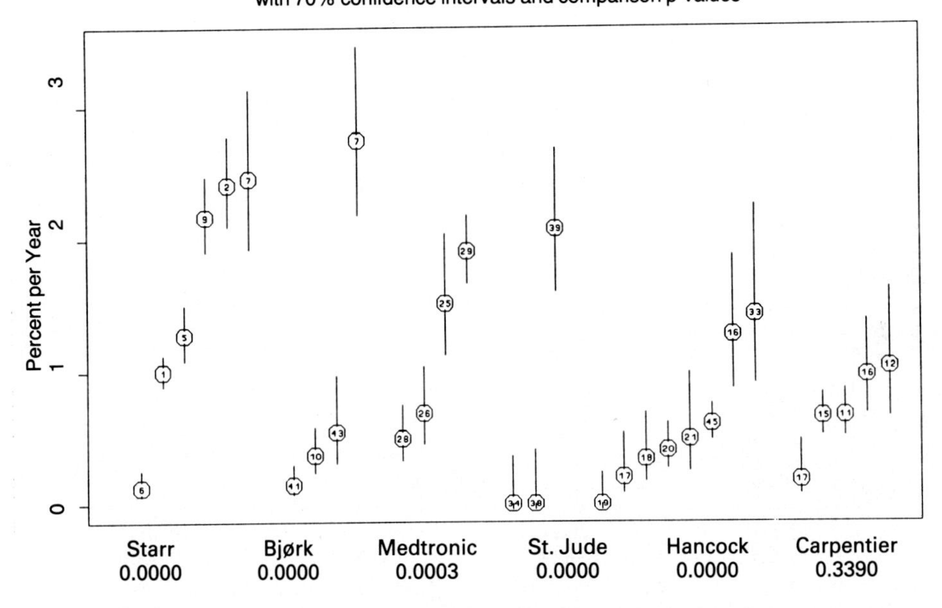

Figure 6.3–4: Comparison of reported bleeding rates for aortic (A) and mitral (B) series. See legend to Figure 6.3–2.

Table 6.3–3
Sources of variability in reported TE results

Patient	*Valve Model*	*Series/Centre*
Age	Tissue vs. mechanical	Patient demographics
Atrial fibrillation	Between tissue	Patient selection
LV thrombus	Among mechanical	Surgical variables
CV disease		Postop anticoagulant management
Hypertension		Data acquisition
Diabetes		Data management
Valve position		Publication bias

relationships between TE and late death (Fig. 6.3–5) and between TE and bleeding (Fig. 6.3–6) could reflect sicker patients having more TE and more difficult medical management (patient factor), or could be related to data acquisition methods (series factor). Postoperative anticoagulant management[53,55] (Chapter 3.4), follow up technique, and methods of data management are important determinants of reported TE results. An attempt to standardise definitions has recently been made[56], but these recommendations still leave much scope for interpretation (Chapter 6.4), and unfortunately they were not in effect in the series analysed here.

The reported data available for analysis (Table 6.3–2) represents only a small fraction (about 2–5%) of the valves implanted, and is certainly not a random subset. There are many types of bias that affect reported results. Selection bias occurs in the collection, the analysis and the decision to report data. One article lists 35 types of bias[57]. A very

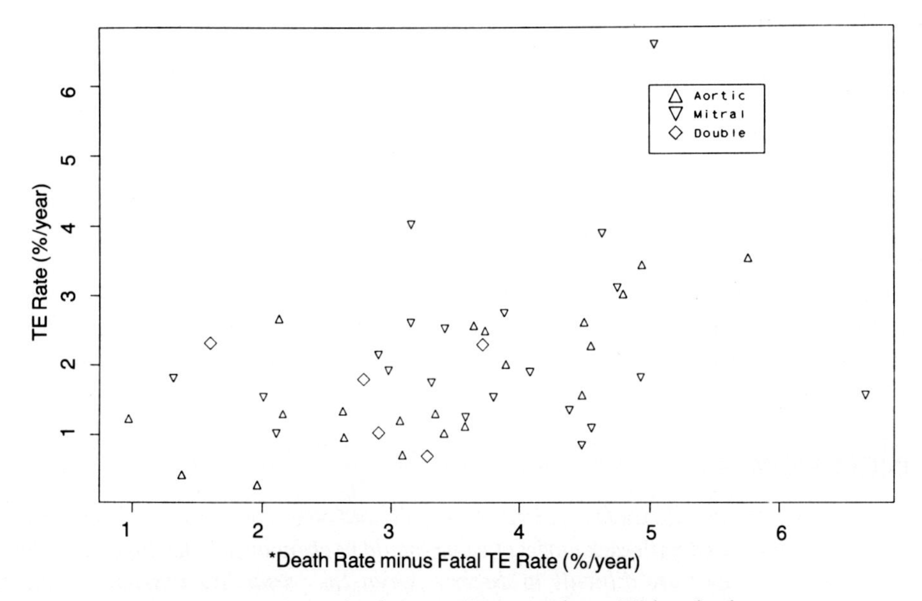

Figure 6.3–5: Relationship between TE rate and non-TE late death rate.

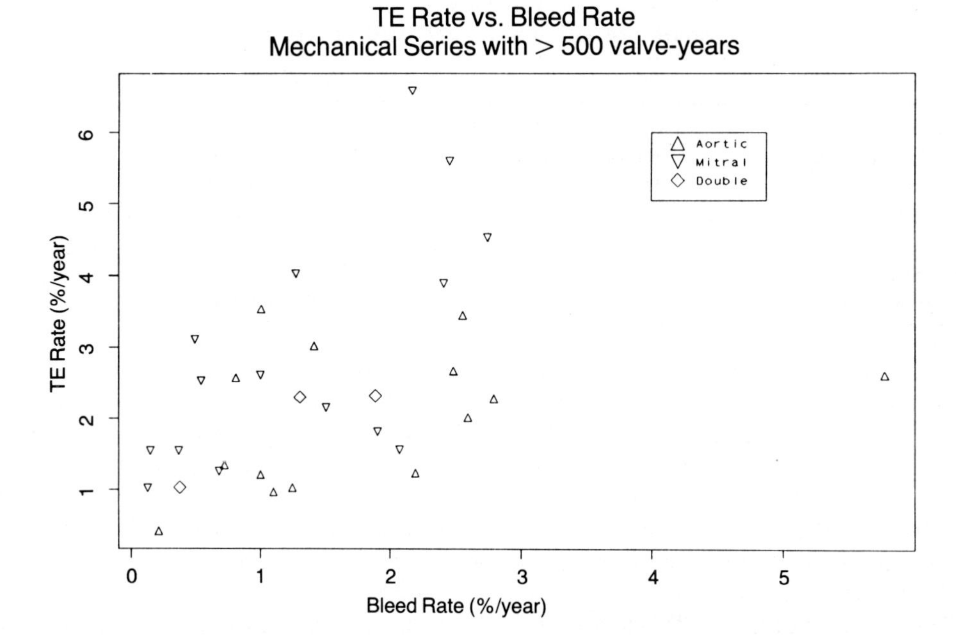

Figure 6.3–6: Relationship between TE rate and bleeding rate.

important example is *publication bias*[58,59]. The series that are published are not necessarily representative. Indeed they may be predominantly those reporting the best or the worst results[59].

It is impossible to separate the effect of valve model from the series/centre factor, since most centres use primarily one type of valve. Even if they use more than one type consistently, patient selection within the centre becomes a source of bias. If a random allocation of valves had been made among patients within a centre, statistical methods could have been used to measure the effect on complication rates due to valve model at that centre. Unfortunately the number of randomised studies of valves is few and those that exist are often too small and short-term to show differences among valves. Those studies which are sufficiently large and long-term often deal with valve models that are obsolete by the time the study is completed. Comparison of complication rates among valve models from the available large observational series is potentially dangerous because a large amount of the observed variation is due to systematic differences associated with uncontrolled factors (other than valve type) which contribute to the observed scatter.

CONCLUSION

On the basis of the variability of reported rates of TE and other complications, the concept of a certain TE rate associated with each model of valve should be abandoned. The differences that may exist between prostheses are difficult to discern, given the variability inherent in literature reports.

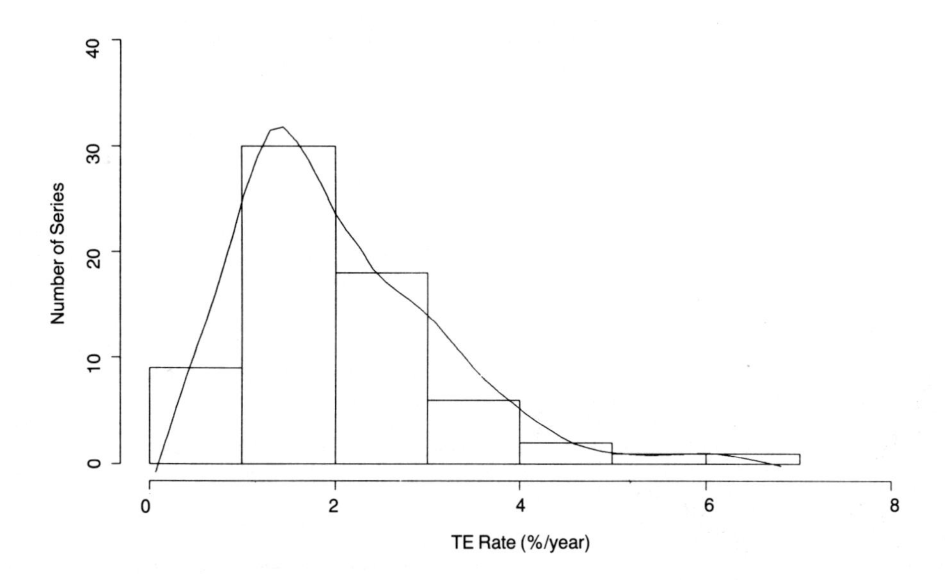

Figure 6.3–7: Heterogeneity among the TE rates from all series, shown as a histogram. A smooth density function is drawn to fit the histogram.

Theoretically, a randomised trial of valve designs would offer the best hope of properly measuring TE rate differences between models. However, the differences may be so small that such a study would take many years, especially with the accrual problems such studies have, and by then valve models or anticoagulant recommendations could change, problems which have already affected randomised valve studies.

This argues for careful collection and use of the mass of observational data that becomes available from ongoing practice data bases[60]. It also argues for collaborative efforts in data collection, using a common protocol and uniform definitions. A national valve registry has been underway for a few years in the UK, and a national Canadian Cardiac Valve Study is currently being planned. The US FDA may enforce new regulations requiring the manufacturer to be responsible for maintaining a valve/patient tracking system. Perhaps, following the model of pacemaker tracking systems, this function could be provided by an independent agent to ensure a controlled protocol for all valve models. Such an independent system would be the highest economy of volume, and may best serve the needs of industry, government, the medical community, and ultimately the patient.

REFERENCES

1. Corcos T, Gandjbakhch I, Pavie A, et al. Long-term results of valve replacement with Starr-Edwards silicone ball prostheses. Circulation 1987;76(Suppl IV):446.
2. Akins CW, Buckley MJ, Daggett WM, Austen WG, Hilgenberg AD, Jacobs ML. Ten-year follow-up of the Starr-Edwards prosthesis. In Rabago G, and Cooley DA (Eds.). Heart Valve Replacement and Future Trends in Cardiac Surgery. Mount Kisco, Futura Publishing Company, 1987:137–143.
3. Hackett D, Fessatidis I, Sapsford R, Oakley C. Ten year clinical evaluation of Starr-Edwards 2400 and 1260 aortic valve prostheses. Br Heart J 1987;57:356–363.

4. Perier P, Bessou JP, Swanson JS, et al. Comparative evaluation of aortic valve replacement with Starr, Bjørk, and porcine valve prostheses. Circulation 1985;72(Suppl II):140–145.
5. Schoevaerdts JC, Buche M, El Gariani A, et al. Twenty years' experience with the Model 6120 Starr-Edwards valve in the mitral position. J Thorac Cardiovasc Surg 1987;94:375–382.
6. Fessatidis I, Hackett D, Oakley CM, Sapsford RN, Bentall HH. Ten-year clinical evaluation of isolated mitral valve and double-valve replacement. Ann Thorac Surg 1987;43:368–372.
7. Perier P, Deloche A, Chauvaud S, et al. Clinical comparison of mitral valve replacement using porcine, Starr and Bjørk valves. J Card Surg 1988;3:359–368.
8. Eberlein U, von der Emde J, Rein J, Esperer HD. Thromboembolic and bleeding complications after mitral valve replacement. Eur J Cardiothorac Surg 1990;4:605–612.
9. Starr A, Grunkemeier GL. Recurrent embolism: significance and management. This book, Chapter 5.2.
10. Fessatidis I, Vassiliadis KE, Monro JL, Ross JK, Shore DF, Drury PJ. Thirteen years evaluation of the Bjørk-Shiley isolated mitral valve prosthesis. The Wessex experience. J Cardiovasc Surg 1989;30: 957–965.
11. Pelletier LC, Carrier M, Leclerc Y, Lepage G, deGuise P, Dyrda I. Porcine versus pericardial bioprostheses: A comparison of late results in 1,593 patients. Ann Thorac Surg 1989;47:352–361.
12. Zussa C. Del Ponte S, Ottino GM, Pansini S, Zattera G, Morea M. Carpentier-Edwards bioprosthesis: A 7-year follow-up in 361 patients. Thorac Cardiovasc Surgeon 1986;34:252–257.
13. Douglas PS, Hirschfeld Jr, JW, Edie RN, Harken AH, Stephenson LW, Edmunds Jr, LH. Clinical comparison of St. Jude and porcine aortic valve prostheses. Circulation 1985;72(Suppl II):135–139.
14. Nashef SAM, Sethia B, Turner MA, Davidson KG, Lewis S, Bain WH. Bjørk-Shiley and Carpentier-Edwards valves. J Thorac Cardiovasc Surg 1987;93:394–404.
15. Jamieson WRE, Allen PA, Miyagishima RT, et al. The Carpentier-Edwards standard porcine bioprosthesis. J Thorac Cardiovasc Surg 1990;99:543–561.
16. Perier P, Deloche A, Chauvaud S, et al. A 10-year comparison of mitral valve replacement with Carpentier-Edwards and Hancock porcine bioprostheses. Ann Thorac Surg 1989;48:54–59.
17. Bolooki H, Kaiser GA, Mallon SM, Palatianos GM. Comparison of long-term results of Carpentier-Edwards and Hancock bioprosthetic valves. Ann Thorac Surg 1986;42:494–499.
18. Hartz RS, Fisher EB, Finkelmeier B, et al. An eight-year experience with porcine bioprosthetic cardiac valves. J Thorac Cardiovasc 1986;91:910–917.
19. Martinell J, Fraile J, Artiz V, Moreno J, Rabago G. Long-term comparative analysis of the Bjørk-Shiley and Hancock valves implanted in 1975. J Thorac Cardiovasc Surg 1985;90:741–749.
20. Cohn LH, Allred EN, Cohn LA, et al. Early and late risk of mitral valve replacement. J Thorac Cardiovasc Surg 1985;90:872–881.
21. Jamieson WRE, Allen P, Janusz MT, et al. First-generation porcine bioprostheses: Valve-related complications in the intermediate term. In Bodnar E, Yacoub M (Eds.). Biologic and Bioprosthetic Valves. New York, Yorke Medical Books, 1986:104–115.
22. Bloomfield P, Kitchin AH, Wheatley DJ, Walbaum PR, Lutz W, Miller HC. A prospective evaluation of the Bjørk-Shiley, Hancock, and Carpentier-Edwards heart valve prostheses. Circulation 1986;73:1213- 1222.
23. Milano AD, Bortolotti U, Mazzucco A, Guerra F, Magni A, Gallucci V. Aortic valve replacement with the Hancock standard, Bjørk-Shiley, and Lillehei-Kaster prostheses. J Thorac Cardiovasc Surg 1989;98:37–47.
24. Vallejo JL, Gonzales-Santos JM, Albertos J, et al. Eight years' experience with the Medtronic-Hall valve prosthesis. Ann Thorac Surg 1990;50:429–436.
25. Beaudet RL, Nakhle G, Beaulieu CL, Doyle D, Gauvin C, Poirier NL. Medtronic-Hall prosthesis: Valve related deaths and complications. Can J Cardiol 1988;4:376–380.
26. Nitter-Hauge S, Abdelnoor M. Ten-year experience with the Medtronic Hall valvular prostheses. Circulation 1989;80(Suppl I):43- 48.
27. Butchart EG, Lewis PA, Grunkemeier GL, Kulatilake N, Breckenridge IM. Low risk of thrombosis and serious embolic events despite low-intensity anticoagulation. Circulation 1988;78(Suppl I):66–77.
28. Antunes MJ, Wessels A, Sadowski RG, et al. Medtronic Hall valve replacement in a third-world population group. J Thorac Cardiovasc Surg 1988;95:980–993.
29. Rabago G, Fraile J, Martinell J et al. Long-term results with double (Mi-Ao) mechanical valve implants. J Cardiovasc Surg 1990;31:24.
30. Arom KV, Nicoloff DM, Kersten TE, Northup, III WF, Lindsay WG, Emery RW. Ten years' experience with the St. Jude Medical valve prosthesis. Ann Thorac Surg 1989;47:831–837.
31. Baudet EM, Oca CC, Roques XF et al. A 5½ year experience with the St. Jude Medical cardiac valve prosthesis. J Thorac Cardiovasc Surg 1985;90:137–144.
32. Burckhardt D, Striebel D, Vogt S et al. Heart valve replacement with St. Jude Medical valve prosthesis. Circulation 1988;78(Suppl I): 18–24.

33. Czer LSC, Matloff JM, Chaux A, DeRobertis MA, Gray RJ. Comparative clinical experience with porcine bioprosthetic and St. Jude valve replacement. Chest 1987;91:503–514.
34. Duncan JM, Cooley DA, Reul GJ et al. Durability and low thrombogenicity of the St. Jude Medical valve at 5-year follow-up. Ann Thorac Surg 1986;42:500–505.
35. Fraedrich G, Hoge R, Fiedler R, Hehrlein FW. Five-years actuarial analysis after heart valve replacement with the St. Jude Medical prosthesis. Z Kardiol 1986;75(Suppl 2):282–285.
36. Kinsley RH, Antunes MJ, Colsen PR. St. Jude Medical valve replacement. J Thorac Cardiovasc Surg 1986;92:349–360.
37. Lund O, Knudsen MA, Pilegaard HK, Magnussen K, Nelson TT. Long-term performance of Starr-Edwards silastic ball valves and St. Jude Medical bileaflet valves. Eur Heart J 1990;11: 108–119.
38. Nair CK, Mohiuddin SM, Hilleman DE et al. Ten-year results with the St. Jude Medical prosthesis. Am J Cardiol 1990;65:217–225.
39. Czer LSC, Chaux A, Matloff JM et al. Ten-year experience with the St. Jude medical valve for primary valve replacement. J Thorac Cardiovasc Surg 1990;100:44–55.
40. Arom KV, Nicoloff DM, Kersten TE, Northrup WF, Lindsay WG, Emery RW. Ten-year follow-up study of patients who had double valve replacement with the St. Jude Medical prosthesis. J Thorac Cardiovasc Surg 1989;98:1008–1016.
41. Sethia B, Turner MA, Lewis S, Rodger RA, Bain WH. Fourteen years' experience with the Bjørk-Shiley tilting disc prosthesis. J Thorac Cardiovasc Surg 1986;91:350–361.
42. Borkon AM, Soule L, Baugham KL et al. Ten-year analysis of the Bjørk-Shiley standard aortic valve. Ann Thorac Surg 1987;43:39- 51.
43. Harjula A, Mattila S, Maamies T et al. Long-term follow-up of Bjørk-Shiley mitral valve replacement. Scand J Thorac Cardiovasc Surg 1986;20:79–84.
44. Flemma RJ, Mullen DD, Kleinman LH, Werner PH, Anderson AJ, Weirauch E. Survival and event-free analysis of 785 patients with Bjørk-Shiley spherical-disc valves. Ann Thorac Surg 1988;45:258- 272.
45. Gallucci V, Mazzucco A, Bortolotti U, Milano A, Guerra F, Thiene G. The standard Hancock porcine biprosthesis: Overall experience at the University of Padova. J Card Surg 1988;3:337–345.
46. McGoon DC. The risk of thromboembolism following valvular operations:How does one know? J Thorac Cardiovasc Surg 1984;88:782- 786.
47. Dunn JK. A stochastic model for the occurrence of transient ischemic attacks. Biometrics 1980;36:91–103.
48. Kalbfleisch JD, Prentice RL. The Statistical Analysis of Failure Time Data. Seattle, John Wiley and Sons, 1980;50.
49. Cox DR. Some simple approximate tests for Poisson variates. Biometrika 1953;40:354–60.
50. Kirklin JW, Surgical concepts, reseach methods and data analysis and use. In Cardiac Surgery. New York, John Wiley & Sons, 1982;183.
51. Bailey KR. Inter-study differences:How should they influence the interpretation and analysis of results? Statist Med 1987;6:351–358.
52. Lawless JF. Statistical Models and Methods for Lifetime Data. Seattle, John Wiley and Sons, 1982;112.
53. Butchart EG, Lewis PA, Kulatilake ENP, Breckenridge IM. Anticoagulation variability between centres: implications for comparative prosthetic valve assessment. Eur J Cardiothorac Surg 1988;2:72- 81.
54. Rahimtoola SH. Lessons learned about the determinants of the results of valve surgery. Circulation 1988;78:1503–1507.
55. Edmunds LH Jr. Thrombotic and bleeding complications of prosthetic heart valves. Ann Thorac Surg 1987;44:430–445.
56. Edmunds LH Jr, Clark RE, Cohn LH, Miller DC, Weisel RD. Guidelines for reporting morbidity and mortality after cardiac valvular operations. Ann Thorac Surg 1988;46:257–259.
57. Sackett DL. Bias in analytic research. J Chron Dis 1979;32:51–63.
58. Pocock SJ, Hughes MD. Estimation issues in clinical trials and overviews. Statist Med 1990;9:657–671.
59. Berlin JA, Begg CB, Louis TA. An assessment of publication bias using a sample of published clinical trials. J Am Statist Assoc 1989;84:381–392.
60. Pryor DB, Lee KL. Methods for the analysis and assessment of clinical databases: the clinician's perspective. Statist Med 1991;10:617–628.

Chapter 6.4

A Critical Assessment of Thrombosis and Embolism Reporting Methods

Endre Bodnar

Published clinical follow up studies fall into two categories. One presents personal or team achievements without any conclusion of general importance being even attempted. The second category contains those papers that report the results of well designed trials or intend to validate, or otherwise, a hypothesis that is based on scientific argument. It includes observational clinical studies that use rigorous scientific methods, conducted so as to yield useful clinical inferences and to assist in formulating testable hypotheses. These publications demand clarity and at least a certain, minimum degree of uniformity in terminology, data collection, management and reporting methods.

This fairly general statement can eminently be applied to clinical science related to thrombosis, embolism and bleeding. However, the onus of achieving the required clarity and uniformity has so far been left mainly to individual efforts, since the generally adopted guidelines for reporting results with replacement heart valves do not contain specific details regarding this subject[1]. The need for a critical assessment of follow up and reporting methods thus emerges and it encompasses terminology as well as data presentation and interpretation.

The first step in this intellectual process is to properly define those events that have been basketed as "thromboembolism" so far, because the grouping of valve thrombosis and systemic embolism together creates a paradox situation and blocks the way to assessing and understanding valve thrombogenicity.

Thrombosis and embolism have to be separated and treated as two different identities, both by definition and empirical argument. It appears that the word 'thromboembolism' has been misinterpreted over the years when applied in an extended way to include embolism and valve thrombosis.

According to the definition in medical dictionaries, thromboembolism is "the occlusion of a blood vessel by the lodgement of a portion of a thrombus". Thrombosis, on the other hand, is defined as "the formation of a thrombus". Nothing can be added to the clarity of these two definitions.

Current clinical experiences seem to confirm the validity of the above two, classical definition. Rigorous statistical analysis of the accumulated data has led to the conclusion that from clinical, pathological and bioengineering points of view, valve thrombosis and embolism are two entirely different identities and should be considered as such (see Chapters 2.4 and 6.2).

The first proposal is, therefore, to define *valve thrombosis* as the development of macroscopical blood clot on the surface of the replacement valve, which is or has been symptomatic. It has to be differentiated from *thrombotic apposition* which is asymptomatic, discovered as an incidental finding at operation or autopsy and which has not given rise to any haemodynamic consequences or embolism. However, under some circumstances the latter definition may merge into the former, since both may be part of the same process and increasingly sophisticated diagnostic methods may be able to detect thrombus on the prosthesis before it becomes symptomatic (see Chapters 2.4, 2.6 and 5.1).

Embolism is the occlusion of a blood vessel by an object that entered the cardiovascular system or developed in it elsewhere. In the vast majority of cases it is caused by the 'lodgement of a portion of a thrombus'. The word 'thromboembolism' is thus acceptable, but a clear statement should be made when it is used that it does not include valve, or any other, thrombosis. However, it is highly recommended that, in the context of replacement heart valves, the less ambiguous term 'embolism' is used as opposed to 'thromboembolism'.

Both the rate of valve thrombosis and that of embolism are confounded in almost all clinical series by several factors other than the true thrombogenicity of the prosthetic valve. Anticoagulation management is probably the most important among the confounding factors (see Chapters 2.4 and 3.4).

When reporting anticoagulation management/experience, it should always be borne in mind that anticoagulation, for both clinical and reporting purposes, is not a categorical but rather a numerical, continuous variable. In clinical practice, well defined goals have to be set and achieved to maintain the required level of anticoagulation. It follows that the statement 'all patients were placed on long term anticoagulation with warfarin' lacks precision.

The second proposal is, therefore, to report the target and the measured range of the level of anticoagulation after heart valve surgery. It is recommended that the results be expressed as International Normalised Ratio (INR) (see Chapter 3.3). Furthermore, the accuracy of the anticoagulation control should be disclosed if substantial inferences are to be made from the assessment of the clinical results.

It certainly gives much food for thought that while a statement on the follow up accuracy is invariably required from clinical follow up studies, the extent of the regular follow up investigations has never been within the scope of accepted or recommended methodology. Therefore, it seems prudent to propose that the frequency of prothrombin tests as well as the measured maximum, minimum and mean INR levels should be accounted for in studies reporting on thrombosis, embolism and bleeding after heart valve surgery. In other terms, the target level of anticoagulation should be stated and that statement accompanied by a clear account of the number (expressed as proportion as well) of patients who remained within the target range during the entire study period. A thorough analysis of the group where this could not be achieved may then lead to new inferences regarding the effect of anticoagulation on thrombosis, embolism and bleeding.

It is apparent from the existing knowledge that the level of anticoagulation has a direct effect on valve thrombosis, embolism and pathological bleeding. It thus confounds the study of thrombogenicity in its entire complexity. There seem to be only two ways of circumventing the problem.

The stratification of thrombosis and embolism incidences according to the actual INR levels is one. There are, however, inherent problems in this approach. While it is possible, though not easy, to maintain identical INR levels in a prospective randomised trial comparing two or more prostheses, retrospective studies will not be comparable unless the INR levels are reported and they coincide.

Theoretically, an empirical curve could be constructed for every single type of replacement valve, depicting the effect of the independent variable INR level on the dependent variable thrombogenicity, be it the rate of valve thrombosis or embolism. If it could be proved that this relation is identical or falls within 95% confidence limits for all types of valvular prostheses, one single curve could be used to 'normalise' clinical results and put individual experiences in perspective. This type of approach has already been started by Eric G. Butchart and his co-workers, using one type of mechanical valve (see Chapter 3.4). Data to construct such curves for other replacement valves are not available, but the importance of the problem warrants clinical research to see if this is possible.

A simpler and more robust method seems to be the calculation of the aggregate of thrombosis, embolism and bleeding, as a TEB index (vide infra). While it would not reveal delicate details on the interaction between thrombogenicity and anticoagulation, it could provide an easy to comprehend number defining the rate, incidence and/or risk imposed by the thrombogenicity of the prosthesis together with other, potentially existing risk factors in the given study group and those of the compulsory preventive measures, that is anticoagulation.

The TEB index could be calculated as the sum of the three complications and/or the individual rate, incidence or hazard of bleeding divided by that of embolism in the same series (Fig. 6.4–1). As a formula for calculating the variance would be readily available, results would become strictly comparable. The informative value could be enhanced further by adapting the concept of weighted events (see Chapter 6.2).

One may argue that misleading information could be generated by this method if patients having a prosthesis of low thrombogenicity are overanticoagulated, resulting in a higher bleeding rate which penalises and confounds the true performance of the valve. In routine clinical situations only two examples fall within the scope of this reasoning.

The first example would be a prospective randomised trial where the tested valves have widely different thrombogenicity and the standard anticoagulation is adjusted in all patients according to the requirements of the worst prosthesis. Such a case, however, is unlikely to exist in real life. As the trial is prospective, the thrombogenicity of the participating valves is unknown and a middle of the range level of anticoagulation would probably be selected for all patients. If the results were to justify it, prosthesis specific anticoagulation could be introduced instead, and the trial regarding thrombogenicity considered as complete.

The second example would be a retrospective follow up study where the INR levels employed were well above the recently introduced internationally recommended standards and grossly above those required for a particular prosthesis of very low thrombogenicity. In such a situation, the TEB index would measure management efficacy rather than valve performance and the results of such an overdosage of anticoagulants could not be accepted for making any inference other than the magnitude of bleeding risk due to overanticoagulation (Fig. 6.4–1).

The remaining group of confounding factors poses a more difficult problem. Atrial fibrillation, left atrial or ventricular thrombus, advanced age, arteriosclerosis, hypertension, diabetes, cigarette smoking and diet factors are all known risk factors for

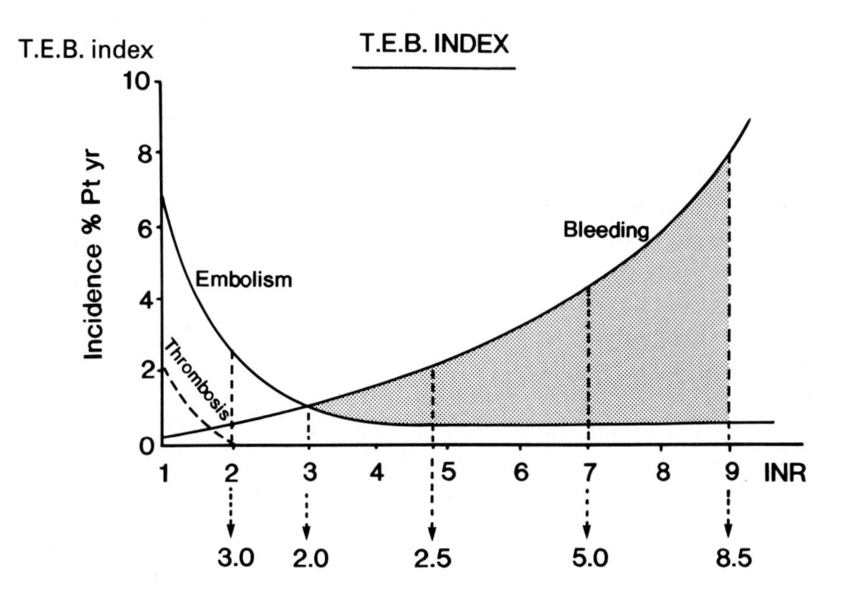

Figure 6.4–1: Graphic representation of TEB index vs. INR level.

embolism (see Chapters 1.1 – 1.5 and Chapter 2.4). If the patient population with heart valve replacement is large enough, all these predisposing factors will be present to a smaller or larger extent. The problem arises because not all factors will be present in all patients and the presence of one factor in a patient does not exclude the presence of one or more others in the same patient. As an example, a 75 year old man with a replacement valve may be in atrial fibrillation, be arteriosclerotic, have diabetes and smoke more than 40 cigarettes a day. This confounding problem is magnified by the fact that the above risk factors may be present without the existence of heart valve disease or even without the existence of any organic cardiac disease in another group selected from the general population.

One convenient way of circumventing the problem is to put all additional risk factors onto a common denominator and call the aggregate, non-valve related risk of embolism the 'background incidence' of the event in the general population. Indeed, it has been proposed to compare all clinical results to that background incidence, eliminating thereby the confounding effect in a summary way. The idea, however, has at least two flaws.

The first arises within the definition of 'general population'. The demographic differences on our globe are such that the proposal of a 'standard' background incidence with a world wide validity must be rejected. The considerable size of racial minority groups in some countries and the widely different living standards within some racial groups prohibit the use of 'general population background' according to individual countries, unless it can be proved statistically that the composition of the valve patient population under consideration is identical to that of the general population in the given country. Patients coming for surgery from another continent would further increase the bias.

The second flaw comes about if one intends to use the general population for comparison with patients after heart valve replacement, because the latter group is not a sample of the former. The bias is introduced by the simple fact that all those receiving a replacement heart valve have had heart valve disease with or without complications prior to surgery. The frequency and importance of the additional risk factors therefore become distorted. One may anticipate that the select group of the general population defined as 'heart valve patients' will have considerably more individuals with atrial fibrillation, for example.

It is therefore suggested that inferences will be more realistic if clinical results after valve replacement are compared to an identical, or closely similar group of heart valve patients who did not have their valve replaced. The problem is not as insurmountable as it appears at first glance.

As has already been established (vide supra), there are two 'background' incidences: general and specific. The former is the stroke and TIA incidence in the general population, the latter is the thrombotic, embolic and bleeding incidence within the study group prior to valve replacement. The embolic and bleeding incidences represent the risk imposed by the valve disease, its complications and those of anticoagulation if used, as well as all other, incremental risk factors present in the study group prior to surgery. It is proposed to use this information to define the specific background incidence regarding postoperative follow up assessment, be it prospective or retrospective.

The number of preoperative emboli in published valve series is often reported but as the number is rarely time related it cannot be used for comparison with postoperative figures. Preoperative bleeding incidence is never reported though there must be at least some, especially because a given number of patients in practically every study group receive anticoagulant treatment prior to heart valve surgery.

Preoperative data can be made time related if a suitable time period is defined within which the events had to occur in order to be counted in the statistics. The time period could be defined in terms of progression of the valve disease, but that would introduce ambiguity. For example, a congenital anomaly is present from birth irrespective of the onset of symptoms, embolism can be the first clinical symptom of valve disease, there may be individual interpretation in pin-pointing the exact start of the disease and so forth.

An arbitrary time limit seems to be more practical and it is proposed to set it at five years prior to surgery. In this way each patient contributes five years of 'preoperative follow up' information. In some cases it will be available from the preoperative patient notes kept by the cardiologist or the general practitioner, in others the patient will have to be asked by the surgeon whether he/she has suffered embolism and/or bleeding, and when, during the last five years leading to heart valve surgery. It should be noted, however, that regular follow up notes and a summary questioning regarding a five year period may not have an identical informative value (vide infra).

The 'total preoperative follow up information' is therefore calculated by multiplying the number of patients in the study group by five (not valid for children younger than five years). The number of events, whether embolism, bleeding or an aggregate of them, divided by the total preoperative follow up years yields the linearised preoperative rate of the given event. Hazard functions can be calculated on a similar basis.

This 'study specific background incidence' ignores the potential of different risk factor combinations being present before and after surgery. Atrial fibrillation, cardiac index and progressive ageing of the patients spring to mind in this respect. Another problematical issue is the number of fatal embolic and/or bleeding complications in patients who never undergo surgery. One solution would be to record fatal events that occur in patients on the waiting list for heart valve surgery, although extremely few patients wait five years for surgery and in some countries there are no waiting lists at all. A method of sampling patients with valve disease under regular cardiological follow-up may be a better alternative. Despite these methodological uncertainties, this type of analysis could have many advantages.

The starting point for follow up studies evaluating long term results after heart valve surgery, the 'time zero', is the date of surgery in all relevant publications. This statistical approach has been uniformly adopted by consensus and it is identical to the method applied in animal experiments when the time related outcome of a single, brief and well defined intervention, whether surgical, pharmacological or other is to be assessed.

There are, however, two major differences between experimental and clinical studies. One is that the former is working with experimental groups that are homogeneous at the start of the experiment and the latter with patient populations that are heterogeneous at the time of surgery, both by definition. The other is that the experimental animals are uniformly normal at the beginning, whereas patients will be at broadly different stages of their valve disease, and therefore definitely not normal when surgery commences.

The realisation of the existence of this heterogenicity led to the introduction of multivariate analysis of operative results and to stratification of long term results in the statistical analysis of the outcome of heart valve replacement. There are several potentials for problems arising from the use of either of these two methods, but they are beyond the scope of this chapter. However, it should be stressed here that the latter is, but the former is not strictly time related.

The proposal to calculate and present time related incidences and/or hazard functions of preoperative thrombosis, embolism and bleeding would provide a means of comparing these complications before and after surgery. It also encompasses the empirical conclusion that heart valve surgery, whether conservative or replacement, is palliative in nature and the surgical intervention(s) is only a single, though significant stage in the long course of the disease. Life curves and/or hazard curves could be constructed accordingly and the effect of operation depicted in accurate terms. In this way, results achieved with widely different patient populations may become more comparable.

To achieve this last goal it is proposed to divide the preoperative rate of event, whether thrombosis, embolism or bleeding by the respective postoperative rate. The resulting 'progress proportion' would be larger than one if the heart valve replacement had a positive effect and decreased the rate of embolism or bleeding. If the progress proportion was found to be smaller than one, the surgical intervention and subsequent postoperative management would have increased the risk of embolism and/or bleeding. Progress proportions from different clinical series could readily be compared and the progress proportion of the thromboembolic complications, together with that of other parameters might reveal important information on timing of surgery and its effect on late postoperative complications.

Thus the third proposal made in this chapter is the introduction of the above defined 'progress proportion', with the recommendation to report the time related incidence of thrombosis, embolism and bleeding that occurred during the five years preceding surgery.

Statistics, however, are only as reliable as the data that were entered into them. Two issues prompting scrutiny arise in this respect. One is the method of data collection, the other relates to the sensitivity and specificity of the methods used to establish the retrospective diagnosis of a thromboembolic or bleeding event.

There are several accepted methods of data collection for a follow up study. They include regular (as opposed to occasional or incidental) out-patient clinics for the entire patient population in the study, contact with the patient by telephone or by questionnaire and questionnaires sent to the GP or referring cardiologist. The contact through correspondence may be regular, for example annual, or it may take place only at the 'closing date' of the study to assess complications that occurred during the last five or ten years. It is generally accepted that equal weight is given to data acquired by any one of the above methods.

There is, however, no evidence in the medical or statistical literature to prove that all of the above methods would yield identical information and thereby be considered as interchangeable. Indeed, the opposite is true.

Horstkotte and Trampisch published the results of a pertinent study in 1986[2]. They applied four different methods to the same patient cohort, which was followed up in a prospective randomised way (Table 6.4–1). Parallel to the regular follow-up at the out-patient clinic, all patients were sent questionnaires at 6 and 18 monthly intervals as well as 36 months after the starting point of the study. As is apparent in Table 6.4–1, about half of the events which were transient or reversible within eight weeks were forgotten and not mentioned by the same patients on the questionnaire sent 18 or 36

Table 6.4–1
Comparison of follow-up methods

Method/Frequency	*OP 6–12 months*	*Q 6 months*	*Q 18 months*	*Q 36 months*
Total follow up	4, 492 months	4,436 months	4,497 months	4,581 months
Transient and/or reversible event	N=14 3.7%/pty	N=13 3.5%/pty	N=8 2.1%/pty	N=6 1.6%/pty
Permanent damage	N=3 0.8%/pty	N=3 0.8%/pty	N=2 0.5%/pty	N=2 0.5%/pty
Lethal event	N=2 0.5%/pty	N=2	N=2	N=2
Valve thrombosis	N=2 0.5%/pty	N=2	N=2	N=2

OP = out-patient clinic, Q = questionnaire
Reproduced after D. Horstkotte and H. J. Trampisch

months after the beginning of the trial. There was, however, no 'loss of memory' regarding events that caused irreversible damage or death, nor in case of prosthetic valve thrombosis.

The conclusion is simple. Reliable follow-up data that includes information on transient and reversible events cannot be collected by any means other than regular follow-up visits to a specialised out-patient clinic at least once a year or by regular questionnaires sent preferably at six monthly intervals. Information derived from occasional questionnaires can be trusted only if it relates to valve thrombosis, lethal events or those causing irreversible damage. It follows that only these three major types of events can be used for comparison between two sets of follow-up information, unless the method of data collection was strictly identical in both studies.

The problem of how to interpret the transient and reversible events is further intensified by the apparent inadequacy of the retrospective diagnostic method applied to them. Usually the patient is asked to answer a specific set of questions in the form of a personal interview or by correspondence, but an internationally accepted and adapted set of relevant questions does not exist and the depth of the interview may vary according to the experience of the physician conducting the out-patient clinic. Furthermore, no attempt has been made so far, to the knowledge of this author, to establish the specificity and sensitivity of these questions in the retrospective diagnosis of cerebral embolism and/or intracranial bleeding.

A study was therefore performed to address this problem. A standard questionnaire was provided by courtesy of Dr. Robert W. M. Frater, who has been using it for many years in his meticulous follow up study at the Albert Einstein College of Medicine, New York (Table 6.4–2). A set of additional questions were added to ascertain or exclude the presence of some major risk factors (Table 6.4–3).

The questionnaire so composed was completed by asking 1,000 people of either sex, all of whom looked apparently normal and were going about their everyday business in London mainline railway terminals during working hours. There was no specific time period set for the study, the standard question being "have you ever had......?".

The male:female ratio was 54.9/45.1, the mean age 36.3 years with a range of 14–97 years. Eighty-five persons had one or more risk factors, 915 had none. A positive answer to at least one of the questions searching for thrombosis, embolism or bleeding

Table 6.4–2
Have you ever had

Temporary weakness or numbness	Temporary memory loss
in your hands	Inability to think clearly
in your legs	to concentrate
your face	to do calculations
Seeing double	to recognize objects
Slurring of your speech	to say what you want
Temporary blindness	Not knowing where you are
Blurring of vision of one eye	Disturbances of balance
or part of one eye	
Blood in your urine	Sharp pain in the sides

Table 6.4–3
Have you had / Do you have

● Heart valve replacement
● Heart disease
● Arterial hypertension
● Diabetes
● Anticoagulant treatment

was given by 69.4% (n = 59) of those with, and by 54.8% (n = 501) without any risk factors. The difference is statistically significant ($p < 0.01$). The total number of reported 'events' was 164 (1.93/person) for those with, and 1331 (1.45/person) for those without any risk factors.

In a sense, the results confirm that the given set of questions are pertinent to the investigation, because the groups with and without a risk factor were separated by a statistically highly significant difference. Nevertheless, the high proportion of presumed false positive responses by those who appeared 'normal' on the grounds of absence of risk factors, dismisses the case for even a tentative specificity of the questionnaire. Furthermore the sensitivity of any questionnaire is also strictly time dependent as shown by the results of the Horstkotte and Trampisch study described above.

The fourth proposal of this chapter is, therefore, to count only valve thrombosis, lethal embolism, lethal bleeding or those events causing permanent damage, when defining and/or comparing the thrombogenicity of replacement heart valves. This should not pre-empt the recording and reporting of minor events as a separate entity, because they may serve in the future for possible further analysis. In general, however, questionnaires should be designed to elicit positive responses that are followed up with more intensive interviews and/or studies.

Finally, the last and perhaps the most important proposal is that we recognize the weaknesses and inherent flaws of the methods that have been used so far, endeavour to set new rules, lay down principles and adhere to them to achieve a better understanding of thrombosis, embolism and bleeding after heart valve replacement.

REFERENCES

1. Edmunds LH, Clark RE, Cohn LH, Miller DC, Weisel RD. Guidelines for reporting morbidity and mortality after cardiac valvular operations. J Thorac Cardiovasc Surg 1988;96:351–353
2. Horstkotte D, Trampisch HJ. Langzeitbeobachgtungen nach Herzklappenersatz. Z Kardiol 1986; 75:641–645

Subject Index

A

ACT see accelerated/activated clotting time, 107
Accelerated clotting time, 109
Activated clotting time, 109
Acute myocardial infarction
  endocardial damage in, 41
ADP secretion
  platelets, by, 249
AFASAK study
  atrial fibrillation, in, 21
Air embolism
  detection by intraoperative echocardiography, 224
Akinetic myocardium
  role in thrombus formation, of, 230
Albumin
  precoating of synthetic surfaces, 167
Amyloidosis, cardiac
  cardioembolism and, 43
Anti-thrombin III
  thromboembolic complications, and, 306
Anticoagulant dose
  computer assisted prediction, 332
  effect on bleeding, 428
  higher vs. lower, 429
Anticoagulants
  co-morbid conditions, in,430
  drug interactions with, 429
  higher vs. lower dose, 429
  pharmacology of, 231
Anticoagulation
  -related haemorrhage, 271, 425, 427, 431, 432
  cardioversion, and, 25
  clinical trials of, 287
  early, value of, 296
  fine tuning of, 303
  ideal level of, 299
  infective endocarditis, in, 76
  infective endocarditis, in the prevention of, 71
  lack of, after valve replacement, 293
  limitations of, 89
  non-cardiac surgery and, 369
  objectives of, 295
  patient compliance, and, 310
  platelet inhibitors and, combined, 255
  pregnancy and, 366
  prosthesis/patient specific, 293
  quality assessment of, 286
  randomised comparison of, 301
  reporting accuracy of, 478
Antiphospholipid antibodies, 72
Anti-endothelial cell antibodies, 188
Antiplatelet drugs
  bioprostheses, and, 309
  caged disc/ball prostheses, and, 308
  coronary artery disease, and, 308
  effect on thrombosis, 163
  indication for, 255, 308
  perioperative use of, 299
  recurrent embolism, and, 308
  release products, and, 164
  thromboprophylaxis, and, 307
Antithrombotic therapy
  atrial fibrillation, in, 20
Aortic atheroma
  detected by intraoperative echocardiography, 224
  source of embolism, as, 187
Aortic stenosis
  thromboembolism, and, 55
Aprotinin
  cardiopulmonary bypass and, 105, 111
  clinical trial of, 113
  dosage of, 112
  extended clinical use of, 114
  mechanism of action, 116
  safety and efficacy of, 114
Arachidonic acid, 164
  metabolism, activation of, 249
  metabolism, inhibitors of, 250
Arrhythmia (see also specific arrhythmias)
  cardioembolism and, 44
Arterial thrombosis
  haemostatic function and, 82
Arteriosclerosis
  cardioembolism and, 32
Artificial materials
  interaction with blood, 160
  passivation of, 162

platelet, interaction with, 163
protein absorption of, 162
Aspirin
platelet inhibitor, as, 250
postoperative use of, 308
Atrial contraction
loss of, 52
Atrial fibrillation
aetiology of, 45
antithrombotic therapy and, 20
BAATAF study in, 23
CAFA study in, 24
cardioembolism and, 45
carotid artery disease, and, 17
cerebral embolism, due to, 34
coagulation factors, and, 17
echocardiographic features of, 18
embolism, and, 190
heart valve disease, in, 46
incidence of, 93
lone, 19
mechanism of, 93
pathogenesis of thromboembolism, in, 16
randomised clinical trials in, 20
SPAF study, in, 22
systemic emboli, and, 17, 189
thromboembolism, and, 95
thyrotoxicosis, and, 19
warfarin vs. aspirin, in, 17
Atrial septal aneurysm
echocardiographic detection of, 235
Auscultatory findings
valve thrombosis, of, 388
Autotransfusion
cardiac surgery and, 105

B

BAATAF study
atrial fibrillation, in, 23
Background incidence of embolism
general vs. specific, 481
statistical analysis, in, 480
Bacterial effect
platelets, on, 161
Ball thrombus
left atrial, 229
Betathromboglobulin
level of anticoagulation, and, 306
Bi-leaflet valves
presentation of valve thrombosis, in, 196
thrombus deposition in, 184
without anticoagulation, 293
Bicuspid aortic valve
endocardial damage with, 44
Biological valves
embolism with, 179
host endothelialisation of, 178
thrombus organisation on, 177, 181
Bioprosthetic valves
anticoagulation policy, with, 305
embolism with, 181
mechanism of thrombus deposition on, 177
propensity to thrombosis, of, 161
Bjørk-Shiley CC valve
shear stress and, 127
Bleeding (see also Haemorrhage)
Bleeding, anticoagulant-related, 271, 425
demographic factors and, 431
management of, 427
overall risk of, 427
Bleeding sites
anticoagulated patients, in, 426
Blood conservation
cardiac surgery, during, 105
Blood flow, intracardial
effect on endocardial cell structure, of, 39
Blood/material interaction
modification of, 166
British Corrected Ratio (BCR)
measuring anticoagulation, for, 301
British Ratio (BR)
measuring anticoagulation, for, 301
Bucolome
warfarin, and, 310

C

CAFA study
atrial fibrillation, in, 24
Caged ball valves
propensity to thrombosis, of, 161
thrombus deposition in, 183
without anticoagulation, 293
Cardiac catheterisation
valve thrombosis, and, 393
Cardiac disease
stroke and, 12
Cardiac pathology
influence on embolic risk, 31
Cardiac surgery

haemostasis, during, 105, 106
platelet function, and, 110
Cardiac tumors
echocardiographic detection of, 237
Cardiff Valve Study
comparing different INR levels, 302
Cardioembolism (see also embolism and thromboembolism)
acute infective endocarditis, in, 37
aetiology of, 32, 34
arrhythmia and, 42
arteriosclerosis and, 32
atrial fibrillation and, 45
Chagas' heart disease, in, 35
cardiac amyloidosis and, 43
cardiac chamber dimension, and, 47
cardiac tumors and, 237
cerebral vs. peripheral, 34
chronic vs. intermittent atrial fibrillation, 46
endocardial damage and, 37
incidence of, 32
left ventricular function and, 55
mitral valve prolapse, in, 236
myocardial contusion and, 41
myocardial function and, 51
right ventricular function and, 54
risk factors for, 20
subendocardial ischaemia and, 41
supraventricular arrhythmia and, 47
ventricular arrhythmia, in, 47
viral myocarditis and, 43
Cardiomyopathy
cerebral embolism due to, 34
Cardiopulmonary bypass
aprotinin and, 105, 111
complement pathways and, 109
desmopressin acetate and, 111
epsilon-amino-caproic-acid and, 110
fibrinolysis and, 109
heparin and, 105
kallikrein and, 109
prostacyclin and, 111
tranexamic acid and, 111
Cardioversion
anticoagulation, and, 25
Carotid arterial flow
effect on endothelium, of, 40
Carotid artery disease
atrial fibrillation, and, 17
Carpentier-Edwards pericardial valve
shear stress and, 140
Carpentier-Edwards porcine valve
shear stress and, 136, 139
Cavitation
clinical consequences of, 145
mechanical valves, in, 141
threshold values of, 145
thrombogenicity of, 186
Cellular morphology
endocardium, of, 39
Central nervous system see CNS
Cerebral cardioembolism
prevalence of risk factors for, 34
Cerebral infarction
anatomical classification of, 8
asymptomatic, in atrial fibrillation, 18
haemorrhagic transformation of, 10
subtype of, 6
Chagas' heart disease
cardioembolism in, 35
Chondrodysplasia punctata
warfarin-induced, 272, 341
Cigarette smoking (see Smoking)
CNS embolism
infective endocarditis, in, 74
Coag-I-System
home prothrombin estimation, for, 327
Coagulability
ethnic differences in, 188
Coagulation factors
atrial fibrillation, and, 17
Coagulometer KC 1A
home prothrombin estimation, for, 326
Collagen
platelet activator, as, 249
Comparison of clinical results
statistical methods of, 460
Complement pathways
cardiopulmonary bypass and, 109
Computer database
drug interactions, of, 331
valve follow-up, for, 439
Computer program
anticoagulant dose prediction, for, 332
Coumatrac Protime Monitor
home prothrombin estimation, for, 327
Cumulative hazard function
definition of, 454
Cyclo-oxygenase
inhibitors, 250

D

DDAVP see desmopressin acetate
Desmopressin acetate
  cardiopulmonary bypass, and, 111
Dextran
  anticoagulant, as, 299
Diabetes
  hypercoagulability in, 188
  stroke and, 12
Dietary fat
  atrial thrombosis, and, 189, 310
  factor VII and, 86
  fibrinogen and, 88
  postoperative management and, 310
Dipyridamole
  platelet inhibitor, as, 251
Disturbed flow
  definition of, 151
Doppler echocardiography
  valve thrombosis, in, 389
Drug interactions
  computer database of, 331

E

EACA see epsilon-amino-caproic-acid
Echo-contrast spontaneous (see Spontaneous echocardiographic contrast)
Echocardiography
  atrial fibrillation, in, 18
  detecting embolic risk, 223
  detecting intracardiac thrombus, 227
  detecting prosthetic valve thrombosis, 231, 389
  intraoperative use of, 223
Eddy viscosity
  Reynolds stress, and, 155
Edwards-Duromedics valve
  shear stress and, 135
Embolic risk
  cardiac pathology, influence of, 31
Embolism (see also Cardioembolism and Thromboembolism)
  atrial fibrillation and, 190
  biological valves, with, 179
  bioprosthetic valves, with, 181
  definition of, 478
  detection of, 218
  hazard function of, 448
  infective endocarditis, in, 73
  intracardiac vegetations, from, 73
  mechanisms of, 183
  microangiography, and, 218
  minor vs. major, 191
  pathogenesis of, 247
  pre- and postoperative, 191
  prevention in atrial fibrillation, 26
  rates of, 193
  risk factor adjusted analysis of, 448
  statistical perception of, 447
  valve vs. non-valve origin of, 189
  versus thrombosis, 172
Embryopathy
  warfarin-induced, 272, 341
Endocardial cell structure
  effect of blood flow on, 39
Endocardial damage
  acute myocardial infarction, in, 41
  cardioembolism and, 37
Endocardial infection
  initiation of, 70
Endocarditis vegetation
  size of, 74
Endocardium
  cellular morphology of, 39
Endocardium, valvular
  effect of flow on, 40
Endothelial damage
  cardiac catheter, and, 71
Endothelial structure
  effect of arterial flow on, 40
Endothelium
  effect of disease processes on, 188
  nitric oxyde synthesis and, 38
  thromboresistance of, 161
Endothelium derived relaxing factor (EDRF) see nitric oxyde
Epsilon-amino-caproic-acid
  cardiopulmonary bypass and, 110
Ethnic differences
  coagulability, in, 188
  tissue ingrowth, in, 175
External Quality Assessment (EQA)
  prothrombin time, of, 283

F

Factor VII
  age and sex relation of, 86

dietary fat, and, 86
hypercoagulability and, 85
plasma lipids, and, 85
Factor XIII, 185
Fat embolism
detection by intraoperative echocardiography, 225
Federation of Dutch Thrombosis Services, 285
Fibrinogen
age and sex relation of, 88
dietary fat and, 88
level of anticoagulation, and, 307
plasma lipids and, 88
platelets and, 87
seasonal variation of, 188
thrombotic risk, and, 87
Fibrinogen level
stroke risk, and, 82
Fibrinolysis
aprotinin and, 116
cardiopulmonary bypass and, 109
Fibrinopeptide A
thrombin activity, and, 306
Fish oil
effect of, 310
platelet inhibitor, as, 250
Follow up by questionnaire
limitations of, 483

H

Haematological detection
thrombosis, of, 215
thrombotic risk, of, 206
Haemolysis
shear stress and, 123
stress threshold for, 153
valve replacement, after, 161
Haemophilia
bleeding vs. thrombosis in, 425
Haemophiliac patient, iatrogenic
definition of, 425
management of, 426
Haemorrhage
background incidence of, 196
heparin, caused by, 265
warfarin-related, 271
Haemostasis
cardiac surgery, during, 105, 106
secondary, 162
Haemostatic function
arterial thrombosis, and, 82
Hancock II valve
shear stress and, 138
Hancock MO valve
shear stress and, 137
Hazard function
embolism, of, 448
valve thrombosis, of, 450
Heparin
adverse effects of, 265
bound to synthetic surfaces, 168
cardiopulmonary bypass and, 105
dosage of, 109
during pregnancy, 340
general description of, 263
low molecular weight, 107
mechanism of action, 263
osteoporosis, induced by, 266
pharmacokinetics of, 264
protamine, and, 107
thrombin inhibitor, as, 252
thrombocytopenia, induced by, 265
variability in activity, 107
Heparin vs. warfarin
pregnancy, during, 343
Hirudin
thrombin inhibitor, as, 252
Histology
valve thrombus, of, 161
Home prothrombin estimation
clinical experiences with, 327
methods of, 326
patient training for, 329
rationale for, 325
Homografts (see Biological valves)
Hydrated dynamic surfaces, 167
Hypercoagulability, 81, 84
diabetes, in, 186
factor VII and, 85
infective disease, in, 188
malignant diseases, in, 188
nephrotic syndrome, in, 188
rebound, 294
surface related, 84
Hypertension
stroke, and, 11
Hyperthyroidism
warfarin and, 271

I

Imidazole
platelet inhibitor, as, 251
INR see International Normalised Ratio
Indium labelling
platelets, of, 208
Infective disease
hypercoagulability in, 188
Infective endocarditis
anticoagulation, in the prevention of, 71
cardioembolism in, 37
early diagnosis of, 77
Interaction
blood/material, 160
International Reference Preparation
thromboplastin, for, 278
International Normalised Ratio (INR)
biological variation of, 285
definition of, 279
high, management of, 431
inter-laboratory variation of, 284
precision of, 285
vs. prothrombin time, 301
International Sensitivity Index
definition of, 279
Intracardiac bacterial vegetation
embolism, and, 73
Intracardiac flow
replacement heart valves and, 44
velocity and pattern of, 44
Intracardiac thrombosis
diagnosis of, 31
echocardiographic detection of, 223, 227
mitral valve disease, in, 228
Intraoperative echocardiography
detecting air embolism, 224
detecting aortic atheroma, 224
detecting fat emboli, 225
detecting intracardiac thrombi, 223
Ionescu-Shiley valve
shear stress and, 140
Ischaemic heart disease
cerebral embolism due to, 34

J

Jet lesion
endocardial damage in, 41

K

Kallikrein
cardiopulmonary bypass and, 109
Karnovsky scale
assessing thromboembolism, in, 455

L

Lacunar infarct, 8, 9
Laminar flow
definition of, 149
target organ of, 456
Late events
changing incidence over time, 448
linearised rate of, 448
target organ of, 456
variable sequelae of, 454
Left atrial size
embolic risk and, 238
thromboembolic complications and, 45
Left ventricular function
cardioembolism and, 55
global vs. regional impairment, 55
Left ventricular thrombus
echocardiographic detection of, 229
Linearised rate
late events of, 448
Lipids
stroke and, 12
Lone atrial fibrillation, 19

M

M-mode echocardiography
valve thrombosis, in, 389
Malignant diseases
hypercoagulability in, 188
Malondialdehyde
valve replacement, after, 164
Martingale theory, 445
Mechanical valves
thrombogenicity of, 182
Medtronic Hall valve
anticoagulation recommendations for, 302
shear stress and, 129
Microangiography
embolism, and, 218
Microcavitation
spontaneous echocardiographic contrast, and, 234
Microthrombus

aortic stenosis, in, 70
biological and bioprosthetic valve cusps, on, 177, 182
Mitral valve prolapse
cerebral embolism due to, 34
echocardiographic diagnosis of, 236
Monoclonal antibodies
thrombosis detection, in, 212
Multivariate analysis
risk factors, of, 456
Mycotic aneurysm
cerebral, in endocarditis, 75
Myocardial contusion
cardioembolism and, 41
Myocardial function
cardioembolism and, 51
Myocarditis, viral
cardioembolism and, 43

N

Nephrotic syndrome
hypercoagulability in, 188
Neutrophils
thrombus formation and, 39
Nitric oxyde
endothelial synthesis of, 38
spontaneous echocardiographic contrast and, 234
Non-bacterial thrombotic vegetation
stroke, and, 72
Non-cardiac surgery
during anticoagulation, 369, 431

O

Obesity and coagulability, 189
Occluder impact
embolism, and, 183
Omnicarbon valve
shear stress and, 131
Opening angles
bi-leaflet valves, of, 393
tilting disc valves, of, 392
Osteoporosis
heparin-induced, 266
Outcome events
point processes, as, 446
Overall thromboembolic hazard
modulated renewal process, as, 452

P

Paediatric heart surgery
aprotinin in, 115
Paradoxical embolism
infective endocarditis, in, 76
patent foramen ovale and, 226
Paroxysmal arrhythmia
intracardiac thrombus formation and, 45
Partial anterior circulation infarct, 9
Passivation
artificial surfaces, of, 162
Patent foramen ovale
echocardiographic diagnosis of, 226
heart valve disease and, 227
paradoxical embolism and, 226
Patient compliance
anticoagulation, and, 310
Patient-specific anticoagulation, 293
PGI2 see prostacyclin
Plasma gas discharge
surface modification, in, 167
Plasma lipids
factor VII and, 85
fibrinogen, and, 88
Platelet
activation by collagen, 249
activation by thrombin, 249
activity after valve replacement, 307
adhesion to artificial surfaces, 164
adhesion, physiology of, 248
aggregation after valve replacement, 166
aggregation, physiology of, 248
aprotinin and, 116
artificial surfaces, and, 248
cAMP level, 251
effect of bacteria on, 161
effect and fibrinogen, 87
function during cardiac surgery, 110
indium-labelled, 208
inhibition by fish oil, 250
inhibition by imidazole, 251
inhibition by prostacyclin, 252
inhibition by sulfinpyrazone, 252
inhibition by ticlopidine, 253
inhibition by triflusal, 251
inhibitors, 247
inhibitors, anticoagulants and, 255
inhibitors, heart valve replacement, after, 254
inhibitors, pharmacology of, 249

interaction with artificial surfaces, 163
kinetics after valve replacement, 166
release products of, 164
scintigraphy after heart valve replacment, 210
sheer stress tolerance of, 153
Polyurethane
thrombogenicity of, 168
Posterior circulation infarct, 8
Predictions
statistical methods of, 459
Pregnancy
anticoagulation during, 341, 366
heparin and, 340
heparin vs. warfarin, 343
replacement valves, and, 340
rheumatic heart disease and, 340
venous thrombosis, during, 339
Preoperative events
time related reporting of, 481
Primary thrombogenicity
replacement heart valves, of, 173
Pro-coagulant activity
basal, 83
Progress proportion
statistical analysis, in, 482
Prostacyclin, 161
cardiopulmonary bypass and, 111
platelet inhibitor, as, 252
Prosthesis specific anticoagulation, 293
Prosthetic valve thrombosis
echocardiographic detection of, 231
measurement of thrombogenicity, as, 193
Protamine
dosage of, 109
heparin and, 107
Protein absorption
artificial materials, of, 162
Protein C
role in skin necrosis, 272
Prothrombin
conversion to thrombin, 83
Prothrombin activity
definition of, 277
Prothrombin level
home estimation of, 325
Prothrombin time
definition of, 277
Pulmonary embolism
right ventricular function and, 54

Q

Quick method
definition of, 277

R

Radiological signs
valve thrombosis, of, 392
Recurrence of events
statistical perception of, 451
Recurrent embolism, 402
management of, 402
patient management after, 413
reoperation for, 411
risk factors for, 406
Release products
platelets, of, 164
Renal embolism
infective endocarditis, in, 74
Replacement heart valves
pregnancy and, 340
primary thrombogenicity of, 173
secondary thrombogenicity of, 186
Reporting methods
standardisation of, 445
Reynold's number, 150
Reynold's stress
eddy viscosity, and, 155
Rheumatic heart disease
cerebral embolism due to, 34
pregnancy and, 340
RIND
definition of, 4
Right ventricular function
cardioembolism and, 54
pulmonary embolism and, 54
Risk factors
cardioembolism, for, 34
confounding effect of, 479
modification of, 307, 458
multivariate analysis of, 456

S

Scintigraphic detection
thrombosis, of, 208
thrombotic risk, of, 206
Secondary haemostasis, 162
Secondary thrombogenicity
replacement valves, of, 186
Sewing ring

normal healing of, 173
thrombogenicity of, 174
Shear rate
spontaneous echocardiographic contrast and, 234
Shear stress (in vivo)
clinical consequences of, 141
haemolysis , and, 123
Shear stress (in vitro)
Bjørk-Shiley CC valve and, 127
Carpentier-Edwards porcine valve and, 136
Carpentier-Ewards porcine valve and, 139
Carpentier-Edwards pericardial valve ands, 140
Edwards-Duromedics valve and, 135
Hancock II valve and, 138
Hancock MO valve and, 137
Ionescu-Shiley valve and, 140
Medtronic Hall valve and, 129
Omnicarbon valve and, 131
St.Jude Medical valve and, 133
Starr-Edwards valve and, 126
Skin reactions
warfarin-related, 272
Smoking
antiplatelet drugs and, 308
effect on fibrinogen, 88
postoperative management and, 309
risk factor for embolism, as, 312
stroke, and, 12
SPAF study
atrial fibrillation, in, 22
Splenic infarct
infective endocarditis, in, 74
Spontaneous echocardiographic contrast
blood, of, 232
in vitro, 234
left atrial, 31, 233, 391
mechanism of, 233
microcavitation and, 234
nitric oxyde (EDRF) and, 234
risk factor, as, 234
shear rate and, 234
St. Jude Medical valve
anticoagulation recommendations for, 304
shear stress and, 133
Standardisation
anticoagulation, of, 277
reporting methods of, 445
Starr-Edwards valve
mechanism of embolism with, 183
recurrent embolism with, 183, 402
shear stress and, 126
Statistical analysis
limitations of, 446
Statistical methods
comparing thromboembolic rates, 465
Stratification
thrombosis and embolism incidences, of, 478
Stroke
aetiology of, 8
athero-thrombotic, 8
cardiac disease, and, 12
cardio-embolic, 8
definition of, 3
diabetes and, 12
epidemiology of pathological subgroups, 6
hypertension and, 11
incidence in the community, 5
lipids and, 12
mechanism in atrial fibrillation, 17
non-bacterial thrombotic vegetation, and, 72
prevention in atrial fibrillation, 26
risk factors, 11
smoking and, 12
Stroke incidence
geographic comparison of, 6
Subendocardial ischaemia
thrombogenic effect of, 41
Sulfinpyrazone
platelet inhibitor, as, 252
Supraventricular arrhythmia
cerebral embolism, due to, 34
thromboembolism in, 47
Surgical technique
thrombogenicity of, 97

T

TEB index
definition of, 479
Thrombin
activity and fibrinopeptide A, 306
conversion from prothrombin, 83
inhibitors, 252
platelet activator, as, 249
Thrombocytopenia
cardiopulmonary bypass, after, 164

heparin-induced, 265
Thromboembolic rates
relation to other factors, 466
variation in, 467
Thromboembolic risk
increase, identification of, 89
population vs. individual, 410
pregnancy, during, 339
stratification of, 19
Thromboembolism
atrial fibrillation and, 95
definition of, 477
pathogenesis in atrial fibrillation, of, 16
prosthesis size and, 98
recurrent, 402
Thrombogenic milieu
early postoperative period, in, 247
Thrombogenicity
artificial materials, of, 160
cavitation, of, 186
clinical assessment of, 192
flow conditions, and, 160
homografts, of, 177
measurement of, 191
mechanical valves, of, 182
patient safety, and, 195
replacement valves, of, 172
secondary, 186
sewing ring, of, 173
xenograft valves, of, 177
Thrombolytic treatment
valve thrombosis, of, 395
Thrombomodulin, 161
Thromboplastin
instrument-specific values of, 283
standards, selection of, 280
Thromboresistance
endothelium, of, 161
Thrombosis
definition of, 477
detection by monoclonal antibodies, 212
haematological detection of, 215
intracardiac, diagnosis of, 31
intracardiac, Chagas' heart disease in, 35
of replacement valves, pathogenesis, 247
of replacement valves, rates, 193
scintigraphic detection of, 208
versus embolism, 172
Thrombotic apposition
definition of, 477
Thrombotic disease
inherited, 84
Thrombotic risk
blood viscosity and, 87
fibrinogen, and, 87
haematological detection of, 206
scintigraphic detection of, 206
Thromboxane
valve replacement, after, 164
Thromboxane synthase
inhibitors of, 251
Thrombus
friability of, 185
Thrombus deposition
bi-leaflet valves, in, 184
caged ball valves, in, 183
occluder impact, and, 183
tilting disc valves, in, 184
Thrombus formation
mechanism of, 206
vs. systemic embolism, 16, 189, 193
Thrombus organisation
biological valves, on, 181
Thyrotoxicosis
atrial fibrillation, and, 19
TIA see Transient Ischaemic Attack
Ticlopidine
platelet inhibitor, as, 253
postoperative use of, 308
Tilting disc valves
opening angles of, 392
presentation of valve thrombosis with, 196
propensity to thrombosis, of, 161
thrombus deposition in, 184
without anticoagulation, 293
Time-varying covariables, 458, 459
Time-varying hazard functions, 451
Tissue ingrowth
replacement valves and, 174
Total anterior circulation infarct, 9
Tranexamic acid
cardiopulmonary bypass, and, 111
Transient ischaemic attack (TIA)
diagnosis by questionnaire, 484
differential diagnosis of, 4
incidence in the community, 5
Transoesophageal echocardiography
valve thrombosis, in, 390
Trasylol see Aprotinin
Triflusal
platelet inhibitor, as, 251
Turbulent flow

definition of, 149
haematological effect of, 149
in vitro effect on blood cells, 153
prosthetic valves, and, 155
Two-dimensional echocardiography
valve thrombosis, in, 389

V

Valve thrombosis
auscultatory findings of, 388
cardiac catheterisation, and, 393
clinical findings in, 387
consequences of, 160, 183
diagnosis of, 394
echocardiographic findings of, 389, 391
hazard function of, 450
radiological findings of, 392
rapidity of presentation, 196
scintillographic diagnosis of, 394
statistical characterisation of, 446
surgical management of, 398
thrombolytic treatment of, 395
Venous thrombosis
pregnancy, during, 339
Ventricular arrhythmia
thromboembolism in, 47
Viral myocarditis 43
Virchow's triad, 160
atrial fibrillation, and, 16
immediate postoperative period, and, 297
Viscosity (blood)
thrombotic risk, and, 87
Vitamin K
warfarin and, 271

W

Warfarin
adverse effects of, 271
drug interactions with, 273
fixed mini-dose, 309
general description of, 266
genetic factors and, 271
hyperthyroidism and, 271
intravenous administration of, 299
liver disease and, 271
mechanism of action, 266
pharmacokinetics of, 267
pregnancy and, 341
teratogenic effect of, 272, 341
vitamin K and, 271
Warfarin vs. aspirin
atrial fibrillation, in, 17
Weibull distribution
definition of, 403